OKU 4

Orthopaedic Knowledge Update

Hip and Knee Reconstruction

AAOS

AMERICAN ACADEMY OF
ORTHOPAEDIC SURGEONS

Orthopaedic Knowledge Update:

Hip and Knee Reconstruction

4

EDITORS:

Andrew H. Glassman, MD, MS
Chief of Adult Reconstructive Surgery
Department of Orthopaedic Surgery
Ohio State University Medical Center
Columbus, Ohio

Paul F. Lachiewicz, MD
Consulting Professor
Department of Orthopaedic Surgery
Duke University School of Medicine
Durham, North Carolina
Attending Surgeon
Chapel Hill Orthopedics Surgery and
Sports Medicine
Chapel Hill, North Carolina

Michael Tanzer, MD, FRCSC
Professor and Jo Miller Chair
Division of Orthopaedic Surgery
McGill University Health Center
Montreal, Quebec, Canada

DEVELOPED BY
THE HIP SOCIETY AND
THE KNEE SOCIETY

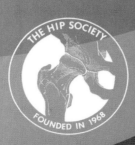

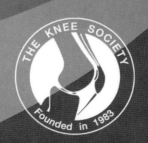

AAOS
AMERICAN ACADEMY OF
ORTHOPAEDIC SURGEONS

AAOS

AMERICAN ACADEMY OF ORTHOPAEDIC SURGEONS

The material presented in *Orthopaedic Knowledge Update: Hip and Knee Reconstruction 4* has been made available by the American Academy of Orthopaedic Surgeons for educational purposes only. This material is not intended to present the only, or necessarily best, methods or procedures for the medical situations discussed, but rather is intended to represent an approach, view, statement, or opinion of the author(s) or producer(s), which may be helpful to others who face similar situations.

Some drugs or medical devices demonstrated in Academy courses or described in Academy print or electronic publications have not been cleared by the Food and Drug Administration (FDA) or have been cleared for specific uses only. The FDA has stated that it is the responsibility of the physician to determine the FDA clearance status of each drug or device he or she wishes to use in clinical practice.

Furthermore, any statements about commercial products are solely the opinion(s) of the author(s) and do not represent an Academy endorsement or evaluation of these products. These statements may not be used in advertising or for any commercial purpose.

Published 2011 by the
American Academy of Orthopaedic Surgeons
6300 North River Road
Rosemont, IL 60018

Fourth Edition
Copyright 2011
by the American Academy of Orthopaedic Surgeons

ISBN 978-0-89203-735-3
Printed in the USA

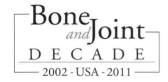

Acknowledgments

Contributors

David Backstein, MD, Med, FRCSC
Associate Professor and Director
Department of Surgery Undergraduate
*   Education*
Mount Sinai Hospital
University of Toronto
Toronto, Ontario, Canada

Robert L. Barrack, MD
Chief of Service
Department of Orthopaedic Surgery
Washington University School of Medicine
St. Louis, Missouri

Paul E. Beaulé, MD, FRCSC
Associate Professor and Head of Adult
*   Reconstruction*
Department of Orthopedics
University of Ottawa
Ottawa, Ontario, Canada

Hany S. Bedair, MD
Attending Orthopedic Surgeon
Department of Orthopedic Surgery
Massachusetts General Hospital
Boston, Massachusetts

James Benjamin, MD
University Orthopedic Specialists
Tucson, Arizona

J. Dennis Bobyn, PhD
Professor
Departments of Surgery and Biomedical
*   Engineering*
McGill University
Montreal, Quebec, Canada

Michael P. Bolognesi, MD
Assistant Professor, Director of Adult
*   Reconstruction Section, and Adult*
*   Reconstruction Fellowship*
Division of Orthopaedic Surgery
Duke University Medical Center
Durham, North Carolina

James A. Browne, MD
Clinical Fellow in Adult Lower Extremity
*   Reconstruction*
Department of Orthopaedic Surgery
Mayo Clinic
Rochester, Minnesota

J.W. Thomas Byrd, MD
Nashville Sports Medicine Foundation
Nashville, Tennessee

Patricia A. Campbell, PhD
Associate Professor
Department of Orthopaedic Surgery
Orthopaedic Hospital/UCLA
Los Angeles, California

John C. Clohisy, MD
Professor of Orthopaedic Surgery, Co-Chief of
*   Adult Reconstructive Surgery, and Director*
*   of Adolescent and Young Adult Hip Service*
Department of Orthopaedic Surgery
Washington University School of Medicine
St. Louis, Missouri

Fred D. Cushner, MD
Director
ISK Institute
Chairman
Division of Orthopedics
Southside Hospital
Bay Shore, New York

Gregory K. Deirmengian, MD
Fellow, Hip and Knee Reconstruction
Rothman Institute Orthopedics
Thomas Jefferson University Medical School
Philadelphia, Pennsylvania

Craig J. Della Valle, MD
Associate Professor, Orthopaedic Surgery
Midwest Orthopaedics at Rush
Rush University Medical Center
Chicago, Illinois

Thomas K. Fehring, MD
OrthoCarolina Hip and Knee Center
Charlotte, North Carolina

Donald Garbuz, MD, MPH, FRCSC
Associate Professor and Head of Division for
*   Lower Limb Reconstruction*
Department of Orthopaedics
University of British Columbia
Vancouver, British Columbia, Canada

Kevin L. Garvin, MD
L. Thomas Hood, MD Professorship
Professor and Chair
Department of Orthopaedic Surgery and
* Rehabilitation*
University of Nebraska Medical Center
Omaha, Nebraska

Mark R. Geyer, MD
Duke University Medical Center
Chapel Hill, North Carolina

Elie Ghanem, MD
Department of Orthopedics
Thomas Jefferson University Hospital
Philadelphia, Pennsylvania

William L. Griffin, MD
OrthoCarolina Hip and Knee Center
Charlotte, North Carolina

Allan E. Gross, MD, FRCSC, O.Ont
Professor of Surgery
Faculty of Medicine
University of Toronto
Department of Orthopaedic Surgery
Mount Sinai Hospital
Toronto, Ontario, Canada

Nadim J. Hallab, BS, MS, PhD
Associate Professor
Department of Orthopaedic Surgery
Rush University
Chicago, Illinois

Curtis W. Hartman, MD
Assistant Professor
Department of Orthopaedic Surgery
University of Nebraska Medical Center
Omaha, Nebraska

Mark A. Hartzband, MD
Senior Attending Physician
Department of Orthopaedic Surgery
Hackensack University Medical Center
Hackensack, New Jersey

William J. Hozack, MD
Professor of Orthopaedic Surgery
Rothman Institute Orthopedics
Thomas Jefferson University Medical School
Philadelphia, Pennsylvania

Joshua J. Jacobs, MD
William A. Hark, MD/Susanne G. Swift
* Professor and Chairman*
Department of Orthopaedic Surgery
Rush University Medical Center
Chicago, Illinois

William A. Jiranek, MD, FACS
Professor and Chief of Adult Reconstruction
* Section*
Department of Orthopaedic Surgery
Virginia Commonwealth School of Medicine
Richmond, Virginia

Norman A. Johanson, MD
Professor and Chairman
Department of Orthopaedic Surgery
Drexel University College of Medicine
Philadelphia, Pennsylvania

Gregg R. Klein, MD
Attending Physician
Department of Orthopaedic Surgery
Hackensack University Medical Center
Hackensack, New Jersey

Yona Kosashvili, MD, MHA
Orthopaedic Surgeon of Lower Extremity
* Reconstruction*
Orthopedic Division
Assaf Harofeh Hospital
Zerifin, Israel

Michal Kozanek, MD
Research Fellow
Department of Orthopedic Surgery
Massachusetts General Hospital
Boston, Massachusetts

Jeffrey Aaron Krempec, MD
Department of Orthopaedics
Carolinas Medical Center
Charlotte, North Carolina

Paul F. Lachiewicz, MD
Consulting Professor
Department of Orthopaedic Surgery
Duke University School of Medicine
Durham, North Carolina
Attending Surgeon
Chapel Hill Orthopedics Surgery and Sports
* Medicine*
Chapel Hill, North Carolina

Carlos J. Lavernia, MD
Chief of Orthopedic Surgery
Mercy Hospital
Miami, Florida

Paul T.H. Lee, MB BCh, MA, FRCS(Eng), FRCS(Orth)
Consultant Trauma and Orthopaedic Surgeon (locum)
Leeds Teaching Hospitals NHS Trust
Leeds, United Kingdom

Michael Leunig, MD
Head of Orthopaedics
Schulthess Clinic and University of Berne
Zurich, Switzerland

David G. Lewallen, MD
Professor of Orthopaedic Surgery and Chair of the Division of Adult Reconstruction
Department of Orthopaedic Surgery
Mayo Clinic
Rochester, Minnesota

Guoan Li, PhD
Director of Bioengineering Lab
Department of Orthopedic Surgery
Massachusetts General Hospital
Boston, Massachusetts

Jay R. Lieberman, MD
Director
New England Musculoskeletal Institute
Professor and Chairman
Department of Orthopaedic Surgery
University of Connecticut Health Center
Farmington, Connecticut

Jess H. Lonner, MD
Associate Professor of Orthopaedic Surgery
Thomas Jefferson University
Rothman Institute
Bryn Mawr Hospital
Philadelphia, Pennsylvania

Steven J. MacDonald, MD, FRCSC
Professor of Orthopaedic Surgery
University of Western Ontario
London, Canada

Henrik Malchau, MD, PhD
Associate Professor
Harvard Medical School
Vice-Chief of Research and Co-Director of the Harris Orthopaedic Lab
Massachusetts General Hospital
Boston, Massachusetts

William J. Maloney, MD
Elsbach-Richards Professor and Chair
Department of Orthopaedic Surgery
Stanford University School of Medicine
Stanford, California

Anthony Marchie, MD, MPhil, FRCSC
Harris Hip Fellow
Department of Orthopaedic Surgery
Massachusetts General Hospital
Boston, Massachusetts

John L. Masonis, MD
OrthoCarolina Hip and Knee Center
Charlotte, North Carolina

Joel M. Matta, MD
Founder and Director
Hip and Pelvis Institute
Santa Monica, California

Harry A. McKellop, PhD
Professor In-Residence
Department of Orthopaedic Surgery
UCLA and Orthopaedic Hospital
Los Angeles, California

Dana C. Mears, MD, PhD
Clinical Professor of Orthopaedic Surgery
University of Pittsburgh Medical Center
Greater Pittsburgh Orthopaedic Associates
Pittsburgh, Pennsylvania

Morteza Meftah, MD
Orthopaedic Research Fellow
Weill Medical College of Cornell University
Department of Orthopaedics
Hospital for Special Surgery
New York, New York

R. Michael Meneghini, MD
Director of Joint Replacement
Indiana Clinic
Clinical Assistant Professor
Department of Orthopaedic Surgery
Indiana University School of Medicine
Indianapolis, Indiana

Stephen B. Murphy, MD
Clinical Assistant Professor of Orthopaedic
  Surgery
Center for Computer Assisted and
  Reconstructive Surgery
New England Baptist Hospital
Tufts University School of Medicine
Boston, Massachusetts

Soheil Najibi, MD, PhD
Attending Surgeon
Hip and Pelvis Institute
Santa Monica, California

Michael P. Nett, MD
Orthopedic Surgeon
Department of Orthopedics
Southside Hospital
Bay Shore, New York

Michael T. Newman, MD
Adult Reconstruction Fellow
Booth, Bartolozzi, Balderston
Pennsylvania Hospital
Philadelphia, Pennsylvania

Ryan M. Nunley, MD
Assistant Professor
Department of Orthopaedic Surgery
Washington University School of Medicine
St. Louis, Missouri

Jeremy M. Oryhon, MD
Lake Cook Orthopedic Associates
Barrington, Illinois

Douglas E. Padgett, MD
Chief of Adult Reconstruction
Department of Orthopaedic Surgery
Hospital for Special Surgery
New York, New York

Mark W. Pagnano, MD
Professor of Orthopedics
Mayo Graduate School of Medicine
Mayo Clinic
Rochester, Minnesota

Wayne G. Paprosky, MD
Department of Orthopaedic Surgery
Rush University Medical Center
Chicago, Illinois

Javad Parvizi, MD
Department of Orthopedics
Rothman Institute at Thomas Jefferson
  University
Philadelphia, Pennsylvania

Andrew D. Pearle, MD
Assistant Attending Orthopedic Surgeon
Shoulder and Sports Medicine Service
Hospital for Special Surgery
New York, New York

Hollis G. Potter, MD
Chief of Division of MRI and Professor of
  Radiology
Department of Radiology and Imaging
Hospital for Special Surgery/Weill Medical
  College of Cornell University
New York, New York

Amar S. Ranawat, MD
Assistant Profesor
Weill Medical College of Cornell University
Department of Orthopaedics
Hospital for Special Surgery
New York, New York

Chitranjan S. Ranawat, MD
Professor of Orthopaedic Surgery
Weill Medical College of Cornell University
Department of Orthopaedics
Hospital for Special Surgery
New York, New York

Michael Ries, MD
Professor and Chief of Arthroplasty
Department of Orthopaedic Surgery
University of California, San Francisco
San Francisco, California

Harry E. Rubash, MD
Chief of Orthopedic Surgery
Department of Orthopedic Surgery
Massachusetts General Hospital
Boston, Massachusetts

Erik Paul Severson, MD
Orthopaedic Instructor
Mayo Clinic
Department of Orthopaedic Surgery
Cuyuna Regional Medical Center
Crosby, Minnesota

Andrew John Shimmin, MD, MBBS, FAOrthA, FRACS
Consultant Orthopedic Surgeon and Director of the Melbourne Orthopedic Research Foundation
Melbourne Orthopedic Group
Windsor, Victoria, Australia

Scott M. Sporer, MD, MS
Assistant Professor of Orthopaedic Surgery
Rush University Medical Center
Chicago, Illinois

Venessa Stas, HonBSc, MD, FRCSC
Clinical Fellow of Adult Reconstructive Surgery
Department of Orthopaedic Surgery
Rush University Medical Center
Chicago, Illinois

Simon D. Steppacher, MD
Hip Faculty Member
Department of Orthopaedic Surgery
University of Bern, Inselspital
Bern, Switzerland

Moritz Tannast, MD
Hip Faculty Member
Department of Orthopaedic Surgery
University of Bern, Inselspital
Bern, Switzerland

Jesse E. Templeton, MD
Clinical Fellow of Adult Reconstructive Surgery
Department of Orthopaedic Surgery
Rush University Medical Center
Chicago, Illinois

Thomas Parker Vail, MD
Professor and Chairman
Department of Orthopaedic Surgery
University of California, San Francisco
San Francisco, California

Kartik Mangudi Varadarajan, BTech, MS
Research Associate
Department of Orthopedic Surgery
Massachusetts General Hospital
Boston, Massachusetts

Fabian von Knoch, MD, PhD
Consultant
Department of Adult Hip and Knee Reconstruction
Schulthess Clinic
Zurich, Switzerland

Steven H. Weeden, MD
Fellowship Director
Department of Orthopaedic Surgery
Texas Hip and Knee Center
Fort Worth, Texas

Richard E. White Jr, MD
Director of Research
New Mexico Center for Joint Replacement Surgery
New Mexico Orthopaedics
Albuquerque, New Mexico

Preface

Orthopaedic Knowledge Update: Hip and Knee Reconstruction 4 complements and updates information that was published in the three previous editions. The first edition was published in 1995, the second in 2000, and the third in 2006. The current edition encompasses knowledge current through the first 10 months of 2010. The current editors have tried to fashion the fourth edition as an update that can stand on its own.

This edition should provide residents, fellows, and practicing orthopaedic surgeons with a clear understanding of the state-of-the-art knowledge relevant to adult hip and knee reconstruction. As with the previous three publications, it can be used as a resource for both general orthopaedic surgeons and hip and knee specialists.

The fourth edition is more focused than the previous edition and is composed of three distinct sections: basic and applied science relevant to both knee and hip arthroplasty; specific total knee arthroplasty topics; and specific total hip arthroplasty topics. There is updated material related to the controversial topics of computer navigation and robotic-assisted surgery, patient-specific knee instrumentation, alternative bearing surfaces and total hip and knee revision arthroplasty. All of the chapters have been written by experts in each subject, with a concerted effort to reflect the current state of hip and knee reconstruction knowledge with objectivity and a minimal amount of personal bias.

We, the editors, would like to thank all of the authors for their efforts to complete their chapters, and putting up with our relentless constructive criticism. We also gratefully acknowledge the invaluable assistance of Marilyn Fox, PhD, Director, Lisa Claxton Moore, Managing Editor, and the other members of the Publications Department of the American Academy of Orthopaedic Surgeons. Their work and diligence helped to make this book of the highest quality.

Andrew H. Glassman, MD, MS
Paul F. Lachiewicz, MD
Michael Tanzer, MD, FRCSC
Editors

Table of Contents

Section 3: Hip

Basic Science and General Knowledge

SECTION EDITORS:
ANDREW H. GLASSMAN, MD, MS
PAUL F. LACHIEWICZ, MD
MICHAEL TANZER, MD, FRCSC

Chapter 1

Imaging of the Hip and Knee

Hollis G. Potter, MD   Robert L. Barrack, MD

Imaging

Despite continued advances in imaging technology, plain radiography remains the standard modality for assessing total hip arthroplasty (THA) and total knee arthroplasty (TKA). Plain radiographic views are routinely obtained preoperatively as a crucial part of accurate diagnosis and preoperative planning (templating). Radiographs are used postoperatively to assess the technical quality of the reconstruction and at follow-up intervals, as surveillance for the major failure modes: loosening, wear/osteolysis, and infection. Radiographic assessment of loosening or failure of ingrowth is improved by the addition of oblique views (**Figure 1**). Detection of lysis is also improved by views in multiple projections, but more advanced imaging modalities such as CT or MRI are far more accurate in detecting the presence and extent of lysis. There are no findings on plain radiographs that are both highly sensitive and highly specific for infection, and this diagnosis is also more accurately made with serologic tests, joint aspiration (image guided for the hip), and judicious use of more advanced imaging modalities.

Radiographs should be screened for general features such as bone mineral density as a potential sign of osteopenia or osteoporosis, which could impact implant choice. A preoperative dual-energy x-ray absorptiometry (DEXA) scan may be considered in some cases, and preoperative and postoperative treatment of osteoporosis may be advisable to minimize the risks of fracture and implant-related pain.

Dr. Potter or an immediate family member is a paid consultant for or an employee of Histogenic Corporation, Stryker, and the Musculoskeletal Transplant Foundation and has received research or institutional support from GE Healthcare. Dr. Barrack or an immediate family member is a board member, owner, officer, or committee member for the American Association of Hip and Knee Surgeons and the American Orthopaedic Association; has received research or institutional support from Medtronic Sofamor Danek and Smith & Nephew; and has received nonincome support (such as equipment or services), commercially derived honoraria, or other non-research–related funding (such as paid travel) from Wolters Kluwer Health and Lippincott Williams & Wilkins.

Digital Templating

Digital imaging is an aspect of the trend toward paperless electronic medical records, which are an important aspect of health care reform. Digital images are easily archived and allow data sharing, portability, and manipulation with several software programs, including those allowing preoperative templating. Disadvantages include somewhat decreased spatial resolution, the cost of the software and site licenses, and the inconsistency of magnification of printed images because many programs rescale to the radiographic film when printing. This inconsistency in magnification can be overcome to some degree by using a magnification marker. Advantages of digital imaging and templating include lower radiation, less toxic waste in production and disposal of film, and potentially less cost in printing and storing films. Despite the advanced technology applied to digital templating, the accuracy has not been shown to be better than the use of traditional acetate overlays in predicting component size for THA or TKA. The results from numerous centers have been extremely variable, but in general, digital templating has been deemed adequate and comparable in accuracy or slightly less accurate than traditional manual methods.[1-3]

Total Hip Arthroplasty

John Charnley is generally credited with describing the goal of restoring normal joint biomechanics by accurate placement of total hip components. This requires careful reproducible measurements preoperatively and postoperatively to achieve the goals of obtaining near-equal limb length and restoring offset and center of rotation as closely as possible. An AP pelvis radiograph should be centered over the pubic symphysis and the limbs should be internally rotated 10° to 15° to reproduce normal femoral offset in an average patient (**Figure 2**). Patients with degenerative arthritis tend to hold the limb in external rotation, which decreases the offset, decreases the intertrochanteric area (and thus the predicted stem size), and changes the profile of the lesser trochanter (making limb-length estimates less accurate). With a tube-to-film distance of 1 m and a film cassette location 5 cm below the patient, magnification averages 20% ± 6% depending on patient size, particularly the thickness of soft tissue posterior to the plane

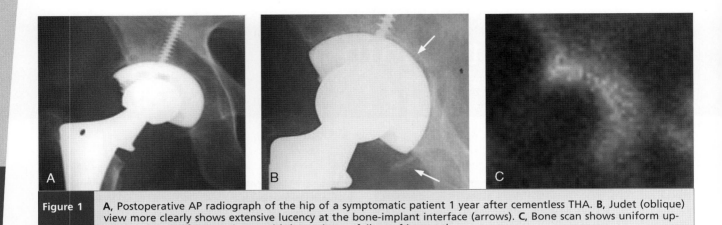

Figure 1 **A,** Postoperative AP radiograph of the hip of a symptomatic patient 1 year after cementless THA. **B,** Judet (oblique) view more clearly shows extensive lucency at the bone-implant interface (arrows). **C,** Bone scan shows uniform uptake at the interface consistent with loosening or failure of ingrowth.

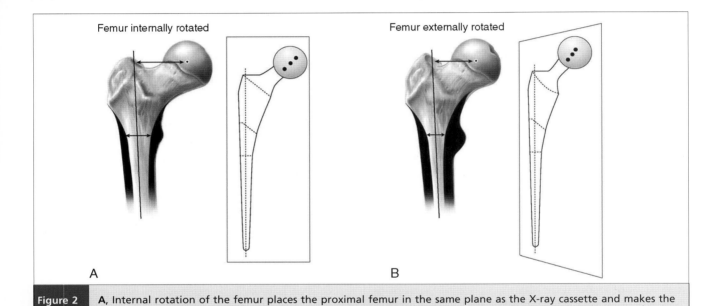

Figure 2 **A,** Internal rotation of the femur places the proximal femur in the same plane as the X-ray cassette and makes the lesser trochanter appear less prominent. **B,** External rotation makes the lesser trochanter appear more prominent as well as decreasing both the apparent intertrochanteric area and the femoral offset. (Reproduced with permission from Barrack RL, Burnett RSJ: Preoperative planning, in Callaghan J, Rosenberg A, Rubash H, eds: *The Adult Hip*, ed 2. Philadelphia, PA, Lippincott Williams & Wilkins, 2007, pp 884-910.)

of the proximal femur and hip joint. True magnification can be more accurately estimated with a magnification marker, but the acetate overlays of most manufacturers have a fixed 20% magnification factor. The quality of the film should be judged for pelvic rotation by comparing the symmetry of the obturator foramina, pelvic tilt by assessing the distance of the coccyx from the symphysis, and pelvic obliquity, which can change apparent limb length.

Limb-length equalization is a crucial goal and the interischial line should be compared to a fixed point on the femur, usually the top or mid position of the lesser trochanter. Radiographic measurement should be compared to the patient's perception and clinical measurement (such as with the use of blocks). The acetabular template is placed adjacent to the teardrop (which cor-

responds anatomically to the base of the cotyloid notch) at a 45° angle in a position that achieves bony contact. If achieving bony contact moves the template proximal to the teardrop, the center of rotation can be measured compared to the normal contralateral side by measuring the horizontal and vertical distance from the teardrop.

Equally important is noting the amount of the template that is uncovered laterally, which should be reproduced at the time of surgery. Obtaining complete bony coverage on a postoperative radiograph when lateral uncoverage was predicted frequently results in a vertical component (> 45°). This is particularly important with metal-on-metal components in which cup angles greater than 55° have been associated with high metal ion levels.[4] Restoring femoral offset is also clinically important. Failure to restore femoral offset has been associated with a limp, weakness, and instability. In one recent study, restoring offset within 5 mm of the native offset and obtaining a cup inclination of less then 45° was associated with less polyethylene wear.[5]

Recently, acetabular anteversion has assumed more clinical importance. Suboptimal anteversion has been associated with both squeaking and increased wear of ceramic-on-ceramic THAs,[6] and increased anteversion has also been suggested as a factor in increased metal ion levels in metal-on-metal surface replacement.[7] Anteversion is usually measured on the cross-table lateral radiograph. This view also allows assessment of the anterior rim of the acetabular component relative to the bony margin. A prominent anterior edge has been associated with symptomatic psoas irritation[8] and should be avoided when possible. The shoot-through lateral view is prone to variability based on patient position, and CT is more accurate for assessing true acetabular component version.[9]

The introduction of new hip component technologies such as advanced bearing surfaces, surface replacement, and modular stems increases the importance of preoperative radiographic assessment. Ceramic-on-ceramic components systems generally have fewer head and liner options, so depth of reaming and level of neck resection must be accomplished with a greater degree of accuracy based on the preoperative plan. Excessive anteversion can cause impingement, subluxation, stripe wear, lysis, and possibly squeaking.[3]

Acetabular dysplasia is often associated with excessive femoral anteversion. Cementless stem rotation is often dictated by the anatomy of the proximal femur placing the femoral neck in excessive anteversion and thus increasing the risk of impingement, instability, and wear. In one recent study, CT of total hips determined that 15% of stems were either anteverted greater than 10% or retroverted.[10] Modular necks are currently available that would allow adjusting neck version independently of the stem. This requires, however, that surgeons be able to judge stem version intraoperatively with precision, which was questioned in this recent study.[10]

Total hip resurfacing is indicated for a relatively small percentage of patients with end-stage osteoarthritis of the hip. There are numerous relative contraindications, most of which can be detected from scrutiny of plain radiographs, including limb-length discrepancy greater than 1 cm, cysts larger than 1 cm, osteoporosis, osteonecrosis involving more than 50% of the femoral head, neck-shaft angle less than 120°, severe coxa breva, head-neck ratio less than 1.2, and severe deformity of the femoral head or neck.[11]

Total Knee Arthroplasty

As in THA, the goal of TKA is to restore normal biomechanics to maximize function and longevity of the implant. The traditional target is to align the components perpendicular to the mechanical axis, defined as a line from the center of the femoral head, through the middle of the knee joint, to the center of the ankle (middle of the talus). Traditionally, this alignment has been obtained by cutting the tibia perpendicular to the tibial shaft (with posterior slope of 3° to 6° depending on the patient's anatomy and the choice of tibial liner) and cutting the femur in 5° to 6° of valgus relative to an intramedullary guide presumed to be in the neutral axis of the femur. One recent study determined that the mechanical axis could not be consistently restored with a fixed valgus cut because variations in femoral anatomy produced an offset between anatomic and mechanical axis on the femoral side of 2° to 9° rather than 5° to 6°.[12] Based on this information, it would be logical to presume that long hip-knee-ankle films could result in more accurate alignment of the mechanical axis by allowing a more accurate valgus angle on the distal cut. A randomized study of 124 primary TKAs did not show a difference in postoperative mechanical axis (defined as those passing through the central third of the knee) in patients whose cut was based on preoperative long radiographs compared to those with short radiographs and a fixed 5° valgus cut.[13]

Although the traditional goals of TKA have been to achieve neutral mechanical alignment, a tibiofemoral angle in the 5° to 7° range, and a neutral tibial cut specifically avoiding varus, half of total knee failures occurring before 10-year follow-up in one series occurred in those knees in the normal alignment range.[14] It has long been held that alignment is the major factor influencing postoperative loosening and instability.[15] This concept has been challenged by a recent study from the Mayo Clinic, which examined the 15-year survival of a modern cemented condylar total knee and determined that survival was not better when a mechanical axis of 0° ± 3° was achieved.[16] The opposite view was expressed by a radiographic review of more than 6,000 TKAs. The failure rate was only 0.5% in those with neutral coronal alignment (2.4° to 7.2°), but more than three times higher in those on the varus or valgus side of that range.[17] Achieving good coronal, sagittal, and rotational alignment in TKA was correlated with faster recovery and better function in one recent study.[18] Multislice CT of the entire extremity was used to more accurately define component alignment in this study.

The ability of traditional total knee alignment guides to consistently achieve coronal or rotational alignment targets measured radiographically has long been questioned.[19] One issue is the variability in the identification of anatomic landmarks. This has led to interest in computer navigation to improve consistency and accuracy of TKA component placement. The end result has been extremely variable and controversial. One meta-analysis of 29 studies comparing computer-assisted surgery (CAS) with conventional TKA concluded CAS achieved better coronal alignment and tibial and femoral slope.[20] Conversely, a study of bilateral simultaneous TKAs in 160 patients, one CAS versus one standard, showed no clinical or radiographic difference.[21] A functional study of conventional versus CAS TKA showed no difference in stability between the two groups.[22]

The inconsistency of traditional cutting guides and CAS in achieving accurate, reproducible alignment, especially rotational alignment, has led to the application of more advanced preoperative imaging (MRI and CT) to produce disposable prefabricated guides customized to each patient's anatomy. Most guides use traditional landmarks such as the mechanical and epicondylar axes to plan cuts, whereas one system uses the flexion-extension or cylindrical axis, which differs from the epicondylar axis by approximately 5°.[23] Custom guides add the additional expense of a preoperative scan and the cost of the cutting guide. They offer potential advantages of increased efficiency and lower cost in the operating room and possibly quicker recovery and better clinical outcomes. Early clinical results have been promising,[24,25] but series are small and follow-up is short. Larger scale, longer term, prospective studies by groups other than those of the designers will hopefully determine whether this approach represents a significant clinical advance.

Bone Scintigraphy

Technetium diphosphonate radionuclide bone scanning, when performed in a three-phase technique, provides a nonspecific assessment of bone turnover surrounding arthroplasty. Although no specific pattern of radionuclide uptake is characteristic of infection, more diffuse radiotracer activity is more likely seen with infection than with aseptic loosening. The classic appearance of prosthetic loosening on a radionuclide scan is generally denoted by moderately increased radiotracer activity in more than two radiographic zones. When combined with indium-111 labeled white blood cell scintigraphy, higher sensitivity and specificity have been reported; however, limitations include the labor-intensive handling of autologous white blood cells, expense, and additional quality assurance issues.[26]

More recent interest has been directed toward the use of fluorodeoxyglucose positron emission tomography (FDG-PET), often combined with CT. Diagnosis for periprosthetic infection using FDG-PET is based on increased FDG uptake at the prosthetic bone interface that is not limited to the soft tissue or neck of the arthroplasty.[26,27] When combined with CT, FDG-PET produces high-resolution imaging in a relatively short acquisition time, allowing for combination of anatomic evaluation of the arthroplasty-bone interface and metabolic assessment based on the cellular metabolic rate and number of glucose transporters.[28] Using a combination of histology, intraoperative findings, and clinical follow-up as the standard, reported sensitivity and specificity for FDG-PET has been 85% and 93%, re-

spectively, with an overall accuracy of 91%.[29] The use of scintigraphic techniques to distinguish periprosthetic loosening from infection should be made based on the regional availability of imaging techniques as well as the confidence of the laboratory to provide consistently good labeling of cells. Of note, the highest diagnostic accuracy for detecting aseptic loosening has been reported with plain radiographs, when combined with either bone scintigraphy or subtraction arthrography; however, considerable interobserver variability exists, even with experienced radiologists.[30]

Scintigraphic techniques also have been used to evaluate bone metabolism, assessing patella viability after knee arthroplasty and lateral release, as well as allograft assessment after grafting of osteolysis in the setting of revision arthroplasty.[31,32] Allogeneic bone grafts have been noted to induce a higher rate of local periprosthetic bone formation in comparison with primary hip arthroplasty, likely because of the induction of higher osteoblastic activity.[32] Technetium 99 (Tc99) bone scanning can be used to examine an unresurfaced patella to ascertain if it is a likely source of pain. The presence of markedly increased uptake supports the diagnosis of osteonecrosis, fracture, or stress reaction as an etiology for symptoms. Unfortunately, patellar resurfacing in this scenario does not lead to predictable resolution of anterior knee pain (**Figure 3**).

Bone Density Assessment

DEXA provides assessment of bone mineral density over specific target areas of the arthroplasty. This technique can be combined with high-quality radiographs or CT and provide information regarding regional alterations in periprosthetic osteoporosis. DEXA analysis has disclosed that progressive shortening of the femoral stem produces more proximal loading, leading to increased periprosthetic bone mineral density over time.[33] Careful attention to technique is essential with regard to patient position, given the sensitivity of DEXA to rotation of the femur. Several studies have examined the impact of hip or knee arthroplasty on the periprosthetic bone density. The presence of a femoral stem is invariably associated with some degree of bone loss. Stems that are less stiff (more isoelastic) seem to be associated with less stress shielding.[34] Studies show that hip resurfacing does not result in bone loss of the femoral neck or proximal femur, presumably because of the different loading pattern from absence of an intramedullary stem.[35,36] Loss of bone density has also been described in the acetabulum adjacent to cementless acetabular components. One recent report has noted less bone loss adjacent to acetabular shells with lower modulus and stiffness,[37] whereas a postmortem study showed the degree of bone loss was substantially less around the acetabulum than the femur and questioned its clinical significance.[38]

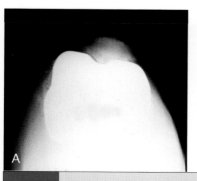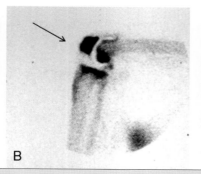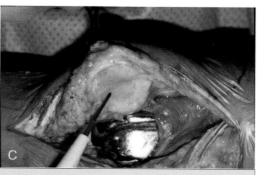

Figure 3 **A,** Sunrise view more than 3 years after TKA, without patella resurfacing, shows apparent erosion of the patella. **B,** Technetium 99 bone scan confirms dramatically increased uptake of the patella (arrow). **C,** Complete cartilage erosion was confirmed intraoperatively. However, revision to a subsequent resurfaced patella provided only temporary relief of anterior knee pain.

1: Basic Science and General Knowledge

Osteoporosis is a contraindication for hip resurfacing. Preoperative DEXA can be used to screen for osteoporosis or osteopenia in patients who have the appearance of diminished bone mineral density on plain radiographs or in postmenopausal women.

Computed Tomography

CT has been a useful adjunct to conventional radiographic assessment for both hip and knee arthroplasty.[39] The advent of multidetector scanners and helical acquisition has allowed for rapid acquisition of imaging data and superior quality coronal and sagittal reformations from axial acquired data sets (**Figure 4**). Helical CT with a metal artifact reduction protocol has been more effective than radiographs in detecting the extent of periacetabular osteolysis following hip arthroplasty.[40] In a preclinical model of simulated osteolysis, CT was more accurate than radiographs in assessing the magnitude of osteolysis, with a slight tendency to overestimate lesion volume.[41] A retrospective review of concurrently acquired CT and radiographic data has shown marked underestimation of the magnitude of osteolysis in the pelvis.[42] Imaging strategies to reduce hardening artifact and hollow data points during the filtered back rejection reconstruction of CT data result in typical parameters of 300 mA-second (mAs) and 140 peak kilovoltage (kVp), which pose a cumulative radiation burden for serial examinations. CT scanning with artifact reduction can be helpful in more accurately determining the extent of osteolysis and need for graft material, the presence of medial wall integrity, and the likelihood of pelvic discontinuity, all of which are helpful in preoperative surgical planning. Recently, CT has also been used to assess bone healing after grafting of lytic lesions.[43] Plain radiographs may be difficult to interpret after a grafting procedure and give the appearance of some degree of healing (**Figure 5, A**), whereas a corresponding CT scan frequently demonstrates clear absence of healing (**Figure 5, B and C**).

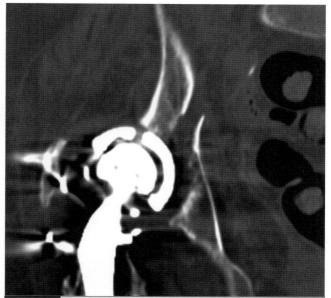

Figure 4 A coronal CT image from an 80-year-old woman after THA shows a transversely oriented, mildly displaced fracture through the acetabulum

In addition to assessment of wear and osteolysis, CT has been used to assess component version as well as the incorporation of bone graft after revision arthroplasty with modular liner exchange.[44,45] Further, CT densitometry has been used to gather information about the load transfer mechanism to the pelvis after cup implantation, allowing for a minimally invasive assessment of the stress shielding phenomenon in vivo.[46]

In an ex vivo analysis of retrieved uncemented metal-backed acetabular cups, CT was accurate and reliable for assessment of linear wear.[47] These techniques rely on fairly labor-intensive analysis of a CT volume set using a distribution of coordinate points to compute the orientation of the cup and require further processing algorithms to reduce metal artifact.[47] In an additional cadaver model, CT has been used to analyze the

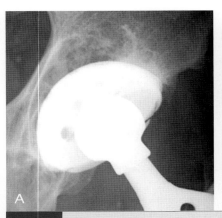 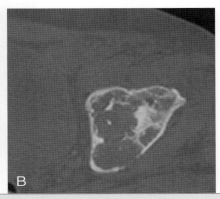 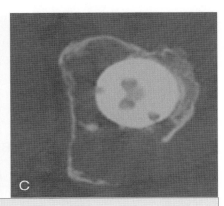

Figure 5 **A,** Plain radiographs at 4 years after surgery with head and liner change, and calcium sulfate/demineralized bone matrix grafting through holes in the shell give the appearance of some degree of bone healing. **B,** CT appearance at 4 years shows limited graft incorporation. **C,** CT appearance not supportive of healing of defect, reconstitution of bone, or alteration of the course of lysis.

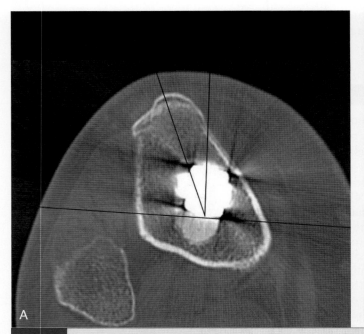 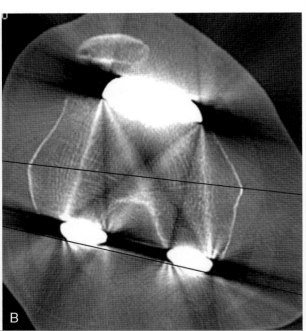

Figure 6 Postoperative CT scans of a patient with a symptomatic patellar subluxation immediately after primary TKA show significant internal rotation of both the tibial (**A**) and femoral (**B**) components.

cement mantle and alignment of the stem, which may have implications for selection of size of the stem and the development of radiolucent regions.[48]

CT has also been used to evaluate total knee component malrotation as a potential cause of total knee failure. Mild combined internal rotation (1° to 4°) was reportedly associated with patellar tilt and lateral tracking, moderate degrees (3° to 8°) with patellar subluxation, and large degrees (7° to 8°) with patellar dislocation or late patellar prosthesis failure[49] (**Figure 6**). The association of combined component internal rotation reportedly had a significantly higher incidence of anterior knee pain in comparison with TKAs without

this finding.[50] There was a high clinical success rate with revision TKA that corrected the component malrotation.

Magnetic Resonance Imaging

Because of its superior soft-tissue contrast, direct multiplanar capabilities, and lack of ionizing radiation, MRI has proven helpful in evaluating painful joint arthroplasty. Protocol modification is necessary to reduce the frequency shift and distortion in the slice profile induced by the close anatomic juxtaposition of ferromagnetic orthopaedic hardware and diamagnetic soft tissue. Strategies include the use of fluid-sensitive pulse sequences with acquisition of images with a wide receiver bandwidth. The wide receiver bandwidth acts to reduce the frequency shift.[51] MRI has been shown to be more sensitive than radiographs in detecting the magnitude of bone loss, as well as detecting intracapsular deposits of wear-induced synovitis in both hip and knee arthroplasty.[51,52] The signal characteristics of the synovial deposits in the setting of particle disease and component wear are variable, but are typically intermediate to low signal intensity, bulky deposits within the higher signal intensity fluid. Bone loss ranges from expansion of the pseudocapsule, creating an indolent erosion of bone to more particulate deposits of intermediate signal intensity osteolysis, surrounded by a low-signal-intensity rim and demarcated from the high signal intensity of the surrounding fatty marrow (**Figure 7**). The presence of periprosthetic fluid collections in the greater trochanteric bursa can easily be discerned, often communicating through a dehiscence in the posterior capsule, and these fluid collections have been described in both metal-on-polyethylene and metal-on-metal arthroplasty.[53]

Given the concerns of ionizing radiation burden in CT, it has been compared with MRI and plain film in a cadaver model of simulated osteolysis. MRI demonstrated superior accuracy in detecting periacetabular bone loss in conventional metal-on-polyethylene implants, with reported sensitivity for optimized MRI of 95.4% compared with optimized CT of 74.7% and radiographs at 51.7%.[54,55] Clear benefits of MRI include the ability to detect and serially follow intracapsular burden of wear-induced synovitis as well as more accurate assessment of bone loss that may not be discernible on either optimized CT or radiographs (**Figure 8**).

In addition to assessment of wear-induced synovitis and osteolysis, the remaining surrounding soft-tissue envelope can be assessed, including the integrity of the

hip abductors, short external rotators, posterior capsule, and iliopsoas tendon.[56,57] Concern exists about the integrity of the short external rotator tendons and posterior capsule repair in patients at risk for dislocation or after dislocation has occurred. In a prospective MRI assessment of patients after hip arthroplasty, 43% of piriformis tendon repairs and 57% of conjoined tendon repairs were dehiscent, whereas the posterior capsule remained intact in 90% of patients.[57] Of note, the "gap" filled in with scar tissue, suggesting that there is

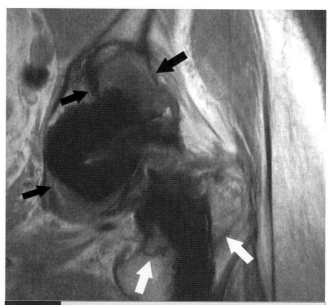

| Figure 7 | Coronal proton density MRI of an 87-year-old man with THA done 21 years previously demonstrates severe periacetabular osteolysis (black arrows), with circumferential involvement and suspected loosening of the acetabular component. Additional osteolysis is noted in Gruen zones 1 and 7 (white arrows). |

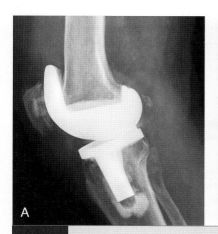
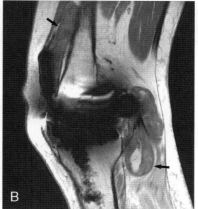
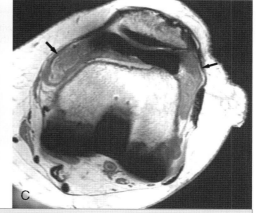

| Figure 8 | Imaging studies from a 60-year-old woman with TKA done 10 years previously. **A,** Lateral radiograph demonstrates well-aligned arthroplasty components with minimal osteolysis. Sagittal (**B**) and axial (**C**) proton density MRIs demonstrate massive intracapsular burden of particle disease (arrows), without component loosening. |

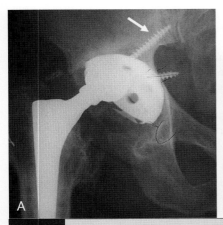
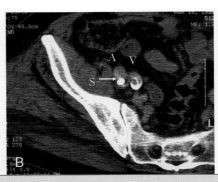
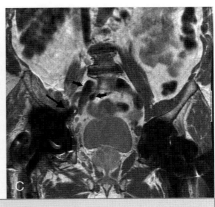

Figure 9   **A**, Plain radiograph shows dramatic polyethylene wear and a THA that was associated with dramatic blood loss during the original procedure. The prominent screw in the pelvis (arrow) was likely the source of the bleeding. **B**, Axial noncontrast CT demonstrates the proximity of the screw (S) to the artery and vein (A and V). **C**, Coronal MRI demonstrates the screw (long arrow) and adjacent artery and vein (short arrows).

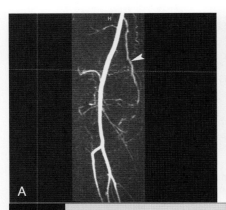
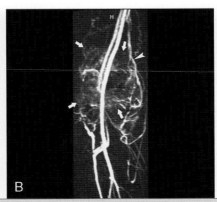
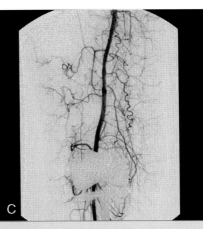

Figure 10   Imaging studies from a 63-year-old woman who has undergone TKA and has recurrent hemarthroses. **A**, The initial run of a contrast-enhanced magnetic resonance angiogram (MRA) demonstrates prominence of the superomedial geniculate artery (arrowhead). **B**, Delayed MRA image demonstrates synovial hyperemia (arrows) with persistent prominence of the superomedial geniculate artery (arrowhead). **C**, Preembolization conventional angiogram confirms the findings seen on MRA.

a scar-filled scaffold that restores the posterior soft-tissue envelope.[57]

Further, preliminary data using MRI to assess kinematics after knee arthroplasty were obtained, specifically to evaluate the effect of posterior tibial translation to medial patella tilt and inferior patella translation, suggesting that MRI might be efficacious in the in vivo longitudinal and dynamic assessment of component rotation following arthroplasty.[58]

Both MRI and CT data have been used to provide patient-specific templates for custom cutting blocks in knee arthroplasty. These techniques require a three-dimensional data set and some assessment of the mechanical axis for implementation. Recent data from a preclinical model suggest that MRI data were associ-

ated with increased error and variability of results compared with CT.[59]

Magnetic Resonance Angiography

Magnetic resonance angiography has supplanted traditional arteriography in the assessment of some periprosthetic conditions. It requires an intravenous injection of gadolinium contrast agent but no direct arterial puncture. Conventional noncontrast CT or MRI can accurately detect the proximity of components, cement, or screws to intrapelvic neurovascular structures before revision surgery (**Figure 9**). One condition for which contrast-enhanced magnetic resonance angiogra-

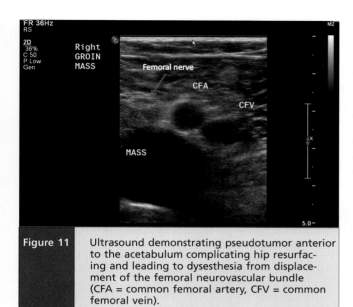

FR 36Hz
RS

2D
36%
C 50
P Low
Gen

Right
GROIN
MASS

Femoral nerve

CFA

CFV

MASS

5.0 —

Figure 11 Ultrasound demonstrating pseudotumor anterior to the acetabulum complicating hip resurfacing and leading to dysesthesia from displacement of the femoral neurovascular bundle (CFA = common femoral artery, CFV = common femoral vein).

phy is useful is the assessment of recurrent hemarthrosis following TKA. Several recent reports have identified subtle arteriovenous malformations of the geniculate vessels as a likely etiology for this rare condition[60] and transcatheter embolization has frequently been successful in treating this condition[61] (**Figure 10**).

Ultrasound

Ultrasound has traditionally been used in orthopaedics to evaluate periarticular soft-tissue structures such as ligaments, tendons, and bursae. In recent years, ultrasound has increasingly been used to identify soft-tissue and fluid collections around hip arthroplasties, especially metal-on-metal hip resurfacings or total hips. One study reported on "pseudotumors" associated with 20 metal-on-metal hip resurfacings in 17 patients using CT, MRI, and ultrasonography.[62] Ultrasound is currently being used for screening and surveillance after THA and hip resurfacing to monitor for development of periarticular fluid or soft-tissue masses that may develop as a result of an adverse local reaction to debris from the bearing surface (**Figure 11**). Ultrasound has advantages of portability, relatively low cost, lack of ionizing radiation, and absence of metal artifact. The contrast resolution, however, is generally inferior to MRI with optimal artifact suppression.

Summary

Although plain radiography will continue to be a mainstay of arthroplasty imaging, the use of digital imaging and templating is likely to increase as part of the electronic medical record mandate. The low incidence of wear and related complications of many standard de-

vices (metal on cross-linked polyethylene) will probably decrease radiographic follow-up intervals. The role of advanced imaging in generating patient-specific instruments and/or implants is a major trend that is likely to be extensively studied in the immediate future. The benefits of MRI include the ability to provide more accurate assessment of the magnitude of periprosthetic bone loss and, more importantly, provide direct, longitudinal assessment of the synovial pattern, located at the origin of the adverse wear-induced synovial reaction that precedes osteoclastic bone resorption.

Annotated References

1. Specht LM, Levitz S, Iorio R, Healy WL, Tilzey JF: A comparison of acetate and digital templating for total knee arthroplasty. *Clin Orthop Relat Res* 2007;464: 179-183.

   Digital templating was found to be at least as accurate as traditional acetate templating for predicting total knee implant size. Level of evidence: II.

2. Iorio R, Siegel J, Specht LM, Tilzey JF, Hartman A, Healy WL: A comparison of acetate vs digital templating for preoperative planning of total hip arthroplasty: Is digital templating accurate and safe? *J Arthroplasty* 2009;24(2):175-179.

   Digital templating was determined to be acceptably safe for preoperative planning for primary THA. Absolute errors were larger for digital compared to acetate templating; however, digital templating was determined to be acceptably safe for preoperative planning. Level of evidence: II.

3. Trickett RW, Hodgson P, Forster MC, Robertson A: The reliability and accuracy of digital templating in total knee replacement. *J Bone Joint Surg Br* 2009;91(7): 903-906.

   Digital templating was found not to predict correct size of total knee components often enough to be of clinical benefit. Level of evidence: II.

4. De Haan R, Campbell PA, Su EP, De Smet KA: Revision of metal-on-metal resurfacing arthroplasty of the hip: The influence of malpositioning of the components. *J Bone Joint Surg Br* 2008;90(9):1158-1163.

   The authors present a retrospective review of 42 patients who had revision metal-on-metal resurfacing. The most common technical errors were excessive abduction (> 55°) or either insufficient or excessive anteversion. Level of evidence: IV.

5. Little NJ, Busch CA, Gallagher JA, Rorabeck CH, Bourne RB: Acetabular polyethylene wear and acetabular inclination and femoral offset. *Clin Orthop Relat Res* 2009;467(11):2895-2900.

   Volumetric and linear polyethylene wear were quantified prospectively in 43 uncemented THAs at 49 months. Reconstruction of femoral offset within 5 mm

1: Basic Science and General Knowledge

of native offset, and acetabular abduction angles less than 45° were associated with less polyethylene wear. Level of evidence: III.

6. Walter WL, O'toole GC, Walter WK, Ellis A, Zicat BA: Squeaking in ceramic-on-ceramic hips: The importance of acetabular component orientation. *J Arthroplasty* 2007;22(4):496-503.

Seventeen patients with THA associated with squeaking were compared to 17 matched control subjects. Patients with squeaking were younger, heavier, taller, and had higher degrees of anteversion compared to those with silent hips. Level of evidence: IV.

7. Langton DJ, Jameson SS, Joyce TJ, Webb J, Nargol AV: The effect of component size and orientation on the concentrations of metal ions after resurfacing arthroplasty of the hip. *J Bone Joint Surg Br* 2008;90(9):1143-1151.

Metal ions were quantified after surface replacement in 76 consecutive patients with a specific recent design. Ion concentrations were significantly higher in patients with smaller components, higher cup abduction angle, and excessive anteversion. Level of evidence: II.

8. Lachiewicz PF, Kauk JR: Anterior iliopsoas impingement and tendinitis after total hip arthroplasty. *J Am Acad Orthop Surg* 2009;17(6):337-344.

Anterior iliopsoas impingement is the cause of groin pain following THA. Release or a resection of the psoas tendon, alone or in combination with acetabular revision for an overhanging anterior component, usually provides relief of symptoms. Level of evidence: V.

9. Ghelman B, Kepler CK, Lyman S, Della Valle AG: CT outperforms radiography for determination of acetabular cup version after THA. *Clin Orthop Relat Res* 2009;467(9):2362-2370.

Cross-table lateral radiographs are associated with variability and the measure of acetabular anteversion, depending on patient position. CT scan is more accurate in measuring anteversion and is independent of patient positioning. Level of evidence: III.

10. Dorr LD, Wan Z, Malik A, Zhu J, Dastane M, Deshmane P: A comparison of surgeon estimation and computed tomographic measurement of femoral component anteversion in cementless total hip arthroplasty. *J Bone Joint Surg Am* 2009;91(11):2598-2604.

CT was used to objectively measure femoral stem version in 109 consecutive THAs (99 patients). Stem version was extremely variable, measuring 10° to 20° in 45%, 0° to 9° (39%), greater than 20° anteversion in 7%, and stem retroversion in 8%. Level of evidence: II.

11. Nunley RM, Della Valle CJ, Barrack RL: Is patient selection important for hip resurfacing? *Clin Orthop Relat Res* 2009;467(1):56-65.

There are numerous selection criteria to consider in incision for total hip resurfacing, including age, sex, obesity, bone density, degree of osteoporosis, renal function, and possible metal sensitivity among others. Level of evidence: V.

12. Bardakos N, Cil A, Thompson B, Stocks G: Mechanical axis cannot be restored in total knee arthroplasty with a fixed valgus resection angle: A radiographic study. *J Arthroplasty* 2007;22(6, Suppl 2):85-89.

The neck-shaft angle of the ipsilateral hip significantly influences the valgus cut angle of a total knee replacement such that a fixed resection angle of 5° or 6° is suboptimal in a substantial portion of patients. Level of evidence: III.

13. McGrory JE, Trousdale RT, Pagnano MW, Nigbur M: Preoperative hip to ankle radiographs in total knee arthroplasty. *Clin Orthop Relat Res* 2002;404:196-202.

14. Tew M, Waugh W: Tibiofemoral alignment and the results of knee replacement. *J Bone Joint Surg Br* 1985;67(4):551-556.

15. Moreland JR: Mechanisms of failure in total knee arthroplasty. *Clin Orthop Relat Res* 1988;226:49-64.

16. Alden KJ, Pagnano MW: Computer-assisted surgery: A wine before its time. *Orthopedics* 2008;31(9):936–939.

Fifteen-year survival of 400 total knees with three modern designs found that survival was not better in those in which mechanical axis was restored within 3° compared with outliers. Level of evidence: Retrospective cohort III.

17. Fang DM, Ritter MA, Davis KE: Coronal alignment in total knee arthroplasty: Just how important is it? *J Arthroplasty* 2009;24(6, Suppl):39-43.

A review of 6,070 total knees in 3,929 patients revealed that those in neutral (defined as 2.4° to 7.2°) alignment had the lowest failure rate (0.5%) compared to those in either varus (1.8%) or valgus (1.5%) alignment. Level of evidence: III.

18. Longstaff LM, Sloan K, Stamp N, Scaddan M, Beaver R: Good alignment after total knee arthroplasty leads to faster rehabilitation and better function. *J Arthroplasty* 2009;24(4):570-578.

One hundred fifty-nine patients underwent postoperative CT for component orientation (sagittal, coronal, and rotational alignment of the femoral and tibial components and femorotibial mismatch). A lower cumulative error score correlated with a better functional outcome. Level of evidence: II.

19. Robinson M, Eckhoff DG, Reinig KD, Bagur MM, Bach JM: Variability of landmark identification in total knee arthroplasty. *Clin Orthop Relat Res* 2006;442:57-62.

Anatomic landmarks used to align total knee guides or to register for computer-assisted navigation are prone to significant interobserver error and were deemed not to be reliable. Level of evidence: III.

20. Mason JB, Fehring TK, Estok R, Banel D, Fahrbach K: Meta-analysis of alignment outcomes in computer-assisted total knee arthroplasty surgery. *J Arthroplasty* 2007;22(8):1097-1106.

A meta-analysis of 29 studies of computer-assisted versus conventional TKA between 1990 and 2007 showed improved alignment for CAS compared to conventional TKA. Level of evidence: III.

21. Kim YH, Kim JS, Choi Y, Kwon OR: Computer-assisted surgical navigation does not improve the alignment and orientation of the components in total knee arthroplasty. *J Bone Joint Surg Am* 2009;91(1): 14-19.

    Sequential simultaneous bilateral TKA was performed in 160 patients (320 knees with 1 knee performed using CAS and the other using conventional techniques). There was no substantial difference in component alignment based on radiographs or CT scans. Level of evidence: II.

22. Song EK, Seon JK, Yoon TR, Park SJ, Cho SG, Yim JH: Comparative study of stability after total knee arthroplasties between navigation system and conventional techniques. *J Arthroplasty* 2007;22(8):1107-1111.

    Mediolateral and anteroposterior laxity using stress radiographs were compared in conventional versus CAS. There was no significant difference between the groups in terms of TKA stability. Level of evidence: II.

23. Eckhoff D, Hogan C, DiMatteo L, Robinson M, Bach J: Difference between the epicondylar and cylindrical axis of the knee. *Clin Orthop Relat Res* 2007;461: 238-244.

    A CT study of 23 cadaver knees demonstrated that the epicondylar axis and the flexion extension axis differed by approximately 5°.

24. Lombardi AV Jr, Berend KR, Adams JB: Patient-specific approach in total knee arthroplasty. *Orthopedics* 2008;31(9):927-930.

    Forty-four TKAs were performed using custom cutting guides with restoration of alignment between 4° and 6° valgus in all cases. Level of evidence: IV.

25. Howell SM, Kuznik K, Hull ML, Siston RA: Results of an initial experience with custom-fit positioning total knee arthroplasty in a series of 48 patients. *Orthopedics* 2008;31(9):857-863.

    Custom cutting guides were used based on a flexion extension axis with removal of osteophytes and limited, if any, ligament release and was associated with rapid return of function, motion, stability, and patient satisfaction. Level of evidence: IV.

26. Parvizi J, Ghanem E, Menashe S, Barrack RL, Bauer TW: Periprosthetic infection: What are the diagnostic challenges? *J Bone Joint Surg Am* 2006;88(Suppl 4): 138-147.

    Data are presented from a scientific exhibit detailing three studies on periprosthetic infection with the use of joint fluid analysis, intraoperative tissue sample, and FDG-PET. A detailed statistical analysis underscores the limitations and value of each test. Level of evidence: III.

27. Pill SG, Parvizi J, Tang PH, et al: Comparison of fluorodeoxyglucose positron emission tomography and (111)indium-white blood cell imaging in the diagnosis of periprosthetic infection of the hip. *J Arthroplasty* 2006;21(6, Suppl 2):91-97.

    Eighty-nine patients with 92 painful hip prostheses were prospectively evaluated with either combined FDG-PET and technetium-99m sulfur colloid (111)indium-labeled white blood cell scintigraphy bone marrow/white blood cell scan or FDG-PET only. FDG-PET demonstrated high predictive values for the diagnosis of infection. Level of evidence: II.

28. Schillaci O: Hybrid imaging systems in the diagnosis of osteomyelitis and prosthetic joint infection. *Q J Nucl Med Mol Imaging* 2009;53(1):95-104.

    This article reviews the currently available literature on the use of hybrid systems in the diagnosis of osteomyelitis and periprosthetic bone infection. Level of evidence: III.

29. Chryssikos T, Parvizi J, Ghanem E, Newberg A, Zhuang H, Alavi A: FDG-PET imaging can diagnose periprosthetic infection of the hip. *Clin Orthop Relat Res* 2008;466(6):1338-1342.

    Investigators evaluated 113 patients with 127 painful hip arthroplasties with FDG-PET. Sensitivity of FDG-PET for infection was reported as 85% (28 of 33 scans) with a specificity of 93% (87 of 94 scans) yielding an overall accuracy of 91% (115 of 127 patients). Level of evidence: II, diagnostic study.

30. Temmerman OP, Raijmakers PG, David EF, et al: A comparison of radiographic and scintigraphic techniques to assess aseptic loosening of the acetabular component in a total hip replacement. *J Bone Joint Surg Am* 2004;86-A(11):2456-2463.

31. Pawar U, Rao KN, Sundaram PS, Thilak J, Varghese J: Scintigraphic assessment of patellar viability in total knee arthroplasty after lateral release. *J Arthroplasty* 2009;24(4):636-640.

    A prospective assessment of Tc-99m bone scans to assess patellar viability in patients undergoing primary knee arthroplasty with/without lateral release is done. A greater incidence of transient patellar hypovascularity was associated with lateral release. Level of evidence: II.

32. Temmerman OP, Raijmakers PG, Heyligers IC, et al: Bone metabolism after total hip revision surgery with impacted grafting: Evaluation using H2 15O and [18F]fluoride PET: A pilot study. *Mol Imaging Biol* 2008;10(5):288-293.

    In a pilot study using H_2 ^{15}O and [^{18}F]fluoride PET, bone grafted revision hip arthroplasty was compared to primary hip arthroplasty; bone metabolism after revision was three times higher, suggesting that bone metabolism in allogeneic grafts may partly rely on blood flow adaptation. Level of evidence: II.

33. Albanese CV, Santori FS, Pavan L, Learmonth ID, Passariello R: Periprosthetic DXA after total hip arthro-

1: Basic Science and General Knowledge

plasty with short vs. ultra-short custom-made femoral stems: 37 patients followed for 3 years. *Acta Orthop* 2009;80(3):291-297.

Bone mineral density was evaluated after hip arthroplasty with progressive shortening of the stem, which produced more proximal loading and increased medial periprosthetic bone mineral density. DEXA may be used to evaluate biologic response to changes in implant shape. Level of evidence: II-2.

34. Glassman AH, Bobyn JD, Tanzer M: New femoral designs: Do they influence stress shielding? *Clin Orthop Relat Res* 2006;453:64-74.

DEXA scanning has been performed on a variety of stem designs preoperatively and postoperatively, and the available evidence indicates that stem stiffness plays a dominant role in the degree of stress shielding that occurs. Level of evidence: III

35. Harty JA, Devitt B, Harty LC, Molloy M, McGuinness A: Dual energy X-ray absorptiometry analysis of periprosthetic stress shielding in the Birmingham resurfacing hip replacement. *Arch Orthop Trauma Surg* 2005; 125(10):693-695.

Twenty-eight patients underwent DEXA analysis for the proximal femur and femoral neck following Birmingham hip resurfacing. Femoral neck bone density did not decrease and is unlikely to be an etiology for femoral neck fractures. Level of evidence: II.

36. Kishida Y, Sugano N, Nishii T, Miki H, Yamaguchi K, Yoshikawa H: Preservation of the bone mineral density of the femur after surface replacement of the hip. *J Bone Joint Surg Br* 2004;86(2):185-189.

37. Meneghini RM, Ford KS, McCollough CH, Hanssen AD, Lewallen DG: Bone remodeling around porous metal cementless acetabular components. *J Arthroplasty* 2010;25(5):741-747.

Quantitative CT was used to compare bone mineral density in the acetabulum at a mean of 7.7 years following cementless THA. Significantly less stress shielding occurred around highly porous metal implants with a lower elastic modulus compared to the traditional porous-coated component. Level of evidence: II.

38. Stepniewski AS, Egawa H, Sychterz-Terefenko C, Leung S, Engh CA Sr: Periacetabular bone density after total hip arthroplasty a postmortem analysis. *J Arthroplasty* 2008;23(4):593-599.

Postmortem analysis was performed on five retrieved pelves, and DEXA scans were performed for comparison with the contralateral side. Much lower degrees of stress shielding were observed in the pelvis than the femur, and the clinical significance of the small degree of stress shielding was expressed. Level of evidence: II.

39. Reish TG, Clarke HD, Scuderi GR, Math KR, Scott WN: Use of multi-detector computed tomography for the detection of periprosthetic osteolysis in total knee arthroplasty. *J Knee Surg* 2006;19(4):259-264.

A retrospective comparison of radiographs and CT for detection of osteolysis surrounding knee arthroplasty demonstrated the superior ability of multidetector CT to detect the magnitude of bone loss. Level of evidence: III.

40. Puri L, Wixson RL, Stern SH, Kohli J, Hendrix RW, Stulberg SD: Use of helical computed tomography for the assessment of acetabular osteolysis after total hip arthroplasty. *J Bone Joint Surg Am* 2002;84-A(4):609-614.

41. Claus AM, Totterman SM, Sychterz CJ, Tamez-Peña JG, Looney RJ, Engh CA Sr: Computed tomography to assess pelvic lysis after total hip replacement. *Clin Orthop Relat Res* 2004;422:167-174.

42. Egawa H, Powers CC, Beykirch SE, Hopper RH Jr, Engh CA Jr, Engh CA: Can the volume of pelvic osteolysis be calculated without using computed tomography? *Clin Orthop Relat Res* 2009;467(1):181-187.

The area of pelvic osteolysis measured on radiographs, heavy patient activity level, and total volume of wear were associated with pelvic osteolysis volume as assessed by CT, but estimates of osteolysis volume deviated from actual CT volume in many cases. Level of evidence: III.

43. Mall NA, Nunley RM, Smith KE, Maloney WJ, Clohisy JC, Barrack RL: The fate of grafting acetabular defects during revision total hip arthroplasty. *Clin Orthop Relat Res* 2010; Epub ahead of print.

CT scans of 40 patients were analyzed for defect healing following either complete revision or head liner change.

44. Wines AP, McNicol D: Computed tomography measurement of the accuracy of component version in total hip arthroplasty. *J Arthroplasty* 2006;21(5):696-701.

Intraoperative version analysis was compared with postoperative CT in 111 primary arthroplasties. Only 71% of femoral and 45% of acetabular components were within the expected version range, raising concerns about the accuracy of intraoperative estimation of version. Level of evidence: II-2.

45. Puri L, Lapinski B, Wixson RL, Lynch J, Hendrix R, Stulberg SD: Computed tomographic follow-up evaluation of operative intervention for periacetabular lysis. *J Arthroplasty* 2006;21(6, Suppl 2):78-82.

Postoperative (minimum 2 years) CT evaluation was performed following revision in a small cohort who had undergone liner exchange and bone grafting for osteolysis. Preoperative and postoperative evaluations were compared, demonstrating substantial decrease in the size of osteolytic lesions. Level of evidence: II-2.

46. Mueller LA, Kress A, Nowak T, et al: Periacetabular bone changes after uncemented total hip arthroplasty evaluated by quantitative computed tomography. *Acta Orthop* 2006;77(3):380-385.

CT-assisted osteodensitometry demonstrated that mean bone density of cortical bone cranial to the cup increased by 3.6%, whereas cancellous bone decreased by 18%. Cancellous bone loss was greater ventral to the cup than dorsally, demonstrating stress shielding phenomenon in vivo. Level of evidence: II-2.

47. Jedenmalm A, Noz ME, Olivecrona H, Olivecrona L, Stark A: A new approach for assessment of wear in metal-backed acetabular cups using computed tomography: A phantom study with retrievals. *Acta Orthop* 2008;79(2):218-224.

A study of explanted acetabular cups demonstrated that CT is able to reliably measure linear wear at clinically relevant levels of accuracy.

48. Scheerlinck T, de Mey J, Deklerck R, Noble PC: CT analysis of defects of the cement mantle and alignment of the stem: In vitro comparison of Charnley-Kerboul femoral hip implants inserted line-to-line and undersized in paired femora. *J Bone Joint Surg Br* 2006; 88(1):19-25.

Charnley-Kerboul stems were implanted in a cadaver model to compare implants inserted line-to-line versus undersized in paired femora. In the line-to-line group, penetration of cement into cancellous bone resulted in a superior mean thickness of cement with fewer cement-deficient regions.

49. Berger RA, Crossett LS, Jacobs JJ, Rubash HE: Malrotation causing patellofemoral complications after total knee arthroplasty. *Clin Orthop Relat Res* 1998; 356 :144-153.

50. Barrack RL, Schrader T, Bertot AJ, Wolfe MW, Myers L: Component rotation and anterior knee pain after total knee arthroplasty. *Clin Orthop Relat Res* 2001; 392:46-55.

51. Potter HG, Nestor BJ, Sofka CM, Ho ST, Peters LE, Salvati EA: Magnetic resonance imaging after total hip arthroplasty: Evaluation of periprosthetic soft tissue. *J Bone Joint Surg Am* 2004;86-A(9):1947-1954.

52. Vessely MB, Frick MA, Oakes D, Wenger DE, Berry DJ: Magnetic resonance imaging with metal suppression for evaluation of periprosthetic osteolysis after total knee arthroplasty. *J Arthroplasty* 2006;21(6):826-831.

The investigators performed a retrospective review of 11 patients referred for MRI with infected periprosthetic osteolysis, noting that the extent of osteolysis was greater on MRI than estimated radiographically. Level of evidence: II-3.

53. Toms AP, Marshall TJ, Cahir J, et al: MRI of early symptomatic metal-on-metal total hip arthroplasty: A retrospective review of radiological findings in 20 hips. *Clin Radiol* 2008;63(1):49-58.

A retrospective review of MRI evaluation of metal-on-metal hip arthroplasties demonstrated a variety of adverse soft-tissue reactions. Level of evidence: IV.

54. Walde TA, Weiland DE, Leung SB, et al: Comparison of CT, MRI, and radiographs in assessing pelvic osteolysis: A cadaveric study. *Clin Orthop Relat Res* 2005;437:138-144.

In a simulated osteolysis model, CT was compared to radiographs and MRI for detection of periacetabular bone loss. Sensitivity was 51.7% for radiography, 74.7% for CT, and 95.4% for MRI with similar specificity, indicating superior accuracy of MRI in detecting and quantifying bone loss.

55. Weiland DE, Walde TA, Leung SB, et al: Magnetic resonance imaging in the evaluation of periprosthetic acetabular osteolysis: A cadaveric study. *J Orthop Res* 2005;23(4):713-719.

A cadaver model of simulated bone loss demonstrated the higher accuracy of MRI in detecting periacetabular bone loss compared with standardized radiographs.

56. Pfirrmann CW, Notzli HP, Dora C, Hodler J, Zanetti M: Abductor tendons and muscles assessed at MR imaging after total hip arthroplasty in asymptomatic and symptomatic patients. *Radiology* 2005;235(3):969-976.

A prospective MRI evaluation of the hip abductors after arthroplasty demonstrated that tendon defects and fatty muscle atrophy were uncommon in asymptomatic patients but more frequent in symptomatic cohorts. Level of evidence: III.

57. Pellicci PM, Potter HG, Foo LF, Boettner F: MRI shows biologic restoration of posterior soft tissue repairs after THA. *Clin Orthop Relat Res* 2009;467(4): 940-945.

Prospective MRI evaluation of the soft-tissue envelope of primary arthroplasties demonstrated that 43% of piriformis and 57% of conjoined tendon repairs showed a gap that filled in with scar tissue, indicating an anatomic scaffold for posterior support. Level of evidence: II-2.

58. Lee KY, Slavinsky JP, Ries MD, Blumenkrantz G, Majumdar S: Magnetic resonance imaging of in vivo kinematics after total knee arthroplasty. *J Magn Reson Imaging* 2005;21(2):172-178.

An MRI pilot study of in vivo kinematics following knee arthroplasty under simulated weight-bearing demonstrates the ability of MRI to potentially evaluate in vivo kinematics. Level of evidence: III.

59. White D, Chelule KL, Seedhom BB: Accuracy of MRI vs CT imaging with particular reference to patient specific templates for total knee replacement surgery. *Int J Med Robot* 2008;4(3):224-231.

The investigators studied 10 ovine knees using MRI and CT parameters generating bone models from each three-dimensional data set, disclosing that the bone models generated from MRI were less accurate than those generated from CT data.

60. Ibrahim M, Booth RE Jr, Clark TW: Embolization of traumatic pseudoaneurysms after total knee arthroplasty. *J Arthroplasty* 2004;19(1):123-128.

61. Given MF, Smith P, Lyon SM, Robertson D, Thomson KR: Embolization of spontaneous hemarthrosis post total knee replacement. *Cardiovasc Intervent Radiol* 2008;31(5):986-988.

1: Basic Science and General Knowledge

Three cases of recurrent hemarthrosis following total knee replacement were successfully treated with angiography and microembolization of the geniculate branches. Level of evidence: IV.

62. Pandit H, Glyn-Jones S, McLardy-Smith P, et al: Pseudotumours associated with metal-on-metal hip resurfacings. *J Bone Joint Surg Br* 2008;90(7):847-851.

Soft-tissue masses developed in 20 hips (17 patients) following metal-on-metal hip resurfacings that were detected using CT, MRI, or ultrasonography. All of the patients were women. Thirteen of 20 hips required revision to THA. A 1% incidence of pseudotumors is estimated in patients treated with metal-on-metal hip resurfacing.

Chapter 2

Bearing Surfaces for Total Hip and Total Knee Arthroplasty

William J. Maloney, MD   Harry A. McKellop, PhD   Patricia A. Campbell, PhD

Paul F. Lachiewicz, MD   Mark R. Geyer, MD

Highly Cross-Linked Polyethylene in Total Hip Arthroplasty
William J. Maloney, MD
Harry A. McKellop, PhD
Patricia A. Campbell, PhD

Polyethylene is a long chain hydrocarbon. When exposed to radiation, carbon-hydrogen and carbon-carbon bonds can be broken. As a result, chain scission or free-radical formation can occur. Oxygen can bind at the free radical site, leading to oxidation. Both chain scission and oxidation have negative consequences for wear and are detrimental to the mechanical properties of the material.

Cross-linking involves the formation of a carbon-carbon bond between two adjacent polyethylene molecules. The cross-linking process involves two main steps. The first step is irradiation, which produces the free radicals. Free radicals then react to cross-link polymer chains. Cross-linking density is proportional to the radiation dose. Doses of 50 to 100 kGy (5 to 10 Mrads) are typically used in commercially available products. The second step is heating (thermal stabilization). The purpose of this step is to reduce free radicals and thus the risk of oxidation in vivo. Heating can be performed below or above the melting point (annealing or remelting, respectively). The type of radiation, radi-

ation dose, and the method of thermal stabilization, machining, and terminal sterilization differs among commercially available products and makes each product unique, thereby requiring each be studied individually.

Prior to commercial release, highly cross-linked polyethylene underwent extensive laboratory testing. Simulators have been used to study the impact of cross-linking on wear. It is important to note that laboratory studies assessing wear measure weight loss of the material being tested. In contrast, clinical studies measure femoral head penetration. Volumetric wear must then be calculated. Wear simulator studies demonstrate a marked reduction in wear for cross-linked polyethylene in both hip and knee replacement applications when compared with conventional polyethylene.[1-7] In general, wear reduction is proportional to the radiation dose, with diminishing benefits seen when the dose exceeds 100 kGy. Wear studies have also demonstrated that highly cross-linked polyethylene is relatively insensitive to head size, at least when compared with conventional polyethylene. Conventional polyethylene demonstrates a significant increase in volumetric wear with increasing femoral head size. Thin polyethylene does not appear to negatively impact wear of highly cross-linked polyethylene in the hip, but thin polyethylene is at higher risk for fracture, especially if unsupported by

Dr. Maloney or an immediate family member has received royalties from Wright Medical Technology and Zimmer; serves as an unpaid consultant for ISTO Technologies and Moximed; owns stock or stock options in Abbott, Gillead, ISTO Technologies, Johnson & Johnson, Merck, Moximed, and Pfizer; has received research or institutional support from AO, Biomet, DePuy Spine, DePuy, Nuvasive, Smith & Nephew, Stryker, and Zimmer; and is a board member, owner, officer, or committee member for the American Joint Replacement Registry and the Hip Society. Dr. McKellop has received royalties from DePuy; is a member of a speakers' bureau or has made paid presentations on behalf of DePuy; is a paid consultant for or an employee of DePuy; and has received research or institutional support from Aircase, Biomet, Corin USA, DePuy, Encore Medical, Exactech, Mathys Ltd, Medtronic Sofamor Danek, National Institutes of Health, Stryker, Wright Medical Technology, and Zimmer. Dr. Campbell has received research or institutional support from DePuy, Smith & Nephew, Wright Medical Technology, Stryker, Zimmer, and Biomet. Dr. Lachiewicz or an immediate family member serves as a board member, owner, officer, or committee member of the Hip Society, Southern Orthopaedic Association, and the Orthopaedic Surgery and Trauma Society; has received royalties from Innomed; is a member of a speakers' bureau or has made paid presentations on behalf of Zimmer, Covidien, and Rush-Copley Hospital; serves as a paid consultant to or is an employee of Leerink Swann, Gerson Lehrman Group, GuidepointGlobal, and the Center for Healthcare Education LLC; and has received research or institutional support from Zimmer. Neither Dr. Geyer nor any immediate family member has received anything of value from or owns stock in a commercial company or institution related directly or indirectly to the subject of this chapter.

The second half of this chapter is reprinted from Lachiewicz PF, Geyer MR: The use of highly cross-linked polyethylene in total knee arthroplasty. J Am Acad Orthop Surg 2011;19:143-151.

metal. As a result of the improved wear resistance of highly cross-linked polyethylene against larger femoral heads in vitro, 36-mm, 38-mm, and 40-mm femoral heads are commercially available for hip replacement.

Wear studies are usually done under conditions that optimize lubrication, counterface roughness, and implant position. In vivo, adverse conditions including scratches on the counterface and three-body wear occur. To accurately characterize the wear performance of highly cross-linked polyethylene, wear testing has been performed under adverse conditions. In one study, alumina grit was introduced into the articulation simulating three-body wear.[3] The wear performance of highly cross-linked polyethylene was superior to conventional polyethylene. Another study evaluated the effect of artificially scratched counterfaces on wear.[6] Against moderately rough femoral heads, highly cross-linked polyethylene was again superior to conventional polyethylene. A recent study characterized the surface roughness of femoral heads retrieved at revision surgery.[4] These femoral heads of varying roughness resulting from in vivo use were then used in a simulator test. Again, highly cross-linked polyethylene performed better than conventional polyethylene against clinically relevant damaged femoral heads.

Increasing radiation dose above 100 kGy has potential disadvantages because it diminishes important mechanical properties of the polyethylene, including fatigue resistance and yield strength, ultimate strength, and elongation to failure. In vitro testing has demonstrated that resistance to fatigue crack propagation declined with increasing radiation dose. Despite an overall reduction in mechanical properties related to the cross-linking process, the commercial products remain above ASTM International standards for use in patients. In addition, highly cross-linked polyethylene is mechanically superior to conventional polyethylene that has undergone significant oxidation.

Commercially available highly cross-linked polyethylene acetabular liners have fractured in vivo. Fracture appears multifactorial.[8-10] Surgical technique certainly plays a role. In the hip, liner fracture has been associated with suboptimally positioned components, leading to edge loading in areas of thin polyethylene. Liner fractures are most commonly associated with femoral heads larger than 32 mm. There is an absence of complete agreement on the relative role played by the reduction in mechanical properties of highly cross-linked polyethylene in fractures seen clinically. Finite element studies performed analyzing suboptimally positioned acetabular components with large femoral heads and relatively thin liners demonstrate that both conventional and highly cross-linked polyethylene would fracture under similar conditions.[11] Particle analysis from in vitro studies demonstrated that although the wear volume was markedly reduced with highly cross-linked polyethylene, the average highly cross-linked polyethylene particle was smaller than the conventional polyethylene wear particle.[12,13] This led to concern that highly cross-linked polyethylene particles may be more bioreactive when compared with conventional polyethylene. Although the data are somewhat conflicting, the consensus is that particle for particle, highly cross-linked polyethylene is more reactive in cell culture. However, because the volume of highly cross-linked polyethylene particles is significantly smaller than that of conventional polyethylene, the overall biologic impact is less for the highly cross-linked material. Highly cross-linked polyethylene was introduced into clinical practice in 1999 in the United States with the hope that the low wear seen in vitro would be reproduced in vivo. It was hypothesized that a significant reduction in wear would result in a reduction in osteolysis and aseptic loosening. Multiple prospective trials have been performed that have evaluated wear with commercially available products. Radiostereometric analysis (RSA) was used in two randomized clinical studies performed in Goteberg, Sweden.[14] In the first study, 60 patients with a median age of 55 years were randomized to either highly cross-linked polyethylene (Durasol, Zimmer, Warsaw, IN) or conventional polyethylene in cemented total hip replacement. In the second study, 32 patients with a median age of 48 years underwent bilateral hybrid total hip replacements. The first hip was randomized to either highly cross-linked polyethylene (Longevity, Zimmer) or conventional polyethylene, with the second hip receiving the other material. Patients were followed for a minimum of 5 years. In both studies, highly cross-linked polyethylene had a significantly lower femoral head penetration rate. With highly cross-linked polyethylene, femoral head penetration tended to plateau at approximately 1 year and thereafter was nearly flat. Overall, wear was reduced by more than 95%. In another RSA study from Oslo, Norway, highly cross-linked polyethylene (Crossfire, Howmedica Osteonics, Mahwah, NJ) was compared with conventional polyethylene over a 5- to 6-year period.[15] After correcting for creep, the annual femoral head penetration rate for the highly cross-linked material was less than 6μm.

In a retrospective study, 182 patients (200 hips) with highly cross-linked polyethylene liners (Longevity) and 28- and 32-mm heads were analyzed at a minimum of 6 years of follow-up.[16] Steady state wear in both groups was negligible and there was no difference in wear with the two head sizes. In a prospective study from the same group, wear was measured using RSA comparing 28-mm and 36-mm heads against highly cross-linked polyethylene.[17] No difference in wear at 3 years was noted. A clinical study comparing conventional femoral heads to large femoral heads also documented equivalent linear wear. However, the calculated volumetric wear was higher with the larger femoral heads.[18] Wear performance of highly cross-linked polyethylene has also been superior in young patients. In one study, a group of patients younger than 50 years with a mean age of 41 years with highly cross-linked polyethylene (Longevity) acetabular liners were followed for a mean of 4 years.[19] After the bedding-in phase, femoral head penetration was not detectable using the Martell method to measure wear.

The goal with the introduction of highly cross-linked polyethylene was to reduce wear. This goal has clearly been met in the hip. The hypothesis was that a reduction in wear would lead to a reduction in osteolysis and loosening. Data are now available to support this hypothesis in hip replacement.

One study compared conventional polyethylene (Enduron, DePuy, Warsaw, IN) with highly cross-linked polyethylene (Marathon, DePuy) by performing CT scans at a minimum of 5 years after the index procedure.[20] The prevalence of osteolysis was significantly greater in patients with the conventional polyethylene (28% versus 8%). In addition, the osteolytic lesions were significantly smaller with the highly cross-linked polyethylene. Another minimum 5-year follow-up study evaluated the same bearing surfaces.[21] Patients with the highly cross-linked polyethylene had significantly lower femoral head penetration rates, volumetric wear, and activity-adjusted wear. No patients in the highly cross-linked polyethylene group had radiographic evidence of osteolysis compared with 33% (8 of 24) in the conventional polyethylene group. Another study retrospectively compared 50 patients age 50 years or younger (mean age 43.2 years) with conventional acetabular liners with 48 patients age 50 years or younger (mean age, 46.5 years) with highly cross-linked polyethylene (Longevity) acetabular liners.[22] There was no difference in body mass index, activity score, sex, preoperative Harris hip score, or acetabular component position between the two groups. Osteolysis was assessed with radiographs and CT. Linear wear was measured using the Martell method. The mean follow-up period was 7.2 years. In the highly cross-linked polyethylene group, no osteolysis was detected on radiographs and one lesion (1 of 48, 2%) was noted on CT. In contrast, 7 of 50 hips (14%) with conventional polyethylene had lysis on plain radiographs and 12 of 50 (24%) on CT.

Metal-on-Metal Hip Bearings in Total Hip Arthroplasty

Modern total hip replacements with metal-on-metal bearings were introduced in the early 1990s, followed by hip resurfacing arthroplasties. Metal-on-metal bearings have provided a low-wear alternative to polyethylene and have had good results in most patients.[23,24] In recent years, however, there has been growing concern regarding patients who require revision because of the adverse reactions in the local tissue and bone to metallic wear products, potentially including osteolysis, the formation of enlarged bursae, tissue masses (often referred to as pseudotumors), and necrosis. Identifying the causes of these failures is the focus of an extensive international research effort.

Hip simulator testing and analysis of retrieved implants have shown that wear in metal-on-metal bearings typically is characterized by higher wear during a "running-in" period (approximately the first million cycles in a simulator, or the first 1 to 2 years in vivo), followed by substantially lower steady-state wear.[25,26] The effects of alloy composition and implant design parameters on the two wear phases have been extensively investigated in laboratory tests, and a recent meta-analysis of the results of 56 independent hip joint simulator studies identified the following trends:[27]

1. For diameters 36 mm or greater, the amount of run-in wear decreased with increasing diameter, but not the amount of steady-state wear.
2. Primarily for diameters 36 mm or greater, wear decreased with decreasing clearance.
3. Wear was less with lower surface roughness and with higher sphericity.
4. Wear was comparable for wrought and cast alloys.
5. The influence of carbon content on wear was inconsistent among studies.
6. After-casting heat treatment, which reduces the size of the carbides, did not substantially affect the amount of wear during wear-in. Although the steady-state wear after heat treatment was greater than with as-cast alloys when averaged across studies, the wear rates were comparable within some individual studies, and it was concluded that additional investigations are needed to clarify the effect of heat treatment on wear.[27]

It should be emphasized that most of the hip simulator wear studies done in the past were conducted with the components in an ideal orientation, that is, with the cup positioned such that the contact zone was well within the intended bearing area.[27] In contrast, in clinical use, the acetabular components are sometimes implanted in excessive abduction and/or anteversion[28,29] such that the contact zone is very near or on the rim of the cup. Hip simulator testing and analysis of retrieved implants[29-32] have shown that such rim contact can markedly increase the rate of wear, and clinically, component malpositioning is emerging as one of the key factors determining the rate of wear and the ion levels. In addition, among current designs of hip surface replacements, the coverage arc ranges from 151° to 170°, and a cup with less coverage will experience edge wear at a lower abduction angle than a cup with greater coverage. Thus, smaller diameter components implanted at high abduction angles and/or excessive anteversion are at greater risk of edge wear and elevated ions, and their incidence increases as the coverage arc of the acetabular component decreases.[32-35]

Wear Particles, Corrosion, and Cytotoxicity
Metallic ions are released from the bulk implant and the wear particles. Because they tend to accumulate in the periprosthetic tissues, the local concentration of particles and ions may increase substantially with time, potentially reaching toxic levels. Moreover, studies

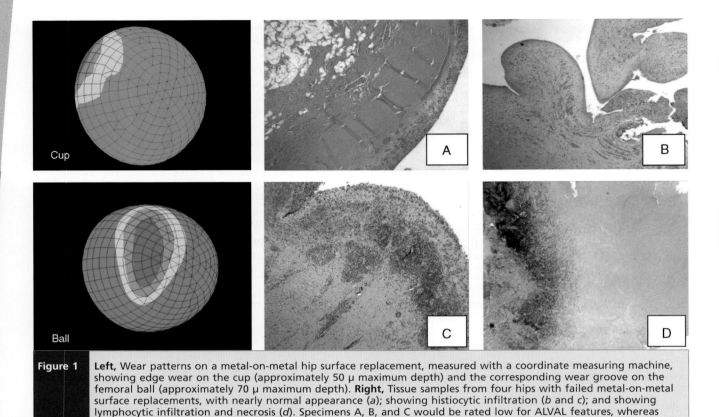

Figure 1   **Left,** Wear patterns on a metal-on-metal hip surface replacement, measured with a coordinate measuring machine, showing edge wear on the cup (approximately 50 μ maximum depth) and the corresponding wear groove on the femoral ball (approximately 70 μ maximum depth). **Right,** Tissue samples from four hips with failed metal-on-metal surface replacements, with nearly normal appearance (*a*); showing histiocytic infiltration (*b* and *c*); and showing lymphocytic infiltration and necrosis (*d*). Specimens A, B, and C would be rated low for ALVAL features, whereas changes in D warrant a high ALVAL score.

have shown that internalized particles enter an acidified phagosomal microenvironment, with pH as low as 4.6,[36] which may accelerate the corrosion process, creating a cycle of necrosis, recruitment of macrophages and rephagocytosis, and leading to an expanding necrotic zone. Extensive necrosis is a common feature of periprosthetic masses or pseudotumors.

Because consistently elevated ion levels may be an indication of a malfunctioning implant, and there is evidence that hips with elevated ion levels are at higher risk for adverse soft-tissue reactions, including pseudotumors, periodic measurement of metal ions in the blood or urine has been advocated to detect early clinical malfunction of metal-on-metal hip replacements.[37,38] Interestingly, although some controversy exists, patient activity does not appear to be a major factor influencing wear and ion levels, and extreme levels of activity do not lead to outlier levels of ions.[39,40]

Is Hip Pain Caused by Wear or Allergy?
Although there is a clear association between component malpositioning and poor clinical performance, it remains unclear if the adverse biologic reactions are a function simply of the amount of wear, or if they also depend on the morphology and composition of the resultant wear debris and the type of ions generated. Recent reports from a large-volume teaching hospital specializing in metal-on-metal hip surgery have described

painful pseudotumors in the hip joints of female patients with metal-on-metal hip surface replacements.[41] Initially, this was thought to be a result of metal hypersensitivity (allergy), primarily because of the presence of extensive lymphocytic infiltrates in the tissues, and because the pseudotumors occurred only in female patients, who might be predisposed to metal allergy due to a higher incidence of jewelry sensitivity. However, pseudotumors have since been reported in male patients.[42]

Metal allergies in response to metal-on-metal hip implants have long been reported, but were considered to be rare until a form of type IV delayed hypersensitivity response was described that was prevalent in patients with modern-generation metal-on-metal hips.[43] This response is referred to as aseptic lymphocytic vasculitis associated lesion (ALVAL), a histologic term describing the features of tissues from metal-on-metal joints (**Figure 1**), although now often used to describe unexplained pain around metal-on-metal hip replacements. However, it is not yet clear whether pseudotumors, ALVAL, and other forms of painful periprosthetic tissue reactions reflect variations over a spectrum of metal sensitivity or are a dose-related immune response to wear particles and/or ions.[44,45] The question of whether patients with preexisting metal allergies are predisposed to problems with metal-on-metal hip replacements is the subject of current research.[42,46]

Highly Cross-linked Polyethylene in Total Knee Arthroplasty
Paul F. Lachiewicz, MD
Mark R. Geyer, MD

Polyethylene wear, with resultant particle-induced osteolysis, is a major cause of late failure of total knee arthroplasty (TKA) and of the need for revision.[47,48] The prevalence of osteolysis after TKA has been reported at 5% to 20%, at follow-up periods of less than 5 years to 15 years.[49,50] Polyethylene wear and osteolysis after TKA are multifactorial and associated with implant design, patient factors, and technical issues. The implant factors include the polyethylene locking mechanism–backside wear, the design of the posterior-stabilized tibial post, and the method of polyethylene fabrication and sterilization.[49,51] Patient factors such as age and activity level have been implicated in excessive polyethylene wear. Technical factors also may contribute to or predispose to excessive polyethylene wear after TKA; these can include excessive flexion of the femoral component or hyperextension of the knee, with resultant impingement and wear of the tibial polyethylene post, and axial malalignment. Previous attempts to improve the knee tibial polyethylene liner with carbon fibers or increased crystallinity adversely affected the results of the arthroplasty, despite in vitro mechanical testing that showed safety and efficacy.[51]

Highly cross-linked polyethylene liners for total hip arthroplasty acetabular components are now widely accepted as providing decreased wear at 5 to 8 years after surgery.[16,52] However, the fabrication techniques varied widely among these highly cross-linked polyethylene products, with resultant differences in measured linear wear and a decrease in mechanical strength; the decrease in mechanical strength has been implicated in the rare instances of liner fracture. So-called second-generation highly cross-linked polyethylenes have recently been introduced to address the issue of decreased material strength. These polyethylenes are sequentially irradiated and annealed or doped with vitamin E.[53,54] The use of highly cross-linked polyethylene in TKA was proposed after its early success in total hip arthroplasty,[55] but it has not been widely accepted for routine use. It is important to be aware of the polyethylene products now available for implantation, the laboratory simulator testing of these devices, the early reported clinical results, and the potential risks and complications of the use of highly cross-linked polyethylenes in TKA.

TKA Polyethylene Products
Information from the 10 manufacturers of TKA products in the United States is presented in Table 1. In regard to sterilization, polyethylene tibial liners in the past were sterilized by gamma irradiation, ethylene oxide, or gas plasma. At present, most TKA tibial and patella polyethylene prostheses are cross-linked (joined by covalent bonds) to some degree because gamma (less

than 5 Mrad) or electron-beam irradiation is done by all manufacturers. Four manufacturers (Aesculap, Center Valley, PA; DJO Surgical, Austin, TX; Exactech, Gainesville, FL; and StelKast, McMurray, PA) do not provide a specific highly cross-linked polyethylene for their TKA components, although most fabricate one for their total hip arthroplasty components. Two manufacturers (DePuy, Warsaw, IN and Wright Medical, Arlington, TN) provide a "moderately" cross-linked (5 Mrad) tibial polyethylene liner. Four manufacturers (Biomet, Warsaw, IN; Smith & Nephew, Memphis, TN; Stryker Orthopaedics, Mahwah, NJ; and Zimmer, Warsaw, IN) (five products) provide different highly cross-linked tibial polyethylene liners (6.5 to 10 Mrad). One manufacturer, Wright Medical, does not fabricate a moderately cross-linked tibial polyethylene for a posterior-stabilized knee prosthesis. Two of these four manufacturers (Stryker and Zimmer) also provide a highly cross-linked polyethylene patella prosthesis.

These products differ in the type of polyethylene resin used, the method of irradiation, and the amount of radiation. There are also major differences in the thermal treatments after irradiation. In addition, each manufacturer has a different proprietary method of polyethylene fabrication, sterilization, and packaging. Thus, the clinical results of these TKA polyethylene liners cannot be grouped together, and the results may have significant differences in their in vivo wear, prevalence of osteolysis, and complications.

The amount of radiation and method of irradiation have an important effect on the wear and mechanical properties of the tibial polyethylene liner in vitro. One laboratory reported significant decreases in wear of 5 (54%), 7.5 (78%), and 10 Mrad (95%).[55,56] There was no improvement in wear with higher doses of irradiation. However, the mechanical properties (toughness, as measured by small-punch tests) were improved from 5 to 7.5 Mrad only, then decreased with increasing doses of irradiation.

The thermal treatment and terminal method of sterilization and packaging of these TKA polyethylenes may be just as important for the long-term performance of these materials in vivo. Different thermal treatments are used to form crosslinks and extinguish free radicals. Some polyethylenes are remelted (heated above the melting temperature), and some are annealed (heated to just below the melting temperature). With radiation doses at or near 10 Mrad, remelted highly cross-linked polyethylene exhibits reduced mechanical and fatigue properties compared with those of conventional and annealed polyethylene. However, annealed highly cross-linked polyethylene has a higher level of free radicals, and with increased oxidation in vivo after implantation, there may be reduced mechanical strength and increased wear with long-term follow-up. One manufacturer has developed a method to eliminate the remelting process and maintain oxidative resistance by sequential irradiation and annealing. This polyethylene is reported to have oxidation resistance similar to

Table 1

Cross-linked Polyethylene for TKA

Manufacturer	Product Name	Prosthesis	Tibia/Patella	Radiation Dose (Mrad)	Fabrication/Sterilization	Resin
Aesculap (Center Valley, PA)	—	Columbus Knee System	Y/Y	3 ± 2	Gamma, in nitrogen	GUR 1020
Biomet (Warsaw, IN)	E 1	Vanguard (CR, CR lipped, anterior stabilized, PS, PS+)	Y/N	10	Gamma, vitamin E doping at < 130°C, packaged in argon, terminal 3 Mrad sterilization	GUR 1020
DePuy (Warsaw, IN)	XLK	Sigma (CR, PS, HF)	Y/N	5	Gamma, remelted at 155°C, packaged in vacuum, gas plasma	GUR 1020
DJO Surgical (Austin, TX)	—	Foundation, 3D Knee System	Y/Y	2.5 to 4 (both)	Gamma, no oxygen; nitrogen flush packaging (both)	GUR 1050 GUR 1020
Exactech (Gainesville, FL)	—	Optetrak (PS, CR, HF)	Y/Y	2.5 to 4	Gamma, vacuum	GUR 1020 (tibia) GUR 1050 (patella)
Smith & Nephew (Memphis, TN)	XLPE Verilast (with Oxinium femur)	Legion (CR, PS) Genesis II (CR, PS)	Y/N	7.5	Gamma, vacuum, full remelt, packaged in air, gas plasma	GUR 1020
StelKast (McMurray, PA)	—	Proven Gen-Flex (CR, PS, HF)	Y/Y	2.5 to 4	Gamma, in argon	GUR 1050
Stryker Orthopaedics (Mahwah, NJ)	X3	Triathlon (uni, CR, PS) Scorpio (CR, PS)	Y/Y	9 (3 × 3)	Sequential radiation, annealing below melt temperature ×3, packaged in air, gas plasma	GUR 1020
Wright Medical (Arlington, TN)	A -Class	Advance Medial Pivot (CR only)	Y/N	5	Gamma, remelted >140°C, packaged in air, ETO	GUR 1020
Zimmer (Warsaw, IN)	Prolong	NexGen (CR, PS, HF)	Y/Y	6.5	Electron-beam, remelted at 150°C, packaged in air, gas plasma	GUR 1050
	Durasul	Natural (CS)	Y/Y	9.5	Electron-beam, remelted at 150°C, packaged in air, ETO	GUR 1050

CR = posterior cruciate retaining, CS = cruciate substituting, ETO = ethylene oxide, GUR = granular, PS= posterior stabilized, HF = high flexion, Mrad = megarad (kGy), N = no, uni = unicompartmental, XLPE = cross-linked polyethylene, Y = yes

that of virgin polyethylene, with maintained mechanical strength and significantly reduced wear for both cruciate-retaining and posterior-stabilized knee designs.[53] The method of final sterilization and packaging may also be important because terminal irradiation or packaging in the presence of oxygen may also lead to late oxidation in vivo.

Polyethylene Wear in TKA

Polyethylene wear of the tibial component liner of TKA occurs by two methods: fatigue damage (pitting and delamination) and adhesive and abrasive wear[51,54] (**Figure 2**). Wear of the polyethylene patella component presumably occurs through the same mechanisms. Polyethylene pitting and delamination are accelerated by oxidation secondary to residual free radicals produced through the sterilization of the polyethylene by gamma irradiation. At present, most manufacturers sterilize their components by gamma irradiation in a vacuum or an inert gas (ie, nitrogen, argon), by gas plasma, or by ethylene oxide gas. However, the rate and severity of oxidation of the polyethylene in vivo and thus the rate and severity of future delamination are not known.

Adhesive and abrasive wear of the tibial polyethylene remains the major source of particulate debris from modern TKA and the predominant late cause of osteolysis and loosening. Adhesive wear is caused by the orientation and strain hardening of the polyethylene surface. Abrasive wear is caused by the rubbing action of the surface of the femoral component and third-body particles, such as bone cement and bone fragments. Abrasive wear produces larger polyethylene debris particles than does adhesive wear because of the cutting action on the polyethylene surface. These processes may also occur on the backside of a tibial liner with both mobile-bearing and modular fixed-bearing prostheses.

Thermal treatment, when performed above the melt temperature (>140°C), reduces or eliminates the concentration of free radicals in the polyethylene, thereby possibly preventing oxidation and its resultant embrittlement in vivo.[54] Thus, higher cross-linking of the tibial (and patella) polyethylene and melting to eliminate free radicals should decrease delamination and adhesive and abrasive wear in vivo over the long term.

Two approaches to reduce wear that have limited effect on the mechanical properties include sequential irradiation and annealing or doping with vitamin E below the melting temperature.

Laboratory Simulator Wear Testing

In the absence of extensive clinical data, the results of in vitro testing of highly cross-linked polyethylene liners in a knee simulator may provide some insight or useful information for the practicing surgeon who is considering the use of these materials. Several of these moderately or highly cross-linked tibial polyethylene liners have been tested in knee simulator models; however, the studies reveal numerous limitations.

At least three different models of knee simulator are reported on. The complex motion pattern of the knee, which includes rolling, sliding, and rotation, may not be accurately reproduced by these knee simulators. In addition, the absolute wear measurements in the different studies may not be comparable. The studies also differ in the number of specimens tested, number of million-cycles, and load and gait conditions. In several studies, the polyethylene is experimentally "aged" by heat treatment or exposure to oxygen for a certain number of days. Most of the studies assume that the knee alignment and ligament balance are optimal and that there is no third-body debris (for example, cement, bone particles) in the lubricating solution.

The strengths of the knee simulator studies are the comparisons of the highly cross-linked polyethylene to the control conventional polyethylene and the ability to

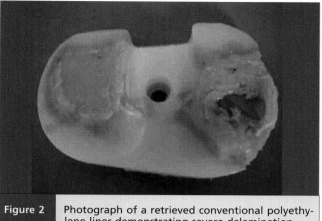

Figure 2 Photograph of a retrieved conventional polyethylene liner demonstrating severe delamination.

study adverse clinical situations (for example, axial malalignment, ligament imbalance, scratched femoral components) in a relatively large number of specimens.

One study tested GUR 1050 compression-molded polyethylene treated by electron beam irradiation of 9.5 Mrad, followed by melting at 150°C for 2 hours (Durasul; Zimmer) with a cruciate-retaining total knee femoral component (Natural-KneeII, Zimmer).[57] The control group was GUR 4150 compression-molded polyethylene sterilized by gamma irradiation of 2.5 to 4 Mrad in an oxygen-free package. These tibial liners were also aged and oxidized in an air convection oven for 35 days to simulate 5 years of aging oxidation. Three groups of tibial liners (unaged and aged conventional polyethylene and aged highly cross-linked polyethylene) were tested in a knee simulator under so-called normal gait conditions for 5 million cycles. Wear was measured by both gravimetric (weight loss) and volumetric (coordinate measuring) methods. During 5 million cycles of simulated gait, the aged conventional tibial polyethylene had large areas of delamination; however, the unaged and aged highly cross-linked polyethylene liners showed no delamination. The gravimetric analysis showed 9.6 ± 3.6 mg per million cycles for aged conventional and 8.8 ± 1.5 mg per million cycles for unaged conventional polyethylene (*P* value not stated). The aged highly cross-linked polyethylene showed a weight gain (bovine serum fluid absorption) for the first 3 million cycles, followed by wear of 0.7 ± 1 mg per million cycles (**Figure 3**). The total (medial and lateral) volumetric wear measurements showed that the aged highly cross-linked polyethylene liner had approximately one third the wear of the aged and unaged conventional polyethylene liners. The limitations of this study included the small number of liners tested and the operation of the knee simulator at a nonphysiologic frequency.

This highly cross-linked polyethylene was also studied in two "adverse" wear condition models. In one study, four explanted, artificially roughened femoral components were tested against unaged polyethylenes

1: Basic Science and General Knowledge

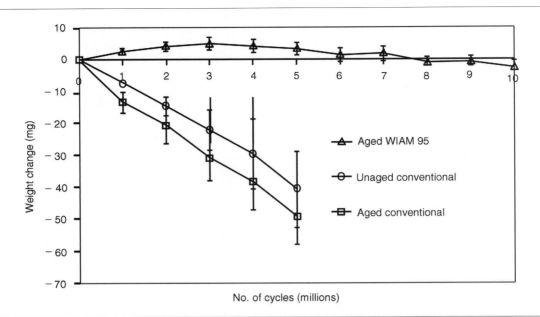

Figure 3 A graph demonstrating the average gravimetric change in the three groups for the duration of the study. The aged and unaged conventional inserts displayed a steady wear rate, with an average weight loss at 5 million cycles of 49 ±12 mg and 40 ± 9 mg, respectively. The highly cross-linked polyethylene inserts showed an initial average weight gain of 4 mg for the first 3 million cycles and remained relatively unchanged thereafter. WIAM = warm-irradiation by means of adiabatic melting. (Reproduced with permission from Muratoglu OK, Bragdon CR, Jasty M, O'Connor DO, Von Knoch RS, Harris WH: Knee-simulator testing of conventional and cross-linked polyethylene tibial inserts. *J Arthroplasty* 2004;19(7):887-897.)

in the same knee simulator for 2 million cycles.[58] The wear rate was 80% lower for the eight highly cross-linked liners than for the conventional liners. This study attempted to simulate in vivo wear when the femoral component may become scratched or roughened with use. In another study, the femoral component was positioned in the knee simulator to mimic a tight unbalanced posterior cruciate ligament.[59] The aged highly cross-linked and unaged conventional polyethylene liners showed no delamination at 0.5 million cycles, whereas the aged conventional polyethylene liners showed delamination at 50,000 cycles.

Another study compared the wear of electron beam 6.5 Mrad irradiated and melted GUR 1050 polyethylene (Prolong, Zimmer) to 2.5 to 4 Mrad gamma irradiated-in-nitrogen GUR 1050 polyethylene with a posterior cruciate–retaining knee prosthesis (NexGen CR, Zimmer) in a knee simulator model for 7 million cycles.[2] Both polyethylenes were unaged, the tibial base plate had four screw holes, and backside wear was allowed. By gravimetric analysis, the combined articular and backside wear was significantly less for the highly cross-linked polyethylene (4.6 ± 2 mm^3 per million cycles) than for the conventional polyethylene (23 ± 6 mm^3 per million cycles). This highly cross-linked polyethylene has not been tested in a posterior cruciate–substituting design or when severe axial (5° to 7° varus) or coronal malalignment of the components exists.

One study compared polyethylene gamma irradiated in air with sequentially irradiated and annealed (9 Mrad) highly cross-linked polyethylene (X3; Stryker Orthopaedics) and 6.5 Mrad (Prolong; Zimmer) electron-beam, remelted and gas plasma–sterilized polyethylene in the same knee simulator after accelerated aging (oxygen bomb for 14 days) under two malalignment conditions (7° varus, 80:20 medial/lateral load distribution, 9° tibial internal rotation; and 5° varus, 70:30 medial/lateral load distribution, 4° tibial internal rotation).[60] None of the highly cross-linked aged liners showed visible delamination or severe wear over 5 million cycles of testing. Both types of highly cross-linked polyethylene wore significantly less than did the control polyethylene. However, the overall wear rates for the electron-beam, remelted polyethylene were higher than those for the sequentially irradiated and annealed polyethylene (4.13 ± 0.8 versus 1.83 ± 0.4 mg/million cycles; $P < 0.01$).

At least three other knee simulator studies of the sequentially irradiated and annealed highly cross-linked polyethylene tibial liner (X3) have been published. One laboratory studied both 9-mm cruciate-retaining and posterior-stabilized tibial liners to 5 million cycles and measured gravimetric and volumetric wear, visual damage, and tensile properties before and after aging.[53] The cruciate-retaining liner had 68% less wear and the posterior-stabilized liner had 64% less wear than did the conventional unaged polyethylene. Visual wear damage to the tibial post was much less with the highly cross-linked polyethylene. There was no difference in the mean size or morphology of the wear particles produced between the conventional polyethylene (0.31 μm) and the highly cross-linked polyethylene (0.29 μm).

A second study tested the cruciate-retaining liner to 10 million cycles with a different simulator and a different femoral component.[61] The wear rate of the sequentially irradiated and annealed (9 Mrad) polyethylene was reduced by 86% compared with that of the conventional (3 Mrad) polyethylene. The third study compared six different polyethylene liners, including three highly cross-linked liners, in a third, different knee simulator to 5 million cycles.[62] All three highly cross-linked polyethylene liners had significantly lower wear rates compared with the conventional polyethylene; however, the sequentially irradiated and annealed polyethylene had the lowest wear rate.

One laboratory used the Leeds knee simulator (Leeds/Prosim Knee Wear Simulator; Simulation Solutions, Stockport, UK) to test non–cross-linked GUR 1020, moderately (5 Mrad) cross-linked GUR 1050, and highly (10 Mrad) cross-linked GUR 1050 and annealed polyethylene liners with both cruciate-retaining, fixed-bearing prostheses and rotating-platform, mobile-bearing prostheses for 5 million cycles.[63] In lower cross-shear conditions (20° rotation), which are more representative of the knee joint, the highly cross-linked polyethylene had a 33% reduction in gravimetric wear compared with the conventional polyethylene. However, the highly cross-linked polyethylene had higher wear under abrasive conditions, with a deliberately scratched femoral component. This finding conflicts with the results of other studies and may be related to the amount of abrasion of the femoral component and the method of testing. With the Leeds knee simulator, rotating-platform, mobile-bearing knees had a lower wear rate compared to the fixed-bearing knees, and this wear was reduced with a moderately cross-linked polyethylene. This study's conclusions are limited by the use of different molecular weight polyethylenes for the conventional and moderately and highly cross-linked polyethylenes.

One biomechanical study has been published of the fatigue strength of a simulated posterior-stabilized tibial post fabricated from GUR 1050, which was gamma-irradiated to 8.5 Mrad, then doped with vitamin E, which improves the mechanical strength and fatigue crack propagation of highly cross-linked and melted polyethylene.[53] This vitamin E-doped polyethylene showed bending fatigue strength comparable to that of conventional unaged polyethylene and improved strength comparable to that of aged conventional polyethylene. However, this vitamin E-doped polyethylene has not been tested in abrasive conditions or under ligament imbalance or axial malalignment conditions. To date, there are no published reports of fatigue testing of highly cross-linked polyethylene patella components.

Clinical Results

Few reports have been published of the clinical or radiographic results of highly cross-linked polyethylene tibial liners, and none of highly cross-linked patella prostheses in TKA. A reliable, validated method of measuring in vivo wear of tibial polyethylene liners is not presently available.

A highly cross-linked polyethylene tibial liner (Durasul) has been available for use since February 2001. One retrospective cohort study compared a series of 100 cruciate-retaining and -sacrificing (ultra congruent liner) TKAs with a conventional polyethylene liner, sterilized by gamma irradiation in nitrogen, with 100 knees of identical design with Durasul highly cross-linked (9.5 Mrad) polyethylene liners.[64] It was unclear from the study whether the patella prosthesis implanted was also fabricated of highly cross-linked polyethylene. The patient groups were similar, and evaluation was by a physical examination and conventional radiographs only. The mean follow-up time was 91 months (range, 82 to 101 months) for the conventional polyethylene liners and 75 months (range, 69 to 82 months) for the highly cross-linked liners. There was no significant difference between the groups in the number of revisions done for tibial component loosening. However, 20 tibial radiolucent lines were seen (20 patients) with the conventional polyethylene compared with 2 tibial radiolucent lines (2 patients) with highly cross-linked polyethylene (statistical significance not stated). There were no cases of early catastrophic failure related to either polyethylene liner. This study was limited by its retrospective and nonrandomized design, as well as by the absence of a measure of activity level. There were also numerous confounding variables, including mode of fixation (cemented or press-fit), patella resurfacing status, and posterior cruciate ligament status. It is reasonable to assume that this particular TKA with the Durasul highly cross-linked polyethylene tibial liner is safe for use at a mean 6-year follow-up time, but no advantage to conventional polyethylene has been demonstrated by the results of this single study.

Another variety of highly cross-linked polyethylene (6.5 Mrad) (Prolong) has been available since August 2003. Authors of a 2009 study reported a prospective, consecutive series comparing 113 cruciate-retaining knees (99 patients) with conventional polyethylene tibial liners with 89 cruciate-retaining knees (83 patients) with Prolong highly cross-linked polyethylene tibial liners.[65] The groups were comparable in terms of patient age, sex, and preoperative diagnosis, although the conventional polyethylene group had less preoperative range of motion. Patella resurfacing was performed only in patients with rheumatoid arthritis. At 2-year follow-up, there were no clinical or radiographic differences between the two groups. Tibial radiolucent lines were more frequently seen in the conventional polyethylene group (9.7%) than the highly cross-linked polyethylene group (4.5%), but this difference was not statistically significant. This study was limited by lack of randomization and by the short follow-up time.

One study compared 8 retrieved highly cross-linked polyethylene tibial liners (Durasul) with 71 retrieved conventional polyethylene liners.[66] Both polyethylene liners demonstrated substantial surface changes, scuffing, and scratching. No significant difference was seen between the highly cross-linked and conventional polyethylene liners in terms of the total optical damage score. This study evaluated a small number of highly cross-linked liners, most of which were in vivo for less than 1 year. Large-scale surface deformation did not occur in any liner. Additional retrieved specimens with much longer follow-up times will be required to determine the in vivo efficacy of highly cross-linked polyethylenes.

The ultimate advantage of highly cross-linked polyethylene tibial liners or patella prostheses will be demonstrated only in properly designed prospective randomized studies. According to the Website www.ClinicalTrials.gov (a service of the National Institutes of Health), there are at least four prospective randomized trials comparing conventional to moderately or highly cross-linked polyethylene that have started or are about to begin recruitment.

Clinical Risks and Complications of Highly Cross-linked Polyethylene

Potential risks exist with the use of moderately or highly cross-linked polyethylene in TKA. The additional irradiation dose and, in some products, thermal stabilization (remelting), can adversely affect the mechanical properties of the polyethylene, resulting in reduced strength, fatigue resistance, and fracture toughness. In vitro testing of standardized highly cross-linked specimens show reduced fracture toughness and resistance to fatigue crack propagation compared with conventional polyethylene.[67,68] How these factors might clinically affect the locking mechanism of modular tibial components is uncertain. No reports exist of catastrophic failure of two designs of highly cross-linked polyethylene tibial liners in cruciate-retaining or sacrificing (ultracongruent liner) prostheses at short- to medium-term follow-up.

However, concern exists regarding the mechanical strength of tibial posterior-stabilized posts and patella prosthesis cement fixation pegs used with highly cross-linked polyethylene. Doping the polyethylene with vitamin E has been proposed to retain the strength of highly cross-linked polyethylene, but no clinical studies yet document the efficacy of this process.[53] Although numerous case reports have been published of fractures of tibial posts fabricated of conventional polyethylene, only one report describes fracture of a highly cross-linked polyethylene tibial post (X3 Scorpio, Stryker Orthopaedics) in two posterior-stabilized knee prostheses.[10] Both occurred in female patients, one at 8 and the other at 16 weeks after surgery, with the sudden onset of pain, instability, and effusion. In both cases, it was postulated that these post fractures were the result of "subtle" component malposition, with impingement of the femoral component on the tibial post in extension, as well as the result of flexion instability. The tibial liners were revised from 10 to 15 mm and 12 to 18 mm, respectively, but no follow-up was reported. It remains unclear how subtle this malposition was if an increase of 5 mm and 6 mm, respectively, in polyethylene thickness was required. This specific tibial polyethylene is fabricated with three cycles of sequential 3-Mrad irradiation and annealing below the melt temperature.

The scope of the problem of fatigue fracture of the tibial post is unknown, but it could limit the use of highly cross-linked polyethylene to posterior cruciate ligament–retaining or –sacrificing (deep dished) designs. Fracture of one or more fixation pegs of a highly cross-linked cemented polyethylene patella prosthesis has not been reported.

A second concern with the use of moderately and highly cross-linked polyethylene in TKA is the size and biologic activity of the particles produced in a wear simulator study. Reports related to this issue are conflicting. A group of authors studied wear debris produced in the Leeds knee simulator with conventional GUR 1020 polyethylene and moderately cross-linked GUR 1050 polyethylene (5 Mrad), using both fixed-bearing and mobile-bearing knee designs.[63] Although wear rates were lower with the GUR 1020, the wear debris particles were smaller with the moderately cross-linked GUR 1050 polyethylene than with the conventional GUR 1020 polyethylene, with both mobile-bearing and fixed-bearing designs. Analysis of both designs and both polyethylenes showed that more than 95% of particles generated were less than 1 µm. However, the moderately cross-linked polyethylene had a higher number of particles less than 0.1 µm.

In another part of the study, when the wear debris and lubricant from the simulator were co-cultured with human macrophages, the amount of tumor necrosis factor-α (TNF-α) was measured. With moderately and highly (10 Mrad) cross-linked polyethylene, the amount of TNF-α produced was greater than with both the conventional polyethylene and the human macrophages (control group) alone, but this was statistically significant only compared with the human macrophages.[63] However, the clinical significance of these particles in vivo and their relationship to radiographic osteolysis is still unknown.

Another knee simulator study measured wear particle size and morphology and the number of particles produced after 5 million cycles of six different tibial polyethylene liners, including three highly cross-linked products (X3 CR, Durasul ultracongruent, and Prolong CR), one experimental 5-Mrad mobile-bearing liner, and two conventional liners (one mobile-bearing and one congruent).[69] Most particles were round, smooth, and submicron in size. There were small but statistically significant differences in the size and shape description of analyzed wear particles. A significantly lower number of particles per million cycles was reported for the X3, Durasul, and 5-Mrad mobile-bearing liners, and the lowest number of particles produced were with the X3 polyethylene.

In a third knee simulator study of mildly (3.5 Mrad) and highly (7 Mrad) cross-linked polyethylene tested against cobalt-chromium and zirconia femoral components, the particle size, morphology, and number produced were measured.[70] No differences in particle size or morphology were reported, but a fourfold decrease was shown in the number of particles with increased cross-linking. In a 1-year in vivo study of synovial fluid aspirated from four highly cross-linked polyethylene (Prolong) knees and three conventional polyethylene knees, a significantly smaller total number of particles and concentration of particles was reported in the highly cross-linked knees.[71]

Summary

First-generation highly cross-linked polyethylene acetabular liners have performed well in vivo. Wear simulator studies have predicted the in vivo performance. At intermediate follow-up of highly cross-linked polyethylene in the hip, wear is significantly lower when compared to conventional polyethylene. As a result of this wear reduction, several studies have documented a significant reduction in periprosthetic osteolysis. Fracture of highly cross-linked acetabular liners have been reported. Risk of fracture is multifactorial. Surgical technique, implant design and polyethylene thickness all play a role. The actual role of the altered mechanical properties of highly cross-linked polyethylene in implant fracture is less clear. New polyethylenes that maintain wear resistance while improving fracture toughness are currently under development and in clinical evaluation.

Most modern metal-on-metal hip replacements, including conventional hips and surface replacements, have performed well in clinical use. The incidences of excessive wear, and of adverse local tissue reactions, appear to be functions of the specific design parameters and the surgical positioning of the components. For example, smaller diameter bearings and those with reduced coverage appear to be more sensitive to malpositioning, leading to edge wear, increased levels of particles and ions in the tissues, and an increased incidence of adverse reactions. Ongoing research by tribologists and materials engineers should lead to improvements in the materials and designs of metal-on-metal hip replacements to provide even lower rates of wear and ion release. Detailed research into the nature of the biologic responses to wear particles and ions will help surgeons to identify those patients who are at high risk for adverse reactions and, therefore, would be candidates for alternative bearings. In the meantime, it has become increasingly clear that the most important factor in achieving clinical success with metal-on-metal hip replacements is for the surgeon to implant the components in the appropriate anatomic orientation.

In an effort to reduce polyethylene wear and periprosthetic osteolysis, moderately and highly cross-linked polyethylene tibial liners are now available for use in a wide variety of modular TKA prostheses. Some laboratory wear simulator testing has demonstrated a significant reduction in wear under normal and accelerated wear kinematics, but results are somewhat conflicting. However, data show that the highly cross-linked polyethylene wear particles are smaller and possibly more biologically active. Two early clinical studies have demonstrated the safety of at least two types of highly cross-linked polyethylene at 2 and 5 years. The results of appropriately powered prospective randomized trials with sufficient follow-up will be required to demonstrate efficacy.

Catastrophic fracture of one design of a posterior-stabilized tibial post has been reported. Although a cautious approach to the use of these highly cross-linked tibial and patellar polyethylene components is recommended, their use in younger or more active patients may be considered. Cruciate-retaining and ultra-congruent designs may be more appropriate for use with highly cross-linked polyethylene tibial liners. Although knee simulator testing of some highly cross-linked products has shown excellent wear reduction and fracture resistance, particular caution with the use of posterior-stabilized components and thick liners is recommended because their use may place increased stress on the locking mechanism and tibial post. Surgeons should be cognizant of the importance of axial alignment and ligament balance to help prevent overload and possible failure of these polyethylene liners.

Annotated References

1. Estok DM II, Burrough BR, Muratoglu OK, Harris WH: Comparison of hip simulator wear of 2 different highly cross-linked ultra high molecular weight polyethylene acetabular components using both 32- and 38-mm femoral heads. *J Arthroplasty* 2007;22(4):581-589.

    This simulator study demonstrated that 9.5-Mrad material wore less than the 5-Mrad material with both 32-mm and 38-mm femoral heads.

2. Muratoglu OK, Rubash HE, Bragdon CR, Burroughs BR, Huang A, Harris WH: Simulated normal gait wear testing of a highly cross-linked polyethylene tibial insert. *J Arthroplasty* 2007;22(3):435-444.

    A simulator study demonstrating superior wear with highly cross-linked polyethylene tibial inserts compared with conventional polyethylene is presented.

3. Laurent MP, Johnson TS, Crowninshield RD, Blanchard CR, Bhambri SK, Yao JQ: Characterization of a highly cross-linked ultrahigh molecular-weight polyethylene in clinical use in total hip arthroplasty. *J Arthroplasty* 2008;23(5):751-761.

    This simulator study demonstrated that the relative

wear improvement of highly cross-linked polyethylene was maintained in the presence of bone cement or alumina particles. More than 90% fewer particles in all size ranges were produced with the highly cross-linked material. Average particle size was significantly smaller with the highly cross-linked material.

4. Ito H, Maloney CM, Crowninshield RD, Clohisy JC, McDonald DJ, Maloney WJ: In vivo femoral head damage and its effect on polyethylene wear. *J Arthroplasty* 2010;25(2):302-308.

    Highly cross-linked polyethylene was more wear resistant compared with conventional polyethylene against roughened femoral heads retrieved at revision surgery.

5. Shen FW, Lu Z, McKellop HA: Wear versus thickness and other features of 5 MRAD crosslinked UHMWPE acetabular liners. *Clin Orthop Relat Res* 2011;469(2): 395-404.

    The authors found that wear reduction with 5 Mrad of cross-linking was not offset when ball diameter was increased from 28 mm to 36 mm or when a thin liner was used.

6. McKellop H, Shen FW, DiMaio W, Lancaster JG: Wear of gamma-crosslinked polyethylene acetabular cups against roughened femoral balls. *Clin Orthop Relat Res* 1999;369:73-82.

7. McKellop HA, Shen FW, Lu B, Campbell P, Salovey R: Effect of sterilization method and other modifications on the wear resistance of acetabular cups made of ultra-high molecular weight polyethylene: A hip simulator study. *J Bone Joint Surg Am* 2000;82:1708-1725.

8. Tower SS, Currier JH, Currier BH, Lyford KA, Van Citters DW, Mayor MB: Rim cracking of the cross-linked longevity polyethylene acetabular liner after total hip arthroplasty. *J Bone Joint Surg Am* 2007; 89(10):2212-2217.

    This study evaluated fractured acetabular liners retrieved at revision surgery. The multifactorial nature of liner fracture is discussed. Fractures were attributed to thin polyethylene at the cup rim, vertical cup alignment, and a reduction in the mechanical properties of the highly cross-linked polyethylene liners.

9. Furmanski J, Anderson M, Bal S, et al: Clinical fracture of cross-linked UHMWPE acetabular liners. *Biomaterials* 2009;30(29):5572-5582.

    This study emphasized the effect of implant design on fracture risk. A notched elevated rim design was a common design feature in all four fractured liners. Fracture was also associated with suboptimal implant position.

10. Jung KA, Lee SC, Hwang SH, Kim SM: Fracture of a second-generation highly cross-linked UHMWPE tibial post in a posterior-stabilized scorpio knee system. *Orthopedics* 2008;31(11):1137.

    Fracture of a highly cross-linked polyethylene tibial post was reported.

11. Crowninshield RD, Maloney JU, Wentz DH, Humphrey SM, Blanchard CR: Biomechanics of large femoral heads: What they can and can't do. *Clin Orthop Relat Res* 2004;429:102-107.

12. Illgen RL II, Forsythe TM, Pike JW, Laurent MP, Blanchard CR: Highly crosslinked vs conventional polyethylene particles: An in vitro comparison of biologic activities. *J Arthroplasty* 2008;23(5):721-731.

    Highly cross-linked polyethylene was significantly more inflammatory compared with conventional polyethylene as assessed by release of inflammatory cytokines in cell culture.

13. Galvin AL, Tipper JL, Jennings LM, et al: Wear and biological activity of highly crosslinked polyethylene in the hip under low serum protein concentrations. *Proc Inst Mech Eng H* 2007;221(1):1-10.

    Functional biologic activity, which takes into account wear volume, was lower with highly cross-linked polyethylene when compared with conventional polyethylene.

14. Digas G, Kärrholm J, Thanner J, Herberts P: 5-year experience of highly cross-linked polyethylene in cemented and uncemented sockets: Two randomized studies using radiostereometric analysis. *Acta Orthop* 2007;78(6):746-754.

    The results of two prospective, randomized clinical trials comparing highly cross-linked polyethylene to conventional polyethylene. RSA was used to measure polyethylene wear. In both trials, the highly cross-linked polyethylenes had significantly lower wear in comparison with conventional polyethylene. Level of evidence: I.

15. Röhrl SM, Li MG, Nilsson KG, Nivbrant B: Very low wear of non-remelted highly cross-linked polyethylene cups: An RSA study lasting up to 6 years. *Acta Orthop* 2007;78(6):739-745.

    Two cohorts of patients were followed for a minimum of 6 years. One group had conventional polyethylene and the second group highly cross-linked polyethylene. Polyethylene wear was measured using RSA. Despite concerns over in vivo oxidation with the highly cross-linked polyethylene, it had significantly lower wear.

16. Bragdon CR, Kwon YM, Geller JA, et al: Minimum 6-year followup of highly cross-linked polyethylene in THA. *Clin Orthop Relat Res* 2007;465:122-127.

    This is a retrospective study demonstrating no difference in wear of highly cross-linked polyethylene comparing 28-mm and 32-mm femoral heads.

17. Bragdon CR, Greene ME, Freiberg AA, Harris WH, Malchau H: Radiostereometric analysis comparison of wear of highly cross-linked polyethylene against 36- vs 28-mm femoral heads. *J Arthroplasty* 2007;22(6, Suppl 2):125-129.

    This clinical study demonstrated no difference in wear comparing 28-mm and 36-mm femoral heads with highly cross-linked polyethylene.

18. Lachiewicz PF, Heckman DS, Soileau ES, Mangla J, Martell JM: Femoral head size and wear of highly cross-linked polyethylene at 5 to 8 years. *Clin Orthop Relat Res* 2009;467(12):3290-3296.

    Although the linear wear rate was not affected by head size, volumetric wear was significantly greater with 36-mm and 40-mm femoral heads.

19. Shia DS, Clohisy JC, Schinsky MF, Martell JM, Maloney WJ: THA with highly cross-linked polyethylene in patients 50 years or younger. *Clin Orthop Relat Res* 2009;467(8):2059-2065.

    Clinical studies listed in this article demonstrate superior wear performance of a variety of highly cross-linked polyethylenes compared with conventional polyethylene acetabular liners in total hip arthroplasty.

20. Leung SB, Egawa H, Stepniewski A, Beykirch S, Engh CA Jr, Engh CA Sr: Incidence and volume of pelvic osteolysis at early follow-up with highly cross-linked and noncross-linked polyethylene. *J Arthroplasty* 2007;22(6, Suppl 2):134-139.

    This is a retrospective study comparing 40 hips with conventional polyethylene and 36 hips with highly cross-linked polyethylene. At a minimum of 5 years, patients with highly cross-linked polyethylene had a significantly lower risk of osteolysis. In addition, the patients with highly cross-linked polyethylene in whom osteolysis developed had significantly smaller lesions.

21. Bitsch RG, Loidolt T, Heisel C, Ball S, Schmalzried TP: Reduction of osteolysis with use of Marathon cross-linked polyethylene: A concise follow-up, at a minimum of five years, of a previous report. *J Bone Joint Surg Am* 2008;90(7):1487-1491.

    In this retrospective study, radiographic analysis demonstrated that patients with highly cross-linked polyethylene had significantly lower wear rates, significantly lower adjusted volumetric wear, and significantly reduced risk of developing osteolysis (0% versus 33%) compared with patients with conventional polyethylene at a minimum 5-year follow-up period.

22. Mall NA, Nunley RM, Zhu JJ, Maloney WJ, Barrack RL, Clohisy JC: The incidence of acetabular osteolysis in young patients with conventional versus highly crosslinked polyethylene. *Clin Orthop Relat Res* 2011;469(2):372-381.

    Studies document a marked reduction in periprosthetic osteolysis for patients with highly cross-linked polyethylene liners when compared with patients with conventional polyethylene liners.

23. Weber BG: Experience with the Metasul total hip bearing system. *Clin Orthop Relat Res* 1996;(329, Suppl):S69-S77.

24. Amstutz HC: Hip resurfacing arthroplasty. *J Am Acad Orthop Surg* 2006;14(8):452-453.

    Based on experience with approximately 1,000 cases, the author reviews some key concepts important to the success of metal-on-metal hip surface replacements, including patient selection and surgical techniques.

25. Chan FW, Bobyn JD, Medley JB, Krygier JJ, Tanzer M: The Otto Aufranc Award: Wear and lubrication of metal-on-metal hip implants. *Clin Orthop Relat Res* 1999;369:10-24.

26. Rieker C, Konrad R, Schön R: In vitro comparison of the two hard-hard articulations for total hip replacements. *Proc Inst Mech Eng H* 2001;215(2):153-160.

27. Kretzer JP, Kleinhans JA, Jakubowitz E, Thomsen M, Heisel C: A meta-analysis of design- and manufacturing-related parameters influencing the wear behavior of metal-on-metal hip joint replacements. *J Orthop Res* 2009;27(11):1473-1480.

    The authors compile the results of 56 published studies using hip simulators to assess the influence on wear of ball-cup clearance, diameter, carbon content, and manufacturing method (for example, heat treating).

28. Onda K, Nagoya S, Kaya M, Yamashita T: Cup-neck impingement due to the malposition of the implant as a possible mechanism for metallosis in metal-on-metal total hip arthroplasty. *Orthopedics* 2008;31(4):396.

    The authors discuss a 60-year-old woman with an acetabular component in excessive anteversion that leads to neck-socket impingement, severe metallic wear, and metallosis. Failure was caused by fracture of the trochanter.

29. De Haan R, Campbell PA, Su EP, De Smet KA: Revision of metal-on-metal resurfacing arthroplasty of the hip: The influence of malpositioning of the components. *J Bone Joint Surg Br* 2008;90(9):1158-1163.

    Among 42 patients (30 female) with metal-on-metal hips revised between 1 and 76 months, 27 revisions were caused by malpositioning of the components and featured metallosis and a high level of serum ions. Twelve malpositioned hips had a large, metal-stained bursa (pseudotumor) containing copious amounts of brown or creamy fluid.

30. Williams S, Leslie I, Isaac G, Jin Z, Ingham E, Fisher J: Tribology and wear of metal-on-metal hip prostheses: Influence of cup angle and head position. *J Bone Joint Surg Am* 2008;90(Suppl 3):111-117.

    In a hip simulator, wear of 39-mm diameter metal-on-metal hip surface replacements was fivefold greater when the angle between the applied force and the face of the cup was 55° rather than 45° and was fivefold greater with microlateralization of 0.4 to 0.5 mm. When the two factors were present together, wear increased tenfold.

31. Leslie IJ, Williams S, Isaac G, Ingham E, Fisher J: High cup angle and microseparation increase the wear of hip surface replacements. *Clin Orthop Relat Res* 2009;467(9):2259-2265.

    In a hip simulator, wear of 39-mm metal-on-metal surface replacements with an inclination of 60° was ninefold greater than with 45°, and wear with 55° inclination plus 0.5-mm medial-superior translation (microseparation) was 17-fold greater than with normal cup positioning and no microseparation.

32. De Haan R, Pattyn C, Gill HS, Murray DW, Campbell PA, De Smet K: Correlation between inclination of the acetabular component and metal ion levels in metal-on-metal hip resurfacing replacement. *J Bone Joint Surg Br* 2008;90(10):1291-1297.

    In 214 patients with metal-on-metal resurfacings 1 year after surgery, high wear and ion levels were more likely to occur if the acetabular cups were implanted steeply and when the component was small and the design was low profile, as these factors are associated with increased risk of edge loading. There was no correlation of wear or ion levels with activity.

33. Langton DJ, Jameson SS, Joyce TJ, Webb J, Nargol AV: The effect of component size and orientation on the concentrations of metal ions after resurfacing arthroplasty of the hip. *J Bone Joint Surg Br* 2008;90(9): 1143-1151.

    In 76 patients with metal-on-metal resurfacings, cobalt ions in the blood were higher in components with a diameter 51 mm or less than 53 mm or greater. With components 51 mm or less in diameter, ion concentration was higher with greater inclination and greater anteversion, indicating the importance of component positioning, particularly with small diameter hips.

34. Langton DJ, Joyce TJ, Mangat N, et al: Reducing metal ion release following hip resurfacing arthroplasty. *Orthop Clin North Am* 2011;42(2):169-180.

    Comparing the metal ion levels in 610 patients with one of three hip resurfacing designs with varying coverage arc, size, and cup orientation, the authors reported that one design was more vulnerable to the effects of cup malposition.

35. Langton DJ, Sprowson AP, Joyce TJ, et al: Blood metal ion concentrations after hip resurfacing arthroplasty: A comparative study of articular surface replacement and Birmingham Hip Resurfacing arthroplasties. *J Bone Joint Surg Br* 2009;91(10):1287-1295.

    For 90 articular surface replacements (ASRs) and 70 Birmingham resurfacings, the levels of cobalt and chromium blood ions were lower with larger diameters. With ASRs, ions were higher with inclination of 45° or greater and with anteversion less than 10° or greater than 20°. With Birmingham resurfacings, ion levels were higher for inclination greater than 55°, and anteversion less than 10° or greater than 20°. For males, whole blood and serum chromium were lower with ASRs, possibly because of their smaller diametral clearance.

36. Thiele L, Merkle HP, Walter E: Phagocytosis and phagosomal fate of surface-modified microparticles in dendritic cells and macrophages. *Pharm Res* 2003; 20(2):221-228.

37. Kwon Y, Ostlere S, McLardy-Smith P, et al: "Asymptomatic" Pseudotumors After Metal-on-Metal Hip Resurfacing Arthroplasty Prevalence and Metal Ion Study

Arthroplasty 2011;26(4):511-518.

    The authors studied 158 patients with hip resurfacing who underwent ultrasound and had metal ion measurements after a mean of 61 months. Those with any cystic or solid mass had an aspiration or biopsy. Pseudotumors were found in seven patients (4%) and were associated with significantly higher cobalt and chromium levels and inferior functional scores. Pseudotumors were present in 6 of 61 female patients and 1 of 97 male patients. The authors suggested that periprosthetic pseudotumors are associated with abnormal wear, rather than with metal allergy.

38. De Smet K, De Haan R, Calistri A, et al: Metal ion measurement as a diagnostic tool to identify problems with metal-on-metal hip resurfacing. *J Bone Joint Surg Am* 2008;90(Suppl 4):202-208.

    This study examined 3,300 radiographs from more than 2,000 patients, up to 9 years postoperatively, along with 300 patient ion measurements and 47 retrieval findings (most for component malpositioning). The results demonstrated that high ion levels can indicate the need for a timely revision.

39. Heisel C, Silva M, Skipor AK, Jacobs JJ, Schmalzried TP: The relationship between activity and ions in patients with metal-on-metal bearing hip prostheses. *J Bone Joint Surg Am* 2005;87(4):781-787.

    In seven patients with metal-on-metal hips, the levels of cobalt and chromium ions in serum and of chromium in urine were not substantially affected by activity levels, which included 1 week of limited activity, 1 hour on a treadmill, and 1 week of maximum activity. Level of evidence: II.

40. De Haan R, Campbell P, Reid S, Skipor AK, De Smet K: Metal ion levels in a triathlete with a metal-on-metal resurfacing arthroplasty of the hip. *J Bone Joint Surg Br* 2007;89(4):538-541.

    Serum cobalt and chromium levels did not vary in a triathlete during 2 weeks of prerace training, during the triathlon, and during 2 weeks postrace. Urinary chromium increased immediately after the race, but returned to the prerace level in 6 days.

41. Pandit H, Glyn-Jones S, McLardy-Smith P, et al: Pseudotumours associated with metal-on-metal hip resurfacings. *J Bone Joint Surg Br* 2008;90(7):847-851.

    From 0 to 60 months, pain and conditions including dislocation, nerve palsy, swelling, clicking, and a rash developed in 17 female hip resurfacing patients. All were found to have a soft-tissue mass with necrosis, metal particles, macrophages, and lymphocytes. The authors estimated that pseudotumors would develop in 1% of patients within 5 years, but the actual percentage has proven to be higher (see Kwon et al, reference 37).

42. Hart AJ, Sabah S, Henckel J, et al: The painful metal-on-metal hip resurfacing. *J Bone Joint Surg Br* 2009; 91(6):738-744.

    Metal artifact reduction MRI, three-dimensional CT, and metal ion measurements were performed on 26 patients (9 men, 17 women) with unexplained pain around metal-on-metal hip replacements. Seven men and eight women had periprosthetic masses. Ion levels were higher in painful joints than in malfunctioning joints.

43. Willert HG, Buchhorn GH, Fayyazi A, et al: Metal-on-metal bearings and hypersensitivity in patients with artificial hip joints: A clinical and histomorphological study. *J Bone Joint Surg Am* 2005;87(1):28-36.

    Periprosthetic tissues from 19 consecutive revisions of modern metal-on-metal total hip replacements showed diffuse and perivascular infiltrates of T and B lymphocytes and plasma cells, which suggested a delayed type hypersensitivity response. A new term, ALVAL, was coined to describe these histologic features.

44. Hallab NJ, Caicedo M, Epstein R, McAllister K, Jacobs JJ: In vitro reactivity to implant metals demonstrates a person-dependent association with both T-cell and B-cell activation. *J Biomed Mater Res A* 2010; 92(2):667-682.

    Lymphocyte proliferation and activation were compared in patients with metal sensitivity, either with no implant, with a well performing metal-on-metal total hip replacement, or with a poorly performing metal-on-polymer joint. There was no direct correlation ($R^2 < 0.1$) between lymphocyte proliferation and T cell or B cell activation, and the hypothesis that early lymphocyte expression of activation is exclusively T cell mediated was not supported.

45. Campbell P, Ebramzadeh E, Nelson S, Takamura K, De Smet K, Amstutz HC: Histological features of pseudotumor-like tissues from metal-on-metal hips. *Clin Orthop Relat Res* 2010;468:2321-2327.

    The authors characterized the integrity of the synovial lining, inflammatory cell infiltrates, tissue organization, necrosis, and metal wear particles of pseudotumor-like tissues from metal-on-metal hips revised for suspected high wear reaction or metal hypersensitivity, using a 10-point ALVAL score. The tissues from patients revised for suspected high wear had a lower ALVAL score and fewer lymphocytes, but more macrophages and metal particles than tissues from hips revised for pain and suspected metal hypersensitivity, which had the highest ALVAL scores.

46. Thomas P, Braathen LR, Dörig M, et al: Increased metal allergy in patients with failed metal-on-metal hip arthroplasty and peri-implant T-lymphocytic inflammation. *Allergy* 2009;64(8):1157-1165.

    Patch testing (PT) and lymphocyte transformation testing (LTT) were performed in 16 patients with a revised metal-on-metal arthroplasty and lymphocytic inflammation of the tissues. Thirteen of 16 patients (81%) had positive results by PT and/or LTT to one or more metals. Based on these results, the authors suggested that allergic reactions should be included as a differential diagnosis in failed metal-on-metal arthroplasty.

47. Sharkey PF, Hozack WJ, Rothman RH, Shastri S, Jacoby SM: Insall Award paper: Why are total knee arthroplasties failing today? *Clin Orthop Relat Res* 2002;404(404):7-13.

48. Lachiewicz MP, Lachiewicz PF: Are the relative indications for revision total knee arthroplasty changing? *J Surg Orthop Adv* 2009;18(2):74-76.

    The authors attempted to determine if the indications for revision have changed over the past decade. Demographic data and indications for revision in two cohorts of patients were retrospectively reviewed and results indicate that relative indications for revision TKA have changed.

49. Fehring TK, Murphy JA, Hayes TD, Roberts DW, Pomeroy DL, Griffin WL: Factors influencing wear and osteolysis in press-fit condylar modular total knee replacements. *Clin Orthop Relat Res* 2004;428(428): 40-50.

50. Berry DJ: Recognizing and identifying osteolysis around total knee arthroplasty. *Instr Course Lect* 2004;53:261-264.

51. Wright TM: Polyethylene in knee arthroplasty: What is the future? *Clin Orthop Relat Res* 2005;440:141-148.

    Early clinical results in hip arthroplasty show significant improved wear with the use of highly cross-linked polyethylene as a bearing surface, indicating that the use of polyethylene in knee arthroplasties may improve wear performance.

52. Geerdink CH, Grimm B, Vencken W, Heyligers IC, Tonino AJ: Cross-linked compared with historical polyethylene in THA: An 8-year clinical study. *Clin Orthop Relat Res* 2009;467(4):979-984.

    The authors compared cross-linked polyethylene with historical polyethylene to confirm longer-term reductions in wear. Level of evidence: I.

53. Wang A, Yau SS, Essner A, Herrera L, Manley M, Dumbleton J: A highly crosslinked UHMWPE for CR and PS total knee arthroplasties. *J Arthroplasty* 2008; 23(4): 559-566.

    The authors found that wear and mechanical integrity of sequentially processed posterior-stabilized knee inserts were not affected by aging. Conventional ultrahigh molecular weight polyethylene showed increased delamination, wear, and cracking.

54. Oral E, Malhi AS, Wannomae KK, Muratoglu OK: Highly cross-linked ultrahigh molecular weight polyethylene with improved fatigue resistance for total joint arthroplasty: Recipient of the 2006 Hap Paul Award. *J Arthroplasty* 2008;23(7):1037-1044.

    The authors found that the improved fatigue properties for alpha-tocopherol-doped, irradiated ultra-high molecular weight polyethylene may be an advantage under high stresses.

55. Akagi M, Asano T, Clarke IC, et al: Wear and toughness of crosslinked polyethylene for total knee replacements: A study using a simulator and small-punch testing. *J Orthop Res* 2006;24(10):2021-2027.

Study results indicate that there may be an optimal irradiation dose for cross-linked polyethylene in total knee replacement.

56. Asano T, Akagi M, Clarke IC, Masuda S, Ishii T, Nakamura T: Dose effects of cross-linking polyethylene for total knee arthroplasty on wear performance and mechanical properties. *J Biomed Mater Res B Appl Biomater* 2007;83(2):615-622.

   Study results indicate that some degree of irradiation is beneficial for wear performance and toughness of polyethylene tibial inserts.

57. Muratoglu OK, Bragdon CR, Jasty M, O'Connor DO, Von Knoch RS, Harris WH: Knee-simulator testing of conventional and cross-linked polyethylene tibial inserts. *J Arthroplasty* 2004;19(7):887-897.

58. Muratoglu OK, Burroughs BR, Bragdon CR, Christensen SC, Lozynsky A, Harris WH: Knee simulator wear of polyethylene tibias articulating against explanted rough femoral components. *Clin Orthop Relat Res* 2004;428:108-113.

59. Muratoglu OK, Bragdon CR, O'Connor DO, Perinchief RS, Jasty M, Harris WH: Aggressive wear testing of a cross-linked polyethylene in total knee arthroplasty. *Clin Orthop Relat Res* 2002;404:89-95.

60. Hermida JC, Fischler A, Colwell CW Jr, D'Lima DD: The effect of oxidative aging on the wear performance of highly cross-linked polyethylene knee inserts under conditions of severe malalignment. *J Orthop Res* 2008;26(12):1585-1590.

   Study results indicate the presence of low levels of free radicals and preservation of mechanical properties in knees that had second-generation cross-linked ultra-high-molecular-weight polyethylene.

61. Tsukamoto R, Williams PA, Shoji H, et al: Wear of sequentially enhanced 9-Mrad polyethylene in 10 million cycle knee simulation study. *J Biomed Mater Res B Appl Biomater* 2008;86(1):119-124.

   The authors found that sequentially enhanced polyethylene in tibial inserts was beneficial because of reduced wear rates.

62. Utzschneider S, Harrasser N, Schroeder C, Mazoochian F, Jansson V: Wear of contemporary total knee replacements: A knee simulator study of six current designs. *Clin Biomech (Bristol, Avon)* 2009;24(7):583-588.

   The authors found that the combination of fixed-bearing Scorpio knee design with a sequential irradiated and annealed cross-linked polyethylene tibial insert was advantageous in wear generation.

63. Fisher J, McEwen HM, Tipper JL, et al: Wear, debris, and biologic activity of cross-linked polyethylene in the knee: Benefits and potential concerns. *Clin Orthop Relat Res* 2004;428(428):114-119.

64. Hodrick JT, Severson EP, McAlister DS, Dahl B, Hofmann AA: Highly crosslinked polyethylene is safe for use in total knee arthroplasty. *Clin Orthop Relat Res* 2008;466(11):2806-2812.

   This clinical study retrospectively reviewed 100 patients with highly cross-linked polyethylene tibial inserts compared with 100 patients with conventional polyethylene inserts. With a minimum follow-up of 82 months, knees with highly cross-linked polyethylene had fewer radiolucencies and a lower rate of tibial loosening.

65. Minoda Y, Aihara M, Sakawa A, et al: Comparison between highly cross-linked and conventional polyethylene in total knee arthroplasty. *Knee* 2009;16(5):348-351.

   No difference in loosening or osteolysis was seen in a comparison of the two materials at 2 years.

66. Muratoglu OK, Ruberti J, Melotti S, Spiegelberg SH, Greenbaum ES, Harris WH: Optical analysis of surface changes on early retrievals of highly cross-linked and conventional polyethylene tibial inserts. *J Arthroplasty* 2003;18(7, Suppl 1):42-47.

67. Bradford L, Baker D, Ries MD, Pruitt LA: Fatigue crack propagation resistance of highly crosslinked polyethylene. *Clin Orthop Relat Res* 2004;429(429):68-72.

68. Cole JC, Lemons JE, Eberhardt AW: Gamma irradiation alters fatigue-crack behavior and fracture toughness in 1900 Hand GUR 1050 UHMWPE. *J Biomed Mater Res* 2002;63(5):559-566.

69. Utzschneider S, Paulus A, Datz JC, et al: Influence of design and bearing material on polyethylene wear particle generation in total knee replacement. *Acta Biomater* 2009;5(7):2495-2502.

   The authors analyzed the effect of different knee designs combined with cross-linked polyethylenes on the amount, size, and shape of wear particles.

70. Williams PA, Brown CM, Tsukamoto R, Clarke IC: Polyethylene wear debris produced in a knee simulator model: Effect of crosslinking and counterface material. *J Biomed Mater Res B Appl Biomater* 2010;92(1):78-85.

   Study results showed that the amount of polyethylene cross-linking and the selection of counterface material were important in polyethylene wear debris production in knee replacement simulator models.

71. Iwakiri K, Minoda Y, Kobayashi A, et al: In vivo comparison of wear particles between highly crosslinked polyethylene and conventional polyethylene in the same design of total knee arthroplasties. *J Biomed Mater Res B Appl Biomater* 2009;91(2):799-804.

   In a comparison of in vivo polyethylene wear particle generation of highly cross-linked polyethylene with conventional polyethylene in TKAs, the highly cross-linked insert had fewer, smaller, and rounder wear particles.

1: Basic Science and General Knowledge

Chapter 3

Venous Thromboembolism Guidelines and Prophylaxis

Norman A. Johanson, MD

1: Basic Science and General Knowledge

What Is a Guideline?

Clinical guidelines are created as educational tools that help to guide decision making for the purpose of improving the quality and efficiency of patient care. Guidelines are not exhaustive descriptions of all variables involved in making a clinical decision and therefore should not be treated as dogmatic formulas. The ultimate judgment regarding any specific intervention should be made in light of each patient's unique presentation and the context created by other patient needs, resources, and local or institutional factors.

The prevention of venous thromboembolism (VTE) after hip and knee replacement is a good example of a widely acknowledged problem for which guidelines are appropriately created. The representative ingredients of a well-constructed guideline are defined in the following ways: (1) the patient population should be specifically described; (2) the interventions, such as hip and knee replacement, should be standardized; (3) the various treatments that are being compared, in this case the individual prophylactic agents or regimens, should be studied well enough so that published results may yield meaningful quantitative comparisons; and (4) the outcomes of interest, symptomatic or asymptomatic deep venous thrombosis (DVT), pulmonary embolism (PE), and mortality, are measurable and may be ranked in order of their relative importance. In addition, the complications or patient harm that is potentially caused by any prophylactic regimen must be properly attributed to arrive at an accurate risk-benefit ratio.

How and Why Do Specific Guidelines Differ?

Guidelines written to address the same populations and interventions may differ according to the outcome of primary interest, the evidence that is allowed to be used for evaluation, and the methods (qualitative and quan-

titative) by which the comparisons of different regimens are made. There are several real and apparent conflicts between the American College of Chest Physicians (ACCP) Guidelines for VTE prophylaxis[1] and the American Academy of Orthopaedic Surgeons (AAOS) Guideline for the Prevention of Symptomatic Pulmonary Embolism Following Hip and Knee Replacement.[2] The ACCP first published guidelines in 1986, and in 2008 released its eighth edition. The AAOS guideline was released in May 2007 after being initiated and approved by the AAOS Board of Directors. A comparison of the two guidelines demonstrates how different approaches to the same problem may result in conflicting recommendations (Table 1). The most prominent disagreements pertain to the following issues: (1) the significance of asymptomatic DVT and the appropriateness of combining the rates of asymptomatic and symptomatic VTE to determine superiority of prophylactic regimens; (2) the necessity of promoting individualized patient risk stratification; (3) the value of evidence other than randomized drug trials in supporting the strongest recommendations; and (4) the frequency and importance of postoperative bleeding complications caused by aggressive pharmacologic prophylaxis. Conflict of interest is another serious issue that has been raised by the orthopaedic critique of the ACCP guideline.[3] The critical question is whether the ACCP guideline can claim legitimacy when most of the publications supporting the guideline recommendations have been primarily funded by the pharmaceutical industry (for example, the manufacturers of the recommended products). In addition, can the many individuals responsible for producing the guideline who received financial compensation from the pharmaceutical industry be sufficiently free of important bias?

Asymptomatic DVT: How Important Is It?

The 2004 ACCP guideline states, "Without prophylaxis, the incidence of objectively confirmed, hospital-acquired DVT is approximately 10% to 40% among medical or general surgical patients and 40% to 60% following major orthopedic surgery."[4] This statement, which relies on historic data garnered from compari-

Table 1

Comparison Between AAOS and ACCP Guidelines on Key Issues

Issue of Disagreement	ACCP Guideline	AAOS Guideline
Role of asymptomatic DVT in discriminating among prophylactic agents	Essential	Not important
Method of patient risk assessment	Group (all orthopaedic patients are high risk; no consideration for stratifying bleeding risk)	Individual stratification of symptomatic VTE and bleeding risk
Use of evidence from other than randomized drug trials	Not used	Used because of inconclusive level 1 evidence for symptomatic VTE prevention
Importance of postoperative bleeding	Not emphasized	Emphasized
Potential for conflict of interest	Significant	Minimal

sons of treated and untreated populations, forms the basis of the argument that implies that all VTE is a serious problem for orthopaedic patients in general. Hip and knee replacement patients have been most commonly studied because of the high volumes of these procedures. Hip and knee replacements have become the focus of one of the Surgical Care Improvement Process (SCIP) Guidelines, which require hospitals to document the initiation of VTE prophylaxis within 24 hours of surgery. These recommendations, including the prophylactic agents, arose directly from the 2004 ACCP guidelines.

More contemporary studies comparing preventive regimens have shifted to comparisons of prophylactic agents, which have not shown significant differences in prevention of symptomatic events. Therefore, regardless of the true importance of asymptomatic DVT, this event has been deemed appropriate as a proxy measure for the risk of more serious and life-threatening events such as PE. This logic naturally favors the use of any agent that shows a clear advantage in lowering DVT rates by virtue of its proposed direct impact on reducing PE. An additional argument in favor of aggressively managing asymptomatic DVT rates is the hypothetical correlation between asymptomatic DVT and postphlebitic syndrome. Both arguments are compromised by a lack of contemporary high-level scientific evidence. Although current appropriately powered clinical trials have demonstrated statistically significant differences in DVT rates among selected agents, the concurrently reported PE rates for all prophylactic modalities are not statistically different.[2]

The most recently reported rates of PE following total hip or knee replacement in large populations demonstrate the very low incidence of this complication. In total hip replacement, the 90-day rate of nonfatal PE has been reported to be 0.93% in 58,521 Medicare patients who underwent primary total hip replacement with or without prophylaxis during 1995-1996.[5] Death occuring after PE in total hip replacement is very rare. One study reported a 90-day PE-related death rate of 0.22% in 44,785 hip replacement patients in the Scottish Morbidity Record from 1992 to 2001.[6] Nonfatal and fatal PE after total knee replacement are even less common. A California discharge database comprising 222,684 patients who had undergone total knee replacement from 1991-2001 was surveyed. The 90-day nonfatal PE rate was reported as 0.41%.[7] A 0.15% rate of fatal PE was reported in 27,000 total knee replacement patients in the Scottish Morbidity Record.[6] In addition, it has been shown that despite significant changes in VTE prophylaxis and surgical techniques over the past 10 to 15 years, the rates of PE and PE-related mortality have been remarkably stable.[6]

When performing drug trials for the purpose of proving superiority of one agent or regimen over another, it is necessary to include patients with asymptomatic DVT to achieve adequate statistical power. The clinical rationale for this inclusion is that asymptomatic DVT may lead to more serious morbidity. The 2004 ACCP guidelines specifically state, "While most asymptomatic DVT's are not clinically relevant, there is strong concordance between the "surrogate" outcome of asymptomatic DVT and clinically important VTE."[4] The assertion is also made that, "With few exceptions, interventions that reduce asymptomatic DVT also convey similar relative risk reductions in symptomatic VTE."[4] These claims have not been substantiated for hip and knee replacement using contemporary data. Orthopaedic surgeons who perform total hip and knee replacements are not in a position to detect any significant compromise in clinical outcomes as a result of undetected VTE. For a high level of evidence regarding this issue to be established, routine screening for DVT in a massive number of contemporary patients would have to be instituted, and both the AAOS and ACCP guidelines recommend against this measure.[1,2] The only serious concern that is uniformly voiced by hip and knee surgeons relates to the risk of symptomatic VTE and mortality. However, there is no agent or regimen that has been established as superior in the prevention of mortality or symptomatic VTE. In a contested meta-analysis, however, it was concluded that aggressive thromboprophylaxis with "potent" pharmacologic agents leads to significantly elevated 3-month all-cause mortality.[8] The potential for patient harm that is inherent in strongly recommended prophylactic regimens for reducing the incidence of asymptomatic DVT has not received adequate attention. One study's strong criticism of the AAOS guideline's lack of regard for asymptomatic DVTs as an outcome of interest is noteworthy for its absence of any mention of patient harm as a critical issue.[9]

Individual Patient Risk Stratification for VTE

There are three basic reasons cited by the ACCP for not seeking an individualized patient risk stratification strategy for VTE in hip and knee replacement: (1) the inability to confidently identify individual patients who do not require prophylaxis; (2) the lack of contemporary rigorous clinical evaluations to support an individualized approach; and (3) "individualizing is logistically complex and is likely associated with suboptimal compliance."[4] The first argument is not currently applicable because of the high level of utilization by orthopaedic surgeons of some form of prophylaxis. Second, the lack of rigorous clinical evaluations to support individualization is an appropriate indictment of contemporary research in this area and should be the foundation of a research agenda going forward. It is not, however, a reason for not pursuing this goal as the ACCP seems to favor. Third, logistic complexity is poorly defined and compliance is a term that begs the question as to the appropriate standard to which compliance is demanded. In this sense, the ACCP guideline discourages the AAOS recommendation for individualization for risk of PE or bleeding.[2] It is ironic that randomized trials, which are required by the ACCP for a strong 1A recommendation, exclude the perceived high-risk patients without providing a high level of evidence to justify such exclusions. In its most recent guideline, the ACCP acknowledges that most studies have excluded patients who are at particularly high risk for either VTE or adverse outcomes. Results are not applicable to all patients, such as those with a history of VTE or an increased risk of bleeding. Clinical judgment may appropriately warrant the use of alternative strategies to the "recommended approach."[1]

There is currently no scientifically valid risk stratification method for VTE in hip and knee replacement. Randomized drug trials systematically exclude perceived high-risk patients and therefore have limited usefulness in risk stratification. Therefore, alternative strategies should be used for this purpose, such as large cohort studies and registry analysis. This concept has been embraced by the AAOS guideline for planning future research.[2]

What Is the Value of Nonrandomized Studies in Constructing Guidelines?

The applicability of guidelines in which the strongest (1A) ACCP recommendations are based solely on randomized drug trials is seriously limited, particularly in patients who may have one or more risk factors for either VTE or adverse effects such as bleeding. To advance beyond this state of affairs it will be necessary to allow for an evolving understanding of the true risk-benefit relationship among patient groups. Large cohort studies and registry data have been helpful in promoting a "real-world" approach to VTE prophylaxis. The usefulness of large databases and registries has already been cited as capable of tracking trends in the incidence of VTE, thus more realistically and efficiently updating the actual health problem that exists.[5-7] Large cohort studies are valuable because of the potential for tracking outcomes in a more inclusive patient population from the standpoint of risk and comorbidity. Large cohort studies are generally less expensive and therefore more broadly undertaken than randomized controlled trials and therefore promise a more representative picture of contemporary trends in clinical practice. Good examples of such studies are those demonstrating the results of multimodal VTE prophylactic strategies. These approaches use regional anesthesia, aspirin, and intermittent pneumatic compression (IPC). In a 2007 study, 1,179 hip and knee replacements were performed on patients deemed not to be at high risk for VTE.[10] There were no fatal PEs, and the rate of nonfatal PE was 0.25%. Another study reported a fatal PE rate of 0.09% and a nonfatal PE rate of 0.7% in 1,032 hip replacements treated postoperatively with thigh-calf pneumatic compression.[11] Fatal and nonfatal PE rates were reportedly 0.04% and 0.54%, respectively, in 2,037 "low-risk" patients with total hip replacement performed under hypotensive epidural anesthesia receiving postoperative aspirin and early mobilization.[12] Similar results were found in patients who had knee replacement. One study found a fatal PE rate of 0.06% to 0.14% and a nonfatal PE rate of 0.26% in 3,473 knee replacements.[13] No fatal PEs and a nonfatal PE rate of 0.5% was reported in 856 consecutive knee replacements.[14] The results of these studies support the use of less aggressive prophylaxis in selected groups of lower-risk patients. The question regarding which patients should be considered at elevated risk for PE or bleeding has yet to be fully answered. Patients with a documented history of symptomatic VTE or thrombophilia, patients on bed rest or unable to mobilize rapidly, and those with other factors based on the surgeon's clinical judgment are currently identified as at risk for PE.[2] Risk of bleeding has usually been related to a history of bleeding at or remote from the surgical site. This may include extensive surgical dissection such as revision procedures and a history of gastrointestinal bleed or hemorrhagic stroke.[2] There is evidence that current orthopaedic practice, particularly relating to hip and knee replacement, already includes some form of risk stratification. Administrative data from more than 300 hospitals were analyzed in more than 93,840 patients who underwent total knee replacement. Patients who received aspirin (n = 4,719) as VTE prophylaxis had lower preoperative risk of VTE, shorter length of hospital stay, lower risk of surgical site bleeding, and lower rates of VTE than patients treated with warfarin (n = 51,923) or low-molecular-weight heparin (LMWH) or fondaparinux (n = 37,198).[15] Unfortunately, under the current ACCP guideline policy, which exclusively relies on randomized controlled trials for strong recommendations, the findings from nonrandomized studies are not admissible for consideration in formulating 1A recommendations.

Bleeding Complications: How Important Are They?

The occurrence of major bleeding complications after elective total hip or knee replacement may lead to adverse patient outcomes such as chronic joint stiffness and infection. The AAOS systematic literature review found a reported rate of major bleeding episodes after total hip and knee replacement using conventional pharmacologic prophylaxis such as that recommended by the ACCP to be between 1% and 3%.[2] Another study reported on the complications encountered in a prospective cohort study of 234 patients (129 total hip arthroplasties, 105 total knee arthroplasties) who received the ACCP 1A recommended 10-day course of enoxaparin (30 mg twice daily).[16] There was a 9% major complication rate, including 4.7% readmissions, 3.4% return to the operating room, and 1.3% incidence of heparin-induced thrombocytopenia. All of these complications were sustained without any apparent VTE prophylactic benefit (symptomatic DVT, 3.8%; nonfatal PE, 1.3%).

A retrospective study of more than 500 knee replacements found that mandated compliance with ACCP guidelines beginning in July 2005 resulted in an increased complication rate (hematoma, seroma, and hemorrhage) from 1.4% before the hospital mandate to 9.6% after the mandate. In addition, the rate of readmission increased from 2.2% to 4.4%.[17]

There is no contemporary study that adequately describes the incidence of major surgical bleeding in patients who have not received prophylaxis, but all reports of mechanical antithrombotic devices are noteworthy for an incidence of major bleeding of less than 1%.[2] The literature is nonstandardized with regard to identification and confirmation of major postoperative bleeding. There is significant variability in operationally defining major bleeding and the appropriate treatment options. The result has been a substantial likelihood of underestimating the bleeding risks of aggressive thromboprophylaxis. Studies that do report on bleeding-related complications do not usually have a follow-up period long enough to link bleeding to the serious development of deep infection or joint stiffness. Recent studies have demonstrated an important relationship between early postoperative wound hematoma or drainage and prosthetic joint infections.[18,19]

The Joint Commission has recently called attention to the risk of anticoagulation-related patient harm. A 2008 study reported on a survey of anticoagulant-related bleeding complications at Saint Joseph HealthCare, a network of three Kentucky hospitals.[20] There was an 18.3% incidence of anticoagulant-related hematoma and seroma among hospitalized patients. The Joint Commission proceeded to issue the National Patient Safety Goal 3E: Reduce the likelihood of patient harm associated with the use of anticoagulant therapy, implemented in January 2009. (http://www.jointcommission.org/PatientSafety/National PatientSafetyGoals/). In September 2008, the Joint Commission issued a Sentinel Event Alert for anticoagulant use emphasizing the dangers of anticoagulants. Thus, the harmful adverse effects of potent anticoagulants are beginning to come into national focus such that the risk-benefit model for all prophylactic agents should be continually reevaluated. This may ultimately lead to the redefinition of appropriate anticoagulation in the normal-risk hip and knee replacement patient.

What Is the Role of Conflict of Interest in Guideline Formation?

An analysis of the ACCP guideline set forth the following critique of that guideline process: (1) randomized controlled trials without venography were excluded from consideration; (2) the studies that were cited had inadequate outcome measures in that there was not a requirement for distinguishing symptomatic and fatal DVT and PE and major surgical and nonsurgical site bleeding; (3) there were no quantitative estimates of event rates for symptomatic and fatal DVT and PE and major surgical and nonsurgical site bleeding; and (4) "potential conflicts of interest" were embedded in the process.[3]

The methodology of this analysis of the ACCP guideline included the following: quantitative systematic review (pooled analysis); inclusion of aspirin, warfarin, LMWH, and pentasaccharides in the analysis; analysis of 14 randomized controlled trials cited by the ACCP dealing with total hip and total knee replacement and hip fracture surgery; two studies rejected by the ACCP because of no venography; and pooled data analysis comparing event rates for venographic DVT, symptomatic DVT and PE, fatal PE, and major surgical and nonsurgical site bleeding. The results of the analysis demonstrated no significant differences in clinically significant VTE outcomes except that warfarin was associated with an increased symptomatic DVT rate compared with aspirin, and an increased bleeding risk was identified with warfarin, LMWH, and pentasaccharides compared with aspirin.[3]

The analysis of the ACCP guideline underscores a critical issue that is emerging from the guideline creation process: The values that exist in every clinical trial as well as the funding support may significantly determine the conclusions and recommendations that flow from the study. Because the analysis included two studies that were rejected by the ACCP, doubt was cast on the justification of risk and benefit implied by the 1A recommendations. The issue of postoperative bleeding was shown to be more rather than less important, this being in line with the current concerns of the Joint Commission and other organizations. The 2004 ACCP guideline specifically stated, "abundant data have demonstrated little or no increase in the rates of clinically important bleeding"...with prophylactic doses of low-dose unfractionated heparin, LMWH, and vitamin K antagonist.[4] Would this statement be as dogmatic today in light of current knowledge, and if not, how might the ACCP guideline be modified?

The power of slight changes in the values and priorities in guideline development can be observed in a recent trans-Atlantic controversy over the treatment of acute coronary syndromes. The North American and European guideline counterparts examined the exact same data set and came to differing opinions regarding the use of aggressive anticoagulation. The critical issue was concern over the tendency for aggressive anticoagulation to lead to bleeding complications. The conflict was described as follows: "The disagreements in the recommendations for enoxaparin and fondaparinux seem to stem from differences in both the interpretation of the trial data and from differences in the application of nearly identical criteria used by both committees to classify the evidence."[21] It therefore appears to be very likely that in "close call" situations the operative power of conflict and bias has the potential for significant influence. A recent report on relationships between professional medical associations and industry made the strong statement that "the establishment of guidelines and registries must be independent of all industry influence, actual or perceived. Under no circumstances should PMAs accept funding from industry to develop practice guidelines or outcome measures"[22]. It is therefore not surprising that the most recent formation of panels to update the ACCP guideline has been accompanied by a meticulous conflict of interest disclosure policy. The practical outworking of this policy remains to be seen.

Summary

Although the ACCP guideline is already into its preparations for the ninth edition, the AAOS guideline process is still in its early phase. The AAOS processes are methodologically sophisticated and free of conflict of interest. The prophylactic strategy advocated for hip and knee replacement uses individual risk stratification and gives the clinician the opportunity to modify the prophylactic regimen for patients according to risk of PE and bleeding. The literature does not provide as definitive decision-making guidance as one would hope, and this represents a challenge for proceeding with a research agenda that will better address the needs of clinicians and their patients.

Annotated References

1. Geerts WH, Bergqvist D, Pineo GF, et al: Prevention of venous thromboembolism: American College of Chest Physicians evidence-based clinical practice guidelines (8th edition). *Chest* 2008;133(6, suppl):381S-453S.

   This is the ACCP's most recent compendium of recommendations for VTE prophylaxis in patients with surgical and nonsurgical conditions, including patients undergoing hip and knee replacements. The hip and knee replacement sections have some changes from the previous edition (2004) such as increased acknowledgment of the benefits of mechanical prophylaxis and potential harms such as bleeding.

2. Johanson NA, Lachiewicz PF, Lieberman JR, et al: American Academy of Orthopaedic Surgeons clinical practice guideline on: Prevention of symptomatic pulmonary embolism in patients undergoing total hip or knee arthroplasty. *J Bone Joint Surg Am* 2009;91(7):1756-1757.

   This is a summary of the 2007 AAOS guideline. The recommendations underscore the need for prevention of symptomatic PE and death rather than asymptomatic DVT, which is the emphasis of the ACCP guideline. Other important recommendations include the need to risk stratify patients for PE and bleeding. Full text and rationales for the AAOS guideline may be found online at: http://aaos.org/research/guidelines/PE_guideline.pdf.

3. Brown GA: Venous thromboembolism prophylaxis after major orthopaedic surgery: A pooled analysis of randomized controlled trials. *J Arthroplasty* 2009;24(6, suppl):77-83.

   This is a report on the quantitative analysis of 14 randomized controlled trials that were cited by the ACCP guidelines plus two that were rejected. No significant differences were found in prophylactic regimens in preventing symptomatic VTE except for an advantage of aspirin over warfarin. The danger of increased bleeding was noted. Conflict of interest was cited as a potential influence on the recommendations of the ACCP guidelines.

4. Geerts WH, Pineo GF, Heit JA, et al: Prevention of venous thromboembolism: The Seventh ACCP Conference on Antithrombotic and Thrombolytic Therapy. *Chest* 2004;126(3, suppl):338S-400S.

   This guideline for VTE prophylaxis issued 1A recommendations for aggressive anticoagulation for both hip and knee replacement patients. The SCIP guidelines, which are actually performance measures extracted from the 2004 ACCP guidelines, were enforced by the Centers for Medicare and Medicaid Services in October 2006, with potential modifications in case of an increased risk of bleeding. The recommendation against individual risk stratification as well as the justification of using asymptomatic DVT as a proxy measure for symptomatic VTE and PE are also contained in this guideline.

5. Katz JN, Losina E, Barrett J, et al: Association between hospital and surgeon procedure volume and outcomes of total hip replacement in the United States medicare population. *J Bone Joint Surg Am* 2001; 83(11):1622-1629.

6. Howie C, Hughes H, Watts AC: Venous thromboembolism associated with hip and knee replacement over a ten-year period: A population-based study. *J Bone Joint Surg Br* 2005;87(12):1675-1680.

   This report from the Scottish Morbidity Record documents the rarity of fatal PE over a 10-year period. It serves as a benchmark against which all prophylactic regimens may be measured, regardless of the demonstrated rates of asymptomatic DVT. The 90-day incidence of fatal PE after total hip replacement was 0.22% and after total knee replacement was 0.15%.

7. SooHoo NF, Lieberman JR, Ko CY, Zingmond DS: Factors predicting complication rates following total knee replacement. *J Bone Joint Surg Am* 2006;88(3): 480-485.

   Using a California hospital administrative data set for knee replacements spanning the decade from 1991 through 2001, the 90-day rates of complications, including PE, were determined and related to hospital volume, comorbidity, and age. Age and comorbidity were shown to influence the probability of adverse outcomes as much as or more than the effect of hospital volume of knee replacement.

8. Sharrock NE, Gonzalez Della Valle A, Go G, Lyman S, Salvati EA: Potent anticoagulants are associated with a higher all-cause mortality rate after hip and knee arthroplasty. *Clin Orthop Relat Res* 2008;466(3):714-721.

   Twenty studies were identified by the authors that were published between 1998 and 2007 and reported the incidence of all-cause mortality as well as prophylactic regimens for VTE. A total of 15,839 patients received LMWH, heparin, ximelagatran, fondaparinux, or rivaroxaban (group A). A total of 7,193 patients received regional anesthesia, pneumatic compression, and aspirin (group B). There were 5,006 patients who received warfarin (group C). All-cause mortality was least frequent in group B.

9. Eikelboom JW, Karthikeyan G, Fagel N, Hirsh J: American Association of Orthopedic Surgeons and American College of Chest Physicians guidelines for venous thromboembolism prevention in hip and knee arthroplasty differ: What are the implications for clinicians and patients? *Chest* 2009;135(2):513-520.

   In this summary of the differences between the two guidelines, the authors argue that asymptomatic DVT is a valid proxy measure for symptomatic VTE. Relative risk is compared using both arthroplasty and nonarthroplasty studies on prophylaxis versus placebo or no treatment.

10. Dorr LD, Gendelman V, Maheshwari AV, Boutary M, Wan Z, Long WT: Multimodal thromboprophylaxis for total hip and knee arthroplasty based on risk assessment. *J Bone Joint Surg Am* 2007;89(12):2648-2657.

    This study used multimodal thromboprophylaxis in selected hip and knee replacement patients that were not believed to be at elevated risk for VTE. With calf compression and aspirin there were no fatal PEs in 1,179 consecutive patients. Nonfatal PEs were identified in 0.25%.

11. Lachiewicz PF, Soileau ES: Multimodal prophylaxis for THA with mechanical compression. *Clin Orthop Relat Res* 2006;453:225-230.

    This series of 1,032 consecutively performed total hip replacements were treated with mechanical prophylaxis; if a postoperative duplex scan was negative, the patient was discharged on aspirin therapy, 325 mg twice daily for 6 weeks. Only one PE-related death was observed, and seven other patients (0.7%) had symptomatic PE.

12. Westrich GH, Farrell C, Bono JV, Ranawat CS, Salvati EA, Sculco TP: The incidence of venous thromboembolism after total hip arthroplasty: A specific hypotensive epidural anesthesia protocol. *J Arthroplasty* 1999; 14(4):456-463.

    This study on unilateral total hip replacement divided patients into high-, and low-risk groups. The lower-risk group (n = 2,037) received hypotensive epidural anesthesia, aspirin, and early mobilization. The PE rate was 0.54% (11 of 2,037), and the fatal PE rate was 0.04%.

13. Lotke PA, Lonner JH: The benefit of aspirin chemoprophylaxis for thromboembolism after total knee arthroplasty. *Clin Orthop Relat Res* 2006;452:175-180.

    This consecutive total knee replacement series included 3,813 knees in 3,473 patients treated with aspirin, 325 mg twice per day, and pneumatic foot pumps. The all-cause mortality rate was 0.26%, proven fatal PE rate was 0.06% (best case) and 0.14% (worst case), and nonfatal PE rate was 0.26%. The adverse bleeding event rate was 0.3%.

14. Lachiewicz PF, Soileau ES: Mechanical calf compression and aspirin prophylaxis for total knee arthroplasty. *Clin Orthop Relat Res* 2007;464:61-64.

    This consecutive series of 856 knee replacements in 599 patients treated with regional anesthesia (97%), aspirin, and pneumatic compression devices resulted in no fatal PEs and a nonfatal PE rate of 0.5%.

15. Bozic KJ, Vail TP, Pekow PS, Maselli JH, Lindenauer PL, Auerbach AD: Does asprin have a role in venous thromboembolism prophylaxis in total knee arthroplasty patients? *J Arthroplasty* 2010;25(7):1053-1060.

    Evidence is presented for surgical risk stratification of VTE using a database of more than 93,840 knee replacement patients hospitalized between October 2003 and September 2005. Patients who were given aspirin for VTE prophylaxis had fewer risk factors for VTE and a lower VTE rate than patients treated with warfarin, LMWH, or fondaparinux.

16. Burnett RS, Clohisy JC, Wright RW, et al: Failure of the American College of Chest Physicians-1A protocol for lovenox in clinical outcomes for thromboembolic prophylaxis. *J Arthroplasty* 2007;22(3):317-324.

    A consecutive cohort study on the bleeding complications associated with utilization of 1A ACCP recommendations is presented. A surprisingly elevated bleeding rate was associated with no real VTE prophylactic benefit.

17. Novicoff WM, Brown TE, Cui Q, Mihalko WM, Slone HS, Saleh KJ: Mandated venous thromboembolism prophylaxis: Possible adverse outcomes. *J Arthroplasty* 2008;23(6, suppl 1):15-19.

    This retrospective study of bleeding-related complication rates before and after the institution of hospital-mandated anticoagulation in 2005, in accordance with SCIP guidelines, revealed a dramatic rise (1.4% to 9.6%) in bleeding and readmission rate (2.2% to 4.4%).

18. Patel VP, Walsh M, Sehgal B, Preston C, DeWal H, Di Cesare PE: Factors associated with prolonged wound drainage after primary total hip and knee arthroplasty. *J Bone Joint Surg Am* 2007;89(1):33-38.

    This is a retrospective study on 1,211 primary hip replacements and 1,226 knee replacements. The use of LMWH was found to be associated with prolonged hip wound drainage, which leads to a higher probability of wound infection. Obesity was the only independent predictor of postoperative infection.

19. Saleh K, Olson M, Resig S, et al: Predictors of wound infection in hip and knee joint replacement: Results from a 20 year surveillance program. *J Orthop Res* 2002;20(3):506-515.

20. Jennings HR, Miller EC, Williams TS, Tichenor SS, Woods EA: Reducing anticoagulant medication adverse vents and avoidable patient harm. *Jt Comm J Qual Patient Saf* 2008;34(4):196-200.

    In this Codman Award–winning study, the authors identified a substantial bleeding complication rate in hospitalized patients who were treated with anticoagulation therapy. Most of the report focuses on the monitoring process that was set up to reduce these complications. There is no emphasis in this report on the reevaluation of the actual indications for aggressive prophylaxis.

21. Eikelboom J, Guyatt G, Hirsh J: Guidelines for anticoagulant use in acute coronary syndromes. *Lancet* 2008;371(9624):1559-1561.

    The authors discuss technical issues surrounding a disagreement between European and North American guidelines based on analysis of identical data sets. This demonstrates how, given a defined benefit of a treatment, elevating the importance of associated bleeding complications may alter recommendations in favor of less aggressive anticoagulation.

22. Rothman DJ, McDonald WJ, Berkowitz CD, et al: Professional medical associations and their relationships with industry: A proposal for controlling conflict of interest. *JAMA* 2009;301(13):1367-1372.

    This article presents a comprehensive rationale for the incremental reduction of financial relationships between professional medical associations and industry. Of note is the call for the elimination of industry's influence, either real or perceived, over clinical practice guideline production.

1: Basic Science and General Knowledge

Chapter 4
Biologic Response to Implants

Curtis W. Hartman, MD   Nadim J. Hallab, PhD   Joshua J. Jacobs, MD   J. Dennis Bobyn, PhD

Introduction
Curtis W. Hartman, MD
Nadim J. Hallab, PhD
Joshua J. Jacobs, MD

Total hip arthroplasty (THA) and total knee arthroplasty have become highly effective treatment options for patients with debilitating hip and knee arthrosis. It has become clear with mid- and long-term data that wear and the biologic response to wear debris is the primary mode of failure for these implants.[1] This response, while originally termed cement disease,[2] is now known to be unrelated to cement, but rather a complex, multifactorial biologic response to wear and corrosion debris, both particulate and ionic[3,4] (**Figure 1**).

Although the biologic response to implants is multifactorial, the generation of debris is certainly an important factor influencing the biologic response. To fully understand the biology, one should have an understanding of the sources of the particulate debris: wear and corrosion. Wear is defined as the removal of material, with the generation of wear particles, that occurs as a result of the relative motion between two opposing surfaces under load.[5,6] Wear occurs via three mechanisms: adhesion, abrasion, and fatigue. Adhesive wear occurs when the strength of adhesion between the two articulating surfaces exceeds the local cohesive strength of the material. Material is usually removed from the weaker surface.[6] Abrasive wear occurs when a hard projection, or asperity, on one surface cuts into the opposing surface.[6] Fatigue wear occurs when particles are released as a consequence of the propagation and coalescence of subsurface cracks that were induced by cyclic loading.[6] Beyond the mechanisms of wear, distinct

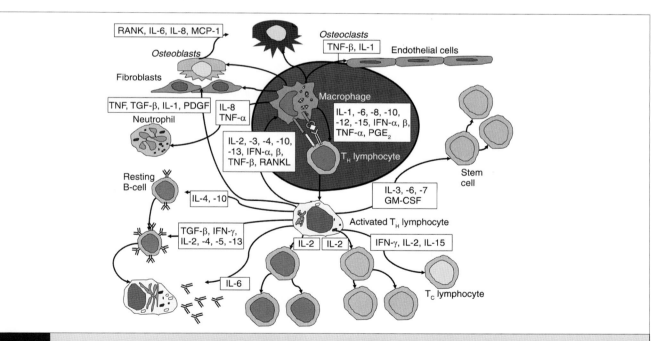

Figure 1	Complex interrelationship between wear products and cells of the innate and adaptive immune systems. (Reproduced from Jacobs JJ, Campbell PA, Knottinen Y; Implant Wear Symposium 2007 Biologic Work Group: How was the biologic reaction to wear particles changed with newer bearing surfaces? *J Am Acad Orthop Surg* 2008; 16 (suppl 1):S49-S55.) GM-CSF = granulocyte monocyte-colony stimulating factor, IFN = interferon, IL = interleukin, MCP = monocyte chemoattractant protein, PDGF = platelet-derived growth factor, PGE$_2$ = prostaglandin E$_2$, RANK = receptor activator of nuclear factor κ B, RANKL = receptor activator of nuclear factor κ B ligand, T$_C$ = cytotoxic T lymphocyte, TGF = transforming growth factor, T$_H$ = T helper lymphocyte, TNF = tumor necrosis factor.

wear modes also have been described.[7] Mode 1 describes wear that occurs between two bearing surfaces where motion was intended. Mode 2 describes wear that occurs when a primary bearing surface articulates with a secondary surface not designed for articulating motion. Mode 3 describes wear that occurs when a third body becomes interposed between the two primary bearing surfaces. Mode 4 describes wear that occurs with motion between two secondary surfaces that are not designed for articulating motion.[5-7] Corrosion is defined as an electrochemical process during which metal ions are released from an implant surface.[5] Although corrosion products can originate from any metal surface, the modular metallic interfaces of modern arthroplasty implants are often the most common sources.[8]

Significant effort has been directed at reducing the volume of particulate wear debris generated by the classic bearing couple of a metallic head articulating against an ultra-high molecular weight polyethylene (UHMWPE) bearing. This research has led to the development of several alternative bearing surfaces, such as highly cross-linked UHMWPE, ceramics, and the so-called second-generation metal-on-metal bearings.

Hip simulator and implant retrieval data have found remarkably low volumetric and linear wear rates with metal-on-metal hip replacements. Following initial wear-in rates of 20 to 25 µm per year, steady-state wear rates are reported to range from 2 to 5 µm per component per year.[9,10] However, a lower wear rate does not necessarily imply fewer biologically active particles.[11] Current data have demonstrated that the size of the particles released from metal-on-metal articulations is an order of magnitude smaller (less than 50 nm) than the particles released from UHMWPE bearings.[12,13] Therefore, even though the linear and volumetric wear rates are lower with metal-on-metal bearings, the number of particles released is significantly higher, and the resulting specific surface area (surface area/mass) is extensive, providing much more surface area available for corrosion and subsequent metal ion release.[5]

In vitro studies have determined that the cell response to particulate debris is a function of the size, composition, and dose of the particles.[14] This response has been described as a fundamental precept of cell/particle biology.[4] Additionally, a particle's aspect ratio, surface roughness, and adsorbed proteins may also influence its biocompatibility.[15] The presence of particulate debris generated from metal-on-metal bearings in the periarticular environment leads to corrosion and the subsequent release of metal ions, which can be detected in the serum, urine, and erythrocytes.[16-19] There is considerable variability in the size, stability, and solubility of the metal corrosion products, and consequently their bioreactivity is equally variable. An increasing number of reports are emerging in the literature detailing pelvic and groin "pseudotumors," osteolysis, periprosthetic necrosis, and lymphocytic infiltrates associated with metal-on-metal prostheses.[20-23] Histologic analysis in many of these reports have revealed prominent lymphocytic aggregates, suggestive of an immunologic response.

Metal Ions

Scientists have studied the effect of metal ions since the introduction of metallic implants. Reports as far back as 1973 have evaluated blood and urine metal ion levels associated with metal-on-metal THA.[24] The resurgence of the second-generation metal-on-metal implants has led to a renewed interest in the physiologic effects of metal ion generation. Multiple published studies examining metal ion levels associated with contemporary metal-on-metal bearings have found elevated levels of serum chromium and cobalt.[16,18,25,26]

A randomized, prospective study evaluated erythrocyte and urine metal ion levels in patients with metal-on-metal or metal-on-polyethylene THAs.[16] At a minimum 2-year follow-up, patients with metal-on-metal hip implants had significantly elevated erythrocyte and urine metal ion concentrations compared with patients receiving metal on polyethylene implants. In addition, 41% of patients with metal-on-metal bearings had increasing metal ion levels at the most recent follow-up. A more recent randomized, prospective study evaluated 91 patients, comparing erythrocyte, serum, and urine metal ion levels.[19] Patients in this study were randomized to receive either a 28-mm metal-on-polyethylene hip implant, a 28-mm metal-on-metal hip implant, or a 36-mm metal-on-metal hip implant. The metal-on-polyethylene arm served as the control group. Using a testing protocol identical to that in the previously described study, these authors found significant increases in serum cobalt and chromium in patients with metal-on-metal bearings in comparison to patients with metal-on-polyethylene bearings.

Authors have also evaluated head size and material to determine its impact on metal ion release.[17,19,26] These results are not conclusive, because data are con-

Dr. Hartman or an immediate family member has received research or institutional support from Smith & Nephew. Dr. Hallab is a member of a Speakers' bureau or has made paid presentations on behalf of Medtronic Sofamor Danek, Smith & Nephew, and Biomet; serves as a paid consultant for or is an employee of Medtronic Sofamor Danek, Biomet, Smith & Nephew, and Invibio; and has received research or institutional support from Smith & Nephew and Zimmer. Dr. Jacobs or an immediate family member serves as a paid consultant for or is an employee of Johnson & Johnson, Medtronis Sofamor Danek, Smith & Nephew, Spinal Motion, and Zimmer; serves as an unpaid consultant for Implant Protection; owns stock or stock options in Implant Protection; and has received research or institutional support from Medtronic Sofamor Danek, Spinal Motion, and Zimmer. Dr. Bobyn or an immediate family member is a paid consultant for or is an employee of Osteotech.

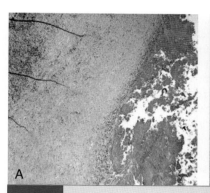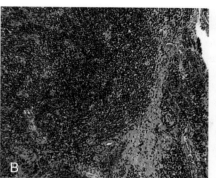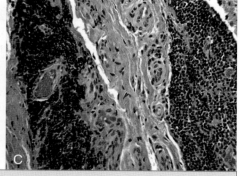

Figure 2 Diffuse and perivascular lymphocytic infiltrates. **A,** Low-power overview of periprosthetic tissue from a patient with a metal-on-metal hip replacement revised for suspected metal sensitivity. Note the adherent fibrin and focal accumulation of lymphocytes deep to the surface, separated by a wide zone of partially necrotic material. **B,** Very dense accumulations of lymphocytes that typify the periprosthetic tissues of patients revised for metal sensitivity. **C,** Higher-power micrograph showing dense aggregates of diffuse and perivascular lymphocytes that are also a common feature of tissues from patients revised for metal sensitivity. Plasma cells are often present in these aggregates. (Reproduced from Jacobs JJ, Campbell PA, Knottinen Y; Implant Wear Symposium 2007 Biologic Work Group: How was the biologic reaction to wear particles changed with newer bearing surfaces? *J Am Acad Orthop Surg* 2008;16(suppl 1):S49-S55.)

1: Basic Science and General Knowledge

flicting. Early reports suggested that larger bearings resulted in higher serum metal ion levels.[26] However, these authors compared two resurfacing arthroplasty implants with 28-mm metal-on-metal THA implants and did not control for differences in metallurgy between the two groups. Other authors have attempted to assess the effect of these variables by comparing an "as cast" high carbon resurfacing arthroplasty implant to a forged high carbon THA.[27] The authors found no statistically significant difference in the whole blood metal ion levels. A more recent study compared 36- and 28-mm metal-on-metal THAs with identical manufacturing and found no differences in the serum, urine, or erythrocyte metal ion levels.[19]

Activity level has been evaluated as a potentially important variable in systemic metal ion loads.[28] Recent data have found that serum and urine chromium and cobalt concentrations are independent of patient activity level in a cohort of patients with unilateral metal-on-metal THA, bilateral metal-on-metal THA, and unilateral metal-on-metal resurfacing arthroplasty. The systemic ion levels remained constant in spite of a mean 16-fold increase in short-term activity levels.

Histopathology

The renewed interest in metal-on-metal hip implants is partially related to the periprosthetic tissue response to polyethylene wear debris. Histopathology from metal-on-metal periprosthetic tissues has confirmed the relative absence of particle-laden macrophages known to be responsible for osteolysis. However, a dramatic cellular response not typically observed with metal-on-polyethylene bearings has been described. An intense lymphocytic infiltrate, typical of autoimmune disorders and inflammatory arthritides, has been identified in the periprosthetic tissues of some patients[20-23,29-31] (Figure 2). These infiltrates have been described as an aseptic lymphocyte-dominated vasculitis-associated lesion (ALVAL) or as a lymphocyte-dominated immunologic answer (LYDIA).[23] In an early report documenting these findings associated with second-generation metal-on-metal bearings, the authors described histomorphologic characteristics of the periprosthetic tissues from a consecutive cohort of revised hips.[23] The patients had persistent or recurrent pain and/or osteolysis. Histologic examination found a diffuse lymphocytic infiltrate and perivascular lymphocytic cuffing. The authors also described extensive fibrin exudation and areas of necrosis. Using an immunohistochemical analysis, the authors made a compelling argument for a cell-mediated immune response to the continuous, periarticular metal ion exposure. Other authors have compared histopathologic findings of periprosthetic tissues from metal-on-metal articulations with those from metal-on-polyethylene articulations.[21] The tissues from metal-on-metal articulations had more extensive and severe surface ulceration. The extent and severity of the surface ulceration was also associated with perivascular lymphocytic cuffing. The authors compared these findings with previous skin[32] and animal studies[33] and suggested support for the hypothesis that ulceration secondary to metal debris is the primary insult and the lymphocytic infiltration is a secondary phenomenon. However, another recent study questions this hypothesis by finding diffuse lymphocytic infiltrates and perivascular cuffing regardless of the extent of superficial necrosis.[29] All of these studies support the hypothesis that diffuse lymphocytic infiltrates with perivascular lymphocytic cuffing are a characteristic histologic pattern associated with symptomatic metal-on-metal bearings.

Hypersensitivity

The relationship between the immune system and particulate debris is complex and continues to stimulate investigation. The role of the immune system in the failure of contemporary metal-on-metal implants has generated particular interest. The phenomenon of metal hypersensitivity and allergy is well documented in the literature.[34] The reported incidence of dermal hypersensitivity to metal is 10% to 15% in the general population.[4,34]

Metallic degradation products can activate the immune system by acting as haptens, forming metal-protein complexes with native proteins. These complexes are considered candidate antigens for eliciting a hypersensitivity response.[34-36] Metals that are frequently cited as sensitizers include nickel, beryllium, cobalt, and chromium. Occasional responses to tantalum, titanium, and vanadium have also been reported. Nickel is the most common sensitizer, followed by cobalt and chromium.[34,35] Hypersensitivity to metallic implants is generally the cell-mediated type IV delayed-type hypersensitivity (DTH) response.

Delayed-type hypersensitivity is characterized by antigen activation of sensitized T lymphocytes (T-DTH). T-DTH lymphocytes subsequently release various cytokines responsible for the recruitment and activation of macrophages, monocytes, neutrophils, and other inflammatory cells. Within a fully developed DTH response, the T-DTH lymphocytes represent only 5% of the population, whereas most cells participating in the response are macrophages. Activated macrophages can trigger the activation of more T-DTH cells due to their increased presentation of interleukin-1 and the class II major histocompatibility complex molecules. The activated T-DTH lymphocytes recruit and activate more macrophages, which in turn activate more T-DTH lymphocytes, setting up a destructive, self-perpetuating cellular response.[34,35] In addition, authors have discovered significant crossover between the cytokine cascade responsible for the DTH response and that responsible for osteolysis associated with larger particulate debris (polyethylene).[36] These findings may help explain the reports of osteolysis associated with failed metal-on-metal THAs.[37-39]

Testing for implant-related metal hypersensitivity continues to be a developing science, and as of yet, no gold standard for diagnosis exists.[35] Several testing modalities have been described. Patch testing, which is performed in vivo, has been historically the most common modality to assess metal hypersensitivity. Although this is a useful test to assess cutaneous hypersensitivity, it is currently unclear how cutaneous responses to metal challenge agents relate to the response seen in the periprosthetic tissues. The haptenic potential of metals in open dermal contact is likely quite different from that of a closed periprosthetic environment. For instance, the skin is exposed to a potential antigen for hours while the periprosthetic tissues are exposed for months to years. There is no consensus on which metal challenge agents (such as metal salts, specific metal-protein complexes) are most appropriate for skin patch testing.[4,34]

In vitro testing can be performed with the lymphocyte transformation test (LTT). The LTT takes advantage of the fact that sensitized lymphocytes proliferate and secrete specific cytokines when challenged with an appropriate antigen. A stimulation index can be calculated by comparing [^{3}H]-thymidine uptake in challenged cells with those that have not been antigen challenged. The stimulation index therefore provides a quantitative measure of lymphocyte proliferation as opposed to the qualitative results of skin patch testing. The use of the LTT has been well established as a method for testing metal sensitivity in a variety of clinical settings.[34,40]

Several recent studies have sought to evaluate the role of the immune system in implant performance. Patients with elevated serum cobalt and chromium levels secondary to metal-on-metal hip implants were found to have significantly elevated lymphocyte reactivity.[41] These authors reported the first direct link between in vivo metal exposure and lymphocyte reactivity. Another study found that lymphocyte reactivity to chromium was significantly higher in patients with THA compared with that of control subjects, and that lymphocyte reactivity to cobalt was significantly higher in patients demonstrating moderate osteolysis compared with those without osteolysis.[36] Unfortunately, the LTT has been limited as a diagnostic tool because, like patch testing, the optimal challenge agent has yet to be identified, methods and results have not been standardized, and the threshold for a positive stimulation index has not been determined.[4,35]

Malignancy

The carcinogenic potential of metallic implants has interested researchers for decades. Animal models have documented the carcinogenic potential of cobalt, chromium, molybdenum, and nickel.[42-44] The first known case of a malignancy associated with a total joint arthroplasty was reported in 1984.[45] The authors described a large malignant fibrous histiocytoma that developed adjacent to a Vitallium (Howmedica, Mahwah, NJ) all-metal McKee-Farrar prosthesis that had been implanted in 1969. A recent review documented at least 25 cases of malignancy occurring in association with a hip or knee prosthesis.[46] Given this relatively small number compared with the large number of prosthetic joints implanted on an annual basis, it has been suggested that the occurrence of malignancies at the site of a metallic implant is likely coincidental.[5] However, these authors cautioned that because many of these cases go unreported, and these tumors may have long latency periods, further study is warranted.

Several large epidemiologic studies have been performed to investigate the incidence of cancer after total hip or knee arthroplasty with conflicting results. At least five studies examining nearly 200,000 patients have found no increase in the risk of developing cancer following total hip or knee replacement.[47-51] Another study examining the Finnish national registry found substantially fewer cancers among recipients metal-on-polyethylene THAs when compared with the general population.[52] A cohort study evaluating cancer risks in Stockholm County, Sweden, found a decreased risk of developing leukemia or lymphoma following THA,[47] whereas others found the risk of leukemia or lymphoma increased after THA,[49,51,53] especially if a metal-on-metal implant was used.[51] Interestingly, several of these studies have found a significantly decreased incidence of certain cancers in patients with hip or knee arthroplasty, including breast, colon, rectum, stomach, and lung.[48-53]

The authors of a study on the risk of cancer following total hip or knee arthroplasty have highlighted the limitations of these data. Citing insufficient periods of follow-up, insufficient data regarding dose-response, population bias, and confounding variables, these authors found that the available data did not support a causal link between total hip or knee arthroplasty and the development of cancer.[46] However, such an association has not been ruled out because of these limitations.

Summary

The use of metallic implants to treat debilitating arthrosis of the hip and knee has resulted in generally excellent results. In an attempt to make these implants more durable, modifications are constantly being proposed. Unfortunately, these modifications can have unintended outcomes. Although adverse biologic responses to metallic implants are rare, surgeons should carefully consider the risks and benefits of decisions they make in an effort to improve the outcomes of patients with hip and knee disease.

Next-Generation Porous Metals for Biologic Fixation
J. Dennis Bobyn, PhD

Most of the basic science underlying the creation and understanding of porous coatings for the 'biologic fixation' of joint arthroplasty implants was completed in the 1970s.[54,55] Initially this involved the sintered beaded cobalt-chromium alloy and the fiber metal titanium types of coatings. These pioneering developments were later followed by hip and knee designs with coarser sintered beaded surfaces made of cobalt-chromium alloy, titanium-based alloy implants with plasma-sprayed textured surfaces, and cancellous structured titanium hip and knee designs, all of which were conceived with the

goal of allowing mechanical attachment to the skeleton through new bone formation on and within the implant surface.

The clinical success of biologic fixation was initially somewhat variable and unpredictable, mostly because of inadequate understanding of and provision for the need to establish an extremely tight interference fit of the implant within bone to provide sufficient initial stability for bone healing at the interface. Once second- and third-generation implant designs addressed the issues of adequate instrumentation, surgical technique, and placement and extent of porous coating, the reliability of 'bone ingrowth' increased to the point where it is presently the most common method of noncemented implant fixation, at least within North America. In other parts of the world there remains strong interest in the use of noncemented implants with corundum-blasted or hydroxyapatite-coated surface treatments that rely on bone apposition for fixation rather than porous materials.

The common theme of the first generation of porous metals was their use as simple surface coatings on solid implant substrates. This has the advantage of combining the bone ingrowth properties of the surface with the required mechanical strength of the substrate. It would be more than 20 years before this design philosophy changed with the development of the first of several foam-like metal materials that could be used as either coatings on a solid substrate or, more importantly, as stand-alone structures for certain applications in reconstructive implant surgery, better optimized for volumetric porosity and frictional properties.

New Porous Structures
Trabecular Metal
Based on a unique and complicated manufacturing process, the material initially referred to as Hedrocel (Implex, Allendale, NJ) and now referred to as Trabecular Metal (Zimmer, Warsaw, IN) was the original new-generation highly porous metal.[56] It starts as soft, open-pored polyurethane foam that is heated at high temperature in a furnace to reduce the polymer to its vitreous carbon backbone. This serves as an inert, rigid scaffold onto the interconnected struts of which is progressively deposited a coating of commercially pure crystalline tantalum by chemical vapor infiltration in a vacuum reactor. At 50 µm thick, the tantalum coating provides the mechanical strength to the construct without excessively occluding the pores of the carbon scaffold. This results in a material with a volume porosity of approximately 75%, a mean compressive strength of 60 MPa, a compressive bulk elastic modulus of approximately 3 GPa, and dodecahedron-shaped interconnecting pores with a mean size of 430 µm, within the optimum pore size range for bone ingrowth[57] (Figure 3, Table 1). The chemical vapor infiltration process used to create the final product is more conducive to using elemental tantalum as opposed to titanium or cobalt-based alloy. The high price of the raw material and the complexity

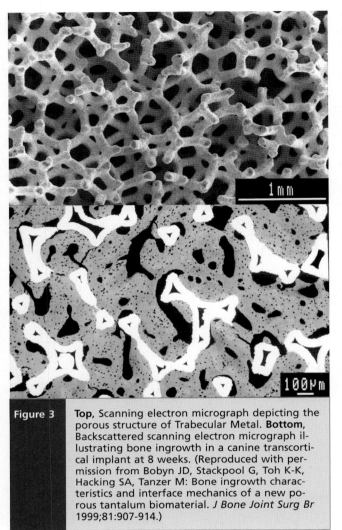

Figure 3 **Top,** Scanning electron micrograph depicting the porous structure of Trabecular Metal. **Bottom,** Backscattered scanning electron micrograph illustrating bone ingrowth in a canine transcortical implant at 8 weeks. (Reproduced with permission from Bobyn JD, Stackpool G, Toh K-K, Hacking SA, Tanzer M: Bone ingrowth characteristics and interface mechanics of a new porous tantalum biomaterial. *J Bone Joint Surg Br* 1999;81:907-914.)

the range shown in vitro and in vivo to be osteoconductive, or to promote bone apposition.[58,59] Individual struts at the surface of the material aid in creating a substantially higher coefficient of friction against bone compared with traditional porous coatings, especially for net-shaped parts.[60] This is an important attribute because it adds to the initial mechanical stability of the implant after insertion or impaction into bone, a factor known to increase the reliability of bone ingrowth.[54,55] The geometry of the pores is highly ordered and dimensionally uniform, providing controlled and reproducible porosity that yields isotropic and consistent mechanical properties of the parts. The process enables the manufacture of bulk implants such as hip and knee augments, wedges, or cones that do not require a solid substrate. This is important because the elastic modulus of the material is much lower than that of porous-coated implants with solid substrates and hence allows for more physiologic load sharing with bone, providing the opportunity for reduced peri-implant stress shielding and therefore improved retention of peri-implant bone density. The porous structure of Trabecular Metal enables direct compression molding of UHMWPE for the fabrication of low-stiffness monoblock acetabular cups or tibial plateaus without the need for an intervening solid metal backing. Trabecular Metal does not have sufficient inherent strength, however, for the manufacture of bulk implants that must withstand high bending moments; in these instances it is applied to the substrate and serves as a porous coating, albeit one with the aforementioned advantages of higher porosity, strut microtexture and geometry, and interface friction. Animal studies have demonstrated quite rapid and complete bone or fibrous tissue ingrowth resulting in higher interface strength compared with sintered beaded coatings.[61-63]

Trabecular Metal has by far the longest clinical history of any of the newer porous metals, having been first used in 1995 in a monoblock acetabular cup. A wide variety of implant designs has since been developed for primary and revision hip and knee arthroplasty and for the treatment of osteonecrosis. Of particular interest in revision surgery are Trabecular Metal augments, wedges, and cones used as bone graft substitutes for filling voids or defects. There are many reports describing the clinical results with Trabecular Metal; these have uniformly been positive and strongly support the design rationale of the material.[64-79] Also of importance is a radiostereometric analysis showing significantly greater mechanical stability of cementless porous tantalum tibial components compared with cemented tibial components 24 to 48 months postoperatively.[80] Little human retrieval histology has been reported to date, although bone ingrowth has been verified in several devices, mostly acetabular cups removed for recurrent dislocation or infection.[64] A study of harvested osteonecrosis implants described very little overall bone growth within the pores of the material, in contrast to earlier animal studies, although this is more

of the manufacturing add to the total cost of production of trabecular metal implants.

One advantage of the Trabecular Metal process is tight control over dimensional tolerances of the parts. These can be shaped after tantalum deposition using wire electrical discharge machining or made net-shape, when tantalum is deposited onto a preformed carbon template to produce the final part, a process that retains greater surface roughness. Traditional machining of the material is avoided because this tends to smear the relatively soft tantalum and occlude surface pores (this is also the case with all of the foam-like titanium porous metals). Compared with the 35% to 45% volume porosities of traditional porous coatings such as sintered beads or fiber metal, the much higher porosity of the new-generation materials such as Trabecular Metal allows for more bone to form at the interface and therefore higher ultimate fixation strength per unit area, a factor that is particularly crucial in the early postoperative period. By serendipity, the tantalum deposition process leaves a microtexture on the struts in likely to have been related to the healing potential of host bone than to the material itself.[81]

Tritanium

There are simpler methods for making highly porous foam-like metal structures that involve mixing a sacrificial material such as polymer particles together with an appropriate fraction and size of metal particulate, compacting the conglomerate into a 'green' preform, and heating the part in a high temperature vacuum furnace to eliminate the unneeded filler. The result is a metallic construct with interconnected, fairly regular pores and high-volume porosity.

Tritanium (Stryker, Mahwah, NJ) is one such material developed to provide similar properties and advantages as described above for Trabecular Metal. Tritanium is manufactured from commercially pure titanium and possesses 72% ± 5% volume porosity, a correspondingly low elastic modulus of 2.7 GPa, and interconnected pores characterized by a biomodal structure, the major pore diameter averaging 546 ± 100 μm and the interconnecting portal size averaging 311 ± 50 μm (**Figure 4, Table 1**). As with Trabecular Metal, the manufacturing process of Tritanium results in a distinct microtexture on the walls and struts of the material and its overall geometry creates a coefficient of friction against bone of 1.01 ± 0.18, higher than measured for most other porous surfaces. Preclinical studies have confirmed extensive bone ingrowth of Tritanium implants used in a canine THA model.[82]

Although Tritanium has the same type of overall advantages as Trabecular Metal for bone ingrowth, at this time it is primarily used commercially as a 1.5-mm-thick coating on the metal backing of primary and revision acetabular implants. Future development includes acetabular revision augments such as wedges and spacers that are made entirely of Tritanium, much in the same fashion as some of the Trabecular Metal implants. These bulk Tritanium implants do not require a solid metal substrate and hence offer the additional advantage of better load sharing with bone because of

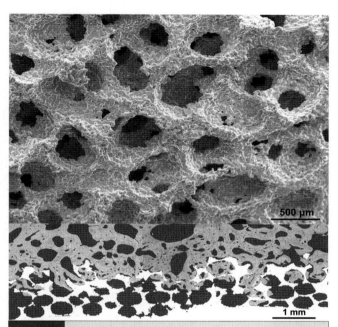

Figure 4 **Top,** Scanning electron micrograph depicting the porous structure of Tritanium. **Bottom,** Backscattered scanning electron micrograph illustrating bone ingrowth in a canine acetabular cup implant at 16 weeks.

Table 1

Physical and Mechanical Characteristics of the Next-Generation Porous Metals*

Porous Metal	Porosity	Mean Pore Size	Compressive Strength	Elastic Modulus	Porous Coating	Monoblock Implant
Trabecular Metal	75%	430 μm	60 MPa	3.0 GPa	Yes	Yes
Tritanium	72%	546 μm (major pores) 311 μm (interconnecting)	NA	2.7 GPa	Yes	Yes
Biofoam	69%	530 μm (major pores) 200 μm (interconnecting)	86 MPa	2.7 GPa	Yes	Yes
Regenerex	67%	300 μm	157 MPa	1.9 GPa	Yes	Yes
Gription	64%	220 μm	NA	NA	Yes	No
Stiktite	60%	215 μm	NA	NA	Yes	No

* All materials have received FDA clearance for use in specific implants.
NA = not available or not applicable

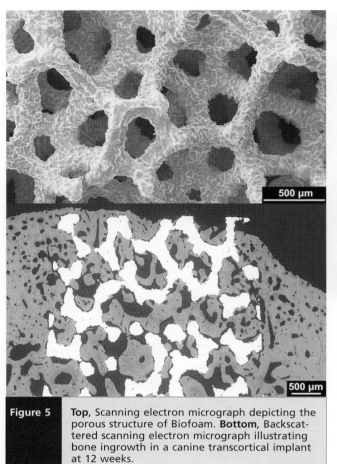

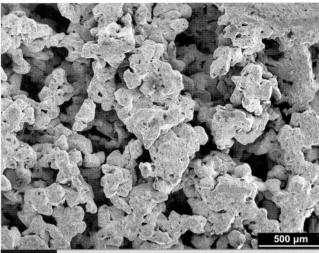

Figure 6   Scanning electron micrograph depicting the porous structure of Regenerex.

Figure 5   **Top**, Scanning electron micrograph depicting the porous structure of Biofoam. **Bottom**, Backscattered scanning electron micrograph illustrating bone ingrowth in a canine transcortical implant at 12 weeks.

the low elastic modulus of the material. An advanced version of Tritanium is also being developed using selective laser melting technology that will permit the direct fabrication of both entirely porous implants and porous-coated implants, in the latter case without the need for a secondary step to bond the coating to the substrate. This promises to enable the manufacture of both standard and complex parts, adding the latitude to vary the implant porosity according to strength and tissue ingrowth requirements. Clinical follow-up of Tritanium devices is relatively short term with few published data to date.[83]

Biofoam

The most similar in appearance to Trabecular Metal, Biofoam (Wright Medical Technology, Arlington, TN) is made of commercially pure titanium and also possesses a dodecahedral structure, with the larger pores averaging 530 µm and the smaller interconnecting portals averaging approximately 200 µm[84] (**Figure 5, Table 1**). The volume porosity can range between 60% and 70%; at 69% porosity the mean compressive strength is 86 MPa and the bulk material has a compressive elastic modulus of 2.7 GPa. The material possesses a noticeable microtexture on all of the strut surfaces, and the friction coefficient against bone is higher than for ti-

tanium plasma spray or sintered beaded surfaces. Transcortical implants placed in metaphyseal and diaphyseal sites have demonstrated substantial bone ingrowth and attachment strength, more than with sintered beaded surfaces. Biofoam is used as a coating on tibial base plates and acetabular shells and as a standalone bulk material for implants used in foot fusion and osteotomy surgery. It also has the capacity to be used in a similar manner for bone defect augments in the hip and knee. Clinical follow-up currently is limited.

Regenerex

Regenerex (Biomet, Warsaw, IN) is another form of highly porous metal made of titanium alloy.[85] The volume porosity of Regenerex averages 67%, the pore size averages 300 µm (range, 100 to 600 µm), and the elastic modulus is 1.9 GPa (**Figure 6, Table 1**). Because the porosity is somewhat lower than that of either Tritanium or Trabecular Metal, the strength of the bulk material is substantially greater at 157 MPa. This material has been incorporated into the design of a fairly wide variety of implants for the hip, knee, and shoulder. It is used both as a porous coating and as a bulk material (for hip and knee augments in revision surgery), the latter once again taking advantage of the low stiffness for better potential load sharing with bone. Animal studies with transcortical implants have confirmed the suitability of Regenerex for bone ingrowth, with comparably high percentage filling with new bone as reported for Tritanium and Trabecular Metal. Regenerex appears to have a somewhat coarser and a more uneven surface structure than the other highly porous metals. This could reduce contact area with bone and create a wider tolerance band of part size that would require careful registry with instrumentation and surgical technique to ensure control over initial implant fixation. Clinical follow-up is short because of the recent development of the material.

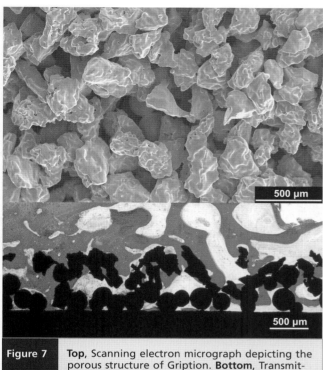

1: Basic Science and General Knowledge

Figure 7 **Top**, Scanning electron micrograph depicting the porous structure of Gription. **Bottom**, Transmitted light micrograph of a stained histologic section illustrating bone ingrowth in a canine transcortical implant at 16 weeks. Note the layer of spherical particles beneath the aspherical particles of the porous coating.

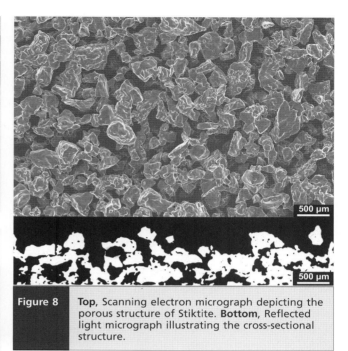

Figure 8 **Top**, Scanning electron micrograph depicting the porous structure of Stiktite. **Bottom**, Reflected light micrograph illustrating the cross-sectional structure.

Modified Porous Coatings

Separate from the innovative developments in the manufacture of entirely new three-dimensional porous structures with high porosity and low stiffness are two variations on the traditional method of sintering particles together in a high-temperature furnace to create a beaded type of porous coating. Both variations involve using aspherical instead of spherical particles to create a coating with rougher surface features that increase the friction coefficient against bone.

Gription

A simple modification in the geometry of the outer layer of sintered titanium particles led to the creation of Gription (DePuy, Johnson & Johnson, Warsaw, IN), a traditional type of porous coating with higher porosity and rougher surface features. Aspherical particles of commercially pure titanium are metallurgically bonded to a layer of spherical titanium beads on a solid implant base in a typical high-temperature vacuum furnace to produce a surface with a volume porosity of 64% ± 3%, a pore diameter of 220 ± 20 μm, and a static coefficient of friction against simulated bone material of 1.2 ± 0.1[86] (Figure 7, Table 1). Gription cannot be manufactured in bulk form for the fabrication of stand-alone implants, but a similar structure could likely be made in cobalt-

based alloy instead of titanium. Currently, Gription is applied only to acetabular cups and a short femoral stem. Clinical follow-up is too short to enable comment or comparisons with other porous metals.

Stiktite

A similar innovation using asymmetric particles to create a sintered porous coating resulted in Stiktite (Smith & Nephew, Memphis, TN), a titanium surface with a porosity of 60% and an average pore size of approximately 215 μm (Figure 8, Table 1). Friction testing using an inclined plane apparatus showed the surface to have friction coefficients against bovine cortical and cancellous bone that were 40% and 19% greater, respectively, than those of a spherical beaded coating.[87] Using a friction and wear testing machine, linear dynamic friction tests against a bone analog material demonstrated the maximum friction coefficient of Stiktite (1.14 ± 0.07) to be equivalent to that of Trabecular Metal (1.11 ± 0.03) and twice that of conventional sintered spherical beads (0.55 ± 0.08).[88] The benefit of higher interface friction was demonstrated in a radiostereometric analysis of 20 Stiktite acetabular cups that quantified substantially less implant migration in the early postoperative period compared with implants of the same design coated with spherical beads.[89] Preclinical study in an ovine tibial metaphyseal implant model confirmed extensive bone growth into the asymmetric coating and substantial mechanical fixation at 6 and 26 weeks, although not to a significantly greater extent compared with implants having a spherical beaded coating.[90] Like Gription, Stiktite is strictly a coating, and clinical follow-up is too short to enable comment.

Summary

After more than two decades of substantial clinical success with early-generation porous coatings, the new porous metals were all designed with similar properties in mind and incorporate, to somewhat varying degrees, increased friction coefficient against bone, increased volume porosity, and distinctly textured or microtextured surfaces. These features have raised the level of opportunity and increased the chance for and reliability of implant fixation by improving initial implant stability and the rate and extent of mechanical fixation by bone ingrowth. It is believed that the surface microtexture present on some of the materials may also promote osteoconduction and osseointegration in much the same manner as does the time-proven corundumized surface on titanium hip stems.[91,92] This concept is supported by a study that showed the benefit to bone ingrowth of superimposing an acid-etched microtexture on sintered titanium beaded surfaces.[93]

Given the excellent clinical results and the high likelihood of obtaining bone ingrowth with many conventional porous coatings, it could be argued that enhanced biologic fixation is not really required, at least not in routine primary cases with strong, viable bone stock. However, it is of certain value in revision cases where initial implant stability can be tenuous because of defects and/or fragile peri-implant host bone. Improving immediate implant fixation and enabling earlier and stronger biologic fixation to develop could never be a disadvantage, regardless of the procedure, and likely extends the indications in which porous devices can be reliably used.[94] In acetabular revision for instance, Trabecular Metal shells and augments have been used in far more challenging mechanical constructs and with greater success than before.[69,71,76,78] Any of the stand-alone porous augments, spacers, and wedges that are used as bone graft substitutes have enabled new options for hip and knee revision surgery. In these situations, the low structural stiffness of the high-porosity material provides the added theoretic advantage of better load sharing with peri-implant bone, less stress-related bone resorption, and consequently more reliable long-term mechanical implant support.[95] It remains to be demonstrated with certainty that this is actually the case; a carefully planned, long-term prospective study and quantitative peri-implant bone density measurements would be required for proper validation. Noteworthy in this context is the recent quantitative study that showed greater bone retention around porous tantalum monoblock cups compared with traditional metal-backed cups.[96]

Although there are some differences in the various strength measurements among the various porous metals, all have met or exceeded ASTM International and Food and Drug Administration (FDA) guidelines for adequate bond strength to the implant substrate in the case of coatings and bulk compressive strength in the case of stand-alone implants. All but one of the newer porous materials are made of titanium or titanium alloy. The exception is Trabecular Metal, which is made of commercially pure tantalum because of the particularity of the manufacturing process. Tantalum has more than six decades of history of use as a medical implant material, possessing excellent chemical stability and proven utility for bone ingrowth; in terms of biocompatibility, all evidence indicates it to be on par with titanium from biologic and clinical perspectives.[97-100] The elastic moduli of the stand-alone structures such as Trabecular Metal, Tritanium, Biofoam, and Regenerex are all within the low range of 2 to 3 GPa, and small differences are unlikely to be clinically meaningful. The same can probably be said about the cited differences in friction coefficient against bone; the test methods are not always consistent from one study to the next, some tests using real bone and others using simulated bone, and different test methods can yield different results. Marketing claims of superiority due to small differences in strength, elastic modulus, or friction coefficient should be assessed judiciously. The essential message from the data is that the higher porosity structures with modified three-dimensional geometries have measurably and substantially less stiffness and greater friction coefficients than the early-generation porous coatings. Higher-porosity structures that are bonded to solid implant substrates lose almost all of the stiffness advantage because the much greater substrate stiffness dictates the overall implant behavior in terms of load sharing and stress shielding. This concept is also true of modified porous materials such as Gription and Stiktite that only exist as coatings on substrates.

Regarding the actual strength of the bone-implant interface that develops by bone ingrowth, there is no absolute value that determines success or failure of implant fixation. In other words, it is not possible to describe or ascertain a threshold of fixation below which is inadequate or above which is sufficient for adequate clinical function. This is because bone strength varies considerably with density, mechanical demands vary considerably with patient weight and activity level, and biologic fixation is affected by the viability of host bone, the extent of initial fixation, and the early postoperative load-bearing regimen, all of which are patient specific. For this reason it is difficult to interpret cited values of interface strength derived from animal implant studies (transcortical implant model) that are not particularly germane to hip or knee replacement. As with other measurement parameters, small differences between the various materials in terms of interface fixation strength are probably not clinically meaningful, especially in view of variations in implant type and methodology from one study to another. All that can be reasonably said is that faster and greater fixation strength is better; this is the crux of what the new generation of porous metals provides. Also worth emphasizing is that only the very superficial portion of any porous surface is necessary for establishing mechanical fixation by bone ingrowth, only the outermost 100 to 200 μm. Bone growth deep inside the pores does not add to interface strength, and thus the bulk porosity of stand-alone implants does not provide additional opportunity for attachment strength. The fully porous augments, spacers, and wedges are primarily low-stiffness constructs that are relatively simple to manufacture and also enable some degree of custom shaping or drilling for screw fixation at the time of surgery (although this is not usually an FDA-approved procedure).

The most extensive clinical follow-up, as stated earlier, has been obtained with the groundbreaking Trabecular Metal because it preceded by almost a decade the more recent porous metals. As evident from **Figures** 3 to 8 there are differences in pore geometry and overall physical structure between the various materials. However, provided there is ample mechanical strength, appropriate quality control over manufacturing tolerances, and proper dimensional registry with instrumentation, there is every reason to also expect good results with the recent materials in terms of biologic fixation. Bone healing into porous metals is almost certain to occur given a biocompatible material, adequate initial implant stability, and appropriate pore size. The new-generation porous metals satisfy all of these conditions and should only help to increase the reliability of biologic fixation in hip and knee replacement surgery while also providing new tools to address complex reconstructions, especially in revision procedures.

Annotated References

1. Harris WH: The problem is osteolysis. *Clin Orthop Relat Res* 1995;311:46-53.

2. Jones LC, Hungerford DS: Cement disease. *Clin Orthop Relat Res* 1987;225:192-206.

3. Tuan RS, Lee FY, T Konttinen Y, Wilkinson JM, Smith RL; Implant Wear Symposium 2007 Biologic Work Group: What are the local and systemic biologic reactions and mediators to wear debris, and what host factors determine or modulate the biologic response to wear particles? *J Am Acad Orthop Surg* 2008; 16(Suppl 1):S42-S48.

   The authors provide a review of the basic science concerning the biologic response to wear debris.

4. Jacobs JJ, Campbell PA, T Konttinen Y; Implant Wear Symposium 2007 Biologic Work Group: How has the biologic reaction to wear particles changed with newer bearing surfaces? *J Am Acad Orthop Surg* 2008; 16(suppl 1):S49-S55.

   The authors provide a review of the biologic response to wear debris from modern bearings.

5. Meneghini RM, Hallab NJ, Jacobs JJ: The biology of alternative bearing surfaces in total joint arthroplasty. *Instr Course Lect* 2005;54:481-493.

   The authors provide a review of various alternative bearing materials and the biologic response to debris generated from these bearings.

6. Schmalzried TP, Callaghan JJ: Wear in total hip and knee replacements. *J Bone Joint Surg Am* 1999;81(1): 115-136.

7. McKellop HA, Campbell P, Park SH, et al: The origin of submicron polyethylene wear debris in total hip arthroplasty. *Clin Orthop Relat Res* 1995;311:3-20.

8. Urban RM, Jacobs JJ, Gilbert JL, Galante JO: Migration of corrosion products from modular hip prostheses: Particle microanalysis and histopathological findings. *J Bone Joint Surg Am* 1994;76(9):1345-1359.

9. Santavirta S, Böhler M, Harris WH, et al: Alternative materials to improve total hip replacement tribology. *Acta Orthop Scand* 2003;74(4):380-388.

10. Sieber HP, Rieker CB, Köttig P: Analysis of 118 second-generation metal-on-metal retrieved hip implants. *J Bone Joint Surg Br* 1999;81(1):46-50.

11. Ingham E, Fisher J: Biological reactions to wear debris in total joint replacement. *Proc Inst Mech Eng H* 2000;214(1):21-37.

12. Doorn PF, Campbell PA, Worrall J, Benya PD, McKellop HA, Amstutz HC: Metal wear particle characterization from metal on metal total hip replacements: Transmission electron microscopy study of periprosthetic tissues and isolated particles. *J Biomed Mater Res* 1998;42(1):103-111.

13. Firkins PJ, Tipper JL, Saadatzadeh MR, et al: Quantitative analysis of wear and wear debris from metal-on-metal hip prostheses tested in a physiological hip joint simulator. *Biomed Mater Eng* 2001;11(2):143-157.

14. Shanbhag AS, Jacobs JJ, Black J, Galante JO, Glant TT: Human monocyte response to particulate biomaterials generated in vivo and in vitro. *J Orthop Res* 1995;13(5):792-801.

15. Hallab NJ, Skipor A, Jacobs JJ: Interfacial kinetics of titanium- and cobalt-based implant alloys in human serum: Metal release and biofilm formation. *J Biomed Mater Res A* 2003;65(3):311-318.

16. MacDonald SJ, McCalden RW, Chess DG, et al: Metal-on-metal versus polyethylene in hip arthroplasty: A randomized clinical trial. *Clin Orthop Relat Res* 2003;406: 282-296.

17. Vendittoli PA, Mottard S, Roy AG, Dupont C, Lavigne M: Chromium and cobalt ion release following the Durom high carbon content, forged metal-on-metal surface replacement of the hip. *J Bone Joint Surg Br* 2007;89(4):441-448.

    The authors evaluated whole blood, serum, and erythrocyte cobalt and chromium concentrations following hip resurfacing arthroplasty using the Durom implant. The 1- and 2-year mean chromium levels were 1.8 and 1.5 times higher than preoperative levels, whereas cobalt levels were 4.5 and 3.9 times higher.

1: Basic Science and General Knowledge

18. Brodner W, Bitzan P, Meisinger V, Kaider A, Gottsauner-Wolf F, Kotz R: Serum cobalt levels after metal-on-metal total hip arthroplasty. *J Bone Joint Surg Am* 2003;85(11):2168-2173.

19. Engh CA Jr, MacDonald SJ, Sritulanondha S, Thompson A, Naudie D, Engh CA: 2008 John Charnley award: Metal ion levels after metal-on-metal total hip arthroplasty. A randomized trial. *Clin Orthop Relat Res* 2009;467(1):101-111.

    The authors performed a randomized trial to compare 2-year postoperative ion levels in 28-mm metal-on-polyethylene bearings with 28- and 36-mm metal-on-metal bearings. No difference was detected in metal ion concentration between the 28- and 36-mm metal-on-metal bearings.

20. Campbell P, Shimmin A, Walter L, Solomon M: Metal sensitivity as a cause of groin pain in metal-on-metal hip resurfacing. *J Arthroplasty* 2008;23(7):1080-1085.

    The authors present case reports of four patients revised for groin pain following metal-on-metal hip resurfacing. Histology revealed extensive lymphocytic infiltrates in all patients consistent with an ALVAL. All patients had complete resolution of symptoms following revision.

21. Davies AP, Willert HG, Campbell PA, Learmonth ID, Case CP: An unusual lymphocytic perivascular infiltration in tissues around contemporary metal-on-metal joint replacements. *J Bone Joint Surg Am* 2005;87(1):18-27.

    The authors performed a histomorphometric analysis comparing tissue samples from THA using cobalt-chromium (CoCr) on CoCr, CoCr on polyethylene, and titanium on polyethylene. The patterns and types of inflammation seen with metal-on-metal and metal-on-polyethylene were very different.

22. Pandit H, Glyn-Jones S, McLardy-Smith P, et al: Pseudotumours associated with metal-on-metal hip resurfacings. *J Bone Joint Surg Br* 2008;90(7):847-851.

    The authors report 17 patients with symptomatic groin masses associated with metal-on-metal resurfacing arthroplasty. Revision was performed in 13 patients and histology found extensive necrosis and lymphocytic aggregates. The cohort included patients with three different resurfacing prostheses.

23. Willert HG, Buchhorn GH, Fayyazi A, et al : Metal-on-metal bearings and hypersensitivity in patients with artificial hip joints: A clinical and histomorphological study. *J Bone Joint Surg Am* 2005;87(1):28-36.

    The authors performed a histomorphologic analysis of 19 consecutive failed metal-on-metal THAs. The histologic findings were suggestive of an aggressive immune response described as an ALVAL.

24. Coleman RF, Herrington J, Scales JT: Concentration of wear products in hair, blood, and urine after total hip replacement. *Br Med J* 1973;1(5852):527-529.

25. Back DL, Young DA, Shimmin AJ: How do serum cobalt and chromium levels change after metal-on-metal hip resurfacing? *Clin Orthop Relat Res* 2005;438:177-181.

    The authors prospectively studied 20 patients with a Birmingham Hip Resurfacing (BHR; Smith & Nephew) hip arthroplasty and normal renal function to evaluate serum cobalt and chromium levels periodically for 2 years. Serum cobalt levels reached a peak at 6 months, whereas serum chromium peaked at 9 months. Both cobalt and chromium levels gradually declined over the study period but remained elevated over preoperative levels.

26. Clarke MT, Lee PT, Arora A, Villar RN: Levels of metal ions after small- and large-diameter metal-on-metal hip arthroplasty. *J Bone Joint Surg Br* 2003;85(6):913-917.

27. Daniel J, Ziaee H, Salama A, Pradhan C, McMinn DJ: The effect of the diameter of metal-on-metal bearings on systemic exposure to cobalt and chromium. *J Bone Joint Surg Br* 2006;88(4):443-448.

    The authors evaluated whole blood and urine cobalt and chromium levels in patients with either a 50- or 54-mm BHR hip or a 28- mm Metasul hip (Zimmer) to determine if bearing diameter had an important influence on metal ion release. There was no significant difference between blood or urine metal ion levels in any group.

28. Heisel C, Silva M, Skipor AK, Jacobs JJ, Schmalzried TP: The relationship between activity and ions in patients with metal-on-metal bearing hip prostheses. *J Bone Joint Surg Am* 2005;87(4):781-787.

    This study evaluated seven patients with well-functioning metal-on-metal hip prostheses to determine if activity level influenced the serum cobalt and chromium levels. In spite of activity level increases up to 1,621%, no correlation could be found with serum ion levels.

29. Witzleb WC, Hanisch U, Kolar N, Krummenauer F, Guenther KP: Neo-capsule tissue reactions in metal-on-metal hip arthroplasty. *Acta Orthop* 2007;78(2):211-220.

    The authors of this study performed a histopathologic and immunohistochemical analysis of the neocapsule of 46 failed metal-on-metal hip arthroplasties. A distinct lymphocytic infiltration was found in all cases with in situ time of more than 7 months.

30. Grammatopolous G, Pandit H, Kwon YM, et al: Hip resurfacings revised for inflammatory pseudotumour have a poor outcome. *J Bone Joint Surg Br* 2009; 91(8):1019-1024.

    The authors evaluated the outcome of 16 hip resurfacings revised for pseudotumor and compared these with 21 revised for fracture and 16 revised for other reasons. Patients revised for pseudotumor had significantly worse Oxford hip scores compared with those revised for fracture or other reasons.

31. Mahendra G, Pandit H, Kliskey K, Murray D, Gill HS, Athanasou N: Necrotic and inflammatory changes in

metal-on-metal resurfacing hip arthroplasties. *Acta Orthop* 2009;80(6):653-659.

The authors analyzed morphologic and immunophenotypic changes in the periprosthetic tissues of 52 failed metal-on-metal hip arthroplasties. They identified a spectrum of necrotic and inflammatory changes suggesting it may involve both a cytotoxic response and a DTH response.

32. Hartman A, Hoedemaeker PJ, Nater JP: Histological aspects of DNCB sensitization and challenge tests. *Br J Dermatol* 1976;94(4):407-416.

33. Howie DW, Vernon-Roberts B: The synovial response to intraarticular cobalt-chrome wear particles. *Clin Orthop Relat Res* 1988;232:244-254.

34. Hallab N, Merritt K, Jacobs JJ: Metal sensitivity in patients with orthopaedic implants. *J Bone Joint Surg Am* 2001;83(3):428-436.

35. Jacobs JJ, Urban RM, Hallab NJ, Skipor AK, Fischer A, Wimmer MA: Metal-on-metal bearing surfaces. *J Am Acad Orthop Surg* 2009;17(2):69-76.

The authors reviewed the tribology of metal-on-metal prostheses and the biologic response to their wear debris.

36. Hallab NJ, Anderson S, Stafford T, Glant T, Jacobs JJ: Lymphocyte responses in patients with total hip arthroplasty. *J Orthop Res* 2005;23(2):384-391.

The authors used lymphocyte transformation testing and cytokine release to compare lymphocyte reactivity to cobalt, chromium, nickel, and titanium in six subject groups. Subjects with a history of metal sensitivity were the most reactive to nickel. Subjects with THA were more than three times more reactive to chromium than controls. THA subjects with moderate compared with mild osteolysis were more reactive to cobalt. THA subjects with osteolysis demonstrated a more than twofold increased cytokine response to chromium.

37. Korovessis P, Petsinis G, Repanti M, Repantis T: Metallosis after contemporary metal-on-metal total hip arthroplasty: Five to nine-year follow-up. *J Bone Joint Surg Am* 2006;88(6):1183-1191.

The authors reviewed the histology of retrieved periprosthetic tissues in 11 patients with a metal-on-metal THA revised for aseptic loosening. The tissues showed metallosis and extensive lymphocytic and plasma-cell infiltration around the metal debris.

38. Milosev I, Trebse R, Kovac S, Cör A, Pisot V: Survivorship and retrieval analysis of Sikomet metal-on-metal total hip replacements at a mean of seven years. *J Bone Joint Surg Am* 2006;88(6):1173-1182.

The authors reviewed the histology of periprosthetic tissue from 17 patients with a metal-on-metal THA revised for aseptic loosening. Thirteen of the hips demonstrated a hypersensitivity-like reaction with aseptic inflammatory changes accompanied by moderate to extensive diffuse and perivascular infiltration of lymphocytes.

39. Park YS, Moon YW, Lim SJ, Yang JM, Ahn G, Choi YL: Early osteolysis following second-generation metal-on-metal hip replacement. *J Bone Joint Surg Am* 2005;87(7):1515-1521.

The authors performed a retrospective review of 10 of 169 hips with osteolysis following a contemporary metal-on-metal THA. Patients with osteolysis had a significantly higher rate of hypersensitivity via skin patch testing to cobalt compared with controls. Histologic analysis found infiltrating lymphocytes and activated macrophages secreting bone-resorbing cytokines.

40. Everness KM, Gawkrodger DJ, Botham PA, Hunter JA: The discrimination between nickel-sensitive and non-nickel-sensitive subjects by an in vitro lymphocyte transformation test. *Br J Dermatol* 1990;122(3):293-298.

41. Hallab NJ, Anderson S, Caicedo M, Skipor A, Campbell P, Jacobs JJ: Immune responses correlate with serum-metal in metal-on-metal hip arthroplasty. *J Arthroplasty* 2004;19(8, suppl 3)88-93.

42. Heath JC, Freeman MA, Swanson SA: Carcinogenic properties of wear particles from prostheses made in cobalt-chromium alloy. *Lancet* 1971;1(7699):564-566.

43. Memoli VA, Urban RM, Alroy J, Galante JO: Malignant neoplasms associated with orthopedic implant materials in rats. *J Orthop Res* 1986;4(3):346-355.

44. Swanson SA, Freeman MA, Heath JC: Laboratory tests on total joint replacement prostheses. *J Bone Joint Surg Br* 1973;55(4):759-773.

45. Swann M: Malignant soft-tissue tumour at the site of a total hip replacement. *J Bone Joint Surg Br* 1984;66(5):629-631.

46. Tharani R, Dorey FJ, Schmalzried TP: The risk of cancer following total hip or knee arthroplasty. *J Bone Joint Surg Am* 2001;83(5):774-780.

47. Mathiesen EB, Ahlbom A, Bermann G, Lindgren JU: Total hip replacement and cancer: A cohort study. *J Bone Joint Surg Br* 1995;77(3):345-350.

48. Nyrén O, McLaughlin JK, Gridley G, et al: Cancer risk after hip replacement with metal implants: A population-based cohort study in Sweden. *J Natl Cancer Inst* 1995;87(1):28-33.

49. Paavolainen P, Pukkala E, Pulkkinen P, Visuri T: Cancer incidence after total knee arthroplasty: A nationwide Finnish cohort from 1980 to 1996 involving 9,444 patients. *Acta Orthop Scand* 1999;70(6):609-617.

50. Signorello LB, Ye W, Fryzek JP, et al: Nationwide study of cancer risk among hip replacement patients in Sweden. *J Natl Cancer Inst* 2001;93(18):1405-1410.

51. Visuri T, Pukkala E, Paavolainen P, Pulkkinen P, Riska EB: Cancer risk after metal on metal and polyethylene on metal total hip arthroplasty. *Clin Orthop Relat Res* 1996;(329, suppl)S280-S289.

52. Paavolainen P, Pukkala E, Pulkkinen P, Visuri T: Cancer incidence in Finnish hip replacement patients from 1980 to 1995: A nationwide cohort study involving 31,651 patients. *J Arthroplasty* 1999;14(3):272-280.

53. Gillespie WJ, Frampton CM, Henderson RJ, Ryan PM: The incidence of cancer following total hip replacement. *J Bone Joint Surg Br* 1988;70(4):539-542.

54. Bobyn JD, Tanzer M, Miller JE: Fundamental principles of biologic fixation, in Morrey BF, ed: *Reconstructive Surgery of the Joints*. Edinburgh, United Kingdom, Churchill Livingstone, 1996, pp 75-94.

55. Kienapfel H, Sprey C, Wilke A, Griss P: Implant fixation by bone ingrowth. *J Arthroplasty* 1999;14(3):355-368.

56. Cohen R: A porous tantalum trabecular metal: Basic science. *Am J Orthop (Belle Mead NJ)* 2002;31(4):216-217.

57. Bobyn JD, Pilliar RM, Cameron HU, Weatherly GC: The optimum pore size for the fixation of porous-surfaced metal implants by the ingrowth of bone. *Clin Orthop Relat Res* 1980;150(150):263-270.

58. Kieswetter K, Schwartz Z, Hummert TW, et al: Surface roughness modulates the local production of growth factors and cytokines by osteoblast-like MG-63 cells. *J Biomed Mater Res* 1996;32(1):55-63.

59. Hacking SA, Bobyn JD, Tanzer M, Krygier JJ: The osseous response to corundum blasted implant surfaces in a canine hip model. *Clin Orthop Relat Res* 1999;364:240-253.

60. Fitzpatrick D, Ahn P, Brown T, Poggie R: Friction coefficients of porous tantalum and cancellous and cortical bone in *Proceedings from the 21st Annual Meeting of the American Society of Biomechanics*. 1997, p 119.

61. Bobyn JD, Stackpool GJ, Hacking SA, Tanzer M, Krygier JJ: Characteristics of bone ingrowth and interface mechanics of a new porous tantalum biomaterial. *J Bone Joint Surg Br* 1999;81(5):907-914.

62. Bobyn JD, Toh K-K, Hacking SA, Tanzer M, Krygier JJ: Tissue response to porous tantalum acetabular cups: A canine model. *J Arthroplasty* 1999;14(3):347-354.

63. Hacking SA, Bobyn JD, Toh K-K, Tanzer M, Krygier JJ: Fibrous tissue ingrowth and attachment to porous tantalum. *J Biomed Mater Res* 2000;52(4):631-638.

64. Bobyn JD, Poggie RA, Krygier JJ, et al: Clinical validation of a structural porous tantalum biomaterial for adult reconstruction. *J Bone Joint Surg Am* 2004;86(suppl 2):123-129.

65. Nehme A, Lewallen DG, Hanssen AD: Modular porous metal augments for treatment of severe acetabular bone loss during revision hip arthroplasty. *Clin Orthop Relat Res* 2004;429:201-208.

66. Tsao AK, Roberson JR, Christie MJ, et al: Biomechanical and clinical evaluations of a porous tantalum implant for the treatment of early-stage osteonecrosis. *J Bone Joint Surg Am* 2005;87(suppl 2):22-27.

One hundred thirteen porous tantalum implants in 98 patients were studied for treatment of Steinberg stage I or II osteonecrosis. Twenty-two were revised at a mean of 12 months, and overall survivorship at 48 months was 72.5%.

67. Unger AS, Lewis RJ, Gruen T: Evaluation of a porous tantalum uncemented acetabular cup in revision total hip arthroplasty: Clinical and radiological results of 60 hips. *J Arthroplasty* 2005;20(8):1002-1009.

Sixty consecutive revision cases using a porous tantalum nonmodular acetabular cup, 55 without adjuvant screw fixation, were followed for a mean of 42 months. Radiographs showed excellent stability; there was one revision for aseptic loosening.

68. Gruen TA, Poggie RA, Lewallen DG, et al: Radiographic evaluation of a monoblock acetabular component: A multicenter study with 2- to 5-year results. *J Arthroplasty* 2005;20(3):369-378.

Serial radiographs of 414 primary cases with a porous tantalum nonmodular acetabular component were studied at a mean follow-up of 33 months. Postoperative retroacetabular gaps mostly disappeared, and there was no evidence of continuous periacetabular interface radiolucencies or lysis and no revisions for loosening.

69. Sporer SM, Paprosky WG: The use of a trabecular metal acetabular component and trabecular metal augment for severe acetabular defects. *J Arthroplasty* 2006;21(6, suppl 2)83-86.

The use of porous tantalum modular acetabular cups with porous tantalum augments is described in 28 patients treated for a type IIIa defect at a mean of 3.1 years follow-up. One patient required re-revision for recurrent instability whereas the others appeared radiographically stable.

70. Radnay CS, Scuderi GR: Management of bone loss: Augments, cones, offset stems. *Clin Orthop Relat Res* 2006;446:83-92.

Porous tantalum tibial cones were press-fit into the prepared cavitary defect in ten revision knee arthroplasties. Pericone voids were filled with morcellized grafting material; the core tibial component was cemented into the cone. At mean follow-up of 10 months there was no radiographic evidence of loosening.

71. Weeden SH, Schmidt RH: The use of tantalum porous metal implants for Paprosky 3A and 3B defects. *J Arthroplasty* 2007;22(6, suppl 2)151-155.

Porous tantalum acetabular implants were used in 43 revisions, 26 of which included porous tantalum modular augments. At a mean of 2.8 years follow-up there was one failure caused by septic loosening for an overall success rate of 98%.

72. Meneghini RM, Lewallen DG, Hanssen AD: Use of porous tantalum metaphyseal cones for severe tibial bone loss during revision total knee replacement. *J Bone Joint Surg Am* 2008;90(1):78-84.

    The surgical technique is described for using porous tantalum tibial metaphyseal cones in revision total knee reconstruction. In 15 cases followed for a mean of 34 months, there was uniform radiographic evidence of osseointegration with no evidence of loosening or migration.

73. Malkani AL, Price MR, Crawford CH III, Baker DL: Acetabular component revision using a porous tantalum biomaterial: A case series. *J Arthroplasty* 2009; 24(7):1068-1073.

    Twenty-two cases in which porous tantalum acetabular shells were used to reconstruct Paprosky type 2 or 3 defects were retrospectively reviewed at a mean follow-up of 39 months. There was radiographic evidence of stable fixation in 21 cases; 1 case had recurrent infection requiring resection arthroplasty.

74. Holt GE, Christie MJ, Schwartz HS: Trabecular metal endoprosthetic limb salvage reconstruction of the lower limb. *J Arthroplasty* 2009;24(7):1079-1085.

    Custom-made porous tantalum endoprostheses were used to reconstruct seven cases following resection for femur and proximal tibia sarcomas. At minimum follow-up of 6 years the average functional score was 95% of normal. There were no infections or hardware failures. One implant was revised at 98 months for mechanical instability.

75. Long WJ, Scuderi GR: Porous tantalum cones for large metaphyseal tibial defects in revision total knee arthroplasty: A minimum 2-year follow-up. *J Arthroplasty* 2009;24(7):1086-1092.

    Sixteen cases (three postinfection) in which porous tantalum tibial cones were used in revision knee arthroplasty were reviewed at a mean of 31 months follow-up. There were two cases of recurrent sepsis requiring implant removal. Radiographs of the remaining 14 cases indicated stable fixation.

76. Lakstein D, Backstein D, Safir O, Kosashvili Y, Gross AE: Trabecular Metal cups for acetabular defects with 50% or less host bone contact. *Clin Orthop Relat Res* 2009;467(9):2318-2324.

    Fifty-three revision hip arthroplasty procedures using porous tantalum cups for contained defects with 50% or less contact with native bone were prospectively followed for a mean of 45 months. Two cups (4%) were revised and two additional cups (4%) were probably loose.

77. Macheras G, Kateros K, Kostakos A, Koutsostathis S, Danomaras D, Papagelopoulos PJ: Eight- to ten-year clinical and radiographic outcome of a porous tantalum monoblock acetabular component. *J Arthroplasty* 2009;24(5):705-709.

    A porous tantalum nonmodular acetabular component was assessed in 151 cases of primary hip arthroplasty at a follow-up of 8 to 10 years. Clinical scores were excellent; there was no radiographic evidence of gross polyethylene wear, progressive radiolucencies, osteolytic lesions, or component subsidence.

78. Siegmeth A, Duncan CP, Masri BA, Kim WY, Garbuz DS: Modular tantalum augments for acetabular defects in revision hip arthroplasty. *Clin Orthop Relat Res* 2009;467(1):199-205.

    Thirty-four cases in which large acetabular defects were reconstructed with a porous tantalum shell and augment were prospectively followed for a mean of 34 months. Thirty-two cups were radiographically stable and two were re-revised for mechanical loosening.

79. Jafari SM, Bender B, Coyle C, Parvizi J, Sharkey PF, Hozack WJ: Do tantalum and titanium cups show similar results in revision hip arthroplasty? *Clin Orthop Relat Res* 2010;468(2):459-465.

    Clinical outcomes were retrospectively compared for 81 porous tantalum cups and 214 hydroxyapatite-coated cups used in revision hip arthroplasty. The porous tantalum cups showed a lower mechanical failure rate, particularly in hips with major bone deficiency.

80. Wilson DA, Astephen JL, Hennigar AW, Dunbar MJ: Inducible displacement of a trabecular metal tibial monoblock component. *J Arthrop* 2010;25(6):893-900.

    Radiostereometric analysis was used to compare the mechanical stability of 14 uncemented Trabecular Metal monoblock tibial components with 11 cemented tibial components 24 to 48 months postoperatively. The uncemented components showed significantly lower inducible displacements.

81. Tanzer M, Bobyn JD, Krygier JJ, Karabasz D: Histopathologic retrieval analysis of clinically failed porous tantalum osteonecrosis implants. *J Bone Joint Surg Am* 2008;90(6):1282-1289.

    Seventeen porous tantalum osteonecrosis intervention implants were retrieved at the time of conversion to a THA and examined histologically. Bone ingrowth was minimal (mean extent = 1.9%) and subchondral bone appeared to be insufficiently supported by the implant.

82. Frenkel SR, Jaffe WL, Dimaano F, Iesaka K, Hua T: Bone response to a novel highly porous surface in a canine implantable chamber. *J Biomed Mater Res B Appl Biomater* 2004;71(2):387-391.

83. Ramappa M, Bajwa A, Kulkarni A, McMurtry I, Port A: Early results of a new highly porous modular acetabular cup in revision arthroplasty. *Hip Int* 2009; 19(3):239-244.

    A prospective study of 43 acetabular component revisions using an acetabular cup with Tritanium porous coating showed radiographic evidence of cup integration in all but one case at mean follow-up of 18 months. One patient with pelvic discontinuity was revised for symptomatic aseptic loosening.

84. Scholvin D, Obert R, Moseley J, et al: Highly porous reticulated titanium foam for orthopedic implant applications. *Proc Amer Acad Orthop Surg* 2008:SE40.

This abstract summarizes the physical and mechanical properties of a new porous titanium foam biomaterial.

85. Lombardi AV Jr, Berasi CC, Berend KR: Evolution of tibial fixation in total knee arthroplasty. *Arthroplasty* 2007;22(4, suppl 1):25-29.

The status of cementless tibial fixation in total knee arthroplasty is reviewed. Brief information and comments are provided about porous tantalum devices and a recently developed highly porous titanium alloy construct.

86. Minter JO, Rivard K, Aboud B: Characterization of a new rougher porous coating for revision reconstructive surgery. *Trans 54th Orthop Res Soc* 2008;33:1870.

This abstract summarizes the physical and mechanical properties of a new, higher-friction porous coating made by sintering nonspherical titanium particles onto a base layer of spherical titanium alloy beads.

87. Heiner AD, Brown TD: Friction coefficients of a new bone ingrowth structure. *Trans 53rd Orthop Res Soc* 2007;32:1623.

The friction coefficient of a spherical beaded porous coating and an asymmetric titanium particle porous coating were measured using standard test methods. The coefficient was 40% and 19% greater for the asymmetric coating against bovine cortical and cancellous bone, respectively.

88. Gilmour LJ, Jones R, Dickinson J: Mechanical properties of a sintered asymmetric particle ingrowth coating. *Proc Amer Soc Mater Conference* (Materials and Processes for Medical Devices) 2009:11.2.

This abstract summarizes the results of mechanical property and friction coefficient testing of a sintered titanium porous coating made with asymmetric particles.

89. Bourne RB, MCalden RW, Naudie D, Charron KD, Yuan X, Holdsworth DW: The next generation of acetabular shell design and bearing surfaces. *Orthopedics* 2008;31(12, suppl 2).

The migration of 20 modular acetabular cups with a higher friction porous coating was quantified using radiostereometric analysis and compared with migration data from the same implant with sintered spherical beads. The implant with the higher-friction asymmetric particle coating showed substantially less postoperative migration.

90. Heuer DA, Williams M, Moss R, et al: Biologic fixation of an asymmetric titanium particle porous coating in a load-bearing animal model. *Trans Intl Soc for Tech in Arthroplasty (ISTA)* 2008:A-1062.

Porous coatings made with sintered spherical beads or asymmetric particles were compared in an ovine metaphyseal implant model at 6 and 26 weeks. Although immediate implant stability was significantly greater with the asymmetric coating, the interface strength was similar at the later time periods.

91. Delaunay C, Bonnomet F, North J, Jobard D, Cazeau C, Kempf J-F: Grit-blasted titanium femoral stem in cementless primary total hip arthroplasty: A 5- to 10-year multicenter study. *J Arthroplasty* 2001;16(1):47-54.

92. Bhalodiya HP, Singh SP: Results with the cementless Spotorno stem in total hip arthroplasty. *J Arthroplasty* 2009;24(8):1188-1192.

One hundred corundum-blasted titanium Spotorno (CLS) stems were followed in 97 patients with a mean age of 36.7 years for a mean of 5 years (range 2.5-8 years). Ninety-eight hips had stable fixation; two showed marked subsidence that stabilized.

93. Hacking SA, Harvey EJ, Tanzer M, Krygier JJ, Bobyn JD: Acid-etched microtexture for enhancement of bone growth into porous-coated implants. *J Bone Joint Surg Br* 2003;85(8):1182-1189.

94. Meneghini RM, Meyer C, Buckley CA, Hanssen AD, Lewallen DG: Mechanical stability of novel highly porous metal acetabular components in revision total hip arthroplasty. *J Arthroplasty* 2010;25(3):337-341.

Acetabular components with either fiber metal or higher friction porous tantalum surfaces were inserted into hemipelvis specimens with a superolateral defect. Mechanical testing showed significantly superior stability of the porous tantalum components.

95. Bobyn JD, Tanzer M, Glassman AH: Stress related bone resorption, in Shanbhag AS, Rubash HE, Jacobs, JJ, eds: *Joint Replacements and Bone Resorption: Pathology, Biomaterials, and Clinical Practice.* New York, NY, Marcel Dekker, 2006.

96. Meneghini RM, Ford KS, McCollough CH, Hanssen AD, Lewallen DG: Bone remodeling around porous metal cementless acetabular components. *J Arthroplasty* 2010;25(5):741-747.

Quantitative measurements of bone mineral density were made at a mean of 7.7 years around eight titanium metal-backed cups and seven monoblock porous tantalum cups. There was significantly greater bone retention around the lower-stiffness tantalum cups, indicating less stress shielding.

97. Black J: Biological performance of tantalum. *Clin Mater* 1994;16(3):167-173.

98. Findlay DM, Welldon K, Atkins GJ, Howie DW, Zannettino AC, Bobyn D: The proliferation and phenotypic expression of human osteoblasts on tantalum metal. *Biomaterials* 2004;25(12):2215-2227.

99. Welldon KJ, Atkins GJ, Howie DW, Findlay DM: Primary human osteoblasts grow into porous tantalum and maintain an osteoblastic phenotype. *J Biomed Mater Res A* 2008;84(3):691-701.

Human osteoblasts were grown in vitro on disks of porous tantalum, solid tantalum, and tissue culture plastic. The cells attached well to the tantalum struts, underwent extensive cell division, and penetrated into the pores. No substrate-dependent differences were seen in the extent of mineralization.

100. Schildhauer TA, Peter E, Muhr G, Köller M: Activation of human leukocytes on tantalum trabecular metal in comparison to commonly used orthopedic metal implant materials. *J Biomed Mater Res A* 2009; 88(2):332-341.

Leukocyte function and cytokine response of human leukocytes were analyzed for porous tantalum and several other test metals. Several results indicated that leukocyte activation at the surface of porous tantalum induced a microenvironment that may enhance local host defense mechanisms.

1: Basic Science and General Knowledge

Osteonecrosis of the Hip and Knee

Jay R. Lieberman, MD   Kevin L. Garvin, MD

Osteonecrosis of the Hip
Jay R. Lieberman, MD

Osteonecrosis of the hip usually affects young, active patients and can lead to destruction of the joint and loss of function. Each year there are approximately 20,000 to 30,000 new cases of osteonecrosis, and approximately 10% of all total hip arthroplasties (THAs) are performed for this diagnosis.[1,2] Unfortunately, the etiology of osteonecrosis is unknown and therefore there is no definitive treatment modality for this disease.

Etiology and Pathology

The etiology of osteonecrosis of the hip has not been established. However, there are several risk factors that have been associated with the development of this disease, including corticosteroid use, heavy alcohol use, trauma, and coagulation abnormalities. Recently, it has been hypothesized that the pathophysiology of osteonecrosis may be secondary to impaired mesenchymal cell differentiation and direct cellular toxicity.[3] The results of several in vitro studies suggest that dysfunction of mesenchymal stem cells could be responsible for the changes that occur in osteonecrosis of the femoral head. These changes may be attributed to decreased osteogenic differentiation of cells in the femoral head and to alterations in blood flow from increased adipogenic volume in the femoral head. For example, it has been hypothesized that osteogenic and adipogenic differentiation of mesenchymal stem cells may be altered in patients with alcohol-induced osteonecrosis.[3] In one study, bone marrow was collected from the proximal femurs of patients undergoing THA for alcohol-induced osteonecrosis of the femoral head or a femoral neck fracture. The mesenchymal stem cells harvested from patients with alcohol-induced osteonecrosis demonstrated reduced ability to differentiate toward an osteogenic lineage compared with cells obtained from patients with a femoral neck fracture.[4] In another study, the osteogenic differentiation capacity of bone marrow stromal cells in patients with alcohol-induced osteonecrosis was considerably reduced compared with mesenchymal cells harvested from patients with osteoarthritis.[5] In vitro alcohol exposure led to a reduction of osteogenic gene expression and enhanced adipogenic morphologic characteristics in a cloned bone marrow stem cell population.[6]

The relationship between corticosteroids and the development of osteonecrosis has also been analyzed. When bone marrow stromal cells are exposed to dexamethasone in culture, there is increased expression of both the adipogenic gene 422 (aP2) and triglyceride synthesis. In addition, a decrease in cellular proliferation and bone marker gene expression was noted.[7] In a porcine model of vasoconstriction within the femoral head, 24 hours of treatment with methylprednisolone led to an enhanced vasoconstrictive response to endothelin-1 and reduced vasodilatation of the corticosteroid-treated vessels in response to bradykinin.[8] It was hypothesized that the methylprednisolone enhanced contraction of the femoral head arteries, which decreased the femoral head blood flow.

An analysis of these basic science studies suggests that the alteration of specific molecular pathways in some patients may be associated with the development of osteonecrosis of the femoral head. In addition, both alcohol and corticosteroids impair bone marrow stromal cell differentiation and blood supply, which may alter physiologic bone turnover and oxygenation. Unfortunately, it has not been explained why osteonecrosis never develops in most patients who abuse alcohol or receive treatment with steroids. The continuing inability to identify the specific molecular pathways underlying this disease limits surgeons' ability to identify potential targets for pharmacologic intervention or prevention.

As stated previously, most patients with various risk factors associated with osteonecrosis do not develop this disease. Therefore, it has been hypothesized that there must be specific genetic predispositions for the development of osteonecrosis. A gene mutation mapped to chromosome 12Q13 has been associated with type II collagen abnormalities and autosomal dominant osteonecrosis of the femoral head.[9] In addi-

Dr. Lieberman or an immediate family member serves as a paid consultant for or is an employee of DePuy; has received research or institutional support from Amgen and Arthrex; and serves as a board member, owner, officer, or committee member for the American Academy of Orthopaedic Surgeons and the American Association of Hip and Knee Surgeons. Dr. Garvin serves as a paid consultant for or is an employee of Biomet and serves as a board member, owner, officer, or committee member for the American Academy of Orthopaedic Surgeons and the American Orthopaedic Association.

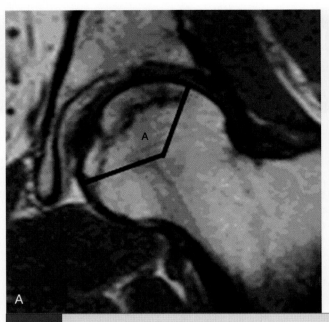
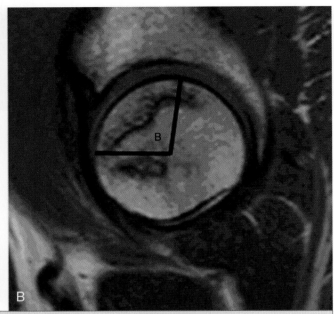

Figure 1 MRIs of the left hip demonstrating midcoronal (**A**) and midsagittal (**B**) images. The modified Kerboul angle is used to determine the extent of femoral head involvement with osteonecrosis by adding angle A and angle B. (Adapted with permission from Ha YC, Jung WH, Kim JR, Seong NH, Kim SY, Koo KH: Prediction of collapse in femoral head osteonecrosis: A modified Kerboul method with use of magnetic resonance images. *J Bone Joint Surg Am* 2006;88(suppl 3):35-40.)

tion, an association between osteonecrosis of the femoral head and an endothelial nitric oxide synthase gene polymorphism has been noted in a cohort of Korean patients compared with age-matched control subjects.[10] These data suggest that some patients in whom osteonecrosis of the femoral head develops may have a genetic predisposition for development of the disease. However, a useful screening test for a specific marker gene associated with osteonecrosis has not been identified.

Update on Imaging and Evaluation

MRI continues to be the gold standard for evaluation of osteonecrosis of the femoral head, with 99% sensitivity and specificity in diagnosing the disease. MRI can now be used to predict collapse of the femoral head. Using a modified Kerboul method, a combined necrotic angle can be calculated from midsagittal and midcoronal MRIs[11] (**Figure 1**). In one study, 37 precollapse hips with osteonecrosis were randomly assigned to a core decompression group or a nonsurgical group. At a minimum 5-year follow-up, none of the hips with a combined necrotic angle 190° or less collapsed, whereas all 25 hips with a combined necrotic angle 240° or greater collapsed. Four of the eight hips with a combined necrotic angle between 190° and 240° collapsed. The outcome was not influenced by the treatment of the hip. These data suggest that the modified Kerboul combined necrotic angle is a useful method to predict future collapse in hips with osteonecrosis of the femoral head.[11]

In another prospective study, 83 asymptomatic or minimally symptomatic hips in 61 consecutive patients were followed prospectively with MRI.[12] At mean follow-up of 60 months, 36 of the 83 hips (43%) were asymptomatic. Bone marrow edema was present in 28 hips (34%), and 27 of the 28 hips with bone marrow edema were symptomatic. The presence of bone marrow edema on MRI was correlated with worsening hip pain. The authors concluded that bone marrow edema was the essential risk factor associated with progression of symptoms.

Treatment

Significant controversy currently exists regarding the appropriate management of patients with precollapse osteonecrosis of the hip. The reasons for this lack of consensus include (1) the etiology of the disease remains unknown; (2) studies include patients with a variety of different risk factors for the disease; and (3) there are no appropriately powered multicenter randomized trials assessing the efficacy of different modalities. **Table 1** delineates a potential treatment algorithm for patients with osteonecrosis, but clearly further work to define optimal treatment is necessary.

Nonsurgical Treatment

A study evaluating the natural history of asymptomatic lesions in the contralateral hip provides some information that can be useful to manage these patients. A prospective study of 40 hips with small asymptomatic lesions diagnosed by MRI during the workup of a symptomatic opposite hip in patients with known risk

Table 1

Treatment Algorithm for Osteonecrosis of the Femoral Head

Radiographic Stage	Symptoms	Treatment Options
I and II	Asymptomatic	Observation, possible core decompression ± vascularized or nonvascularized bone grafting
IA, IB, IC, IIA, IIB, IIC	Symptomatic	Core decompression ± vascularized or nonvascularized bone grafting
IC, IIC, IIIA, IIIB, IIIC, IVA	Symptomatic	Core decompression ± vascularized or nonvascularized bone grafting, osteotomy, resurfacing arthroplasty, THA
IVB, IVC, V, VI	Symptomatic	Resurfacing arthroplasty (depending on extent of femoral head involvement) and THA

factors for osteonecrosis demonstrated that at average follow-up of 11 years, 35 of the 40 hips (88%) were symptomatic.[13] The mean interval between diagnosis and the development of symptoms was 80 months. At average follow-up of 11 years, 29 hips (73%) had collapse of the femoral head. All hips were symptomatic for at least 6 months before collapse. This study provides some critical data to facilitate management of patients with osteonecrosis, including (1) a minimum 5-year follow-up is necessary to truly evaluate the success of surgical treatment of patients with osteonecrosis of the hip; (2) because collapse typically follows the onset of symptoms by at least 6 months, surgical treatment can be delayed in many cases until symptoms are noted; and (3) because small lesions will eventually collapse, close observation and even prophylactic treatment should be considered for the opposite asymptomatic hip with a moderate to large lesion.[3]

Pharmacologic Agents

Recently, several small studies have analyzed the efficacy of pharmacologic agents in delaying progression of osteonecrosis. In a randomized prospective study, the efficacy of the bisphosphonate alendronate (70 mg orally daily for 25 weeks) was compared with placebo for the prevention of femoral head collapse in patients with Steinberg stage II or III atraumatic osteonecrosis of the femoral head.[14] Twenty-seven patients were considered idiopathic and 13 patients had a history of corticosteroid use. At minimum follow-up of 24 months (range, 24 to 28 months), 2 of 29 femoral heads (7%) in the alendronate group had collapsed, whereas 19 of 25 femoral heads (76%) in the control group collapsed. Sixteen hips in the control group underwent THA compared with only one hip in the alendronate group. It has been hypothesized that the bisphosphonates delay bone turnover, which may prevent collapse of the femoral head.

Another prospective study evaluated the efficacy of the low-molecular-weight heparin enoxaparin and its influence on the progression of osteonecrosis in patients who had thrombophilic or hypofibrinolytic disorders. In this study, 16 patients with Ficat stage I or II osteonecrosis (precollapse lesions) of the femoral head and thrombophilic and hypofibrinolytic disorders were compared with 12 patients (15 hips) who had steroid-induced osteonecrosis. Nineteen of 20 hips with primary osteonecrosis were unchanged at final follow-up (≥ 108 weeks), whereas a collapsed hip developed in 12 of 15 hips with steroid-induced osteonecrosis.[15]

Although the results of these studies are encouraging, to truly determine their efficacy, appropriately powered, long-term randomized studies are needed. Both efficacy and safety need to be analyzed and the influence of patient comorbidities on outcomes needs to be assessed.

Biophysical Modalities

Recently, both extracorporeal shock wave and electromagnetic therapies have been evaluated as potential treatment modalities for femoral head osteonecrosis. In a prospective randomized trial, patients with ARCO stage I, II, or III osteonecrosis of the hip were treated with either extracorporeal shock wave therapy (23 patients, 29 hips) or core decompression and nonvascularized fibular bone grafting (25 patients, 28 hips).[16] The risk factors for osteonecrosis were alcohol related in 32 patients, steroid induced in 4 patients, and idiopathic in 12 patients. At average follow-up of 25 months (range, 24 to 35 months) 23 of 30 hips (77%) treated with shock wave therapy were improved when evaluated with respect to Harris hip scores and the ability to carry out activities of daily living. Only 8 of 29 hips treated with a core decompression and a nonvascularized fibular graft had better scores. In the shock wave therapy group, three (10%) went on to THA versus nine (31%) in the core decompression group. A retrospective study was performed to evaluate the efficacy of pulsed electromagnetic field stimulation in 76 patients with Ficat I, II, or III osteonecrosis of the femoral head.[17] Pulsed electromagnetic field stimulation was found to be effective in limiting pain in 35 of 76 patients (46%) after 60 days of therapy. Twenty hips (26%) demonstrated radiographic progression at final follow-up (average follow-up was 28 months).[17] Again, although the short-term results with these modalities are promising, appropriately powered randomized trials are essential to determine their true efficacy.

Surgical Treatment

Traditional surgical treatment of osteonecrotic lesions of the hip can be categorized as either femoral head-sparing or arthroplasty procedures. In general, femoral head-sparing procedures have higher rates of success when they are reserved for patients with precollapse lesions. The different types of femoral head-saving procedures include core decompression, core decompression with nonvascularized or vascularized bone grafting, and rotational osteotomies. Over the years, core decompression using a variety of techniques has been demonstrated to be relatively effective in managing small to moderate-sized lesions.

Novel Therapies

Recently, there has been interest in using mesenchymal stem cells to enhance repair of osteonecrosis of the hip. In a pilot study that included 13 patients (18 hips) with precollapse lesions, the patients were randomized to be treated with either a 3-mm core decompression alone or core decompression with implantation of autologous bone marrow mononuclear cells. Fourteen of the hips had corticosteroid-induced osteonecrosis, two had alcohol-related disease, and two were idiopathic. After 24 months the group treated with bone marrow grafting had a decrease in symptoms and only 1 of 10 hips demonstrated progression of the disease. In contrast, five of the eight hips treated with core decompression alone had radiographic evidence of progression.[18]

In a prospective study, 116 patients (189 hips) with osteonecrosis were treated with core decompression and injection of concentrated autologous bone marrow mononuclear cells.[19] The risk factors for osteonecrosis were corticosteroids in 31 hips (16%), alcohol related in 56 hips (30%), sickle cell disease in 64 hips (34%), and idiopathic in 10 hips (5%). In patients with precollapse lesions, arthroplasty was performed in 9 of 145 hips. THA was needed in 25 of 44 hips with postcollapse lesions. In this study, patients who received a larger number of progenitor cells during bone grafting demonstrated better survival. Patients with steroid- or alcohol-related osteonecrosis received a lower number of transplanted cells and had a greater risk of failure at the later follow-up period. This finding is consistent with the previously mentioned basic science studies.

Another novel therapy has been the use of porous tantalum rods in combination with core decompression. The goal is for the tantalum rod to provide structural support for the necrotic bone to prevent collapse while reducing the complications associated with autograft harvest or allograft bone. Fifty-four consecutive patients with osteonecrosis of the hip were treated with core decompression and porous tantalum rods. Survivorship analysis revealed an overall survival rate of 68.1% at 48 months; 15.5% (9 hips) were converted to THA.[20] In a more recent study of 17 failed porous tantalum implants, retrieval analysis revealed that there was little bone ingrowth and insufficient subchondral bone in the femoral head in the region of the rod. This

group of retrievals represented 17 of 113 hips (15%) that were used to treat precollapse lesions. All failures occurred between 3 and 36 months after implantation. These results raise questions about the potential efficacy of the tantalum implant and the surgical technique used in these cases.[21]

In a pair of retrospective studies, the efficacy of bone graft enhanced with bone morphogenetic protein was evaluated for the treatment of osteonecrosis of the femoral head. In one study,[22] a bone morphogenetic protein bone graft substitute was implanted into the femoral head via a trapdoor at the femoral head-neck junction in 33 patients (39 hips). At minimum follow-up of 24 months (mean, 36 months; range, 24 to 50 months) 25 of 30 hips had a successful clinical result (a Harris Hip score ≥ 80 points and no further surgery). Two of nine hips with a large lesion required more surgery. Although these results are promising, this procedure requires an extensive surgical dissection to expose the femoral neck and it is more difficult to perform than a standard core decompression. In another study, a novel biologic bone graft substitute (an alloimplant of allogenic, antigen-extracted, autolyzed fibula bone perfused with human bone morphogenetic protein and noncollagenous proteins) was used in combination with core decompression to treat 15 patients (17 hips) with osteonecrosis.[23] In 14 of 17 hips there was no evidence of radiographic progression of disease at an average follow-up of 53 months (range, 26 to 94 months). Two of the 13 hips that did progress had collapse of the femoral head before the procedure. The results of these two studies suggest that core decompression may be more effective when combined with an osteoinductive agent.

Although the results of these studies using bone morphogenetic protein or mesenchymal stem cells are promising, randomized trials are necessary to determine if these procedures are more effective than core decompression alone. Core decompression combined with a vascularized or nonvascularized graft has been demonstrated to be effective, but appropriately powered randomized trials are needed to determine which of these modalities is the best and truly superior to a core decompression alone. The results may be influenced by both the size of the lesion and the presence of risk factors.

There is general agreement that most patients with collapse of the femoral head will not do well with a femoral head-saving procedure. Therefore, these patients are candidates for an arthroplasty procedure. A variety of studies have demonstrated the efficacy of THA in patients with osteonecrosis. The use of cementless fixation has led to improved outcomes. Because many of these patients are younger than 50 years, the selection of an appropriate bearing surface remains an area of controversy. Future studies evaluating the outcomes of THA for patients with osteonecrosis need to focus on specific patient populations with osteonecrosis (that is, idiopathic, steroid-induced, or alcohol-induced osteonecrosis, or inflammatory arthritis) to optimize results.

Hip resurfacing has received increased attention for management of osteonecrosis because many of the patients are young and there is an opportunity to preserve femoral bone stock and the large femoral head provides increased stability and range of motion. One retrospective study compared the results of treatment of osteonecrosis of the femoral head with hip resurfacing (39 hips) with a matched cohort of patients with osteoarthritis (42 hips) treated with hip resurfacing.[24] The mean follow-up in both groups was 4 months. There were similar clinical outcomes in both groups with good to excellent outcomes in 93% of the osteonecrosis patients and 98% of the osteoarthritis patients. In each group there were two hips that required conversion to a THA. Another study reported on the results of a single surgeon series of 60 hips (73 patients) undergoing metal-on-metal resurfacing for osteonecrosis.[25] At a mean of 6.1 years (range, 2 to 12 years), the overall survival rate was 93%. In a recent retrospective review, 71 patients (96 hips) with osteonecrosis were treated with a hip resurfacing.[26] At mean follow-up of 4 to 5 years (range, 4 to 8 years) the cumulative survival rate was 95.4%. Overall, three of the hips had failed. These authors stressed the importance of appropriate positioning of the acetabular component combined with a valgus position of the femoral component as being critical for a successful hip resurfacing reconstruction.

Although these results are promising, there are some caveats to using resurfacing in this patient population. First, the results of resurfacing for all diagnoses are better in males with excellent bone stock. Therefore, the results may be compromised in patients using steroids or females with narrow femoral necks. Second, patients with osteonecrosis have variable amounts of dead bone and cysts in the femoral head that can compromise the cement fixation in the femoral head and limit the longevity of the fixation. Third, metal-on-metal articulations should not be used in patients with renal compromise. Randomized trials comparing femoral head resurfacing to results with THA with large femoral heads are necessary to determine the role of resurfacing in patients with osteonecrosis.

A recent study compared the results of cementless THA for osteonecrosis with a matched cohort of patients with osteoarthritis treated with THA[27] (52 hips in each group). The average duration of follow-up was 41 months (range, 24 to 61 months). Good to excellent outcomes were noted in 49 hips (94%) in the osteonecrosis group and 50 hips (96%) in the osteoarthritis group. In another study of 71 patients (73 hips) with osteonecrosis who were younger than 50 years, all patients were treated with an alumina head and a highly cross-linked polyethylene liner.[28] The average follow-up was 8.5 years (range, 7 to 9 years) and there were no revisions for either osteolysis or aseptic loosening.

Osteonecrosis of the Knee
Kevin L. Garvin, MD

Osteonecrosis is an infrequent cause of knee disease. The distal femur is the most common site of knee involvement but represents only 10% of all osteonecrosis.[29] Approximately 2% of all total knee arthroplasties are performed for osteonecrosis.[30,31] The ultimate cause of osteonecrosis of the knee, like that of the hip, is disruption of the blood supply to the affected area, but why it occurs is not known.[32,33] Knowledge about osteonecrosis of the knee derives largely from an understanding of osteonecrosis of the hip.

Types of Osteonecrosis

Spontaneous or primary osteonecrosis of the knee generally affects patients older than 55 years, occurs predominantly in females, and is usually unilateral. Other joints are not affected and only one condyle of the knee is involved.[34-37]

Secondary osteonecrosis of the knee occurs in a population of patients similar to the population of patients with osteonecrosis of the hip. The patients are younger ($\leq$ 55 years), often female (4:1 ratio), and both knees are usually affected (in > 80% of patients). Other major joints such as the hip and shoulder may be involved. Knee involvement is diffuse as both condyles of the distal femur and both condyles of the proximal tibia are likely to be affected.[38-40]

The third type is osteonecrosis in the postoperative knee. It is similar to spontaneous osteonecrosis of the knee in that it affects the medial condyle more frequently than the lateral condyle but, unlike spontaneous osteonecrosis, it occurs equally in males and females. The mean age of affected patients in one study was 58 years (range, 21 to 82 years). The diagnostic radiographic findings in postarthroscopic osteonecrosis have been described. Histologic evidence of a fracture as the cause of the patients' symptoms was reported in a series of eight patients with postoperative osteonecrosis of the knee.[41]

Risk Factors

The risk factors commonly associated with secondary osteonecrosis of the knee are similar to those for the hip and include corticosteroid therapy, alcohol consumption, sickle cell disease, metabolic disorders, and autoimmune disorders (systemic lupus erythematosus, rheumatoid arthritis, Behçet disease).[42] The dose of corticosteroid therapy associated with the onset of osteonecrosis has been a topic of interest. Two hundred four cardiac transplant patients were studied and five patients with osteonecrosis of the hip and one of the knee were identified.[43] The authors of this study were not able to correlate the likelihood of osteonecrosis with the dosage of the corticosteroids given to the patients after organ transplant. Risk factors for spontaneous osteonecrosis have not been identified.

Table 2			
Modified Knee Staging Classification (Ficat and Arlet)			
Stage	Joint Space	Head Contour	Trabecular Pattern
I	Normal	Normal	Osteoporosis mottled areas
II	Normal	Normal	Wedge sclerosis
III	Normal or slightly decreased	Subchondral collapse	Sequestrum appearance
IV	Decreased	Collapse	Extensive destruction

History and Physical Examination

The most common complaint of patients with osteonecrosis of the knee is pain; swelling and stiffness associated with an effusion also are common. Symptoms are usually of gradual onset. As the disease progresses, the symptoms progress from pain only to those of end-stage arthritis. Alternatively, patients can also experience sudden onset of pain associated with the acute collapse of the femoral condyle. The symptoms can include mechanical catching or locking of the knee because of the incongruous condyle.

Differential diagnoses for patients with these symptoms include transient ischemic osteoporosis, bone marrow edema, and the more recently recognized post-arthroscopic osteonecrosis of the knee. Transient ischemic osteoporosis is believed to be a distinct entity with unique features that distinguish it from osteonecrosis.[44,45] The condition has a propensity to affect middle-aged men, or women either during the last trimester of pregnancy or postpartum. The lower extremity is involved exclusively. Risk factors have not been identified. Transient osteoporosis is best diagnosed using MRI, which is both sensitive and specific. Fortunately, the disease is self-limiting but recurrence is possible. Migratory transient osteoporosis can be a challenging diagnostic and therapeutic condition for the patient and physician. Metastatic carcinoma, multiple myeloma, lymphoma, inflammatory arthritis, osteomyelitis, and other serious diseases must be excluded and the patient reassured that the entity is nonprogressive and self-limiting. Supportive treatment includes protective weight bearing, analgesics, and nonsteroidal anti-inflammatory drugs.

Bone marrow edema is a finding that may be seen in the early stages of osteonecrosis or transient osteonecrosis. The term "bone marrow edema syndrome" has been used but can be confusing because bone marrow edema on MRI is a nonspecific signal pattern that may be present in other disease entities.[46,47]

Radiographic Findings

In the early stages of osteonecrosis, radiographs show increased bone density at the involved site. The increased density is caused by new bone formation adjacent to the necrotic bone it is replacing. The density is accentuated by a surrounding area of osteopenia. In the later stages of osteonecrosis, a crescent sign is evident as the necrotic bone segment collapses from the subchondral bone. Finally, the unsupported subchondral bone also collapses, resulting in a flattened condylar surface, ultimately leading to end-stage arthritis.

Bone scintigraphy and MRI have been used to assist with the diagnosis.[48,49] Authors of a 2008 study evaluated 48 patients with 163 osteonecrotic lesions.[50] Each of the 48 patients had a bone scan and an MRI less than 3 months apart. The diagnosis of osteonecrosis was confirmed by histopathology. MRI confirmed the histopathology in all 163 lesions (100%) but the bone scan did so in only 91 of the lesions (56%). The bone scan was least sensitive for early-stage lesions, when ancillary testing modalities are of the most potential value. The study did not support the use of bone scans as a diagnostic or screening tool for osteonecrosis.

Treatment

The treatment of patients with osteonecrosis depends on the symptoms and the stage of disease[51] (Table 2). Symptomatic patients with early-stage osteonecrosis (stage I or stage II) are treated nonsurgically with analgesics, nonsteroidal anti-inflammatory drugs, physical therapy, and protected weight bearing. Small areas of osteonecrosis are more likely to resolve. Spontaneous osteonecrosis is also more likely to improve and resolve compared with secondary osteonecrosis.

Historically, nonsurgical treatment of osteonecrosis of the knee has had a minimal role. The natural history of osteonecrosis has been regarded as a slowly progressive disease, altered only by surgical intervention.[52] However, prostaglandin I2 or synonoma prostacyclin has recently been reported to lessen pain associated with osteonecrosis and bone marrow edema.[53] Another nonsurgical treatment includes the use of bisphosphonates, which function to inhibit bone resorption and have been successfully used to treat patients with metabolic bone disease when osteoclastic activity is increased.[52] Bisphosphonates also have been used successfully to treat patients with osteonecrosis of the hip, but information regarding their use in the knee is limited.[54] Intravenous ibandronate has been used successfully to treat transient osteoporosis of the hip.[55] The role of bisphosphonates in the knee was recently evaluated. In 22 of 28 patients, bisphosphonate treatment using intrave-

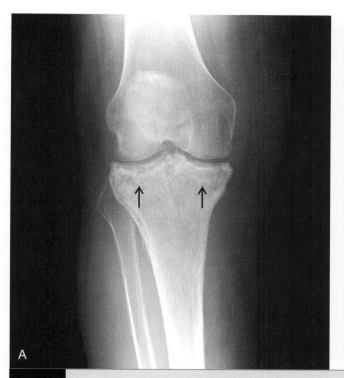
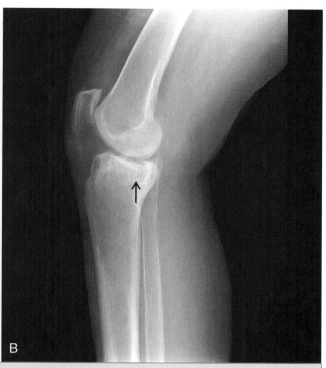

Figure 2   Preoperative AP (**A**) and lateral (**B**) radiographs of the knee of a 54-year-old man taking steroids and immunosuppressive agents after a liver transplant. The patient had stage IV osteonecrosis of the knee and severe pain. The radiographs also show collapse of the tibial plateau (arrows). A total knee arthroplasty using stemmed components was done to assist with implant fixation to bone.

nous pamidronate (120 mg) followed by oral alendronate (70 mg weekly) for 4 to 6 months was effective. Symptoms completely resolved in 15 patients and were improved in 6 patients who reported minimal residual pain. In 18 patients, MRI evaluation confirmed resolution of the bone marrow edema. Based on the information available, further studies are needed to confirm a beneficial effect of bisphosphonate therapy for osteonecrosis of the knee.

Surgical treatment is indicated for those patients in whom nonsurgical treatment has failed. Arthroscopy may be indicated for patients with mechanical symptoms resulting from a loose osteochondral flap which, when excised arthroscopically, may provide symptomatic relief. A high tibial valgus osteotomy can relieve the stress if the medial compartment of the knee is affected. The results of medial opening wedge high tibial osteotomy were reported in 52 patients (57 knees).[56] Twenty-three of the patients (23 knees) had osteonecrosis. In all of the patients, the osteotomy was preceded by arthroscopy and débridement of the regenerated cartilage on the femoral condyle followed by drilling of the avascular medial condyle. All of the patients with osteonecrosis had preoperative collapse of the condyle (10 stage III, 13 stage IV). At mean follow-up of 40 months (range, 24 to 62 months) pain and function were improved and valgus alignment was maintained for all of the patients.

Theoretically, core decompression decreases the intraosseous pressure within the area of affected bone and allows for return of vascularity and hence, new bone formation. The results of 47 knees with 3 months or more of symptoms that were treated with a core decompression have been reported.[57] Good or excellent results were achieved and maintained in 73% of the knees at average follow-up of 11 years. The authors concluded that core decompression may slow the rate of symptomatic progression.

Impaction bone grafting of the osteonecrotic region has been proposed as another treatment option. Six patients (nine knees) with extensive corticosteroid associated osteonecrotic lesions of the femoral condyles were treated with impaction grafting technique. At average follow-up of 51 months (range, 29 to 93 months), all of the patients were clinically improved. None of the patients' knees required replacement, but of six knees with preoperative collapse, three had minimal arthritis with a Kellgren score of 1. One of the knees had radiographic evidence of arthritis before the bone grafting technique.

The role of unicompartmental arthroplasty for osteonecrosis of the knee is controversial. The authors of a 2005 study specifically evaluated the Oxford unicompartmental arthroplasty for focal spontaneous osteonecrosis of the knee.[58] Twenty-nine knees (27 patients) were evaluated 5.2 years (range, 1 to 13 years) after the

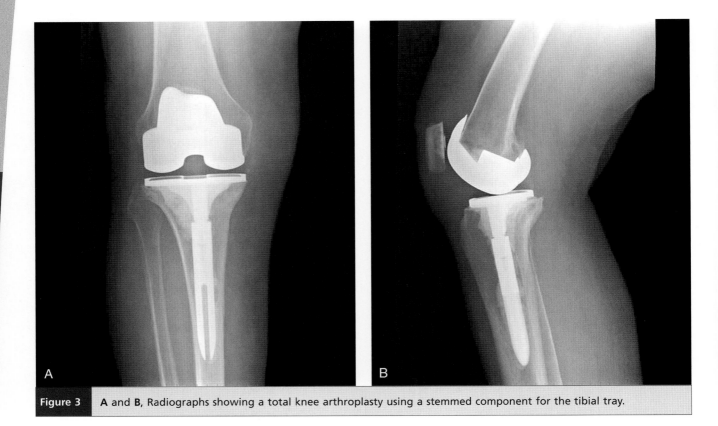

Figure 3   **A** and **B**, Radiographs showing a total knee arthroplasty using a stemmed component for the tibial tray.

surgical procedure. The authors compared this group to a control group of 27 patients with medial compartment arthritis. There were no statistically significant differences between the groups in terms of outcome when using the Oxford Knee Score as a measurement. The long-term results of lateral unicondylar replacement were also reported recently. Of 39 patients with 40 lateral cemented metal-back unicompartmental knee arthroplasties, only 4 patients had osteonecrosis. At mean follow-up of 12.6 years, all 4 patients' knees were in place without revision surgery or loosening.

Total knee arthroplasty has been the gold standard for most patients with stage IV osteonecrosis. Authors of a 2006 study performed a literature review and identified 15 published studies of total knee replacement for osteonecrosis since 1982.[38] The studies were divided to distinguish stages and type (spontaneous versus secondary osteonecrosis) of disease. Several conclusions could be drawn. First, the results of total knee arthroplasty for spontaneous and secondary osteonecrosis of the knee have been excellent since 1985. Second, the use of cement and modern knee designs with the option of ancillary stem extensions for select patients may have contributed to those excellent results (**Figures 2** and **3**). Knees with bone loss or extensive osteonecrotic bone were best treated with the use of ancillary stems. With the implementation of these techniques, the frequency of a good or excellent outcome increased from 55% to 96% and the revision rate dropped from 36% to 4%.

The results are similar to those of total knee arthroplasty for patients with osteoarthritis, but it should be noted that a direct comparison study has not been performed. Using a global knee score, the results of total knee arthroplasty for patients with spontaneous osteonecrosis are slightly better than the results of total knee arthroplasty for patients with secondary osteonecrosis and comparable to the results for patients with osteoarthritis.

Summary

Over the past two decades the results of THA for management of osteonecrosis of the hip has shown improvement in clinical results. The advent of cementless fixation was a critical element in the improved clinical outcomes and decreased failure rates. Although study results are promising, long-term follow-up is needed to determine the optimal acetabular and femoral components and bearing surfaces to treat these young patients with osteonecrosis of the hip. Osteonecrosis of the knee is an infrequent but potentially disabling disease. The treatment of the osteonecrosis is based on the severity of the necrotic lesion. Bisphosphonate treatment is relatively new and may be effective for precollapse lesions. Once the condyle has collapsed, total knee arthroplasty is indicated, and excellent results using stemmed components as necessary have been reported.

Annotated References

1. Lieberman JR, Berry DJ, Mont MA, et al: Osteonecrosis of the hip: Management in the 21st century. *Instr Course Lect* 2003;52:337-355.

2. Mont MA, Jones LC, Hungerford DS: Nontraumatic osteonecrosis of the femoral head: Ten years later. *J Bone Joint Surg Am* 2006;88(5):1117-1132.

   The authors present an excellent review of management of patients with osteonecrosis of the femoral head.

3. Petrigliano FA, Lieberman JR: Osteonecrosis of the hip: Novel approaches to evaluation and treatment. *Clin Orthop Relat Res* 2007;465:53-62.

   A review of new techniques used to manage osteonecrosis of the femoral head is presented.

4. Suh KT, Kim SW, Roh HL, Youn MS, Jung JS: Decreased osteogenic differentiation of mesenchymal stem cells in alcohol-induced osteonecrosis. *Clin Orthop Relat Res* 2005;431:220-225.

   In this in vitro study the authors compared the differentiation ability of mesenchymal stem cells isolated from the bone marrow in patients undergoing THA for osteonecrosis for femoral neck fracture. The cells obtained from patients with osteonecrosis of the femoral head demonstrated a reduced ability to differentiate into osteogenic lineages compared with cells obtained from patients who sustained a femoral neck fracture.

5. Lee JS, Lee JS, Roh HL, Kim CH, Jung JS, Suh KT: Alterations in the differentiation ability of mesenchymal stem cells in patients with nontraumatic osteonecrosis of the femoral head: Comparative analysis according to the risk factor. *J Orthop Res* 2006;24(4):604-609.

   This in vitro study assessed the osteogenic and adipocytic differentiation ability of mesenchymal stem cells that were harvested from patients with either osteonecrosis of the femoral head or osteoarthritis. The authors concluded that there was altered differentiation ability in mesenchymal stem cells that were harvested from osteonecrotic femoral heads.

6. Cui Q, Wang Y, Saleh KJ, Wang GJ, Balian G: Alcohol-induced adipogenesis in a cloned bone-marrow stem cell. *J Bone Joint Surg Am* 2006; 88(suppl 3):148-154.

   In an in vitro study, D1 cells (cloned mouse bone-marrow stem cells) were treated with increasing concentrations of ethanol. The cells treated with ethanol started to accumulate triglyceride vesicles and the levels of alkaline phosphatase decreased. Alcohol treatment decreased osteogenesis and enhanced adipogenesis. These findings support the clinical observation that alcohol-induced osteonecrosis may be associated with increased adipocyte formation.

7. Yin L, Li YB, Wang YS: Dexamethasone-induced adipogenesis in primary marrow stromal cell cultures: Mechanism of steroid-induced osteonecrosis. *Chin Med J (Engl)* 2006;119(7):581-588.

   The purpose of this study was to observe the influence of dexamethasone on the differentiation of bone marrow stromal cells (MSCs) and its potential relationship to steroid-induced osteonecrosis. Dexamethasone induced differentiation of MSCs into adipocytes and inhibited the osteogenic differentiation of these MSCs.

8. Drescher W, Bünger MH, Weigert K, Bünger C, Hansen ES: Methylprednisolone enhances contraction of porcine femoral head epiphyseal arteries. *Clin Orthop Relat Res* 2004;423:112-117.

9. Liu YF, Chen WM, Lin YF, et al: Type II collagen gene variants and inherited osteonecrosis of the femoral head. *N Engl J Med* 2005;352(22):2294-2301.

   The authors identified three families in which there was autosomal dominant inheritance of osteonecrosis and mapped the chromosome position of the gene to 12q13. The authors noted a mutant allele in exon 50 of *Col2A1* gene. All the patients with osteonecrosis of the femoral head carried *Col2A1* mutations. The authors suggested that in families with osteonecrosis haplotype, sequence analysis of the *Col2A1* gene may be used to identify patients at higher risk for developing osteonecrosis.

10. Koo KH, Lee JS, Lee YJ, Kim KJ, Yoo JJ, Kim HJ: Endothelial nitric oxide synthase gene polymorphisms in patients with nontraumatic femoral head osteonecrosis. *J Orthop Res* 2006;24(8):1722-1728.

    Genomic DNA from 103 patients with nontraumatic osteonecrosis of the hip and 103 control subjects matched for sex and age was analyzed for the 27-base pair repeat polymorphism in intron 4 and Glu298Asp polymorphism in exon 7. The distribution of the two polymorphisms was not significantly different between the patients and control subjects. The data suggest that there may be a protective role of nitric oxide in the development of osteonecrosis of the hip.

11. Ha YC, Jung WH, Kim JR, Seong NH, Kim SY, Koo KH: Prediction of collapse in femoral head osteonecrosis: A modified Kerboul method with use of magnetic resonance images. *J Bone Joint Surg Am* 2006; 88(suppl 3):35-40.

    In this study 37 hips (33 patients) with early-stage osteonecrosis were analyzed using the modified method of Kerboul et al. The authors measured the arch of the femoral head surface involved with osteonecrosis on midcoronal and midsagittal MRIs and then calculated the sum of the angles. None of the four hips with a combined necrotic angle of less than 190° collapsed. In contrast, all 25 hips with a combined necrotic angle of greater than 240° collapsed.

12. Ito H, Matsuno T, Minami A: Relationship between bone marrow edema and development of symptoms in patients with osteonecrosis of the femoral head. *AJR Am J Roentgenol* 2006;186(6):1761-1770.

    The authors investigated the significance of risk factors on MRIs to predict the outcome of patients with osteonecrosis of the femoral head. Eighty-three asymptomatic or minimally symptomatic hips (61 patients) were followed prospectively. Thirty-three of the 83 hips (40%) were symptomatic at the last follow-up. Bone marrow edema was present in 28 hips (34%) during the follow-up period and 27 of 28 hips were symptomatic. Bone marrow edema was significantly correlated with increased hip pain ($P < 0.0001$).

13. Hernigou P, Poignard A, Nogier A, Manicom O: Fate of very small asymptomatic stage-I osteonecrotic lesions of the hip. *J Bone Joint Surg Am* 2004;86(12): 2589-2593.

14. Lai KA, Shen WJ, Yang CY, Shao CJ, Hsu JT, Lin RM: The use of alendronate to prevent early collapse of the femoral head in patients with nontraumatic osteonecrosis: A randomized clinical study. *J Bone Joint Surg Am* 2005;87(10):2155-2159.

    Forty patients with stage II or III osteonecrosis were divided into alendronate and control groups. Patients in the alendronate group received 70 mg of alendronate for 25 weeks and the control group received placebo. Only 2 of 29 femoral heads in the alendronate group collapsed. In contrast, 19 of 25 of femoral heads in the control group collapsed. Alendronate may prevent early collapse of the femoral head.

15. Glueck CJ, Freiberg RA, Sieve L, Wang P: Enoxaparin prevents progression of stages I and II osteonecrosis of the hip. *Clin Orthop Relat Res* 2005;435:164-170.

    In this prospective pilot study, the authors assessed the influence of enoxaparin on the progression of stage I and II primary osteonecrosis of the hip associated with thrombophilia or hypofibrinolysis versus corticosteroid-associated secondary osteonecrosis. Nineteen of 20 hips with primary osteonecrosis did not progress from stage I or II disease. In contrast, 12 of 15 hips (80%) with secondary osteonecrosis related to corticosteroid use progressed to stage III or IV osteonecrosis.

16. Wang CJ, Wang FS, Huang CC, Yang KD, Weng LH, Huang HY: Treatment for osteonecrosis of the femoral head: Comparison of extracorporeal shock waves with core decompression and bone-grafting. *J Bone Joint Surg Am* 2005;87(11):2380-2387.

    This study compared the results of treatment of osteonecrosis with either extracorporeal shock waves or core decompression with bone grafting. There were 23 patients (29 hips) in the shock wave group and there were 25 patients (28 hips) in the core decompression group. At average follow-up of 25 months, the shock wave group had decreased pain and higher hip scores compared with the surgical group.

17. Massari L, Fini F, Cadossi R, Setti S, Traina GC: Biophysical stimulation with pulsed electromagnetic fields in osteonecrosis of the femoral head. *J Bone Joint Surg Am* 2006;88:56-60.

    It is hypothesized that the short-term effect of pulsed electromagnetic field stimulation may be to protect articular cartilage from the catabolic effect of inflammation and subchondral bone marrow edema, and the long-term effect may be to promote osteogenic activity in areas of necrosis and prevent trabecular fracture and subchondral bone collapse. Level of evidence: IV.

18. Gangji V, Hauzeur JP, Matos C, De Maertelaer V, Toungouz M, Lambermont M: Treatment of osteonecrosis of the femoral head with implantation of autologous bone-marrow cells: A pilot study. *J Bone Joint Surg Am* 2004;86(6):1153-1160.

19. Hernigou P, Beaujean F: Treatment of osteonecrosis with autologous bone marrow grafting. *Clin Orthop Relat Res* 2002;405:14-23.

20. Veillette CJ, Mehdian H, Schemitsch EH, McKee MD: Survivorship analysis and radiographic outcome following tantalum rod insertion for osteonecrosis of the femoral head. *J Bone Joint Surg Am* 2006;88(suppl 3): 48-55.

    The purpose of this study was to evaluate the clinical and radiographic outcomes with the use of core decompression and a porous tantalum implant for the treatment of osteonecrosis of the femoral head. Overall 9 of 58 hips (15.5%) were converted to a THA at average follow-up of 24 months. The overall survival rate was 92%.

21. Tanzer M, Bobyn JD, Krygier JJ, Karabasz D: Histopathologic retrieval analysis of clinically failed porous tantalum osteonecrosis implants. *J Bone Joint Surg Am* 2008;90(6):1282-1289.

    The authors performed an investigational device exemption study that included 113 porous tantalum implants that were used to treat osteonecrosis of the femoral head with core decompression and implantation of a porous tantalum rod. At average follow-up of 13 months, 17 of 113 implants had already failed.

22. Seyler TM, Marker DR, Ulrich SD, Fatscher T, Mont MA: Nonvascularized bone grafting defers joint arthroplasty in hip osteonecrosis. *Clin Orthop Relat Res* 2008;466(5):1125-1132.

    A retrospective review is presented of 33 patients (39 hips) with osteonecrosis of the hip treated with a trapdoor at the head-neck junction to débride the necrotic bone and with grafting of the femoral head with autogenous graft and osteoprotegerin-1. At minimum follow-up of 24 months, 25 of 30 hips with small or moderate-sized lesions required no further surgery. Two of nine hips with large lesions required additional surgery.

23. Lieberman JR, Conduah A, Urist MR: Treatment of osteonecrosis of the femoral head with core decompression and human bone morphogenetic protein. *Clin Orthop Relat Res* 2004;429:139-145.

24. Mont MA, Seyler TM, Marker DR, Marulanda GA, Delanois RE: Use of metal-on-metal total hip resurfacing for the treatment of osteonecrosis of the femoral head. *J Bone Joint Surg Am* 2006;88:90-97.

    Metal-on-metal total hip resurfacing to treat patients with osteonecrosis of the femoral head had excellent short-term results. Level of evidence: II.

full weight bearing. They concluded that the treatment plan was highly successful for correcting knee malalignment in patients with medial compartment osteoarthritis. Level of evidence: IV.

57. Mont MA, Tomek IM, Hungerford DS: Core decompression for avascular necrosis of the distal femur: Long term followup. *Clin Orthop Relat Res* 1997;334: 124-130.

58. Langdown AJ, Pandit H, Price AJ, et al: Oxford medial unicompartmental arthroplasty for focal spontaneous osteonecrosis of the knee. *Acta Orthop* 2005; 76(5):688-692.

The authors review the literature and discuss the treatment options for spontaneous osteonecrosis of the knee.

Chapter 6

Pain Management and Accelerated Rehabilitation

Gregory K. Deirmengian, MD   William J. Hozack, MD

Introduction

Hip and knee arthroplasty are highly successful surgical procedures that result in pain relief, functional recovery, and improved quality of life for most patients. Yet, many surgical candidates who would otherwise greatly benefit from hip or knee arthroplasty are deterred by the prospect of significant postoperative pain and an extended period of time to functional recovery. These notions have been associated with traditional perioperative approaches such as general anesthesia and patient-controlled intravenous narcotics.

Recently, much focus has been placed on strategies that aim to improve pain management and time to functional recovery. It has become clear that achieving these goals requires a multidisciplinary approach involving the participation of the patient, family, orthopaedic surgeon, nurses, anesthesia team, and rehabilitation team. This chapter will explore the multiple factors that act in concert during the entire perioperative period, leading to optimal pain management and accelerated rehabilitation.

Preoperative Counseling, Education, and Physiotherapy

Success in minimizing postoperative pain and achievement of rapid recovery requires intervention well before the day of surgery. Many patients with degenerative arthritis have physical, emotional, and psychological factors that may hinder successful postoperative recovery.[1] Several measures may be taken to properly set patient expectations, reduce anxiety, and make lifestyle changes that will improve the likelihood of success.

Patient counseling is an essential component of preoperative preparation. Many hip and knee arthroplasty candidates take narcotic medication to control arthritic pain. Such patients build a tolerance to narcotics and may become desensitized to the effects of such pain medication. In this setting, successful postoperative pain management is quite difficult. Discussing these effects and recommending decreasing if not discontinuing all narcotic pain medications could improve the patients' postoperative experience. Similarly, nutritional counseling should take place preoperatively. When appropriate, patients are encouraged to pursue strategies to achieve weight loss and proper nutrition. A list of supplements and alternative medications should be reviewed and patients instructed to discontinue those that may have a negative effect during the perioperative period. Similarly, smoking cessation programs should be initiated when applicable. These measures have been shown to improve wound healing, avoid postoperative complications, and decrease the length of the hospital stay.[2-5]

Preoperative patient education also plays an important role in preparing for surgery. Often, patients are not well informed and may have misconceptions regarding surgery, anesthesia, and postoperative pain and recovery. As a result, patients may have unnecessary fear, anxiety, and false expectations that affect their recovery. For example, a patient who had not been informed about the role of ambulating the day of surgery after a total hip replacement might be reluctant to attempt to achieve the goal. Several educational approaches may be used preoperatively, including audiovisual aids, booklets, Web-based learning, and classes. Focus should also be placed on answering all of the patient's questions. Familiarization with the hospital setting may also be helpful in relieving preoperative anxiety. Such measures have been shown to improve functional outcome and patient satisfaction and to decrease the length of the hospital stay.[6-9]

Physiotherapy also can be used in preparation for surgery. Many patients with hip and knee arthritis develop muscular atrophy secondary to joint pain, stiff-

Dr. Deirmengian or an immediate family member is a member of a speakers' bureau or has made paid presentations on behalf of Angiotech; serves as a paid consultant for or is an employee of Synthes, Angiotech, Zimmer, and Biomet; and owns stock or stock options in CD Diagnostics. Dr. Hozack or an immediate family member has received royalties from Stryker; serves as a paid consultant for or is an employee of Stryker; has received research or institutional support from Stryker; and serves as a board member, owner, officer, or committee member for the Hip Society.

ness, and disuse. Additionally, general deconditioning results from inactivity. These factors may have an impact on the ability to participate in a rapid recovery program. Goals of preoperative physiotherapy include gentle improvement of strength and motion, gait and assistive device training, and patient education. These measures may play a role in improving the time to functional return.[10,11]

Anesthesia

The anesthesiology team has a tremendous influence on the patients' ability to participate in an accelerated rehabilitation program. Although the anesthesiology team often administers several modalities in the perioperative period, it is important to distinguish the team's role in intraoperative anesthesia from their role in postoperative analgesia. For example, regional nerve blocks, such as a femoral nerve block, are commonly placed before surgery, but such measures are insufficient for pain control during the procedure and are placed in an effort to minimize postoperative pain. The role of the anesthesiologist in postoperative pain management will be reviewed in a separate section.

From the standpoint of anesthesia, the two basic options are general anesthesia and neuraxial anesthesia. General anesthesia involves the administration of intravenous and inhalation agents to induce a state of unconsciousness with the absence of pain. Neuraxial anesthesia involves the administration of anesthetic agents within the epidural and/or spinal compartments to eliminate sensation below the level of administration.

Neuraxial anesthesia has several advantages within the realm of rapid postoperative recovery. It allows for a rapid and predictable block of pain perception that persists several hours after completion of the procedure. Furthermore, the anesthesiologist may place an epidural catheter or administer a morphine derivative into the epidural space to provide postoperative analgesia for several days.[12] Neuraxial anesthesia also avoids many of the postoperative effects of general anesthesia such as confusion, drowsiness, and dizziness, which may interfere with participation in early physical therapy, rapid recovery, and timely discharge. Furthermore, recent meta-analyses have shown that neuraxial anesthesia is associated with reduced intraoperative blood loss and need for postoperative transfusion, along with reduced incidence of thromboembolic disease.[13-15] As a result of the benefits of neuraxial anesthesia, patients achieve better satisfaction and reach rehabilitation milestones earlier than patients who receive general anesthesia.[16]

Surgical Factors

Several surgical factors influence the patients' ability to participate in a rapid recovery program.

Total Hip Arthroplasty

One of the most important prerequisites of a successful rapid recovery program is the ability of the patient to bear full weight on the operated extremity immediately after surgery. Weight-bearing limitations mandate the use of assistive devices and preclude patient participation in aggressive early rehabilitation programs. Although often taken for granted, focus on careful technique, avoidance of complications such as intraoperative fracture, and the use of stem designs that provide immediate stable fixation allow for unrestricted postoperative weight bearing.

With accelerated rehabilitation programs, the risk of early hip dislocation is another important consideration. With improved pain control and rapid return of function, patients are likely to test the limits of their motion in the early postoperative period. At the same time, limiting motion through the use of hip precautions (limiting flexion beyond 90° in the early postoperative period) may limit certain functional activities that the patient would otherwise be able to achieve. Hip precautions have been shown to negatively influence time to return to work, quality of sleep, time to driving, and overall patient satisfaction.[17] Technical considerations that influence the risk of dislocation are critical for rapid recovery programs. Obtaining sufficient exposure and visualization of anatomic landmarks allows for an optimal implant position. Maximizing the head-to-neck ratio increases the limits of motion before impingement and increases the excursion distance of the femoral head before dislocation. Restoration of appropriate femoral offset and leg lengths prevents osseous impingement and also establishes favorable soft-tissue tension.[18,19] For patients who participate in accelerated rehabilitation programs, the importance of avoiding technical errors that increase the risk of dislocation cannot be understated.

The choice of surgical approach is another important consideration; the posterior and anterolateral approaches are commonly used. Traditionally, the main disadvantages of the posterior and anterolateral approaches have been increased risk of dislocation and risk of postoperative limp, respectively. Both disadvantages may have a significant effect on patient participation in a rapid recovery program. Recently, it has been shown that the risk of dislocation with the anterolateral approach is exceedingly low and is not influenced by hip precautions.[17] As such, hip precautions are unnecessary for patients after total hip arthroplasty with the anterolateral approach. Furthermore, risk of abductor dysfunction after hip arthroplasty with the use of the anterolateral approach has not been clearly demonstrated in the literature. Regarding the posterior approach, repair of the capsule and short external rotators has been shown to have a significant effect on the risk of dislocation.[20] Although it is possible that a large head-to-neck ratio combined with a posterior repair could eliminate the need for hip precautions with the posterior approach, this theory has not been investigated to date.

Recently, much attention has been placed on minimally invasive techniques in total hip arthroplasty. The definition of minimally invasive has been inconsistent, varying from the size of the skin incision to the extent of trauma to the deeper soft tissues. The common goals of these techniques have included limitation of soft-tissue damage, minimization of postoperative pain, rapid recovery, and improved cosmesis. The most commonly used approaches include the mini-posterior approach, mini-anterolateral approach, direct anterior approach, and two-incision approach. Detailed descriptions of these techniques are discussed in chapter 19. Although public enthusiasm and clinical adoption of minimally invasive techniques have rapidly grown during the last decade, high-quality studies that investigate risks and benefits have lagged behind. A recent systematic review of the literature regarding minimally invasive total hip arthroplasty revealed few high-quality studies that investigate the matter.[21]

Although few surgeons would argue the lack of long-term benefits of minimally invasive total hip arthroplasty, its role in early postoperative recovery has been debated. The size of the hip incision does not seem to have an effect on postoperative analgesia requirement, functional recovery, length of hospital stay, or disposition at discharge.[22] The extent of the deep dissection may play a role in early functional recovery.[23] Proponents of the direct anterior approach advocate the potential benefits of the minimal muscular trauma associated with the technique. A recent clinical comparison of the direct anterior approach to the mini-posterior approach suggested a more rapid recovery of hip function and gait associated with the direct anterior approach.[24] Although such approaches that limit soft-tissue trauma may play a part in rapid recovery programs, the combined influence of factors such as preoperative patient education and preconditioning, contemporary analgesia protocols, and accelerated rehabilitation protocols have shown to be the main influence.[25] Minimally invasive techniques should be used with great caution and appropriate judgment because of the learning curve associated with complications. If used improperly, minimally invasive techniques could have a long-lasting negative effect on surgical outcomes.[26,27]

Total Knee Arthroplasty

Surgical factors that influence recovery after total knee arthroplasty mirror those of total hip arthroplasty. Again, the importance of adequate exposure and visualization to allow for proper positioning and orientation of components and avoidance of complications cannot be understated. Paralleling the trend in total hip arthroplasty, there has been recent interest in less invasive techniques in total knee arthroplasty that aim to minimize pain and hasten recovery in the early postoperative period.

The length of the skin incision does not seem to influence the postoperative level of pain or speed recovery, but may cause more wound complications.[22,28] Any true benefit to minimally invasive total knee arthroplasty likely lies in the deep dissection. Attempts at minimizing deep soft-tissue trauma have included quadriceps-sparing approaches and techniques that avoid patellar eversion and tibial translation. Although high-quality studies are lacking on the matter, the available data suggest that these efforts may improve pain and hasten recovery in the first several postoperative weeks, but they are unlikely to have an effect 6 weeks after surgery.[29-31] Like total hip arthroplasty, it is possible that minimally invasive total knee arthroplasty techniques make a small contribution within a multimodal approach to rapid recovery.

Pain Management

Minimization of postoperative pain is one of the most critical factors allowing for accelerated rehabilitation after total joint arthroplasty. Insufficient pain control and adverse effects related to anesthetic and analgesic agents preclude patient participation in aggressive rehabilitation programs. Successful pain management protocols typically involve combinations of modalities, examples of which are described in the next paragraphs. The multimodal approach to pain control has proved successful in several recent studies.[32,33]

Pain Assessment

Although often taken for granted, successful pain management depends on effective pain assessment, involving the combined efforts of the patient, family, orthopaedic surgeon, nursing staff, rehabilitation team, and anesthesia team. Pain assessment should occur frequently in the preoperative, intraoperative, and postoperative periods. The patient and family must understand their important roles in pain assessment and management. The mainstay of pain assessment should be patient self-reporting, using one of many available tools, such as the visual analog scale. Healthcare professionals should recognize the potential discrepancy between patients' behavior and their actual pain, commonly due to variability in patients' ability to cope with pain. The patients and family should understand and actively participate in adjustments to the pain management plan that occur in response to changes in pain assessment scores.[34]

Regional Anesthesia and Nerve Blocks

In addition to providing general or neuraxial anesthesia, the anesthesiology team plays a key role in providing postoperative analgesia. The administration of local anesthetic agents and/or morphine derivatives into the epidural or intrathecal space is an effective means of postoperative pain control. Additionally, epidural catheter placement allows for continued postoperative administration of such medication in the epidural space. This intervention has been shown to improve patient satisfaction, decrease the use of intravenous morphine, and accelerate recovery.[16] One of the difficulties associated with the use of epidural catheters is the risk of epidural hematoma in conjunction with anticoagulant medications such as enoxaparin and warfarin. A single-dose, extended-release epidural morphine formulation (DepoDur, Pacira Pharmaceuticals, San Diego, CA) was developed as an alternative. The use of DepoDur avoids the need for an epidural catheter while still providing several days of postoperative pain relief. The formulation has been found to be safe and effective for use in total knee arthroplasty with a threefold decrease in patient use of systemic opioids.[12]

Although the use of local anesthetic agents and morphine derivatives in the neuraxial system are excellent pain-relieving modalities, they can be associated with systemic adverse effects, such as hypotension, nausea, pruritus, motor blockade, and respiratory depression. Although these conditions can be addressed from a medical standpoint, they may interfere with participation in physical therapy, slowing patient recovery. The use of regional nerve blocks is a more specific approach that prevents many of these adverse effects. Commonly targeted nerves for total hip and knee replacement include the femoral nerve, sciatic nerve, and lumbar plexus. Local anesthetic can be administered as a single shot or continuously through a temporary catheter. Although continuous nerve blocks need to be carefully titrated to minimize motor blockade, the intervention has been quite successful. Several recent studies have demonstrated the benefits of regional nerve blocks in total hip and knee arthroplasty.[35-37]

Local Periarticular Injections
During both hip and knee arthroplasty, the infiltration of the periarticular tissues with combinations of medication can also be helpful in providing postoperative pain relief. Typical cocktails include mixtures of medications such as local anesthetic agents, morphine sulfate, epinephrine, corticosteroid, and antibiotics. Such agents act through different physiologic mechanisms to provide local anesthesia, analgesia, and anti-inflammatory effects.

For total hip arthroplasty, the cocktail is abundantly infiltrated into periarticular tissues, including the capsule, synovium, iliopsoas tendon, external rotators, abductors, gluteus maximus tendon, and fascia lata. For total knee arthroplasty, the cocktail is copiously infiltrated into tissues including the capsule, posteromedial and posterolateral structures, synovium, extensor mechanism, collateral ligaments, iliotibial band, and pes anserinus. The medication is administered during several aspects of the procedure when the relevant tissues are most accessible. Several recent well-designed studies have shown that as part of a multimodal program, periarticular injections have a significant clinical impact on postoperative pain control, functional recovery, and patient satisfaction.[38,39] One of the main problems with most of these studies is a poor definition of

what tissues are being injected with the exact amount of medication. These studies have failed to evaluate whether fewer medications in each cocktail could be used with the same effect.

Oral and Intravenous Medications
The administration of oral and intravenous medication is one of the most critical elements of a successful pain management protocol. Traditionally, postoperative pain has been treated with patient-controlled intravenous narcotic medications, such as morphine, hydromorphone, and fentanyl. Although potent and effective, patient-controlled intravenous narcotics have several disadvantages, especially in the realm of rapid recovery. Because they are short-acting and administered through an apparatus connected to the patient through intravenous tubing, effective patient mobilization is quite difficult. Additionally, intravenous narcotics are commonly associated with adverse effects, including nausea, somnolence, dizziness, pruritus, urinary retention, and respiratory depression, that often preclude active patient participation in physical therapy sessions.[34]

The recent focus on accelerated rehabilitation has led to the development of approaches that aim to minimize the need for intravenous narcotics. Several oral and intravenous medications are used in combination throughout the perioperative period, with intravenous narcotics reserved for breakthrough pain. For example, cyclooxygenase-2 (COX-2) inhibitors have been shown to reduce opioid consumption, increase patient satisfaction, and decrease adverse effects associated with intravenous narcotics.[40] Table 1 reviews the most common classes of medications used for pain control in rapid recovery programs.

The success of any combination of medications used during the perioperative period relies on a few critical concepts. First, several medications with different mechanisms of action should be administered in conjunction. The most common classes of medications (Table 1) include nonsteroidal anti-inflammatory drugs, opioids, neuromodulatory agents, and centrally acting nonopioids. Second, medications with different durations of action should be used in combination. For example, sustained-release opioids may be used in conjunction with short-acting opioids to better control the balance between pain relief and medication-associated adverse effects. Third, combinations of medications must be administered on a scheduled basis throughout the perioperative period. Recently, the benefits of preemptive analgesia have been recognized. The goal of preemptive analgesia is to pretreat pain to modulate the response of the peripheral and central nervous system to the surgical stimulus. When used as part of a rapid recovery program, preemptive analgesia effectively improves postoperative pain and decreases the length of hospital stay.[41] Fourth, medications that treat the common adverse effects associated with anesthetic and analgesic agents, such as nausea and pruritus, should be administered throughout the perioperative period on a scheduled basis.

Table 1

List of Commonly Used Pain Medications in the Perioperative Period for Hip and Knee Arthroplasty in Accelerated Rehabilitation Programs

Class	Example	Administration	Mechanism of Action	Comments
NSAID	Ketorolac	PO/IV/IM	Nonselective COX inhibition	Potent NSAID, limit to several doses
	Ibuprofen	PO	Nonselective COX inhibition	
	Celecoxib	PO	Selective COX-2 inhibition	COX-2 specificity limits gastrointestinal side effects
Opioid	Morphine sulfate	IV/PCA	Opioid receptor modulation	Short-acting
	Fentanyl	IV/PCA	Opioid receptor modulation	Short-acting, less nausea
	Hydromorphone	PO/IV/PCA	Opioid receptor modulation	Potent, less side effects
	Oxycodone	PO	Opioid receptor modulation	Intermediate-acting
	Oxycodone SR	PO	Opioid receptor modulation	Long-acting
NM	Gabapentin	PO	CNS calcium channel modulation	Targets neuropathic pain
	Pregabalin	PO	CNS calcium channel modulation	Targets neuropathic pain
Other	Tylenol	PO	Unknown	
	Tramadol	PO	Unknown	Some opioid agonistic effect

NSAID = nonsteroidal anti-inflammatory drug; NM = neuromodulation; SR = sustained release; CNS = central nervous system; COX = cyclooxygenase; PO = by mouth; IV = intravenous; IM = intramuscular; PCA = Patient-controlled analgesia

Aggressive Postoperative Physical Therapy and Rehabilitation

With optimal preoperative education, preconditioning, surgical technique, anesthesia, and postoperative pain management, total joint arthroplasty patients are primed for accelerated rehabilitation. In this setting, the nursing staff, physical therapists, and members of the social services team are critical in the achievement of the goals of a rapid recovery program. One of the early goals of accelerated rehabilitation is patient mobilization on the day of surgery. The nursing staff may help mobilize the patient to a chair immediately after surgery. Physical therapists assess the patient the day of surgery and immediately help the patient attempt standing and ambulation.

In the ensuing days, the physical therapy team visits the patient several times each day to facilitate quick achievement of milestones such as independent ambulation and stair climbing. It is important to ensure proper hydration to prevent hypotensive episodes, but all tubes and lines should be removed from the patient as soon as the first postoperative day to allow for frequent mobilization. With these measures as well as encouragement, reassurance, and effective pain control, the motivated patient rapidly reaches functional independence.

After completion of the inpatient phase of recovery, most patients are able to return home and transition to a home-based rehabilitation program involving physical therapy and home nursing visits. Although patients occasionally require admission to an inpatient rehabilitation facility, a randomized controlled trial recently demonstrated equal outcomes between inpatient rehabilitation and a home-based program.[42] Although both options should be considered for each patient on an individual basis, the goal of a rapid recovery program should be to return all patients directly home within the first few postoperative days. With recent advancements in accelerated rehabilitation programs, the possibility of outpatient hip and knee arthroplasty has been considered. Although this approach appears safe in select patients,[43,44] it must be kept in mind that most medical complications have been shown to occur in the first few postoperative days.[45]

Summary

Recent advances in postoperative pain management and accelerated rehabilitation have become standard practices in most institutions. Such programs have significant costs, especially in terms of time and effort, but

1: Basic Science and General Knowledge

lead to improved patient satisfaction and cost savings. As discussed, successful accelerated rehabilitation requires interaction of multiple disciplines. Clinical pathway programs are necessary in coordinating the multiple teams and modalities involved. Total joint arthroplasty has provided excellent long-term outcomes and patient satisfaction. Advances in postoperative pain management and accelerated rehabilitation have recently improved the patient experience in the short-term. This success may open the door to improving the quality of life for patients who have refused the intervention because of fear and anxiety associated with significant postoperative pain and extended time to functional recovery.

Annotated References

1. Dorr LD, Chao L: The emotional state of the patient after total hip and knee arthroplasty. *Clin Orthop Relat Res* 2007;463:7-12.

   The authors present a review of the important role that emotional and psychological factors play in the achievement of patient satisfaction after hip and knee arthroplasty. These factors tend to be unrecognized. Level of evidence: V.

2. Del Savio GC, Zelicof SB, Wexler LM, et al: Preoperative nutritional status and outcome of elective total hip replacement. *Clin Orthop Relat Res* 1996;326:153-161.

3. Patel VP, Walsh M, Sehgal B, Preston C, DeWal H, Di Cesare PE: Factors associated with prolonged wound drainage after primary total hip and knee arthroplasty. *J Bone Joint Surg Am* 2007;89(1):33-38.

   The authors explored the risk factors associated with prolonged wound drainage and found that obesity is one of those factors that increases the risk of prolonged drainage, and this was associated with a higher rate of infection. Level of evidence: II.

4. Møller AM, Villebro N, Pedersen T, Tønnesen H: Effect of preoperative smoking intervention on postoperative complications: A randomised clinical trial. *Lancet* 2002;359(9301):114-117.

5. Hejblum G, Atsou K, Dautzenberg B, Chouaid C: Cost-benefit analysis of a simulated institution-based preoperative smoking cessation intervention in patients undergoing total hip and knee arthroplasties in France. *Chest* 2009;135(2):477-483.

   The authors present evidence that the savings resulting from reduced hospital costs and decreased length of hospital stay outweighs the costs of preoperative smoking cessation intervention.

6. Yoon RS, Nellans KW, Geller JA, Kim AD, Jacobs MR, Macaulay W: Patient education before hip or knee arthroplasty lowers length of stay. *J Arthroplasty* 2010;25(4):547-551.

   The authors report that patients who participate in preoperative educational programs have a significant decrease in the length of hospital stay after hip and knee arthroplasty by approximately 1 day.

7. Lee A, Gin T: Educating patients about anaesthesia: Effect of various modes on patients' knowledge, anxiety and satisfaction. *Curr Opin Anaesthesiol* 2005;18(2):205-208.

   The authors review the important role of preoperative patient education regarding anesthesia. The implementation of such a program can reduce patient anxiety and maximize patient satisfaction.

8. Giraudet-Le Quintrec JS, Coste J, Vastel L, et al: Positive effect of patient education for hip surgery: A randomized trial. *Clin Orthop Relat Res* 2003;414:112-120.

9. McGregor AH, Rylands H, Owen A, Doré CJ, Hughes SP: Does preoperative hip rehabilitation advice improve recovery and patient satisfaction? *J Arthroplasty* 2004;19(4):464-468.

   The authors report that preoperative hip rehabilitation education improved the cost and length of stay associated with the procedure. The intervention also leads to higher patient satisfaction and more realistic expectations of surgery.

10. Wang AW, Gilbey HJ, Ackland TR: Perioperative exercise programs improve early return of ambulatory function after total hip arthroplasty: A randomized, controlled trial. *Am J Phys Med Rehabil* 2002;81(11):801-806.

11. Sharma V, Morgan PM, Cheng EY: Factors influencing early rehabilitation after THA: A systematic review. *Clin Orthop Relat Res* 2009;467(6):1400-1411.

    The authors conducted a systematic review of the literature aimed at identifying the factors that influence early rehabilitation after total hip arthroplasty. The authors concluded that preoperative physiotherapy may facilitate faster postoperative recovery, but better studies are needed. Level of evidence: II.

12. Hartrick CT, Martin G, Kantor G, Koncelik J, Manvelian G: Evaluation of a single-dose, extended-release epidural morphine formulation for pain after knee arthroplasty. *J Bone Joint Surg Am* 2006;88(2):273-281.

    The authors evaluated the use of DepoDur in patients with total knee arthroplasty and found that these patients had a threefold decrease in use of postoperative systemic opioids. Nausea, pyrexia, vomiting, pruritus, and hypotension are common. DepoDur is safe and effective for treating pain after total knee arthroplasty with proper patient selection.

13. Hu S, Zhang ZY, Hua YQ, Li J, Cai ZD: A comparison of regional and general anaesthesia for total replacement of the hip or knee: A meta-analysis. *J Bone Joint Surg Br* 2009;91(7):935-942.

    The authors report the result of a meta-analysis comparing regional and general anesthesia for total hip and total knee replacement. Regional anesthesia reduces time for surgery, need for transfusion, and risk of thromboembolic disease.

14. Macfarlane AJ, Prasad GA, Chan VW, Brull R: Does regional anesthesia improve outcome after total knee arthroplasty? *Clin Orthop Relat Res* 2009;467(9): 2379-2402.

   The authors report the results of a systematic review comparing the results of general and regional anesthesia for total knee arthroplasty. Regional anesthesia facilitated rehabilitation, and reduced postoperative pain, morphine consumption, opioid-related adverse effects, and length of hospital stay. Level of evidence: II.

15. Maurer SG, Chen AL, Hiebert R, Pereira GC, Di Cesare PE: Comparison of outcomes of using spinal versus general anesthesia in total hip arthroplasty. *Am J Orthop (Belle Mead NJ)* 2007;36(7):E101-E106.

   The authors conduct a study comparing general and spinal anesthesia for total hip arthroplasty. Spinal anesthesia showed mean reductions of 12% in surgical time, 25% in estimated intraoperative blood loss, 38% in rate of surgical blood loss, and 50% in intraoperative transfusion requirements.

16. Williams-Russo P, Sharrock NE, Haas SB, et al: Randomized trial of epidural versus general anesthesia: Outcomes after primary total knee replacement. *Clin Orthop Relat Res* 1996;331:199-208.

17. Peak EL, Parvizi J, Ciminiello M, et al: The role of patient restrictions in reducing the prevalence of early dislocation following total hip arthroplasty: A randomized, prospective study. *J Bone Joint Surg Am* 2005;87(2):247-253.

   The authors compared the rate of dislocation with and without postoperative hip precautions for the anterolateral approach. They found no difference in the rate of dislocation. The group without restrictions had better sleep, faster return to driving and work, and better overall satisfaction.

18. Khatod M, Barber T, Paxton E, Namba R, Fithian D: An analysis of the risk of hip dislocation with a contemporary total joint registry. *Clin Orthop Relat Res* 2006;447:19-23.

   The authors report the factors that influence the risk of early hip dislocation using a contemporary total joint registry. Patients with a femoral head size of 32 mm or greater had a significantly decreased rate of dislocation compared with those with a size 28-mm head.

19. Malik A, Maheshwari A, Dorr LD: Impingement with total hip replacement. *J Bone Joint Surg Am* 2007; 89(8):1832-1842.

   The authors review the etiology and clinical effects of impingement in total hip arthroplasty. Combined acetabular and femoral anteversion is one of the important factors that determines the impingement-free zone.

20. Kwon MS, Kuskowski M, Mulhall KJ, Macaulay W, Brown TE, Saleh KJ: Does surgical approach affect total hip arthroplasty dislocation rates? *Clin Orthop Relat Res* 2006;447:34-38.

   The authors report the results of a meta-analysis comparing the risk of dislocation with and without a posterior capsular repair for the posterior approach. Posterior repair reduces the risk of dislocation from 4.46% to 0.49%.

21. Wall SJ, Mears SC: Analysis of published evidence on minimally invasive total hip arthroplasty. *J Arthroplasty* 2008;23(7, suppl):55-58.

   The authors perform a systematic review of the literature regarding minimally invasive total hip arthroplasty and report very few high-quality studies regarding the matter. The miniposterior approach was the most studied and was the only technique with evidence based on randomized controlled studies.

22. Ciminiello M, Parvizi J, Sharkey PF, Eslampour A, Rothman RH: Total hip arthroplasty: Is small incision better? *J Arthroplasty* 2006;21(4):484-488.

   The authors report the results of a matched-pair study of the outcome of total hip arthroplasty performed through classic or small incision. There was no difference between the groups in blood loss, analgesia requirement, functional recovery, length of hospital stay, or disposition at discharge.

23. Dorr LD, Maheshwari AV, Long WT, Wan Z, Sirianni LE: Early pain relief and function after posterior minimally invasive and conventional total hip arthroplasty: A prospective, randomized, blinded study. *J Bone Joint Surg Am* 2007;89(6):1153-1160.

   The authors report the results of a prospective, randomized, blinded study comparing the mini-posterior approach with the classic posterior approach. Of interest, the deep dissection was more extensive for the classic approach and the mini-posterior skin incision was enlarged before closure. The mini-posterior group shows better early pain control, earlier discharge to home, and less use of assistive devices. Level of evidence: I.

24. Nakata K, Nishikawa M, Yamamoto K, Hirota S, Yoshikawa H: A clinical comparative study of the direct anterior with mini-posterior approach: Two consecutive series. *J Arthroplasty* 2009;24(5):698-704.

   The authors report the results of a clinical comparison of early outcomes of the direct anterior and mini-posterior approaches. The results suggest more rapid recovery for hip function and gait ability associated with the direct anterior approach.

25. Pour AE, Parvizi J, Sharkey PF, Hozack WJ, Rothman RH: Minimally invasive hip arthroplasty: What role does patient preconditioning play? *J Bone Joint Surg Am* 2007;89(9):1920-1927.

   The authors report the results of a study that shows factors such as patient education, accelerated rehabilitation, and improved pain control improve time of discharge to home, patient satisfaction, and walking abil-

1: Basic Science and General Knowledge

ity at the time of discharge regardless of the size of the incision.

26. Rittmeister M, Callitsis C: Factors influencing cup orientation in 500 consecutive total hip replacements. *Clin Orthop Relat Res* 2006;445:192-196.

The authors report the results of a case series investigating factors that influence acetabular component positioning outside the optimal range. The minimally invasive technique is associated with acetabular component orientation outside this range. Level of evidence: IV.

27. Woolson ST, Pouliot MA, Huddleston JI: Primary total hip arthroplasty using an anterior approach and a fracture table: Short-term results from a community hospital. *J Arthroplasty* 2009;24(7):999-1005.

The authors report the complications and learning curve of the direct anterior approach used by community surgeons compared with that of the innovator of the procedure. There was a sixfold increased rate of major complications and a twofold increased rate of blood loss and surgical time in the hands of the community surgeon.

28. Kolisek FR, Bonutti PM, Hozack WJ, et al: Clinical experience using a minimally invasive surgical approach for total knee arthroplasty: Early results of a prospective randomized study compared to a standard approach. *J Arthroplasty* 2007;22(1):8-13.

The authors report the results of a prospective, randomized, multicenter study to assess the safety and efficacy of small-incision total knee arthroplasty. No differences were found in blood loss or early functional recovery, but there were more wound complications associated with the small-incision group.

29. Huang HT, Su JY, Chang JK, Chen CH, Wang GJ: The early clinical outcome of minimally invasive quadriceps-sparing total knee arthroplasty: Report of a 2-year follow-up. *J Arthroplasty* 2007;22(7):1007-1012.

The authors report a retrospective matched-group comparison of quadriceps-sparing and standard medial parapatellar approaches. There was improved quadriceps strength, range of motion, and pain control in the quadriceps-sparing group, but the greatest benefit was limited to the first 2 postoperative weeks.

30. King J, Stamper DL, Schaad DC, Leopold SS: Minimally invasive total knee arthroplasty compared with traditional total knee arthroplasty: Assessment of the learning curve and the postoperative recuperative period. *J Bone Joint Surg Am* 2007;89(7):1497-1503.

This retrospective investigation comparing standard and quadriceps-sparing total knee replacement finds a shorter hospital stay, higher rate of discharge to home, less narcotic use, and higher rate of ambulation without assistive devices at 2 and 6 weeks after surgery. The authors did not evert the patella or dislocate the tibia in the quadriceps-sparing group.

31. Dalury DF, Mulliken BD, Adams MJ, Lewis C, Sauder RR, Bushey JA: Early recovery after total knee arthroplasty performed with and without patellar eversion and tibial translation: A prospective randomized study. *J Bone Joint Surg Am* 2009;91(6):1339-1343.

The authors report a prospective randomized study investigating the influence of patellar eversion and tibial translation in early functional recovery after total knee arthroplasty. The results showed no difference in range of motion, quadriceps strength, or patient satisfaction at 6 weeks, 12 weeks, or 6 months after the surgery.

32. Maheshwari AV, Boutary M, Yun AG, Sirianni LE, Dorr LD: Multimodal analgesia without routine parenteral narcotics for total hip arthroplasty. *Clin Orthop Relat Res* 2006;453:231-238.

The authors report the evaluation of a multimodal approach to postoperative pain management after total hip arthroplasty with a goal of eliminating parenteral narcotics. They found the approach improved pain, accelerated recovery, and avoided adverse effects.

33. Peters CL, Shirley B, Erickson J: The effect of a new multimodal perioperative anesthetic regimen on postoperative pain, side effects, rehabilitation, and length of hospital stay after total joint arthroplasty. *J Arthroplasty* 2006;21(6, suppl 2):132-138.

The authors report a study of the effects of a multimodal approach to pain management after total hip and total knee arthroplasty. Shortened length of hospital stay, improved pain control, sooner accomplishment of therapy goals, and less narcotic consumption were associated with the approach.

34. Ekman EF, Koman AL: Acute pain following musculoskeletal injuries and orthopaedic surgery. *J Bone Joint Surg Am* 2004;86(6):1316-1327.

The authors provide a comprehensive review of mechanisms and management of acute pain in the realm of orthopaedics.

35. Shum CF, Lo NN, Yeo SJ, Yang KY, Chong HC, Yeo SN: Continuous femoral nerve block in total knee arthroplasty: Immediate and two-year outcomes. *J Arthroplasty* 2009;24(2):204-209.

The authors report a prospective study of the immediate and 2-year outcomes of continuous femoral nerve blocks in total knee arthroplasty. There was less pain, higher satisfaction, and lower morphine use among patients on continuous femoral nerve blocks.

36. Hunt KJ, Bourne MH, Mariani EM: Single-injection femoral and sciatic nerve blocks for pain control after total knee arthroplasty. *J Arthroplasty* 2009;24(4):533-538.

The authors evaluate the effects of adding a single-shot sciatic nerve block to a single-shot femoral nerve block in total knee arthroplasty. There was improved postoperative pain relief and reduced narcotic consumption associated with the addition of a single-shot sciatic nerve block.

37. Marino J, Russo J, Kenny M, Herenstein R, Livote E, Chelly JE: Continuous lumbar plexus block for postoperative pain control after total hip arthroplasty: A randomized controlled trial. *J Bone Joint Surg Am* 2009;91(1):29-37.

The authors investigated the outcomes of the use of a continuous lumbar plexus block for postoperative pain control after total hip arthroplasty compared with a continuous femoral nerve block and patient-controlled intravenous narcotics. The authors found that continuous lumbar plexus blocks reduced the need for opioids and avoided related adverse effects more so than femoral nerve blocks.

38. Parvataneni HK, Shah VP, Howard H, Cole N, Ranawat AS, Ranawat CS: Controlling pain after total hip and knee arthroplasty using a multimodal protocol with local periarticular injections: A prospective randomized study. *J Arthroplasty* 2007;22(6, suppl 2):33-38.

The authors report the results of a prospective randomized study of the benefits of local periarticular injections in total hip and knee arthroplasty. This modality improves pain control and functional recovery.

39. Busch CA, Shore BJ, Bhandari R, et al: Efficacy of periarticular multimodal drug injection in total knee arthroplasty: A randomized trial. *J Bone Joint Surg Am* 2006;88(5):959-963.

The authors report the results of a randomized study of the efficacy of periarticular multimodal injections in total knee arthroplasty. They found that the injections significantly reduce the requirements for patient-controlled analgesia and improve patient satisfaction.

40. Buvanendran A, Kroin JS, Tuman KJ, et al: Effects of perioperative administration of a selective cyclooxygenase 2 inhibitor on pain management and recovery of function after knee replacement: A randomized controlled trial. *JAMA* 2003;290(18):2411-2418.

41. Mallory TH, Lombardi AV Jr, Fada RA, Dodds KL, Adams JB: Pain management for joint arthroplasty: Preemptive analgesia. *J Arthroplasty* 2002;17(4, suppl 1):129-133.

42. Mahomed NN, Davis AM, Hawker G, et al: Inpatient compared with home-based rehabilitation following primary unilateral total hip or knee replacement: A randomized controlled trial. *J Bone Joint Surg Am* 2008;90(8):1673-1680.

The authors report a randomized controlled trial comparing home-based and inpatient rehabilitation programs after total hip and total knee arthroplasty. They found no difference in pain, functional outcomes, or patient satisfaction between the groups and therefore recommended the home-based program.

43. Berger RA, Kusuma SK, Sanders SA, Thill ES, Sporer SM: The feasibility and perioperative complications of outpatient knee arthroplasty. *Clin Orthop Relat Res* 2009;467(6):1443-1449.

The authors investigate the feasibility of and complications associated with outpatient total knee arthroplasty. Of patients who had surgery completed by noon and agreed to consider discharge the day of surgery, 94% were successful. They have no deaths and no pulmonary or cardiac complications. Level of evidence: IV.

44. Dorr LD, Thomas DJ, Zhu J, Dastane M, Chao L, Long WT: Outpatient total hip arthroplasty. *J Arthroplasty* 2010;25(4):501-506.

The authors investigate the possibility of outpatient total hip arthroplasty with a rapid recovery program. Of patients younger than 65 years who chose to enroll, 77% went home the day of surgery. The patients were followed for 6 months with no reported complications. The authors concluded that the approach is safe in select patients.

45. Parvizi J, Mui A, Purtill JJ, Sharkey PF, Hozack WJ, Rothman RH: Total joint arthroplasty: When do fatal or near-fatal complications occur? *J Bone Joint Surg Am* 2007;89(1):27-32.

The authors investigated the timing of major complications after total hip and knee arthroplasty and found that most occur within the timeframe of typical inpatient admission.

Section 2

Knee

SECTION EDITOR:
PAUL F. LACHIEWICZ, MD

Chapter 7

Biomechanics of the Knee and Total Knee Arthroplasty

Guoan Li, PhD   Hany S. Bedair, MD   Michal Kozanek, MD   Kartik M. Varadarajan, BTech, MS
Harry E. Rubash, MD

Introduction

The success of total knee arthroplasty (TKA) depends to a large extent on the understanding of biomechanical principles of both the normal and TKA knee. New developments and discoveries in biomechanics of knee arthroplasty over the past 5 years include characterization of knee forces in vivo; biomechanics of high-flexion, partial knee replacement designs; and sex-specific differences.

Forces Within the Knee Joint During Dynamic Weight-Bearing Activities

Until recently, in vivo tibiofemoral contact forces could only be estimated via inverse dynamic optimization-based computational models. A fairly in-depth description of this technique was presented in the previous edition of this book. Estimates of knee joint forces based on these analytical methods have varied anywhere from three to six times body weight (BW) depending on the structuring of the mathematical model and the simulated activity.[1] However, direct measurement of these forces in vivo has now become possible with the development of instrumented knee prostheses. The authors of a 2006 study reported on the first in vivo measurement of axial tibiofemoral forces using an instrumented tibial implant.[1] Peak axial forces ranging from 2.0 times BW during chair sitting-standing to 3.5 times BW during stair climbing were reported using this prosthesis in one TKA patient.[1,2] Peak force during walking was measured to be 2.5 times BW.[2] This implant was also used to determine medial-to-lateral axial force ratio during

Dr. Bedair or an immediate family member has received research or institutional support from Zimmer. Dr. Rubash or an immediate family member has received research or institutional support from Zimmer. None of the following authors or any immediate family member has received anything of value from or owns stock in a commercial company or institution related directly or indirectly to the subject of this chapter: Dr. Li, Dr. Kozanek, and Dr. Varadarajan.

different activities, and reported values ranged from 0.7 (golf swing) to 2.7 (squatting), with most activities showing more load on the medial compartment.[2]

A limitation of the first generation of the implant was that it did not allow for measurement of anteroposterior and mediolateral shear forces and axial moments. This was because of the use of only four axial load cells positioned at four quadrants of the tibial tray. The capability of measuring all force/moment components was added in a subsequent version of the instrumented prosthesis that incorporated 12 strain gauges, albeit at the expense of the ability to directly determine medial-lateral load distribution.[3] Net forces (axial and shear forces combined) measured using this prosthesis ranged from 1.9 times BW during chair sitting-standing to 3.0 times BW during stair climbing.[3,4] However, contribution of shear forces to the net contact force was limited, with peak values ranging from 0.13 times BW during single-leg lunge to 0.3 times BW during walking.[3,4] Peak flexion and adduction moments measured at the tibial tray using the instrumented prosthesis (1.7% to 1.9% BW x height (Ht) and 1.1% to 1.3% BW x Ht) were also small compared with the external peak flexion and adduction moments computed using motion analysis (4.3% to 5.7% BW x Ht and 1.8% to 3.4% BW x Ht).[3]

This second generation of the implant was also combined with a dynamic dual plane fluoroscopy technique to determine the tibiofemoral contact locations simultaneously with the measurement of the contact forces.[4] The motivation for doing this was to understand the link between tibiofemoral kinematics and the resulting contact forces, and to determine the distribution of the axial forces between the medial and lateral compartments, which could not be directly measured using this version of the implant. During single-leg lunge and chair rising or sitting, the center of pressure (CoP) moved along anteroposterior and mediolateral directions with knee flexion and extension, as did the tibiofemoral contact points[4] (Figure 1). Additionally, equal mediolateral axial force distribution was associated with minimal mediolateral shifts in tibiofemoral contact locations. However, a nonuniform mediolateral axial force distribution, with greater load on the lateral

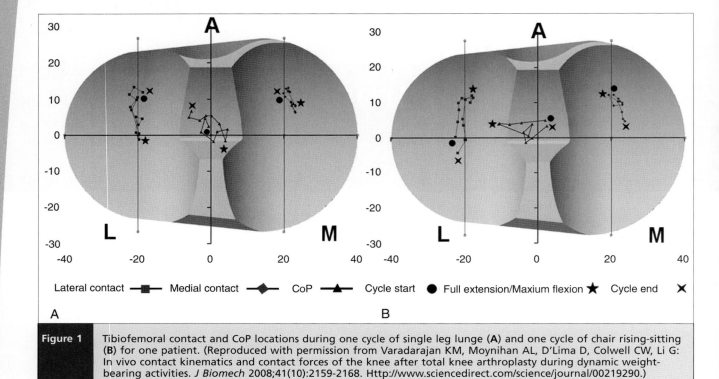

| Lateral contact | ■ | Medial contact | ◆ | CoP | ▲ | Cycle start | ● | Full extension/Maxium flexion | ★ | Cycle end | ✕ |

A   B

Figure 1 Tibiofemoral contact and CoP locations during one cycle of single leg lunge (**A**) and one cycle of chair rising-sitting (**B**) for one patient. (Reproduced with permission from Varadarajan KM, Moynihan AL, D'Lima D, Colwell CW, Li G: In vivo contact kinematics and contact forces of the knee after total knee arthroplasty during dynamic weight-bearing activities. *J Biomech* 2008;41(10):2159-2168. Http://www.sciencedirect.com/science/journal/00219290.)

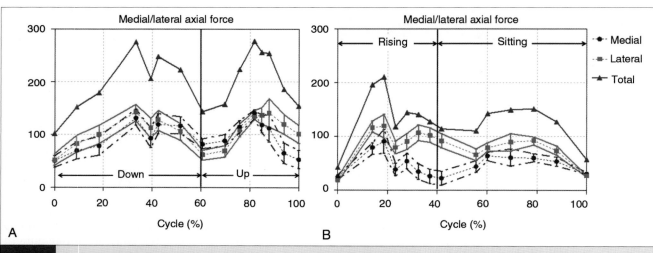

Figure 2 Distribution of axial force on medial and lateral compartments for one patient during one cycle of single-leg lunge (**A**) and one cycle of chair rising-sitting (**B**). The bars and the lines passing through the ends of the bars represent the upper and lower bounds on the estimates of the medial/lateral contact forces. (Reproduced with permission from Varadarajan KM, Moynihan AL, D'Lima D, Colwell CW, Li G: In vivo contact kinematics and contact forces of the knee after total knee arthroplasty during dynamic weight-bearing activities. *J Biomech* 2008;41(10):2159-2168. Http://www.sciencedirect.com/science/journal/00219290.)

compartment, was associated with erratic mediolateral shifts of the lateral contact points. Regarding mediolateral load distribution during different activities, nearly equitable mediolateral force distributions were noted during a single-leg lunge (Figure 2, *A*). However, during the chair activity, higher forces were seen on the lateral compartment (Figure 2, *B*).

High Flexion After TKA

Factors Limiting High Flexion After TKA

Knee flexion is integral to function in many situations of everyday life, and the amount of flexion after TKA has been directly correlated with functional outcome. The human knee is capable of flexion up to 160°. Although most activities occur at flexion angles less than 60°, there are many activities of daily living for which knee flexion near or beyond 90° is necessary; for example, ascending and descending stairs (90°), getting in and out of a vehicle (110°), and climbing out of a bathtub (135°). Kneeling requires more than 140° of flexion. Unfortunately, knee flexion after contemporary TKA rarely exceeds 115°.[5] Initial experiences with the cruciate-sacrificing total condylar prostheses had knee flexion limits ranging from 90° to 95°. During the 30-year evolutionary process of TKA, improved flexion has been achieved with posterior-stabilized as well as posterior cruciate ligament (PCL)–retaining prostheses. A literature review revealed that mean flexion of 100° to 115° is achieved with both TKA designs.[5] Hence, the current prosthetic designs and surgical techniques may not be sufficient to meet the needs of patients who require deep knee flexion for daily activities.

The factors influencing range of motion after TKA can be classified into three major groups.

Preoperative Factors
Although factors such as preoperative diagnosis, degree of deformity, age, sex, and body mass index are important predictors influencing the postoperative range of motion, it is widely agreed that the most important factor in attaining postoperative motion is the patient's preoperative range of motion. Poor long-standing preoperative range of motion may result in tissue changes about the knee such as bony structural changes, periarticular soft-tissue fibrosis, and extensor mechanism stiffness that may lead to limitations to motion.[6] Posterior soft-tissue impingement in obese legs can also limit flexion.

Intraoperative Factors
The most crucial element in restoring kinematic function is creating a well-balanced knee with symmetric and rectangular flexion and extension gaps. Range of motion in flexion may be compromised by an insufficient flexion gap. As the knee flexes, the PCL tightens and this may effectively decrease the dimensions of the flexion gap in cruciate-retaining designs. Therefore, when the PCL is retained, its recession has been suggested to obtain sufficient flexion gap to avoid decreased range of motion. Use of a PCL-substituting design may allow the surgeon to consistently attain a larger and more predictable flexion gap (6 to 8 mm) as the flexion gap increases after PCL removal. A larger flexion gap may translate into improved flexion, but this flexion gap is limited by the tibial post height (to avoid a "jumped post" dislocation wherein the tibial post dislocates out of the femoral box) and also must be balanced with an appropriate extension gap, otherwise laxity in extension and recurvatum will occur. The extensor mechanism is another structure affecting knee flexion. Patella baja will lead to early impingement of the patella on the anterior aspect of the tibial component and will limit flexion.[7] Overhanging osteophytes of the femur and tibia are an additional factor requiring attention; for example, posterior osteophytes cause early posterior impingement and may inhibit full flexion. Finally, component positioning and sizing also may influence knee range of motion. Adequate posterior slope of the tibial component (most current TKA systems use 3° to 7° of posterior slope) may result in a greater range of flexion in some designs, and restoring the posterior femoral condyle offset is critical in reducing posterior femoral shaft impingement on the posterior tibia.

Postoperative Factors
Rehabilitation plays a significant role in achieving deep knee flexion. Despite excellent surgical technique, postoperative soft-tissue contracture can occur, which limits motion. An aggressive rehabilitation protocol accompanied by adequate pain control is necessary to optimize postoperative results.[5] The use of continuous passive motion devices is controversial but may improve ultimate motion.[8]

Biomechanics of High-Flexion TKA
At high knee flexion, the posterior tibial plateau contacts the most proximal aspect of the posterior femoral condyles. In the intact knee, the posterior femoral condylar offset and the menisci, particularly on the lateral side, provide an extended surface that allows rollback of the femoral condyle over the tibia in a stable manner at high knee flexion. However, because the menisci, the anterior cruciate ligament (ACL), and in some designs the PCL are removed in arthroplasty surgery, TKA may not restore the tibiofemoral contact characteristics observed in the native knee. Edge loading at high-flexion angles after TKA may become more dominant, potentially increasing wear at high flexion.

Several recent TKA designs incorporate modifications of various geometric features of existing TKAs to improve range of motion. Some of the motivation for these modifications is to prevent edge loading on the posterior tibial articular surface and increase the tibiofemoral contact area at high degrees of flexion, thus reducing contact stresses. Several such TKA designs have been introduced into the market, each having specific features aimed at improving knee biomechanics at high-flexion angles. These features include proximal/anterior extension of the articulating portion of posterior femoral condyles to provide greater arc of flexion without high-contact stresses (Figure 3); anterior cutout of the tibial polyethylene liner to provide greater clearance for the patella; modified cam-post mechanism in posterior stabilized implants to increase the posterior femoral translation at high flexion; smaller posterior femoral condylar radius; and increased posterior tibial slope to enhance femoral rollback.

The biomechanical research of the past 5 years has focused on investigating whether the theoretic rationales behind the high-flexion TKA designs translate into improved biomechanical performance.[9-15] Using an in vitro robotic experimental setup, a high-flexion

2: Knee

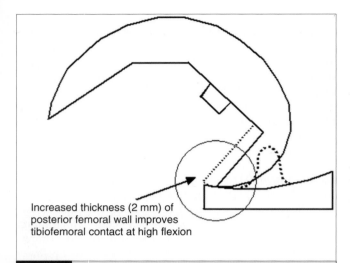

Figure 3 Difference in the sagittal profile of the NexGen (Zimmer, Warsaw, IN) conventional and high-flexion designs. By removing an additional 2 mm of posterior femoral condyles, smooth curvature is maintained at high degrees of flexion. (Reproduced with permission from Li G, Most E, Sultan PG, et al: Knee kinematics with a high-flexion posterior stabilized total knee prosthesis: An in vitro robotic experimental investigation. *J Bone Joint Surg Am* 2004;86(8):1721-1729.)

cruciate-retaining knee was compared with the conventional cruciate-retaining design and with the intact knee in terms of kinematics and PCL force.[14] It was found that both cruciate-retaining TKA designs showed similar kinematics throughout the flexion arc from 0° to 150° (Figure 4). Both tested designs restored approximately 80% of the posterior femoral translation of the intact knee at 150°, with minor differences beyond 150°. The PCL force measured in the high-flexion TKA showed similar patterns to those observed in the intact knee. It is of interest that the PCL force was minimal at low-flexion angles, maximal at 90°, and decreased beyond 90°. This finding underlines the importance of the PCL in the 90° flexion range but perhaps not at high flexion angles.

The fundamental mechanisms that limit further flexion of the knee beyond 120° after TKA have not been clearly identified. It has been suggested that insufficient PCL tension might limit range of knee flexion due to a reduction in posterior femoral translation because it has been shown that below 120°, increases in PCL force coincided with increases in posterior femoral translation.[16] However, at high knee flexion angles, despite the low PCL force in the cruciate-retaining–flexion TKA, posterior femoral translation continued to rise, and almost 80% of intact knee kinematics was restored. The enhanced posterior femoral translation beyond 120°

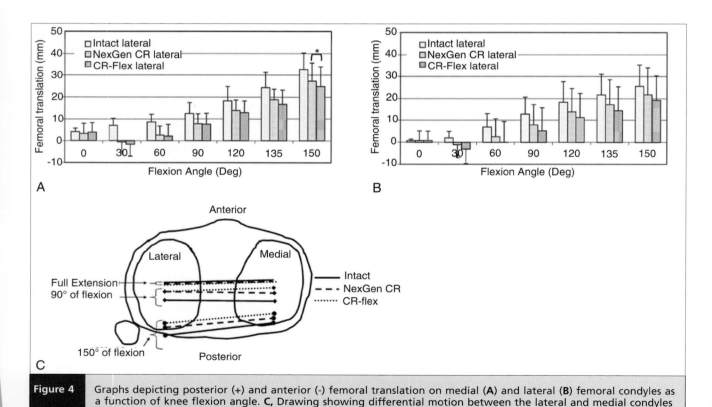

Figure 4 Graphs depicting posterior (+) and anterior (-) femoral translation on medial (**A**) and lateral (**B**) femoral condyles as a function of knee flexion angle. **C,** Drawing showing differential motion between the lateral and medial condyles at selected flexion angles, signifying internal tibial rotation or external femoral rotation with knee flexion. (Reproduced with permission from Most E, Li G, Sultan PG, Park SE, Rubash HE: Kinematic analysis of conventional and high-flexion cruciate-retaining total knee arthroplasties: An in vitro investigation. *J Arthroplasty* 2005;20(4): 529-535. Http://www.sciencedirect.com/science/journal/08835403.)

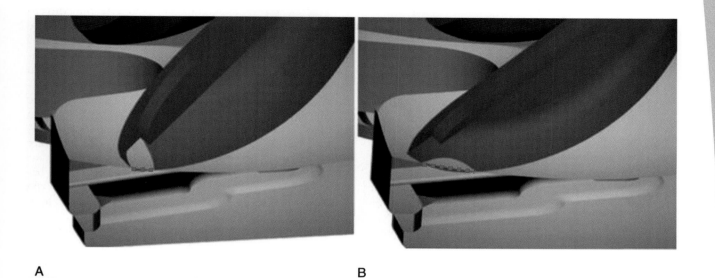

A   B

Figure 5 Cross sections of the tibiofemoral articulation at 130° of flexion in conventional (**A**) and high-flexion (**B**) TKAs. The high-flexion design shows greater contact area between the femoral component and polyethylene (*dotted lines*), while the conventional design has the edge of the posterior femoral condyle contacting the tibial insert. (Reproduced with permission from Suggs JF, Kwon YM, Durbhakula SM, Hanson GR, Li G: In vivo flexion and kinematics of the knee after TKA: Comparison of a conventional and a high flexion cruciate-retaining TKA design. *Knee Surg Sports Traumatol Arthrosc* 2009;17(2):150-156.)

may be caused by the compression of posterior soft tissues between the tibial and femoral shafts, which translates the tibia anteriorly and the femur posteriorly.

With increased posterior femoral translation, the tibiofemoral articular contact tends to reach the posterior edge of the tibial component, which often has an upslope, and may theoretically lead to stress exceeding the known limits of the polyethylene.[17] A subsequent in vitro investigation of tibiofemoral contact behavior revealed earlier posterior edge loading in conventional cruciate-retaining TKA compared with the high-flexion design. At 150°, both designs reached the posterior edge of the polyethylene liner.[13] The in vitro findings have recently been corroborated by in vivo kinematic investigation using the dual fluoroscopic system.[9] No significant difference between the two designs was found in posterior femoral translation; however, at flexion angles greater than 120°, the high-flexion design was more conforming with increased contact area and smaller stress concentrations at the posterior aspect of the polyethylene liner (Figure 5). These data suggest that the high-flexion component may improve contact mechanics and decrease polyethylene stress in patients who can achieve higher flexion, but cannot create higher flexion in a patient.

With regard to the posterior-stabilized, high-flexion TKA, an in vitro study found that it restored 90% of the posterior femoral translation of the intact knee.[12] In addition, it was found that the cam-spine mechanism enhanced posterior femoral translation only at flexion ranges from 90° to 135°. However, despite the absence of cam-spine engagement, the femur continued to

translate posteriorly at high-flexion angles. Again, this is possibly due to compression of the posterior soft tissues translating the tibia anteriorly relative to the femur (Figure 6). The conventional posterior-stabilized TKA was also found to have the cam-spine mechanism engaged at 60° to 90°. However, the posterior femoral translation only reached 60% of the intact knee level.[18]

Partial Joint Arthroplasty
Recently, there has been a renewed interest in partial knee replacements, including unicompartmental and patellofemoral arthroplasties. The attractive theoretic benefits of partial knee replacement over TKA include the replacement of only the diseased compartment, a less invasive procedure, less bone resection, preservation of both cruciate ligaments, increased postoperative range of motion, preserved proprioception resulting in more normal gait, and faster recovery. Unfortunately, knowledge of partial knee replacement biomechanics has been limited to a few studies mostly done in vitro.

Unicompartmental Knee Arthroplasty
Unicompartmental knee arthroplasty (UKA) has the advantage of preserving both cruciate ligaments. From a biomechanical standpoint this should provide for motion that is more similar to that of an intact knee. The role of the ACL in the anteroposterior stability of the knee after UKA was investigated in vitro using a robotic setup.[19] Anteroposterior stability of the knee after UKA with an intact ACL is similar to that of the native knee, but a UKA in the face of ACL deficiency more than doubles the anteroposterior laxity of the knee un-

2: Knee

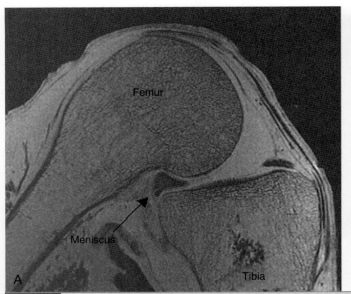
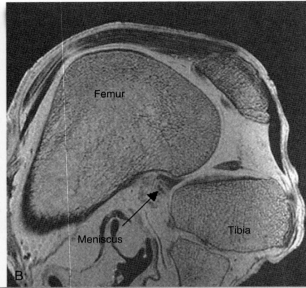

Figure 6 T2-weighted sagittal MRIs with the knee at 150° of flexion showing the articular contact at the medial (**A**) and lateral (**B**) compartments. The menisci help to maintain articular congruency and allow for high flexion to occur. (Reproduced with permission from Li G, Most E, Sultan PG, et al: Knee kinematics with a high-flexion posterior stabilized total knee prosthesis: An in vitro robotic experimental investigation. *J Bone Joint Surg Am* 2004;86(8):1721-1729.)

der anterior tibial load (Figure 7). The ACL-deficient knee after UKA behaved slightly more like the ACL-deficient knee after medial meniscectomy. The fact that the forces in the ACL after UKA are similar to the forces in the ACL of the native knee implies that the ACL plays a role in the knee after UKA similar to the role it plays in the native knee. Moreover, in concert with patients with ACL-deficient native knees, patients with UKA performed in an ACL-deficient knee may report instability. It is important to note that, for the ACL to function after UKA, the surgery must not change the tension in the ACL by altering the flexion and extension gaps. If the implant does not fill or if it overfills the joint space, the ligament tension will be altered and it will not function properly. Although studies have shown that most of the degeneration caused by ACL deficiency takes place in the medial compartment, there is also substantial degeneration that takes place in the lateral and patellofemoral compartments in an ACL-deficient native knee.[20] Because the ACL-deficient UKA displays kinematics similar to that of the ACL-deficient native knee, it seems that the risk of articular degeneration in the lateral and patellofemoral compartments may be increased by the ACL-deficient UKA, but this theory has not been validated.

Patellofemoral Arthroplasty

To date, little is known about the biomechanical performance of current patellofemoral replacement designs. Four patellofemoral replacement designs available in the United Kingdom were compared in vitro in terms of biomechanical parameters, including articular geometry, stability, and tracking.[21] This study showed that al-

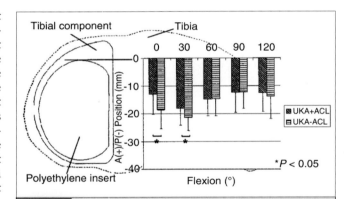

Figure 7 Location of the articular contact was referenced to the anterior edge of the polyethylene insert. Upon transection of the ACL the articular contact moved further posteriorly. (Reproduced with permission from Suggs JF, Li G, Park SE, Sultan PG, Rubash HE, Freiberg AA: Knee biomechanics after UKA and its relation to the ACL: A robotic investigation. *J Orthop Res* 2006;24(4):588-594.)

though most parameters returned within normal limits, problems such as erratic subluxation may occur if the patellar component catches on the edge of the femoral component during flexion-extension of the knee. A subsequent in vivo fluoroscopic analysis showed no difference in sagittal plane patellofemoral kinematics between operated and intact knees of patients undergoing patellofemoral arthroplasty.[22] Certainly, additional biomechanical studies are warranted.

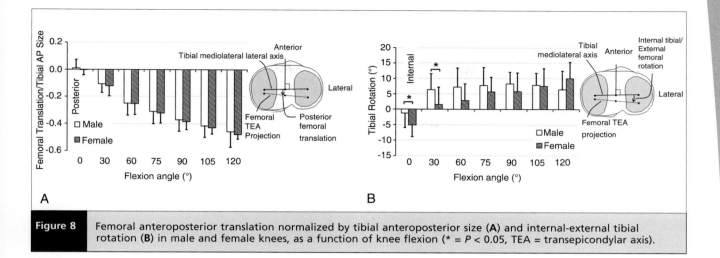

Figure 8   Femoral anteroposterior translation normalized by tibial anteroposterior size (**A**) and internal-external tibial rotation (**B**) in male and female knees, as a function of knee flexion (* = $P < 0.05$, TEA = transepicondylar axis).

Differences Between Male and Female Knee Biomechanics: Myth or Reality?

The question of differences between male and female knee biomechanics has generated much controversy recently,[23] stemming primarily from proposals for sex-specific TKA implants based on three specific anatomic characteristics of female knees:[24] reduced mediolateral to anteroposterior femoral aspect ratio; greater quadriceps (Q) angle; and less prominent anterior femoral condyles. The Q angle has been reported to be 3° to 6° larger in females than in males.[24] One manufacturer has attempted to address this difference by modifying the TKA trochlea to be oriented more laterally for females.[25] However, at least one study has shown that the differences in Q angle disappear if the individual's height is accounted for; that is, shorter people have a larger Q angle, whether male or female.[24] Additionally, there is no evidence to suggest that the trochlear groove in females is actually oriented more laterally. The natural trochlea has an overall medial orientation, while current TKA designs have a laterally oriented trochlea.[26] Female knees also have slightly smaller anterior femoral condyle height (1.1 to 1.7 mm smaller for the medial condyle and 0.5 to 1.5 mm for the lateral condyle). However, even this difference disappears or is further reduced when the smaller size of the female knee is taken into account. A recent review article concluded that among all of these factors only the mediolateral to anteroposterior aspect ratio has been consistently reported to be different between the genders.[24] The mediolateral to anteroposterior aspect ratio has been reported to be in the range of 1.12 to 1.27 for males, and in the range of 1.09 to 1.22 for females.[27] This difference in aspect ratio may warrant a greater range of implant sizes but not necessarily sex-specific implant systems.[23,24]

The focus of most studies relating to male or female sex has been primarily on knee anatomy, but the differences between male and female knee kinematics has not been clearly delineated. However, recent studies have compared the tibiofemoral kinematics,[28] patellar tracking, and patellar tendon orientations[29] in male and female knees using a combination of MRI and dual plane fluoroscopy.

Measurement of tibiofemoral kinematics during a weight-bearing knee flexion activity showed no significant sex differences for femoral anteroposterior and mediolateral translations measured relative to tibia and normalized by tibial anteroposterior or mediolateral size (Figure 8, A). Varus-valgus rotations were also not significantly different between males and females. However, female knees showed significantly greater external tibial rotation at 0° (−5.4° ± 3.6° versus −1.3° ± 4.7°) and smaller internal rotation at 30° flexion (1.7° ± 5.4° versus 6.4° ± 5.2°, Figure 8, B). Females had significantly greater range of tibial rotation (18.2° ± 5.8° versus 12.4° ± 4.1°). Regarding the range of knee motion between 0° and 120° of flexion, there was no significant difference between males and females in the range of anteroposterior translation, mediolateral translation, or varus-valgus rotation.

The tibiofemoral and patellofemoral compartments of the knee joint are closely related through the action of the extensor mechanism. Therefore, based on the differences in the rotational kinematics of the tibiofemoral joint, it was hypothesized that potential sex-related differences in patellar tracking may also exist, particularly through the action of the patellar tendon.[29] A subsequent study conducted to investigate this hypothesis found no significant differences between the patellar tracking parameters of male and female knees.[30] These parameters included patellar anteroposterior, mediolateral, and proximal-distal translations (measured relative to the femur) as well as patellar flexion, tilt, and rotation (Figure 9). However, patellar tendon orientation in sagittal, coronal, and transverse planes was significantly different in males and females. Females showed more anterior patellar tendon orientation in the sagittal plane, particularly at low-flexion angles (Figure 10, A). The average difference in the sagittal plane angle of the female and male patellar tendon

2: Knee

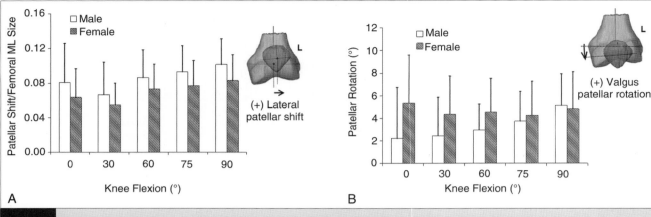

Figure 9 Patellar mediolateral (ML) translation normalized by femoral ML size (**A**) and patellar rotation (**B**) in male and female knees as a function of knee flexion. (Reproduced with permission from Varadarajan KM, Gill TJ, Freiberg AA, Rubash HE, Li G: Patellar tendon orientation and patellar tracking in male and female knees. *J Orthop Res* 2010;28(3):322-328.)

ranged from 4.4° at 0° flexion to 1.3° at 75° flexion. In the coronal plane, all three portions of the patellar tendon were oriented more medially in female knees, with the average difference in orientation ranging from 6.7° at 0° flexion to 2.0° at 75° flexion (Figure 10, *B*). Additionally, female knees also showed greater external tilting of the patellar tendon (Figure 10, *C*), with the average difference in the patellar tendon tilt between males and female knees ranging from 6.6° at 0° flexion to 3.3° at 75° flexion. Another interesting finding from this work was that patellar tendon orientations in the coronal and transverse planes were closely correlated to the tibiofemoral rotation. Based on these results, the authors concluded that there are distinct differences in tibial rotations between male and female knees, which are also associated with differences in patellar tendon orientation. However, the patella itself is effectively constrained with the trochlear groove, which has similar geometries in males and females, and consequently no sex differences in patellar tracking were noted. The increased external tibial rotation and the resultant lateral pull of the patellar tendon could increase contact pressure on the lateral patellofemoral facet in female knees. However, this remains to be investigated.

Summary

The biomechanical research in knee arthroplasty has focused mostly on the following issues: investigation of contact forces after TKA in vivo, issues with high flexion after TKA, evaluation and improvement of partial knee replacement designs such as unicondylar and patellofemoral replacement, and differences between male and female knees. The current literature indicates promising results even though many of these issues remain unresolved. The availability of in vivo joint force data should enable more accurate reproduction of in vivo loads and articular motion patterns in wear simu-

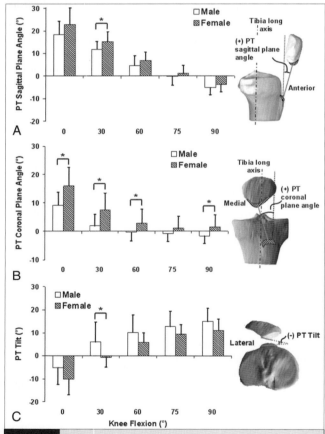

Figure 10 Sagittal plane angle (**A**) and coronal plane angle (**B**) of the central portion of the patellar tendon (PT) and PT tilt (**C**) in male and female knees as a function of knee flexion (* = *P* < 0.05). (Reproduced with permission from Varadarajan KM, Gill TJ, Freiberg AA, Rubash HE, Li G: Patellar tendon orientation and patellar tracking in male and female knees. *J Orthop Res* 2010;28(3):322-328.)

2: Knee

lators, and more accurate computational knee models. The high-flexion TKA designs have been shown to provide biomechanical advantages in terms of improved articular contact at high flexion in patients who can achieve high flexion. The high-flexion TKA, however, does not provide for greater range of motion than a conventional design. Significant progress has also been made in the partial knee replacement designs, and many studies have shown them to be biomechanically comparable to the intact knee. Regarding sex-related differences, the consensus is toward greater range of implant sizes but not necessarily sex-specific implant systems. Few differences in male and female knee kinematics have been discovered and appear to be subtle compared with differences in biomechanics of current TKA systems and the average normal knee.

Annotated References

1. D'Lima DD, Patil S, Steklov N, Slamin JE, Colwell CW Jr: Tibial forces measured in vivo after total knee arthroplasty. *J Arthroplasty* 2006;21(2):255-262.

   The first instrumented prosthesis to measure in vivo tibiofemoral contact forces has been developed. Maximum compressive force of 2.2 times BW during walking and 2.5 times BW during stair climbing were measured in one TKA patient.

2. Mündermann A, Dyrby CO, D'Lima DD, Colwell CW Jr, Andriacchi TP: In vivo knee loading characteristics during activities of daily living as measured by an instrumented total knee replacement. *J Orthop Res* 2008;26(9):1167-1172.

   An instrumented prosthesis was used to measure tibiofemoral joint force during walking, chair rising-sitting, stair ascent-descent, squatting, and golf swings. Total compressive load was highest during stair ascent-descent and lowest during chair rising, and most activities placed a greater load on the medial compartment.

3. D'Lima DD, Patil S, Steklov N, Chien S, Colwell CW Jr: In vivo knee moments and shear after total knee arthroplasty. *J Biomech* 2007;40(suppl 1):S11-S17.

   A second-generation instrumented implant was used to measure all six components of tibiofemoral contact force in one TKA patient during walking, stair climbing, chair-rise and squatting. Peak axial and shear forces ranged from 2.1 to 3.0 times BW and 0.15 to 0.3 times BW, respectively.

4. Varadarajan KM, Moynihan AL, D'Lima D, Colwell CW, Li G: In vivo contact kinematics and contact forces of the knee after total knee arthroplasty during dynamic weight-bearing activities. *J Biomech* 2008;41(10):2159-2168.

   Tibiofemoral contact forces and contact kinematics were measured in three TKA patients. Average axial forces were higher for lunge compared with chair rising-sitting (2.2 versus 1.9 times BW). Peak anteroposterior/mediolateral shear forces averaged 0.13 times BW during lunge and 0.18% BW during chair rising-sitting.

5. Sultan PG, Most E, Schule S, Li G, Rubash HE: Optimizing flexion after total knee arthroplasty: Advances in prosthetic design. *Clin Orthop Relat Res* 2003;416:167-173.

6. Gandhi R, de Beer J, Leone J, Petruccelli D, Winemaker M, Adili A: Predictive risk factors for stiff knees in total knee arthroplasty. *J Arthroplasty* 2006;21(1):46-52.

   This retrospective review of 1,216 primary TKAs evaluated incidence and predictors of arthrofibrosis, defined as flexion less than 90° 1 year after TKA. Preoperative and postoperative relative decreased patellar height and postoperative stiffness were significantly correlated.

7. Maeno S, Kondo M, Niki Y, Matsumoto H: Patellar impingement against the tibial component after total knee arthroplasty. *Clin Orthop Relat Res* 2006;452:265-269.

   Patella baja developed in seven knees in five patients after posterior stabilized TKAs when the patella became impinged against the tibial component.

8. Leach W, Reid J, Murphy F: Continuous passive motion following total knee replacement: A prospective randomized trial with follow-up to 1 year. *Knee Surg Sports Traumatol Arthrosc* 2006;14(10):922-926.

   The authors present a prospective, randomized, single-blind clinical trial to investigate the effect of continuous passive motion on range of knee flexion, lack of extension, pain levels, and analgesic use after total knee replacement surgery. The results substantiate previous findings that short duration, continuous passive motion following TKA does not influence outcome of range of motion or reported pain.

9. Suggs JF, Kwon YM, Durbhakula SM, Hanson GR, Li G: In vivo flexion and kinematics of the knee after TKA: Comparison of a conventional and a high flexion cruciate-retaining TKA design. *Knee Surg Sports Traumatol Arthrosc* 2009;17(2):150-156.

   This study used a dual fluoroscopic system to investigate the six degrees of freedom knee kinematics and tibiofemoral contact in a high-flexion and conventional cruciate-retaining TKA. Both designs produced similar results; however, the use of a high-flexion component improved the tibiofemoral contact environment in patients who could achieve high flexion.

10. Suggs JF, Hanson GR, Park SE, Moynihan AL, Li G: Patient function after a posterior stabilizing total knee arthroplasty: Cam-post engagement and knee kinematics. *Knee Surg Sports Traumatol Arthrosc* 2008;16(3):290-296.

    An in vivo investigation of tibiofemoral kinematics and cam-post engagement during weight-bearing flexion of the knee using a dual fluoroscopic system is presented. It was found that the cam-post engagement corresponded to increased posterior femoral transla-

2: Knee

tion and reduced internal tibial rotation at high flexion. The authors concluded that later cam-post engagement might indicate an environment conducive to greater flexion.

11. Li G, Suggs J, Hanson G, Durbhakula S, Johnson T, Freiberg A: Three-dimensional tibiofemoral articular contact kinematics of a cruciate-retaining total knee arthroplasty. *J Bone Joint Surg Am* 2006;88(2):395-402.

    This study describes the in vivo articular contact kinematics in a cruciate-retaining TKA in nine patients using a dual fluoroscopic system. The current component design did not allow the femoral condyle to roll off the polyethylene edge at high flexion because of the geometry of the posterior lip.

12. Li G, Most E, Sultan PG, et al: Knee kinematics with a high-flexion posterior stabilized total knee prosthesis: An in vitro robotic experimental investigation. *J Bone Joint Surg Am* 2004;86(8):1721-1729.

13. Most E, Sultan PG, Park SE, Papannagari R, Li G: Tibiofemoral contact behavior is improved in high-flexion cruciate retaining TKA. *Clin Orthop Relat Res* 2006;452:59-64.

    This study compared the articular contact characteristics of the high-flexion and conventional cruciate-retaining TKA. The authors reported that articular contact on the conventional TKA reached the posterior edge of the polyethylene liner 15° to 30° earlier than the high-flexion design. It was concluded that the high-flexion design can mechanically better accommodate high flexion in patients who can achieve high flexion.

14. Most E, Li G, Sultan PG, Park SE, Rubash HE: Kinematic analysis of conventional and high-flexion cruciate-retaining total knee arthroplasties: An in vitro investigation. *J Arthroplasty* 2005;20(4):529-535.

    Kinematics and in situ PCL force of conventional and high-flexion cruciate-retaining TKA were compared using a robotic testing setup. Both designs restored almost 80% of the posterior femoral translation of the intact knee. The PCL was found to have greatest in situ forces in the midflexion range and had little effect on kinematics at high flexion.

15. Most E, Li G, Schule S, et al: The kinematics of fixed- and mobile-bearing total knee arthroplasty. *Clin Orthop Relat Res* 2003;416:197-207.

16. Li G, Zayontz S, Most E, Otterberg E, Sabbag K, Rubash HE: Cruciate-retaining and cruciate-substituting total knee arthroplasty: An in vitro comparison of the kinematics under muscle loads. *J Arthroplasty* 2001;16(8, suppl 1):150-156.

17. Morra EA, Greenwald AS: Polymer insert stress in total knee designs during high-flexion activities: A finite element study. *J Bone Joint Surg Am* 2005;87(suppl 2):120-124.

    Finite element modeling was performed to investigate the contact areas and stresses that are associated with polymer insert abrasion. The study concluded that the higher the contact stresses, the greater the propensity for abrasive damage.

18. Li G, Most E, Otterberg E, et al: Biomechanics of posterior-substituting total knee arthroplasty: An in vitro study. *Clin Orthop Relat Res* 2002;404:214-225.

19. Suggs JF, Li G, Park SE, Steffensmeier S, Rubash HE, Freiberg AA: Function of the anterior cruciate ligament after unicompartmental knee arthroplasty: An in vitro robotic study. *J Arthroplasty* 2004;19(2):224-229.

20. Øiestad BE, Engebretsen L, Storheim K, Risberg MA: Knee osteoarthritis after anterior cruciate ligament injury: A systematic review. *Am J Sports Med* 2009;37:1434-1443.

    The authors studied the prevalence of osteoarthritis in the tibiofemoral joint after ACL injury, along with radiologic classification methods and risk factors for the development of osteoarthritis in the knee.

21. Amis AA, Senavongse W, Darcy P: Biomechanics of patellofemoral joint prostheses. *Clin Orthop Relat Res* 2005;436:20-29.

    A cadaver study and a review of the literature on the biomechanics of the patellofemoral joint before and after patellofemoral arthroplasty are presented. Four patellofemoral designs are compared in terms of articular geometry, stability, and tracking. The results showed that most studied parameters were corrected within normal limits; however, problems such as erratic subluxation-reduction may occur.

22. Hollinghurst D, Stoney J, Ward T, Pandit H, Beard D, Murray DW: In vivo sagittal plane kinematics of the Avon patellofemoral arthroplasty. *J Arthroplasty* 2007;22(1):117-123.

    Sagittal plane kinematics was examined in patients who had undergone Avon patellofemoral arthroplasty using a fluoroscopic method. No significant difference existed between the kinematics of knees after patellofemoral arthroplasty compared with normal contralateral knees, except for a uniform elevation in patellar tendon angle throughout the range of motion.

23. Greene KA: Gender-specific design in total knee arthroplasty. *J Arthroplasty* 2007;22(7, suppl 3)27-31.

    Issues surrounding sex-specific TKAs being marketed by some manufacturers are outlined. The authors conclude that there is little evidence regarding inferior results following TKA in females. However, improvements in surgical procedure and prosthetic design are still needed.

24. Merchant AC, Arendt EA, Dye SF, et al: The female knee: Anatomic variations and the female-specific total knee design. *Clin Orthop Relat Res* 2008;466(12):3059-3065.

    This article investigates proposals for female-specific TKA based on increased Q angle, less prominent anterior femoral condyles, and reduced mediolateral-anteroposterior femoral aspect ratio. The authors conclude that the first two differences do not exist and the third may have little clinical significance.

25. Conley S, Rosenberg A, Crowninshield R: The female knee: Anatomic variations. *J Am Acad Orthop Surg* 2007;15(suppl 1):S31-S36.

Three anatomic variations of female knees are highlighted: less prominent anterior condyle, increased Q angle, and reduced mediolateral-anteroposterior femoral aspect ratio. The authors conclude that there is a need for female-specific femoral TKA to lessen intraoperative implant size adjustments and the potential for subtle patellar maltracking.

26. Barink M, Van de Groes S, Verdonschot N, De Waal Malefijt M: The difference in trochlear orientation between the natural knee and current prosthetic knee designs: Towards a truly physiological prosthetic groove orientation. *J Biomech* 2006;39(9):1708-1715.

The coronal plane orientation of a TKA trochlea was compared with that of the natural trochlea. Symmetric (neutral groove orientation) and asymmetric (lateral groove orientation) TKA were different only in the area of the supracondylar pouch. Both differed from normal anatomy by up to 6.4°.

27. Lonner JH, Jasko JG, Thomas BS: Anthropomorphic differences between the distal femora of men and women. *Clin Orthop Relat Res* 2008;466(11):2724-2729.

Distal femoral mediolateral and anteroposterior dimensions for 100 male and 100 female knees were compared intraoperatively after preparation for prosthesis implantation. The mean mediolateral to antero-posterior ratio was larger for men (1.23) compared with women (1.19).

28. Varadarajan KM, Gill TJ, Freiberg AA, Rubash HE, Li G: Gender differences in trochlear groove orientation and rotational kinematics of human knees. *J Orthop Res* 2009;27(7):871-878.

During weight-bearing knee flexion, female knees showed more externally rotated tibia at 0° and 30° flexion and greater range of tibial rotation compared with males. Other tibiofemoral kinematic parameters were not significantly different between the sexes.

29. Varadarajan KM, Gill TJ, Freiberg AA, Rubash HE, Li G: Patellar tendon orientation and patellar tracking in male and female knees. *J Orthop Res* 2010;28(3):322-328.

During weight-bearing knee flexion, patellar tracking in male and female knees was not significantly different. However, the patellar tendon in females was oriented more anteriorly in the sagittal plane, more medially in the coronal plane, and showed greater external tilt in the transverse plane.

30. Yue B, Varadarajan KM, Ai S, Tang T, Rubash HE, Li G: Differences of knee anthropometry between Chinese and white men and women. *J Arthroplasty* 2011;26(1):124-130.

Using three-dimensional knee models, the authors found that knees in Chinese men and women were smaller than those of whites, and tibial aspect ratio differences were probably related to the differences in knee size. These racial differences should be considered in TKA designs for Asian patients.

2: Knee

Chapter 8

Nonarthroplasty Alternatives in Knee Arthritis

David Backstein, MD, Med, FRCSC   Yona Kosashvili, MD, MHA

Medical Therapy

Nonsteroidal anti-inflammatory drugs (NSAIDs) remain the mainstay class of drugs used for alleviating symptoms of knee arthritis. NSAIDs inhibit the conversion of arachidonic acid to prostaglandins, which have a central role in modulating the inflammatory process. Two distinct forms of cyclooxygenase (COX), the prostaglandin synthases, have been identified. COX-1 is generally believed to be responsible for the baseline levels of prostaglandins, whereas COX-2 is responsible for the increased production of prostaglandins in scenarios of inflammation. Both enzymes are located in the stomach, blood vessels, and kidneys. A subtype of COX-1 (COX-1b, also known as COX-3) exists in the brain and may be associated with relief of headaches during NSAID therapy.

Many NSAIDs are currently available on the market, with primary differences in clinical efficacy related to reducing gastrointestinal (GI) and vascular (myocardial infarction and stroke) complications associated with the central role of the COX enzymes in the respective tissues. The adverse effects of COX-2 and COX-1 inhibitors in the US population were compared using data from adult respondents in the 1999 to 2003 Medical Expenditure Panel Survey. Two COX-2 inhibitors were associated with higher rates of complications. Rofecoxib (Vioxx, Merck and Co, White House Station, NJ) had an adjusted odds ratio (OR) of 3.3 for acute myocardial infarction and 4.28 for GI hemorrhage, whereas celecoxib (Celebrex, Pfizer, New York, NY) had an OR of 2.43 for stroke and 4.98 for GI hemorrhage. In comparison, traditional NSAIDs had an OR of 2.38 for GI hemorrhage and no significant adverse effects of acute myocardial infarction (OR 1.47) or

stroke (OR 1.26). Consequently, rofecoxib was associated with 46,783 acute myocardial infarctions and 31,188 GI hemorrhages, whereas celecoxib was associated with 21,832 strokes and 69,954 GI hemorrhages. This resulted in an estimated 26,603 deaths from both coxibs in the study period. The traditional NSAID group was associated with an excess of 87,327 GI hemorrhages and 9,606 deaths in the same time period.[1]

In another study, the GI adverse effects of a newer COX-2 inhibitor (etoricoxib) were compared with those caused by a traditional NSAID (diclofenac) in a multinational study. Although etoricoxib resulted in a lower hazard ratio (0.69, $P = 0.0001$) and fewer uncomplicated events than diclofenac, there was no significant difference in the complicated events in both groups (OR 0.91, $P = 0.561$).[2]

Because COX-1 as well as selective COX-2 have a substantial documented incidence of GI toxicity, one study examined the cost effectiveness of adding a proton pump inhibitor to either traditional NSAIDs (diclofenac, ibuprofen, and naproxen) or COX-2 selective inhibitors (etoricoxib, celecoxib). The addition of a proton pump inhibitor to both COX-2 selective inhibitors and traditional NSAIDs was highly cost effective for all patient groups considered, even for patients at low risk of GI adverse events.[3]

Acetaminophen has been found to result in a very limited reduction in pain (less then 5% improvement) when compared to placebo. NSAIDs have been shown to be superior to acetaminophen in reduction of pain and improvement of functional status in patients with osteoarthritis.[4]

The Glucosamine/Chondroitin Arthritis Intervention Trial (GAIT) evaluated the efficacy of glucosamine and chondroitin sulfate as a treatment of knee osteoarthritis. The primary outcome measure was defined a priori by expert consensus as a 20% decrease in the summed score for the Western Ontario and McMaster Universities (WOMAC) pain subscale from baseline to week 24. Under these terms, glucosamine and chondroitin sulfate alone or in combination did not effectively reduce pain in the overall group of patients. Only the combination of the two was found to be effective in the subgroup of patients with moderate to severe knee pain.[5]

Dr. Backstein or an immediate family member is a member of a speakers' bureau or has made paid presentations on behalf of Stryker, Sanofi-Aventis, and Zimmer and serves as a paid consultant for or is an employee of Stryker and Zimmer. Neither Dr. Kosashvili nor any immediate family member has received anything of value from or owns stock in a commercial company or institution related directly or indirectly to the subject of this chapter.

2: Knee

Injections

Glucocorticoids are potent anti-inflammatory drugs commonly used in intra-articular injections to the knee to avoid systemic adverse effects. Their primary anti-inflammatory mechanism is through synthesis of lipocortin-1 (annexin-1), which inhibits leukocyte inflammatory migration and suppresses the two main products of inflammation, prostaglandins and leukotrienes. Moreover, they also suppress both COX-1 and COX-2 expression much like NSAIDs, potentiating the anti-inflammatory effect.[6,7]

Intra-articular glucocorticoids were more effective than placebo for pain reduction and global assessment of the knee at 1 week after injection. This effect has been demonstrated to last for 2 to 3 weeks (relative risk, 3.1) and subsequently decline, with no benefit evident compared to placebo at 4 to 24 weeks after injection.[7] Intra-articular glucocorticoids had an effect similar to that of arthroscopic lavage, with no differences in any efficacy or safety outcome measures.[8] When triamcinolone hexacetonide (THA) was compared to methylprednisolone acetate (MPA), THA was more effective for pain reduction at 3 weeks, but MPA had a lasting effect that continued up to 8 weeks after injection.[8]

Viscosupplementation therapy with hyaluronic acid (HA) consists of removal of most joint fluid from the affected knee and injection of hyaluronate derivatives once a week for 3 to 5 weeks, depending on the preparation. Currently, a single-dose injection is also available (Synvisc, Genzyme Corporation, Cambridge, MA). A 2005 meta-analysis evaluated the effectiveness of HA injections for knee osteoarthritis compared with saline placebo; a 15% decrease in knee pain was regarded as a clinically significant improvement. HA was not found to be substantially better in relieving knee pain than placebo.[9]

However, in a Cochrane meta-analysis conducted the following year comparing HA to intra-articular glucocorticoids, placebo, and NSAIDs, HA was superior to placebo and steroids in relieving knee pain and restoring function. Pain relief and function improved 28% to 54% and 9% to 32%, respectively, compared to steroids at 5 to 13 weeks after HA injection, suggesting better long-term effects. The benefit, however, was not shown to be better than that of NSAIDs.[6] The most common complication of HA injection is injection site inflammation and pain, with an incidence of 1.2% per injection and 5.2% per patient. No systemic effects or knee infections were reported in any of the studies.[10]

Synovectomy

Synovectomy remains an option for patients with intractable synovitis and limited involvement of the articular cartilage. This situation may be present in the early stages of rheumatoid arthritis and pigmented villonodular synovitis. Surgical indications for synovectomy are severe pain refractory to pharmacotherapy for at least 4 to 6 months, with preserved range of motion and no signs of joint-space narrowing on standing radiographs.

In a recent study comparing early results of open and arthroscopic knee synovectomy, patients had less blood loss, a shorter duration of hospitalization, and fewer flexion contractures after arthroscopic synovectomy at 6-month follow-up.[11] Arthroscopic synovectomy may be performed as an outpatient procedure. Patients are advised to ambulate with crutches or a cane until knee swelling subsides. Physiotherapy for range of motion and muscle strengthening is initiated when symptoms and swelling are adequately controlled.

Synovectomy can also be performed by injecting a radioisotope (yttrium 90). This treatment modality is especially effective in patients with hemophilia or rheumatoid arthritis, with more than 80% excellent results for knee synovitis. However, one study indicated that the results for patients with osteoarthritis are less predictable.[12]

Knee Bracing

Bracing for medial compartment osteoarthritis is intended to provide an opposing valgus force by applying an external three-point bending force via bladders, pads, and straps. Thus, the medial compartment is expected to be less loaded, hopefully alleviating the patient's symptoms. A study that examined the gait of patients before and after brace wear for 6 consecutive weeks demonstrated a significant and substantial improvement in the peak varus moment of the affected knee. The WOMAC scores improved from 50.1 ± 17.6 to 63 ± 18.4, and the visual analog scale pain scores improved from 6.8 ± 2.5 to 4.7 ± 3. This effect was more substantial in patients with increased varus and mediolateral laxity.[13]

However, the mechanical theory regarding the valgus unloading effect of these braces has recently been questioned. In a study comparing the gait of 16 patients wearing an unloader brace for 2 weeks followed by a 2-week washout period and 2 additional weeks wearing the same brace with the unloading effect eliminated after adjusting the brace accordingly, there was no difference. The study examined pain and functional status as well as vastus medialis and vastus lateralis cocontractions as an indirect parameter for instability. The results indicated that compared with baseline levels, both neutral bracing and the 4° valgus bracing reduced the vastus medialis and lateralis concentrations. In addition, there was similar improvement in pain relief and function after use of either the valgus or neutral braces, suggesting that the improvement may be attributed more to the improvement in the mediolateral stability and the ensuing reduction in vastus lateralis and medialis cocontractions rather than the actual unloading effect.[14]

Arthroscopic Lavage and Débridement

Arthroscopic lavage combined with débridement and chondroplasty was intended to provide temporary pain relief for knee osteoarthritis. These procedures theoretically allowed removal of inflammatory mediators, degenerative cartilage, and meniscal fragments. Although many studies published data supportive of this concept, recent literature seriously questions its efficacy.

In a randomized controlled trial at a single center, 92 patients were assigned to arthroscopic lavage and optimized physical and medical therapy compared with 86 patients assigned to physical and medical therapy alone. The primary outcome was the total WOMAC score, whereas the secondary outcome was the Short Form-36 physical component score at 2-year follow-up. Patients were examined at 3, 6, 12, 18, and 24 months after the initiation of treatment. To preserve blinding, a neoprene sleeve was placed over the knee. This study failed to show a benefit of arthroscopic surgery for the treatment of osteoarthritis of the knee at the end of 2 years (WOMAC scores of 874 ± 624 for surgery versus 897 ± 583 for nonsurgical treatment, $P = 0.22$).[15] A recent Cochrane meta-analysis in seven trials including 567 patients found that the arthroscopic lavage had no added benefit in terms of pain relief or improvement in function.[16]

Osteotomies Around the Knee

Realignment osteotomies around the knee for deformity correction and unloading of the arthritic compartment are a well-established treatment alternative for symptomatic knees in young, active patients. Medial compartment arthritis and varus deformity are usually treated by a proximal tibial valgus realignment osteotomy in appropriately selected patients. The subsequent offloading of the medial compartment may ameliorate symptoms, improve knee function, and delay the need for knee arthroplasty.

Conversely, lateral compartment arthritis and valgus deformity are preferably addressed by a femoral varus osteotomy, as proximal tibial varus realignment osteotomy remains controversial. Suboptimal outcomes have been reported, especially when the resulting coronal (mediolateral) tibial slope was in excess of 10°, potentially due to the increased translational forces on intra-articular structures such as the menisci and hyaline cartilage. Thus, only a minor realignment can be reliably executed through the proximal tibia. Instead, a distal femoral varus osteotomy (DFVO) is the preferred procedure and may provide good midterm outcomes even in the presence of moderate patellofemoral arthritis.

High Tibial Osteotomy

Indications for high tibial osteotomy (HTO) include age younger than 60 years, the presence of arthritis primarily involving the medial compartment, less than 15° of flexion contracture, preoperative arc of motion of 90°, and higher physiologic demands. Contraindications to HTO include narrowing of the lateral compartment joint space on standing radiographs with the knees flexed to 30°; ligamentous instability, especially with a high adductor moment (varus thrust); severe and symptomatic patellofemoral arthritis; medial compartment bone loss greater than 2 mm; and inflammatory arthritis. In addition, patients who cannot manage a 3- to 6-month extensive rehabilitation period, are receiving workers' compensation, or had partial/complete meniscectomy may have suboptimal results. HTO may be particularly beneficial for younger individuals with higher physiologic demands and who perform heavy labor. The ensuing alignment asymmetry of the limb should be discussed preoperatively with the patient to avoid dissatisfaction related to its cosmetic appearance.

Preoperative assessment should include a thorough history and physical examination addressing the indications and possible contraindications, including knee range of motion, presence of fixed flexion contracture, and overall limb alignment. Ligamentous instability should be ruled out in a supine position as well as while walking to detect excessive varus thrust, which is associated with poor results and recurrence of varus deformity after HTO.[17]

Full-length AP weight-bearing radiographs of the lower limbs, including the hips, ankles, and knees, are required to establish the mechanical and anatomic axis for preoperative planning. Most authors agree that some overcorrection of the deformity is required. Subsequently, the weight-bearing line (mechanical axis) should pass through the 62% coordinate of the tibial articular surface (medial border of tibia articular surface is 0% and lateral border is 100%), resulting in preferential loading of the lateral tibiofemoral compartment.

The angular correction is calculated by drawing a line from the center of the femoral head to the 62% tibial coordinate. A second line is then drawn from the center of the ankle tibiotalar joint to the 62% tibial coordinate. The angle between these lines represents the angle of correction required. For closing wedge osteotomy (**Figure 1**), once the amount of angular correction required is determined, the size of the wedge planned to be removed from the osteotomy site should be measured directly from properly magnified radiographs. It is recommended that the precise size of wedge to be removed be measured from radiographs, rather than using "rule-of-thumb" estimations such as 1 mm of resection equating to 1° of correction. The closing wedge osteotomy (**Figure 2**) is commonly fixed by two large staples. When a medial opening wedge technique is used, a specially calibrated wedge is tapped into the osteotomy site to match the precalculated corrective angle. Sufficient correction can be verified intraoperatively by fluoroscopy. Opening wedge osteotomy is fixed by a variety of commercially available plates, and bone grafts (autograft from the iliac crest or allograft) also may be used.[18]

2: Knee

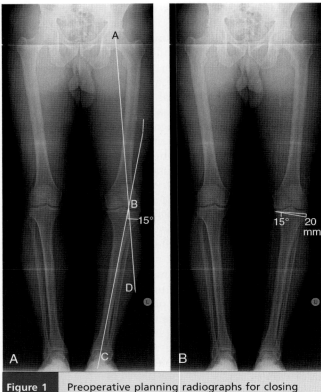

Figure 1 Preoperative planning radiographs for closing wedge osteotomy. **A,** The required angular correction is calculated. Line AD passes from the center of the head to the planned weight-bearing area in the lateral compartment. Line BC passes from the center of the talus to the planned weight-bearing area in the lateral compartment. **B,** The size of the resected wedge is calculated. The 15° correction angle will result in a resection of 20 mm.

Published literature has documented good or excellent results at 10 years in 85% to 90% of the knees treated with osteotomy. In a study of HTO with mean long-term follow-up of 16.4 years (range, 16 to 20 years) including a total of 94 patients (118 knees), the 10-year and 15-year survival rates were 97.6% and 90.4%, respectively, with good or excellent Hospital for Special Surgery knee scores in 73.7% of the knees at most recent follow-up. The study suggests that a preoperative body mass index greater than 27.5 kg/m² and range of movement less than 100° are risk factors for earlier failure.[19] A previous report indicated that an ensuing alignment between 8° and 16° of anatomic valgus is preferable because undercorrection and excessive overcorrection were associated with poor results.[20] The incidence of nonunion is low, occurring in less than 2% of cases in most studies of opening wedge osteotomy when the osteotomy is filled with autologous bone graft from the iliac crest[20,21] or from bone allograft,[22] and the risk of peroneal nerve injury ranges from 0 to 20% when a closing lateral wedge osteotomy is used.[19,23]

Patella baja has been reported frequently with both opening and closing wedge HTO. This phenomenon is believed to be caused by postoperative contracture of the patella tendon.[24] Protracted rehabilitation programs with prolonged immobilization are likely contributing factors. With the use of contemporary rigid fixation techniques and more rapid rehabilitation, patella baja has become less common.[25] It is currently recommended that prophylactic measures be used to prevent deep venous thrombosis.[23]

Pain resulting from recurrence of varus deformity or progression of osteoarthritis may ultimately necessitate conversion to total knee arthroplasty. Soft-tissue scarring and limited range of motion make the surgical approach more difficult. Although exposure can usually be achieved routinely, surgeons should be prepared to use special exposure techniques such as the quadriceps snip. Special attention should be given to appropriate restoration of the rotational alignment of both femoral and tibial components.[26]

Distal Femoral Varus Osteotomy

Patient prerequisites for DFVO are much the same as for HTO. The contraindications include significant osteoarthritis of the medial and/or patellofemoral compartments, poor bone quality, or osteoporosis.[27] In addition, opening wedge femoral varus osteotomy is contraindicated if the width of the opening wedge is greater than 20 mm or in the context of lateral femoral condyle osteonecrosis.[28]

Closing Wedge and Opening Wedge DFVO

Closing wedge DFVO does not require extensive preoperative measurements of angles for correction because appropriate placement of the blade plate will necessarily correct the tibiofemoral angle to 0°, offloading the lateral compartment (**Figure 3**). A subvastus approach through a midline skin incision is used to place a 90° blade plate 2.5 cm proximal and parallel to the joint line monitored by fluoroscopy. The closing wedge osteotomy is performed at the level of the upper border of the trochlea.[27]

For opening wedge DFVO, a lateral approach is used with an osteotomy at the upper level of the trochlea under fluoroscopic control severing the anterior and posterior cortices, while leaving 1 cm of a medial cortex serving as a hinge. A wedge opener is inserted to the desired degree of coronal correction, determined preoperatively, based on long leg standing radiographs similar to HTO. The osteotomy should be gradually opened over several minutes to prevent inadvertent fracture of the medial cortex, especially for corrections larger than 10°. The osteotomy is secured by either a femoral locking plate or a "toothed" T-shaped plate (Arthrex, Naples, FL) and filled with shaped allogenic or tricorticocancellous grafts from the ipsilateral iliac crest.[28]

The results of both DFVO techniques reported in the literature are encouraging. One study reported that 12 of 38 knees (31.6%) were either converted or planned

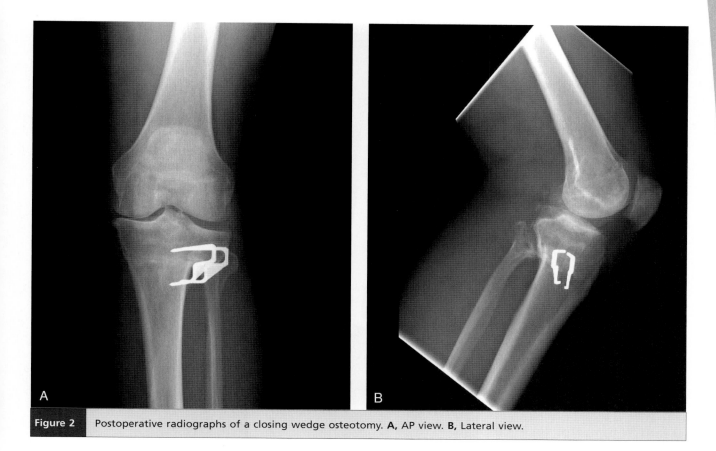

Figure 2   Postoperative radiographs of a closing wedge osteotomy. **A,** AP view. **B,** Lateral view.

to convert to total knee arthorplasty at an average of 123 months (range, 39 to 245 months) after closing wedge DFVO.[27] Excellent results were reported at 4- to 14-year follow-up in 21 patients with marked improvement in pain and knee function.[28]

Isolated Cartilage Lesions

Cartilage defects in the knee joint are common with focal chondral or osteochondral defects found in 19% of 1,000 knee arthroscopies.[29] Because hyaline cartilage receives its nutrition from synovial fluid via hydrostatic pressure gradients produced during joint loading, its healing potential is limited. Consequently, the affected hyaline cartilage is replaced by fibrocartilage produced from stem cells located within the bone marrow. The fibrocartilage has inferior biomechanical properties, which may predispose the involved joint to degeneration. Several new treatment options of cartilage defects have emerged over the past two decades, including marrow stimulation, transplantation of cultured cells or autogenous grafts, (mosaicplasty) and refrigerated allografts.

Marrow Stimulation Techniques

Marrow stimulation can be performed by subchondral drilling or microfracture, which induces the bone marrow stem cells to form fibrocartilage via a fibrin clot at the defect. Subchondral drilling consists of several 2.5-mm drill holes made within the cartilage defect after loose unsupported cartilage is débrided. The same effect can be achieved by using a manual awl to penetrate the subchondral bone. Proper depth of penetration is confirmed when fat droplets are seen emanating from the lesion. Acute osteochondral characteristics following microfracture were compared with drilling in a mature rabbit model of cartilage repair by assessing their effect on subchondral bone using histology and micro-CT at day 1 after surgery.[30] Although microfracture produced fractured and compacted bone around holes, essentially sealing them off from viable bone marrow and potentially impeding repair, drilling cleanly removed bone from the holes to provide access channels to marrow stroma. Drilling was not associated with thermal damage to the surrounding subchondral osteocytes. Drilling deeper to 6 mm rather than 2 mm penetrated the epiphyseal scar in this model and led to greater subchondral hematoma.[30] In a study examining the outcome of microfracture in 24 professional basketball players, all players returned to professional basketball within 30 weeks. The 17 players who continued to play two seasons or more had diminished performance and minutes per game.[31] Despite previously encouraging data, a recently published study cautioned against such treatment of larger defects, which are likely to require treatment with autologous chondrocyte implantation, because they triple the chances for failure of such transplants (26% after drilling ver-

2: Knee

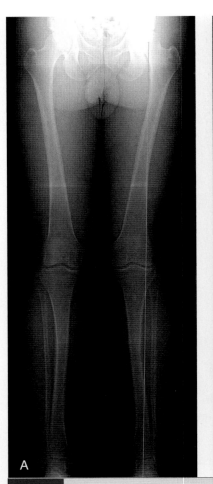 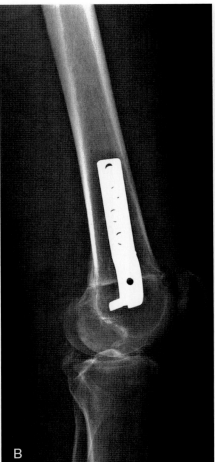 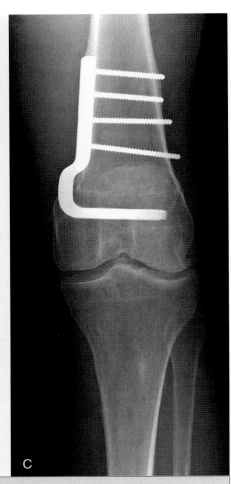

A

B

C

Figure 3   **A,** Preoperative radiograph of a valgus knee. The line connecting the head of the femur to the head of the talus passes lateral to the center of the knee. AP **(B)** and lateral **(C)** postoperative radiographs of a valgus knee treated by DFVO.

sus 8% without drilling).[32] The authors suggested that microfracture should be performed only on smaller defects that have substantial healing potential.

Chondrocyte Transplantation

Autologous Osteochondral Transplantation (Mosaicplasty)

The basic idea behind this concept is to fill the focal defect with multiple cylindrical osteochondral autografts to provide a congruent hyaline-cartilage–covered surface. The use of multiple small cylindrical grafts rather than a single block graft allows more tissue to be transplanted while preserving donor site integrity and achieving better congruency of the new surface. The grafts are usually harvested from the medial and lateral femoral condyle. According to one study, outcome was good to excellent in 92% of femoral condyle defects, 87% of tibial defects, and 79% of patellofemoral defects in a long-term follow-up of 831 patients.[33] In a study evaluating midterm outcomes in 69 patients, significant improvement was demonstrated in 77%. Deterioration of results was observed from 12 months post-

operatively to the most recent follow-up at 5 to 9 years.[34]

Autologous Chondrocyte Implantation

Autologous chondrocyte implantation (ACI) is based on obtaining a 12-mm by 5-mm full-thickness articular cartilage specimen that will supply an estimated 250,000 chondrocytes. These chondrocytes are enzymatically digested and cultured for 3 weeks to obtain an estimated 12 million cells. The cultured chondrocytes are replanted and covered with a periosteal flap harvested from the medial aspect of the proximal tibia. The flap is sutured into place with a 6.0 Vicryl suture after the lesion is débrided of granulation tissue. Special care is taken not to generate bleeding from the subchondral bone bed. Mosaicplasty had superior clinical and histologic outcomes compared with ACI in 40 patients with an articular cartilage lesion of the femoral condyle. Biopsy specimens from representative patients of both groups with histologic staining, immunohistochemistry, scanning electron microscopy, postoperative Lysholm score, and cartilage recovery per arthroscopy

1 year after surgery were used as parameters for comparison. The improvement provided by the ACI in the above parameters lagged behind that provided by mosaicplasty. Histologically, the defects treated with ACI were primarily filled with fibrocartilage whereas the osteochondral cylinder transplants retained their hyaline character, although there was a persistent interface between the transplant and the surrounding original cartilage.[35] However, in posttraumatic lesions, with a mean defect of 4.66 cm², ACI had superior results at 19-month mean follow-up in 100 patients. Arthroscopy at 1 year demonstrated excellent or good repairs in 82% after ACI and in 34% after mosaicplasty, with failure of all five patellar mosaicplasty procedures.[36] Thus, substantial controversy exists regarding the appropriate indications for each technique.

Fresh Stored Osteochondral Allografts

Refrigerated fresh osteochondral allograft transplantation has demonstrated significant clinical success in several centers. Initially, these grafts have been typically implanted less than 1 week from donor asystole. However, the storage time can be increased up to 4 weeks at 4°C, as this does not significantly decrease the clinical benefit of transplantation.[37] Thus, due to infection-related concerns, fresh osteoarticular allografts are currently stored hypothermically for a minimum of 14 days to allow for serologic and microbiologic testing before implantation. The clinical and functional outcomes of 23 consecutive patients receiving refrigerated osteoarticular distal femoral allografts between 15 and 28 days after procurement showed a significant (P < 0.03) improvement in knee scores and function with no graft failure at an average of 3 years.[38] After long-term follow-up, the Kaplan-Meier survivorship of distal femoral refrigerated osteochondral grafts was 95% graft survival at 5 years and 85% at 10 years. Similar findings were reported in a study of 43 patients (23 males patients and 20 females). Twenty-nine patients had involvement of the medial femoral condyle; 13, the lateral femoral condyle; and 1, both condyles. Thirty-eight of the allograft procedures (88%) were considered to be successful (a score of ≥ 15 points on the 18-point modified Merle d'Aubigné and Postel scale) at a mean of 4.5 years postoperatively.[39]

The survivorship of refrigerated osteochondral allografts to reconstruct the tibial plateau was 95% survival at 5 years, 80% at 10 years, and 65% at 15 years.[40] Thus, based on long-term follow-up, osteochondral allografts for large defects of the tibial plateau or distal femur provided a long-lasting and reliable reconstructive solution.

Summary

Several nonarthroplasty options are available for the treatment of patients with symptomatic knee osteoarthritis. COX-1 and COX-2 NSAIDs can be used to relieve pain, preferably with proton pump inhibitors to limit GI adverse effects. Acetaminophen, glucosamine, and chondroitin have limited added value. Intra-articular corticosteroid injections provide short-term (1 to 3 weeks) pain relief, whereas controversy persists regarding the use of HA. Patients need not undergo needle lavage or arthroscopy with débridement or lavage. Partial meniscectomy or loose body removal may be considered as conditions warrant. Braces may be worn when the main complaint is instability. There is no advantage to offloading braces. Osteotomies may be performed in carefully selected patients, especially those with higher physiologic demand and unicompartmental arthritis. ACI is preferable to mosaicplasty or microfracture. Refrigerated fresh allografts are a safe treatment alternative, especially for larger defects, that should be accompanied by an offloading osteotomy.

Annotated References

1. Vaithianathan R, Hockey PM, Moore TJ, Bates DW: Iatrogenic effects of COX-2 inhibitors in the US population: Findings from the Medical Expenditure Panel Survey. *Drug Saf* 2009;32(4):335-343.

   Both COX-2 inhibitors were associated with higher rates of complications. Rofecoxib was associated with 46,783 acute myocardial infarctions and 31,188 GI hemorrhages, whereas celecoxib was associated with 21,832 strokes and 69,954 GI hemorrhages in the same time period.

2. Laine L, Curtis SP, Cryer B, Kaur A, Cannon CP, MEDAL Steering Committee: Assessment of upper gastrointestinal safety of etoricoxib and diclofenac in patients with osteoarthritis and rheumatoid arthritis in the Multinational Etoricoxib and Diclofenac Arthritis Long-term (MEDAL) programme: A randomised comparison. *Lancet* 2007;369(9560):465-473.

   The GI adverse effects of a newer COX-2 inhibitor (etoricoxib) were compared to a traditional NSAID (diclofenac) in a multinational study. Although etoricoxib resulted in a lower hazard ratio (0.69, P = 0.0001), and fewer uncomplicated events than diclofenac, there was no significant difference in the complicated events in both groups (OR 0.91, P = 0.561).

3. Latimer N, Lord J, Grant RL, et al: Cost effectiveness of COX 2 selective inhibitors and traditional NSAIDs alone or in combination with a proton pump inhibitor for people with osteoarthritis. *BMJ* 2009;339:b2538.

   This study found that adding a proton pump inhibitor to either traditional NSAIDs (diclofenac, ibuprofen, and naproxen) or COX-2 selective inhibitors (etoricoxib, celecoxib) was highly cost effective for all patient groups considered, even for patients at low risk of GI adverse events.

4. Towheed TE, Maxwell L, Judd MG, Catton M, Hochberg MC, Wells G: Acetaminophen for osteoarthritis. *Cochrane Database Syst Rev* 2006;1:CD004257.

2: Knee

Acetaminophen had a very limited reduction in pain (less then 5% improvement) when compared to placebo and was substantially inferior to NSAIDs in patients with OA.

5. Clegg DO, Reda DJ, Harris CL, et al: Glucosamine, chondroitin sulfate, and the two in combination for painful knee osteoarthritis. *N Engl J Med* 2006; 354(8):795-808.

The Glucosamine/Chondroitin Arthritis Intervention Trial (GAIT) evaluated the efficacy of glucosamine and chondroitin sulfate as a treatment of knee osteoarthritis. Glucosamine and chondroitin sulfate alone or in combination did not effectively reduce pain in the overall group of patients.

6. Bellamy N, Campbell J, Robinson V, Gee T, Bourne R, Wells G: Intraarticular corticosteroid for treatment of osteoarthritis of the knee. *Cochrane Database Syst Rev* 2006;2:CD005328.

In a Cochrane meta-analysis comparing HA to intraarticular glucocorticoids, placebo, and NSAIDs, HA was found superior to placebo and steroids with a higher improvement in pain and function compared to steroids at 5 to 13 weeks postinjection, suggesting better long-term effects.

7. Richmond J, Hunter D, Irrgang J, et al: Treatment of osteoarthritis of the knee (nonarthroplasty). *J Am Acad Orthop Surg* 2009;17:591-600.

A list of guidelines for nonarthroplasty treatment of knee osteoarthritis is presented. Recommendation 15 suggests that based on several randomized controlled trials, steroid injections provide short-term pain relief and improvement in function.

8. Pyne D, Ioannou Y, Mootoo R, Bhanji A: Intraarticular steroids in knee osteoarthritis: A comparative study of triamcinolone hexacetonide and methylprednisolone acetate. *Clin Rheumatol* 2004;23(2):116-120.

9. Arrich J, Piribauer F, Mad P, Schmid D, Klaushofer K, Müllner M: Intra-articular hyaluronic acid for the treatment of osteoarthritis of the knee: Systematic review and meta-analysis. *CMAJ* 2005;172(8):1039-1043.

A systematic review and meta-analysis of viscosupplementation therapy is presented.

10. Waddell DD, Bricker DC: Clinical experience with the effectiveness and tolerability of hylan G-F 20 in 1047 patients with osteoarthritis of the knee. *J Knee Surg* 2006;19(1):19-27.

The most common complications of HA injections are reviewed.

11. Masłoń A, Witoński D, Pieszyński I, Grzegorzewski A, Synder M: Early clinical results of open and arthroscopic synovectomy in knee inflammation. *Ortop Traumatol Rehabil* 2007;9(5):520-526.

A study comparing early results and complication rates of open versus arthroscopic knee synovectomy is presented.

12. Kavakli K, Aydoğdu S, Omay SB, et al: Long-term evaluation of radioisotope synovectomy with Yttrium 90 for chronic synovitis in Turkish haemophiliacs: Izmir experience. *Haemophilia* 2006;12(1):28-35.

Results of synovectomy by a radioisotope (yttrium 90) are presented.

13. Gaasbeek RD, Groen BE, Hampsink B, van Heerwaarden RJ, Duysens J: Valgus bracing in patients with medial compartment osteoarthritis of the knee: A gait analysis study of a new brace. *Gait Posture* 2007; 26(1):3-10.

The gait of patients before and after wearing an offloading brace for 6 consecutive weeks was studied. Brace wear resulted in a significant and substantial improvement in the peak varus moment of the affected knee.

14. Ramsey DK, Briem K, Axe MJ, Snyder-Mackler L: A mechanical theory for the effectiveness of bracing for medial compartment osteoarthritis of the knee. *J Bone Joint Surg Am* 2007;89(11):2398-2407.

This study questions the mechanical theory regarding valgus unloading. The gait of 16 patients wearing an unloader brace was not found superior to that of patients wearing the same braces without the offloading effect.

15. Kirkley A, Birmingham TB, Litchfield RB, et al: A randomized trial of arthroscopic surgery for osteoarthritis of the knee. *N Engl J Med* 2008;359(11):1097-1107.

In a randomized trial, arthroscopic surgery for osteoarthritis of the knee was compared with physical therapy and medications. No benefit of arthroscopic surgery for the treatment of osteoarthritis of the knee could be demonstrated at the end of 2 years.

16. Reichenbach S, Rutjes AW, Nüesch E, Trelle S, Jüni P: Joint lavage for osteoarthritis of the knee. *Cochrane Database Syst Rev* 2010;5:CD007320.

This meta-analysis in seven trials including 567 patients found no room for arthroscopic lavage in the treatment of knee osteoarthritis.

17. Prodromos CC, Andriacchi TP, Galante JO: A relationship between gait and clinical changes following high tibial osteotomy. *J Bone Joint Surg Am* 1985; 67(8):1188-1194.

18. Takeuchi R, Bito H, Akamatsu Y, et al: In vitro stability of open wedge high tibial osteotomy with synthetic bone graft. *Knee* 2010;17(13):217-220.

A study comparing the fixation alternatives of opening wedge HTO is presented.

19. Akizuki S, Shibakawa A, Takizawa T, Yamazaki I, Horiuchi H: The long-term outcome of high tibial osteotomy: A ten- to 20-year follow-up. *J Bone Joint Surg Br* 2008;90(5):592-596.

Long-term follow-up of 16.4 years of 118 knees is discussed. The 10-year survival rate was 97.6% and the 15-year survival rate was 90.4%, with good or excellent Hospital for Special Surgery knee scores in 73.7% of the knees at most recent follow-up.

20. Sprenger TR, Doerzbacher JF: Tibial osteotomy for the treatment of varus gonarthrosis: Survival and failure analysis to twenty-two years. *J Bone Joint Surg Am* 2003;85-A(3):469-474.

21. Noyes FR, Mayfield W, Barber-Westin SD, Albright JC, Heckmann TP: Opening wedge high tibial osteotomy: An operative technique and rehabilitation program to decrease complications and promote early union and function. *Am J Sports Med* 2006;34:1262-1273.

    The clinical outcomes and surgical technique of opening wedge osteotomy using autograft are discussed.

22. Santic V, Tudor A, Sestan B, Legovic D, Sirola L, Rakovac I: Bone allograft provides bone healing in the medial opening high tibial osteotomy. *Int Orthop* 2010;34:225-229.

    The clinical outcomes and surgical technique of opening wedge high tibial osteotomy using bone allograft for union of the osteotomy site are discussed.

23. Tunggal JA, Higgins GA, Waddell JP: Complications of closing wedge high tibial osteotomy. *Int Orthop* 2010;34:255-61.

    An excellent review of complications related to closing wedge high tibial osteotomy is presented.

24. Backstein D, Meisami B, Gross AE: Patella baja after the modified Coventry-Maquet high tibial osteotomy. *J Knee Surg* 2003;16(4):203-208.

25. Williams A, Natasa D: Osteotomy in the management of knee osteoarthritis and of ligamentous instability. *Curr Orthop* 2006;20:112-120.

    Contemporary rigid fixation techniques and more rapid rehabilitation protocols reduced the incidence of patella baja.

26. Akasaki Y, Matsuda S, Miura H, et al: Total knee arthroplasty following failed high tibial osteotomy: Midterm comparison of posterior cruciate-retaining versus posterior stabilized prosthesis. *Knee Surg Sports Traumatol Arthrosc* 2009;17(7):795-799.

    Although exposure can usually be achieved routinely, surgeons should be prepared to use special exposure techniques such as the quadriceps snip. Moreover, special attention should be given to appropriate restoration of the rotational alignment of both femoral and tibial components.

27. Backstein D, Morag G, Hanna S, Safir O, Gross A: Long-term follow-up of distal femoral varus osteotomy of the knee. *J Arthroplasty* 2007;22(4, Suppl 1)2-6.

    Long-term follow-up and survival analysis of closing wedge DFVO as well as the surgical technique are discussed.

28. Puddu G, Cipolla M, Cerullo G, Franco V, Giannì E: Osteotomies: The surgical treatment of the valgus knee. *Sports Med Arthrosc* 2007;15(1):15-22.

    Clinical outcomes and surgical technique of opening wedge DFVO are discussed.

29. Hjelle K, Solheim E, Strand T, Muri R, Brittberg M: Articular cartilage defects in 1,000 knee arthroscopies. *Arthroscopy* 2002;18(7):730-734.

30. Chen H, Sun J, Hoemann CD, et al: Drilling and microfracture lead to different bone structure and necrosis during bone-marrow stimulation for cartilage repair. *J Orthop Res* 2009;27(11):1432-1438.

    This study compared the outcomes of marrow stimulation by subchondral drilling or microfracture in a mature rabbit model. Drilling was more effective in cleanly removing bone from the holes to provide access channels to marrow stroma.

31. Cerynik DL, Lewullis GE, Joves BC, Palmer MP, Tom JA: Outcomes of microfracture in professional basketball players. *Knee Surg Sports Traumatol Arthrosc* 2009;17(9):1135-1139.

    This study examined the outcome of microfracture in 24 professional NBA basketball players, indicating that although the players returned to professional play, their performance was detrimentally affected.

32. Minas T, Gomoll AH, Rosenberger R, Royce RO, Bryant T: Increased failure rate of autologous chondrocyte implantation after previous treatment with marrow stimulation techniques. *Am J Sports Med* 2009;37(5):902-908.

    The authors cautioned against marrow stimulation in patients with larger defects, which are likely to require treatment with autologous chondrocyte implantation, because they triple the chances for failure of such transplant (26% after drilling versus 8% without drilling).

33. Hangody L, Vásárhelyi G, Hangody LR, et al: Autologous osteochondral grafting: Technique and long-term results. *Injury* 2008;39(Suppl 1):S32-S39.

    This study reports good to excellent outcome in 92% of femoral condyle defects, 87% of tibial defects and 79% of patellofemoral defects in a long-term follow-up of 831 patients.

34. Hegna J, Oyen J, Austgulen OK, Harlem T, Strand T: Osteochondral autografting (mosaicplasty) in articular cartilage defects in the knee: Results at 5 to 9 years. *Knee* 2010;17(1):84-87.

    This study presents midterm results of mosaicplasty.

35. Horas U, Pelinkovic D, Herr G, Aigner T, Schnettler R: Autologous chondrocyte implantation and osteochondral cylinder transplantation in cartilage repair of the knee joint: A prospective, comparative trial. *J Bone Joint Surg Am* 2003;85-A(2):185-192.

    This study reviewed the technique and the outcomes of ACI and indicated that mosaicplasty is superior for ACI.

2: Knee

36. Bentley G, Biant LC, Carrington RW, et al: A prospective, randomised comparison of autologous chondrocyte implantation versus mosaicplasty for osteochondral defects in the knee. *J Bone Joint Surg Br* 2003; 85(2):223-230.

    This study found that in posttraumatic lesions, ACI had superior results. Arthroscopy at 1 year demonstrated excellent or good repairs in 82% after ACI and in 34% after mosaicplasty, with failure of all five patellar mosaicplasty procedures.

37. Davidson PA, Rivenburgh DW, Dawson PE, Rozin R: Clinical, histologic, and radiographic outcomes of distal femoral resurfacing with hypothermically stored osteoarticular allografts. *Am J Sports Med* 2007;35(7): 1082-1090.

    This study reports that the storage time of fresh osteochondral grafts can be increased up to 4 weeks at 4°C without a significant decrease in the clinical benefit of transplantation.

38. LaPrade RF, Botker J, Herzog M, Agel JJ: Refrigerated osteoarticular allografts to treat articular cartilage defects of the femoral condyles: A prospective outcomes study. *J Bone Joint Surg Am* 2009;91(4):805-811.

    The authors reviewed the technique and outcomes of fresh, refrigerated osteochondral allograft transplantation, indicating that they can be used for 4 to 6 weeks after harvesting.

39. Görtz S, Bugbee WD: Allografts in articular cartilage repair. *J Bone Joint Surg Am* 2006; 88:1374-1384.

    The authors present a review of the outcomes of fresh osteochondral refrigerated allograft transplantation in the knee. They elaborate on the indications, contraindications, and the surgical technique of graft harvesting, storage, and transplantation.

40. Gross AE, Shasha N, Aubin P: Long-term followup of the use of fresh osteochondral allografts for posttraumatic knee defects. *Clin Orthop Relat Res* 2005;435: 79-87.

    Long-term follow-up of fresh osteochondral allografts is discussed. The Kaplan-Meier survivorship of distal femoral refrigerated osteochondral grafts was 95% graft survival at 5 years and 85% at 10 years. The survivorship of refrigerated osteochondral allografts to reconstruct the tibial plateau was 95% survival at 5 years, 80% at 10 years, and 65% at 15 years.

2: Knee

Unicompartmental, Patellofemoral, and Bicompartmental Arthroplasty

Michael T. Newman, MD   Jess H. Lonner, MD   Michael Ries, MD

Introduction

Unicompartmental knee arthroplasty (UKA) and patellofemoral arthroplasty are not new concepts. However, revised indications, enhanced instrumentation, and improved designs have stimulated new interest among patients and surgeons. Bone, cartilage, and ligament conservation; rapid recovery; early intervention; and kinematic preservation are advantages that have expanded the adoption of these procedures (in isolation or combined as bicompartmental resurfacing). Candidates for knee arthroplasty are often reluctant to undergo total knee replacement surgery because they fear a painful and lengthy recovery. In one study, approximately 85% of patients were unwilling to undergo total joint arthroplasty.[1] The merits of partial knee arthroplasty can be realized by a larger segment of the population with focal knee arthritis with appropriate educational efforts. This notion is particularly germane when considering the staggering growth of that portion of the population with arthritis of the knee.[2]

Medial UKA

Epidemiology

In the United States it is estimated that between 8% and 10% of knee arthroplasties performed are medial UKAs;[3] those numbers may be as high as 11% to 15% in other countries. The potential for growth of the UKA market is large when considering the growing number of patients with progressive but isolated unicompartmental arthritis (10% to 25% of patients with painful knee arthritis)[4] and the percentage of patients undergoing total knee arthroplasty (TKA) who may be candidates for UKA. The utilization of UKA increased between 1998 and 2005 at an average rate of 32.5% compared to the 9.4% growth in the rate of TKA in the United States.[3]

Indications/Contraindications

The classic indications and contraindications for UKA are well established, although expanding indications for UKA continue to be evaluated.[5-7] Classic recommendations advocated restricting medial UKA to low-demand patients older than 60 years with unicompartmental osteoarthritis (OA) or focal osteonecrosis (**Figure 1**). Additionally, it was recommended that patients weigh less than 82 kg (181 lb), have a minimum 90° flexion arc and flexion contracture of less than 5°, a passively correctable angular deformity less than or equal to 10° of varus, an intact anterior cruciate ligament, and no pain or exposed bone in the patellofemoral or opposite tibiofemoral compartment.[8]

Recently the indications for UKA have expanded to include younger and more active patients, without sub-

Dr. Newman or an immediate family member has received research or institutional support from Zimmer and Genzyme. Dr. Lonner or an immediate family member serves as a board member, owner, officer, or committee member for the Knee Society and the Philadelphia Orthopaedic Society; has received royalties from Zimmer; is a member of a speakers' bureau or has made paid presentations on behalf of Zimmer and MAKO Surgical; is a paid consultant for or is an employee of Zimmer; has received research or institutional support from Zimmer and MAKO Surgical; and owns stock or stock options in MAKO Surgical. Dr. Ries or an immediate family member serves as a board member, owner, officer or committee member for the Foundation for the Advancement of Research in Medicine; has received royalties for Smith & Nephew; is a paid consultant for or is an employee of Smith & Nephew; and has received research or institutional support from Johnson & Johnson, Medtronic, Musculoskeletal Transplant Foundation, National Institutes of Health, Zimmer, AIOD-Assn Intl l'Osteosynthese Dynamique Aleeva Medical, American College of Sports Medicine, American Orthopaedic Society for Sports Medicine, AO Foundation, Arthritis Foundation, Arthrocare Corporation, Arthroscopy Association of North America, Canadian Academy of Sports Medicine, Columbia University Deafness Research Foundation, DePuy, Hacettepe University Harold K.L. Castle Foundation, Histogenic Corporation, International Spinal Injection Society, ISTO Technologies, March of Dimes Birth Defects Foundation, National Institute of Arthritis and Musculoskeletal and Skin Diseases, National Institutes of Dental and Craniofacial Research, North American Spine Society, North Shore-Long Island Jewish Health System, Novo Nordisk Orthologic Corporation, Orthoapedic Research and Education Foundation, Orthopaedic Trauma Association, Scios, Scoliosis Research Society, Spinal Kinetics, SpinalMotion, Spine Solutions, Stryker Corporation, Stryker Howmedica Osteonics, Synthes, TissueLink Medical, Trans1, UC Berkeley United Health Group Company, University of Minnesota, University of Texas at Dallas, Wisconsin Alumni Research Foundation, and Zimmer.

2: Knee

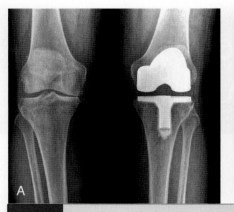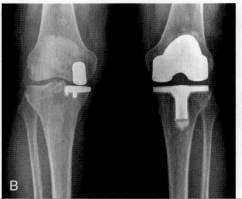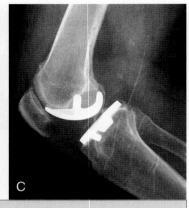

Figure 1 **A**, Preoperative AP radiograph showing isolated medial compartment degenerative disease. **B**, Postoperative AP radiograph after medial unicompartmental joint arthroplasty. **C**, Postoperative lateral radiograph after medial UKA.

stantial compromise in outcomes or implant survivorship,[5-7] making it a legitimate alternative to periarticular osteotomy or TKA in younger patients. Obese patients may have compromised outcomes, although UKA is a reasonable option for patients who are only mildly obese.[5] Incompetence of the anterior cruciate ligament (ACL) may cause abnormal knee kinematics, and anterior tibial subluxation will typically result in posterior tibial wear. However, although ACL insufficiency had historically been considered an absolute contraindication to UKA, it is now considered a reasonable option if there is limited functional instability and the area of femoral contact on the tibia in extension and the location of the tibiofemoral arthritis are anterior.[5] Minimizing the tibial slope in the ACL-deficient knee during UKA is critical, however, to ensure knee stability and implant durability.[9]

Significant subchondral bone loss, due for instance to a large cyst or extensive focal osteonecrosis with structural compromise, may predispose to component subsidence and should thus be considered a contraindication to UKA. Additionally, UKA should be restricted to those without inflammatory arthritis and crystalline arthropathy, although chondrocalcinosis may not be a contraindication if there is no significant inflammation. Grade IV chondromalacia in the lateral compartment of the knee is a contraindication for UKA. Lesser stages of chondromalacia should not be considered contraindications unless the patient reports pain in those compartments.

It is a topic of debate whether the presence of patellofemoral arthritis or grade IV chondromalacia is a contraindication to the performance of UKA. The classic indications suggest that no more than grade III patellofemoral chondromalacia should be present. However, recent studies with a mobile-bearing medial UKA design have suggested that the presence of preoperative patellofemoral arthritis and patellofemoral symptoms are not a contraindication to UKA and do not adversely affect the outcomes.[10] Grade IV chondromalacia of the medial patella or trochlea is better tolerated than lateral patellofemoral wear. Further investigation will

be necessary to determine the role of patellofemoral symptoms or arthritis on UKA outcomes.

Preoperative Evaluation

Pain must be localized to the medial joint. On physical examination, the range of motion, coronal alignment, presence of flexion contractures, and ligament stability should be assessed to determine whether the knee is suitable for unicompartmental arthroplasty.

Routine radiographs should include weight-bearing AP, 45° flexed knee PA, lateral and axial views. Typically, MRI or staging arthroscopy are not indicated and rarely help in clinical decision making. Surgeons should be prepared to convert to TKA or bicompartmental arthroplasty at the time of arthrotomy if other compartments are involved.

Implant Selection/Surgical Technique

Several tibial implant options are available, including fixed-bearing metal-backed, fixed-bearing all-polyethylene, and mobile-bearing components. Equivalent results have been reported, highlighting the requisite emphasis on proper surgical technique and implant design.[11,12]

With conventional techniques there is potential for a wide range of tibial component positioning, and the risk of component malalignment may be greater with minimally invasive surgical approaches.[13] Excessive tibial slope, malalignment, and a varus mechanical axis can predispose to early failure. Computer navigation and robotic-assisted techniques have improved the accuracy of bone preparation in UKA.[14,15]

Outcomes of Medial UKA

Polyethylene wear, component malposition, and progressive opposite and patellofemoral joint degeneration are the most common reasons for revision or reoperation of UKA. Opposite compartment degeneration is uncommon in knees left in slight mechanical varus. Overloading the lateral compartment may be more common with mobile-bearing than fixed-bearing unicompartmental implants. Polyethylene wear is a mechanism of failure for UKAs when polyethylene has a prolonged shelf life or was sterilized by gamma irradiation in air. One study found that shelf life greater than 1.7 years resulted in a 71% survival at 6 years compared to 100% if less than 1.7 years.[16] Another study showed that a tibial slope of less than 7° can protect the ACL from attritional degeneration and rupture.[9]

The results of medial UKA with contemporary designs with at least 10 years of follow-up are available. One study reported a 10-year follow-up with 49 UKAs (38 patients) using a fixed-bearing prosthesis (Miller-Galante implant system (Zimmer, Warsaw, IN)).[17] Implant survival was 98% at 10 years and 95.7% at 13 years. The mean Hospital for Special Surgery knee scores improved from 55 points preoperatively to 92 points postoperatively, with 80% excellent and 12% good results. Progressive patellofemoral joint space loss was observed in 14%. Two knees were revised to TKA because of progressive tibiofemoral arthritis, and no patient had radiographic loosening. The long-term results (average 11.8 years) of the Oxford medial unicompartmental mobile-bearing UKA (Biomet, Warsaw, IN) in 55 knees (51 patients) were reported.[18] The mean postoperative Knee Society knee and function scores were 75 and 90 points, respectively. Six knees were revised to TKA. Survival for any reason at 10 years was 85%; 90% for progression of lateral compartment arthritis as the end point, and 96.3% with component loosening as an end point. The Oxford mobile-bearing UKA was evaluated in patients younger and older than 60 years.[19] The 10-year all-cause survival rate was 90% for those younger than 60 years and 96% for those older than 60 years. Hospital for Special Surgery knee function scores were 94 for patients younger than 60 years and 86 for those older than 60 years, showing that survival is not significantly changed because of age.

The cost-effectiveness of UKA to TKA was recently compared; results indicated that UKAs and TKAs have similar cost-effective profiles in the low-demand, elderly population.[20] Cost analysis was used to determine that the use of UKA is cost-effective when durability and function are similar to that of primary TKA.[21]

Lateral UKA

Isolated lateral compartment OA is associated with lateral joint space narrowing and valgus deformity and is less common than medial compartment OA. Mechanical loads are greater in the medial than lateral compartment, which may favorably affect lateral unicompartmental implant longevity. Valgus alignment is typically corrected to neutral after lateral UKA.[22,23] Mid- to long-term studies demonstrate very low revision rates after lateral unicompartmental arthroplasty.[23-25] However, late failure can occur from progression of disease, loosening, wear, and implant breakage.[26,27]

The indications for lateral UKA include lateral knee

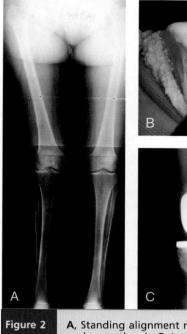
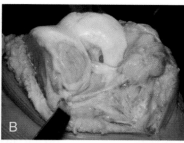
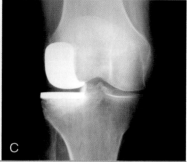

Figure 2 **A,** Standing alignment radiograph showing lateral gonarthrosis. **B,** Lateral arthrotomy for lateral compartment gonarthrosis. **C,** Postoperative radiograph after lateral UKA.

pain associated with isolated lateral tibiofemoral OA limiting activity, an intact ACL, flexion greater than 90°, and flexion contracture less than 10°.[28] Contraindications include a fixed valgus deformity, symptomatic arthrosis of the medial or patellofemoral compartments, and instability. Anterior knee pain should be carefully assessed. Radiographs can underestimate the amount of patellofemoral arthritis that is present.[29] Pain originating from arthrosis of the lateral patellar facet may be improved after lateral UKA by correcting valgus malalignment, which reduces the Q angle and lateral patellofemoral contact. However, medial patellofemoral pain and tenderness indicate pathology on the medial patellar facet that would not be expected to improve after lateral UKA.

Lateral UKA can be performed through either a medial or lateral arthrotomy[28] (**Figure 2**). A highly conservative tibial cut is generally performed first. The flexion and extension gaps are then assessed to determine the distal and posterior position of the femoral component to provide balanced soft-tissue tension throughout the knee's range of motion. The anterior edge of the femoral component is positioned congruent with or below the level of the articular cartilage in the distal trochlear groove to avoid patellar impingement during knee flexion. In lateral UKA, the tibial component should be slightly internally rotated to allow for the greater lateral posterior femoral condylar rollback and femoral external rotation that occurs during normal knee flexion.[23,24]

2: Knee

Both fixed relatively unconstrained or conforming mobile-bearing unicompartmental arthroplasty designs have been used. However, posterior femoral rollback is greater in the lateral than the medial tibiofemoral compartment, which results in greater anteroposterior excursion in the lateral compartment. The increased lateral compartment anteroposterior motion is associated with greater femorotibial sliding motion and risk of dislocation of a mobile-bearing lateral UKA.[30,31] For this reason, a fixed-bearing lateral UKA may be more appropriate than a lateral mobile-bearing prosthesis.

Patellofemoral Arthroplasty

Patellofemoral arthroplasty is an effective treatment of isolated patellofemoral arthritis. Outcomes, however, are impacted by trochlear component design, patient selection, and meticulous surgical technique. Onlay-style trochlear designs have reduced the tendency of patellar instability seen with inlay components due to improved rotational alignment. Isolated patellofemoral arthrosis may occur in 9.2% of patients younger than 40 years.[32] In symptomatic knees, 11% of men and 24% of women may have isolated patellofemoral arthritis.[33] The predilection for patellofemoral arthritis in women may arise from subtle patellar malalignment and an increased incidence of trochlear dysplasia.

Indications/Contraindications

The outcome of patellofemoral arthroplasty can be optimized by limiting it to patients with isolated patellofemoral osteoarthrosis, posttraumatic arthrosis, or severe chondrosis (Outerbridge grade IV). The pain should be restricted to the retropatellar and/or peripatellar areas; provocative activities such as stair or hill climbing, squatting, or prolonged sitting cause an increase in pain. Although it can be most effective for treating patellofemoral dysplasia, patellofemoral arthroplasty should be avoided in patients with considerable patellar maltracking or malalignment, unless these conditions are corrected. Moderate patellar tilt, observed on preoperative tangential radiographs or at the time of arthrotomy, or trochlear dysplasia can easily be corrected with a lateral retinacular recession or release. Patients with excessive Q angles should undergo tibial tubercle realignment before or during patellofemoral arthroplasty (although some trochlear prosthesis shapes may accommodate a slightly increased Q angle). There are no age criteria for patellofemoral arthroplasty provided the other criteria are met.[34]

Contraindications to patellofemoral arthroplasty include inflammatory arthritis, degenerative arthritis, grade III or IV chondromalacia, or chondrocalcinosis involving the menisci or tibiofemoral chondral surfaces. The presence of medial or lateral joint line pain suggests more diffuse chondral disease and should be considered a contraindication to isolated patellofemoral resurfacing. Combining patellofemoral arthroplasty with

medial or lateral UKA (as a modular or monolithic construct) or autologous osteochondral grafting are sound considerations in these situations. Patients with inappropriate expectations and those with unusually excessive pain requiring narcotics may not be suitable candidates. Flexion contractures and limited range of motion are contraindications because they subject the patellofemoral articulation to excessive loads and are indicative of knee pathology that extends beyond the patellofemoral compartment. Although there are intuitive concerns, there are no data available on whether obesity or cruciate ligament insufficiency put the patellofemoral arthroplasty at risk for failure.[35]

Clinical Evaluation

Other causes of anterior knee pain must be excluded, including patella tendinitis, quadriceps tendinitis, prepatellar or pes anserine bursitis, medial or lateral meniscal tears, and concomitant tibiofemoral arthritis. A detailed history and physical examination are usually sufficient to localize the pain to the anterior compartment of the knee. Several key components of the history include determining whether there was previous trauma, a history of subluxation or dislocation, or previous treatments that failed or succeeded in relieving the pain. The pain associated with patellofemoral chondromalacia is almost always directly retropatellar or just medial or lateral to the patella. Typically, patellofemoral pain worsens when walking stairs or hills, squatting, prolonged sitting, and rising from a seated position. Patellofemoral crepitus is also very common.

The physical examination should assess patellar tracking, determine whether the pain is localized to the patellofemoral compartment, and confirm that it is caused by arthritis. Patellar inhibition and compression should produce pain and crepitus. Any associated tenderness along the medial or lateral joint lines should raise the suspicion of more diffuse chondral injury or meniscal pathology and are contraindications to isolated patellofemoral resurfacing. Careful assessment of patellar tracking and the Q angle are extremely important. If there appears to be associated malalignment or evidence of subluxation, patellar realignment may be needed before or during patellofemoral arthroplasty. Range of motion testing should show full extension and a reasonable amount of flexion.

Radiographic evaluation with weight-bearing AP and midflexion PA views is important to rule out tibiofemoral arthritis (Figure 3). Mild squaring of the femoral condyles and small marginal osteophytes are acceptable provided there is no pain or chondromalacia. Lateral radiographs may show patellofemoral osteophytes, joint space narrowing, and the presence of patella alta or baja (Figure 4). Axial films can demonstrate the position of the patella in the trochlear groove and whether there is any trochlear dysplasia or patellar tilt or subluxation (Figure 5). MRI can help determine whether there is cartilage loss in the tibiofemoral compartments. If applicable, previous arthroscopy photo-

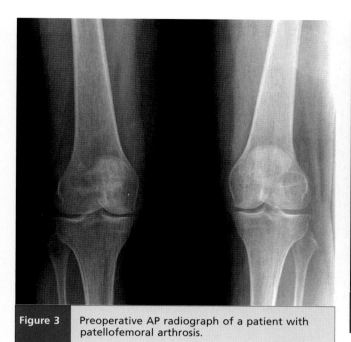

Figure 3 | Preoperative AP radiograph of a patient with patellofemoral arthrosis.

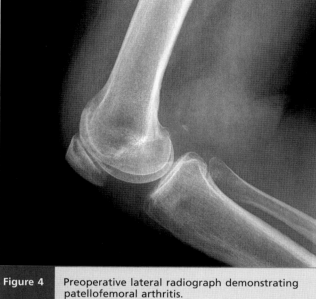

Figure 4 | Preoperative lateral radiograph demonstrating patellofemoral arthritis.

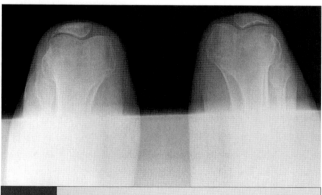

Figure 5 | Preoperative axial radiograph demonstrating bilateral patellofemoral joint arthritis.

graphs should be reviewed to confirm isolated patellofemoral arthritis and rule out associated tibiofemoral pathology.

Surgical Technique

During the arthrotomy, it is important to avoid inadvertent cutting of the articular cartilage of the tibiofemoral compartment or intermeniscal ligament. The tibiofemoral compartments should be assessed. Focal grade IV chondromalacia of a femoral condyle can be treated with autologous osteochondral plug.[36] If diffuse pathology is noted, patellofemoral arthroplasty can be combined with a UKA (modular bicompartmental arthroplasty or monolithic bicompartmental arthroplasty), or a TKA can be performed.

Several key steps in the procedure will enhance surgical outcomes. The first is ensuring that the trochlear component is externally rotated so that it is parallel to the epicondylar axis (or perpendicular to the AP axis of the femur), thus ensuring proper patellar tracking. This prerequisite is impossible with inlay designs, which accounts for the very high incidence of patellar catching and subluxation with those styles.[37-39] Marginal osteophytes bordering the intracondylar notch are removed. The trochlear component should not overhang the medial-lateral femoral margins or impinge the intercondylar notch. Preparation of the trochlear bed should be flush with or recessed approximately 1 mm from the adjacent articular condylar cartilage. Resurfacing the patella should follow the same principles as TKA, with restoration of proper patellar thickness and medialization of the component. The lateral patellar facet should be removed or beveled to avoid lateral impingement and enhance patellar tracking (**Figure 6**).

Patellar tracking is assessed with the trial components in place. If patellar tilt, subluxation, or catching of components is present, proper component position must be ensured and deficiencies corrected. A lateral retinacular recession or release can be performed. In severe cases of subluxation, a proximal realignment may be necessary; if the Q angle is high, a tibial tubercle realignment should be considered.

Immediate weight bearing and range of motion are encouraged. Prophylactic antibiotics are given for 24 hours and thromboembolism prophylaxis is provided for 4 to 6 weeks. Isometric exercises isolating the quadriceps are started immediately. Assistive devices can be discontinued once quadriceps strength has recovered.

Outcomes

The clinical results of patellofemoral arthroplasty are affected by trochlear component shape as well as patient selection and surgical technique.[34,39] Outcomes

2: Knee

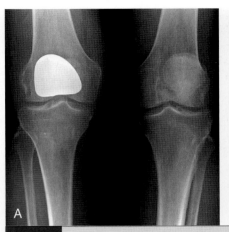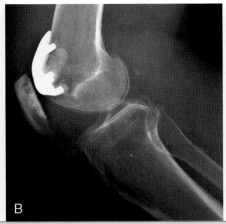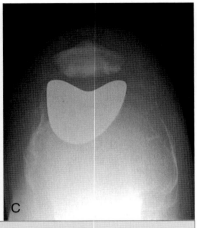

Figure 6 Radiographs of a patient with patellofemoral joint arthroplasty. **A**, Postoperative AP and lateral views. **B**, Postoperative lateral view. **C**, Postoperative axial view.

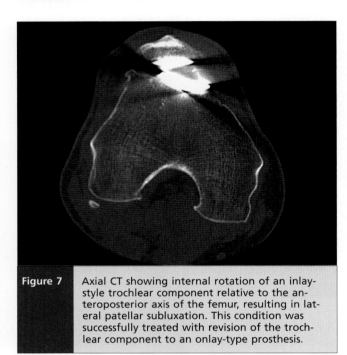

Figure 7 Axial CT showing internal rotation of an inlay-style trochlear component relative to the anteroposterior axis of the femur, resulting in lateral patellar subluxation. This condition was successfully treated with revision of the trochlear component to an onlay-type prosthesis.

have improved, and the need for secondary soft-tissue surgery to enhance patellar tracking after patellofemoral arthroplasty has decreased, due to trochlear design improvements. The radius of curvature, width, thickness, tracking angle, and extent of constraint of the trochlear component impact patellar tracking and outcomes. Contemporary onlay-style designs, which are implanted perpendicular to the anteroposterior femoral axis, have substantially reduced the incidence of patellofemoral complications; however, patella catching and instability remain more common with inlay-style implants, which tend to be internally rotated (except in cases of lateral trochlear dysplasia) (**Figure 7**). Late failures typically occur as a result of progressive tibiofemoral arthritis; loosening and wear are uncommon.

One study reported 85% good or excellent results in 72 first-generation patellofemoral arthroplasties (mean patient age, 60 years) followed for an average of 4 years.[40] There were numerous concomitant surgical procedures performed to enhance patellar tracking, including soft-tissue realignment or tibial tubercle transfer. Longer-term follow-up of those patients, at a mean of 10 years (range, 6 to 16 years) after surgery, found that results deteriorated over time, primarily because of the development of tibiofemoral arthritis. At most recent follow-up, 80% of those who retained their patellofemoral prostheses were pain free and 20% had moderate or severe pain, primarily from tibiofemoral arthritis. Stair climbing was considered normal in 91% of patients. No cases of patellar or trochlear loosening were identified. Early failures peaked at 3 years and were related to inappropriate indications for the surgery and presumably to patellar maltracking problems that could likely be traced to implant design quirks. A secondary peak in failures in the 9th and 10th years postoperatively corresponded to the development of symptomatic tibiofemoral OA, and overall survivorship was 75% at 11 years.[40] An 86% long-term success rate was reported with the same first-generation patellofemoral arthroplasty, even though early secondary soft-tissue surgery was necessary in 18% of patients and revision of the patellofemoral arthroplasty was necessary for catching, imbalance, or malposition in 16%.[41]

In a consecutive series of 30 first-generation implants and 25 second-generation implants, results varied depending on whether an onlay or inlay trochlear design was used.[37] The incidence of patellofemoral dysfunction, subluxation, catching, and substantial pain was reduced from 17% with the inlay design to less than 4% with a more contemporary onlay prosthesis. In another series, 14 inlay design trochlear implants were revised to an onlay implant that had a more favorable topography for patellar tracking.[38] After revision there was statistically significant improvement in knee scores and patellar tracking at a mean 5-year follow-up. Mild femorotibial arthritis (Ahlbach stage I) was predictive of a poorer clinical outcome.

One study reported on 306 second-generation onlay-style patellofemoral arthroplasties; patellar tracking was substantially improved compared to a first-generation inlay-style implant.[42] Patellar subluxation occurred in 3% and residual anterior knee pain was noted in 4% of patients. Four percent required revision to TKA, mostly for tibiofemoral arthritis, but none for mechanical loosening or wear.[42]

Another study reported on 66 second-generation patellofemoral arthroplasties in patients with a mean age of 57 years and mean follow-up of 16 years.[43] Although most patients had substantial and sustained pain relief, 25% were revised to TKA for tibiofemoral arthritis (at a mean of 7.3 years) and 14% for aseptic trochlear component loosening, many of which were uncemented (at a mean of 4.5 years). The best results occurred when the procedure was performed for posttraumatic patellofemoral arthritis or patellar subluxation, and the least favorable results were in patients with primary degenerative arthritis. The development of tibiofemoral arthritis was the most frequent cause of failure. However, at the time of initial patellofemoral arthroplasty, 14% had concomitant tibiofemoral osteotomies for early arthritis, which confounds the results. In those in whom the patellofemoral arthroplasty was retained at most recent follow-up, there were significant improvements in Knee Society scores. The authors continue to advocate for the procedure as an intermediate stage before TKA in the absence of tibiofemoral arthritis or coronal plane malalignment.[43]

Progression of tibiofemoral compartment arthrosis is one of the most common indications for revision to TKA. A 2006 study reported on outcomes of revision to TKA after patellofemoral joint arthroplasty in 12 patients after an average of 3.1 years.[44] None of the patellar components required revision, and standard femoral implants were used without the need for stems, augments, or structural grafts. There were statistically significant improvements of Knee Society clinical and functional scoring and no failures, and it was concluded that TKA is not compromised when revised from patellofemoral joint arthroplasty.

Bicompartmental Arthroplasty

For patients who are not considered suitable candidates for medial UKA as a result of patellofemoral OA, the conventional treatment has been a tricompartmental TKA. TKA is associated with reliable pain relief and excellent survivorship. However, patients who have undergone TKA often do not achieve the level of function of nonarthritic subjects.[45] This result may be related to the altered kinematics of the knee following TKA. During TKA, the ACL and menisci are removed, the joint line is changed, and the geometry of the articular sur-faces is altered. These changes can result in altered kinematics after TKA. "Paradoxical motion" has been observed after posterior cruciate-retaining TKAs in which the femoral condyles contact the posterior tibia in extension and the contact points move anteriorly during knee flexion, while the normal knee exhibits femoral rollback and femoral external rotation during knee flexion.[46] The kinematics after UKA are relatively normal, which is likely related to the retention of the ACL and anatomic structures in the opposite tibiofemoral compartment[47,48]

Bicompartmental (combined medial and patellofemoral) arthroplasty is a relatively new alternative to TKA for the treatment of combined medial and patellofemoral OA. Either the medial or lateral tibiofemoral compartment and the patellofemoral compartment can be simultaneously resurfaced with separate unicompartmental and patellofemoral arthroplasties. The ACL and opposite tibiofemoral compartment are preserved. In a recent report, this approach was associated with excellent pain relief and knee function.[49] Bicompartmental arthroplasty patients could rise independently and ascend stairs leg over leg.

Bicompartmental arthroplasty can also be performed using a single piece femoral component, in combination with a medial tibial unicompartmental component and patellar component (Figure 8). Gait analysis and isokinetic strength tests indicate that normal knee mechanics and gait are restored after bicompartmental arthroplasty.[50] This finding is consistent with previous reports that demonstrate relatively normal kinematics after unicompartmental arthroplasty, which also preserves the ACL.[47,48] Early results using this technique indicate that satisfactory pain relief and function are achieved, and mechanical alignment through the center of the knee is consistently restored.[51] However, because the procedure is relatively new, long-term outcomes have not been reported. In a recent report of 40 bicompartmental knee arthroplasties, a high incidence of pain and early failure was observed.[52] Bicompartmental arthroplasty offers an advantage over TKA by retaining the ACL and restoring more normal knee kinematics.[50] However, it is not clear if clinical outcomes and long-term survivorship will be comparable to TKA.

Summary

Unicompartmental, patellofemoral, and bicompartmental knee arthroplasty are effective treatment alternatives to TKA for more limited knee arthritis. Midterm outcomes may be comparable to those of TKA with proper patient selection, good surgical technique, and implant design. However, kinematic analysis and soft-tissue conservation make partial knee replacement particularly desirable when indicated. Broader adoption of these interventions is likely as data continue to emerge.

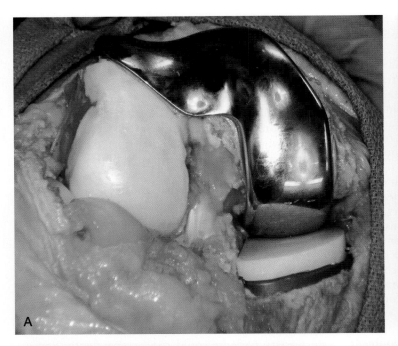
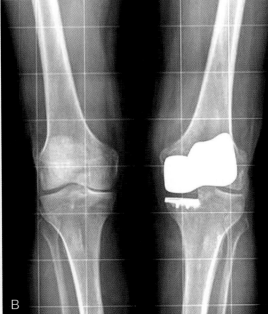
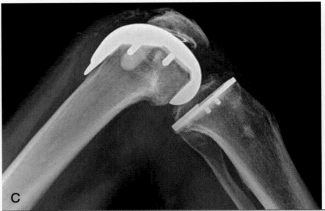
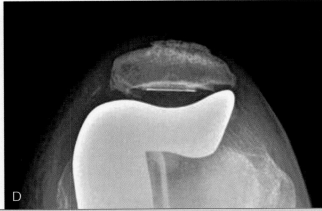

Figure 8 Photograph and radiographs showing monolithic bicompartmental arthroplasty. **A**, Intraoperative photograph (patellofemoral and medial compartments are seen). **B**, Postoperative standing radiographs (medial and patello-femoral compartments are seen). **C**, Lateral postoperative view. **D**, Postoperative axial view.

Annotated References

1. Hawker GA, Wright JG, Coyte PC, et al: Determining the need for hip and knee arthroplasty: The role of clinical severity and patients' preferences. *Med Care* 2001;39(3):206-216.

2. Kurtz S, Ong K, Lau E, Mowat F, Halpern M: Projections of primary and revision hip and knee arthroplasty in the United States from 2005 to 2030. *J Bone Joint Surg Am* 2007;89(4):780-785.

   The authors used Nationwide Inpatient Sample and data from the US Census Bureau to quantify primary and revision arthroplasty rates as a function of age, sex, ethnicity, and region. Estimated increases of 174% in primary total hip arthroplasties and 673% in total knee replacements by the year 2030 were reported.

3. Riddle DL, Jiranek WA, McGlynn FJ: Yearly incidence of unicompartmental knee arthroplasty in the United States. *J Arthroplasty* 2008;23(3):408-412.

   This study evaluated three manufacturers' data in 44 hospitals for the rates of UKA. The authors found an increase of 32.5% in rates of UKA compared to a 9.4% increase in TKA during the same time frame.

4. Ackroyd CE: Medial compartment arthroplasty of the knee. *J Bone Joint Surg Br* 2003;85(7):937-942.

5. Berend KR, Lombardi AV Jr, Adams JB: Obesity, young age, patellofemoral disease, and anterior knee pain: Identifying the unicondylar arthroplasty patient

in the United States. *Orthopedics* 2007;30(5, Suppl)19-23.

The authors evaluated the early outcomes of UKA using the Oxford prosthesis (Biomet, Warsaw, IN) in US patients who did not meet standard inclusion criteria based on weight, age, and isolated pain. Three hundred eighteen UKAs were performed in 270 patients, and it was concluded that currently accepted contraindications had no influence on the successful outcome of the procedure.

6. Pennington DW, Swienckowski JJ, Lutes WB, Drake GN: Unicompartmental knee arthroplasty in patients sixty years of age or younger. *J Bone Joint Surg Am* 2003;85-A(10):1968-1973.

7. Borus T, Thornhill T: Unicompartmental knee arthroplasty. *J Am Acad Orthop Surg* 2008;16(1):9-18.

A review of current approaches to UKA is presented, with a review of advantages to include perioperative mobility and postoperative rehabilitation. Expanding and classic indications with outcomes of both fixed- and mobile-bearing implants are discussed.

8. Kozinn SC, Scott R: Unicondylar knee arthroplasty. *J Bone Joint Surg Am* 1989;71(1):145-150.

9. Hernigou P, Deschamps G: Posterior slope of the tibial implant and the outcome of unicompartmental knee arthroplasty. *J Bone Joint Surg Am* 2004;86-A(3):506-511.

10. Beard DJ, Pandit H, Ostlere S, Jenkins C, Dodd CA, Murray DW: Pre-operative clinical and radiological assessment of the patellofemoral joint in unicompartmental knee replacement and its influence on outcome. *J Bone Joint Surg Br* 2007;89(12):1602-1607.

A review of 100 UKAs in 91 patients between January 2000 and September 2003 is presented. Preoperatively, 54 knees had anterior knee pain and 54 had radiographic evidence of patellofemoral joint degeneration. The authors noted that patients with medial patellofemoral degeneration had outcomes similar to those without and that this condition should not be considered a contraindication for medial or lateral unicompartmental arthroplasty.

11. Hyldahl HC, Regnér L, Carlsson L, Kärrholm J, Weidenhielm L: Does metal backing improve fixation of tibial component in unicondylar knee arthroplasty? A randomized radiostereometric analysis. *J Arthroplasty* 2001;16(2):174-179.

12. Confalonieri N, Manzotti A, Pullen C: Comparison of a mobile with a fixed tibial bearing unicompartmental knee prosthesis: A prospective randomized trial using a dedicated outcome score. *Knee* 2004;11(5):357-362.

13. Hamilton WG, Collier MB, Tarabee E, McAuley JP, Engh CA Jr, Engh GA: Incidence and reasons for reoperation after minimally invasive unicompartmental knee arthroplasty. *J Arthroplasty* 2006;21(6, Suppl 2)98-107.

The authors report on 221 unicompartmental arthroplasties using a minimally invasive technique compared with 514 open medial compartment arthroplasties. Nine failures in 221 knees were reported: 8 for loosening and 1 for infection. Compared to a standard open procedure, the incidence of revision due to aseptic loosening and overall reoperation rates were similar.

14. Keene G, Simpson D, Kalairajah Y: Limb alignment in computer-assisted minimally-invasive unicompartmental knee replacement. *J Bone Joint Surg Br* 2006;88(1):44-48.

A report of 20 consecutive UKAs randomized to either computer navigation or non-navigation is reported. Evaluation of preoperative planned knee alignment was compared. Postoperative assessment of lower limb alignment showed 60% of non-navigated knees were within 2° of planned alignment, whereas 87% of navigated knees were within this range.

15. Lonner JH, John TK, Conditt MA: Robotic arm-assisted UKA improves tibial component alignment: A pilot study. *Clin Orthop Relat Res* 2010;468(1):141-146.

The authors compared 31 consecutive patients undergoing UKA using robotic arm-assisted bone preparation with 27 consecutive patients undergoing UKA using conventional manual instrumentation. Radiographically, the mean square error of posterior tibial slope using manual instrumentation was 3.1° compared to 1.9° using a robotic arm. In the coronal plane the average error was 2.7 +/– 2.1° using manual instruments compared to 0.2 +/– 1.8° with a robotic arm. Level of evidence: III.

16. Collier MB, Engh CA Jr, Engh GA: Shelf age of the polyethylene tibial component and outcome of unicondylar knee arthroplasty. *J Bone Joint Surg Am* 2004;86-A(4):763-769.

17. Berger RA, Meneghini RM, Jacobs JJ, et al: Results of unicompartmental knee arthroplasty at a minimum of ten years of follow-up. *J Bone Joint Surg Am* 2005;87(5):999-1006.

Sixty-two consecutive UKAs with cemented components were followed prospectively for an average of 12 years. Hospital for Special Surgery knee scores improved from 55 preoperatively to 92 postoperatively, with 80% excellent and 12% good results. Only two patients underwent revision during follow-up and no evidence of loosening or osteolysis was found.

18. Emerson RH Jr, Higgins LL: Unicompartmental knee arthroplasty with the oxford prosthesis in patients with medial compartment arthritis. *J Bone Joint Surg Am* 2008;90(1):118-122.

The authors report long-term results of 55 UKAs in 51 patients with respect to outcomes scoring and survivorship. There was an 85% survival rate at 10 years for any reason, 90% for progression of lateral compartment disease, and 96% for loosening. There was substantial sustained improvement of Knee Society

2: Knee

scores and function.

19. Price AJ, Dodd CA, Svard UG, Murray DW: Oxford medial unicompartmental knee arthroplasty in patients younger and older than 60 years of age. *J Bone Joint Surg Br* 2005;87(11):1488-1492.

    The authors present results of Oxford unicompartmental knee arthroplasty in patients younger and older than 60 years. Ten-year all-cause survival rates were reportedly 91% for those younger than 60 years and 96% for those older than 60 years. Hospital for Special Surgery score at 10-year follow-up was 94 for the younger group and 86 for the older patients.

20. Slover J, Espenhaug B, Havelin LI, et al: Cost-effectiveness of unicompartmental and total knee arthroplasty in elderly low-demand patients: A Markov decision analysis. *J Bone Joint Surg Am* 2006;88(11): 2348-2355.

    A model to determine the cost-effectiveness of UKA versus TKA in elderly low-demand patients was developed. It was determined that implantation of UKA was effective in this population if the annual probability of revision is less than 4%. In addition, the cost of UKA needed to be greater than $13,500 or TKA to be less than $8,500 for TKA to become more cost-effective.

21. Soohoo NF, Sharifi H, Kominski G, Lieberman JR: Cost-effectiveness analysis of unicompartmental knee arthroplasty as an alternative to total knee arthroplasty for unicompartmental osteoarthritis. *J Bone Joint Surg Am* 2006;88(9):1975-1982.

    The authors report on a decision model to determine if it is cost-effective to implant single compartment components as opposed to total knee replacement in single compartment disease. They concluded that UKA is a cost-effective choice if costs are less than $50,000 and survival is within 3 to 4 years of anticipated implant survival compared to TKA.

22. Ohdera T, Tokunaga J, Kobayashi A: Unicompartmental knee arthroplasty for lateral gonarthrosis: Midterm results. *J Arthroplasty* 2001;16(2):196-200.

23. Sah AP, Scott RD: Lateral unicompartmental knee arthroplasty through a medial approach: Study with an average five-year follow-up. *J Bone Joint Surg Am* 2007;89(9):1948-1954.

    Forty-nine lateral UKAs were retrospectively reviewed at an average follow-up of 5.2 years. Preoperative alignment averaged 10° of valgus, which was corrected to 6.2° of valgus postoperatively. There were no revisions or soft-tissue complications.

24. Pennington DW, Swienckowski JJ, Lutes WB, Drake GN: Lateral unicompartmental knee arthroplasty: Survivorship and technical considerations at an average follow-up of 12.4 years. *J Arthroplasty* 2006;21(1):13-17.

    Twenty-nine lateral UKAs were performed with the tibial component in 10° to 15° of internal rotation to compensate for the normal "screw home" mechanism of the knee. There were no revisions at an average follow-up of 12.4 years.

25. Argenson JN, Parratte S, Bertani A, Flecher X, Aubaniac JM: Long-term results with a lateral unicondylar replacement. *Clin Orthop Relat Res* 2008;466(11): 2686-2693.

    The authors reviewed 40 lateral unicompartmental arthroplasties at an average follow-up of 12.6 years. Survivorship was 92% at 10 years and 84% at 16 years.

26. Ashraf T, Newman JH, Evans RL, Ackroyd CE: Lateral unicompartmental knee replacement survivorship and clinical experience over 21 years. *J Bone Joint Surg Br* 2002;84(8):1126-1130.

27. Walton MJ, Weale AE, Newman JH: The progression of arthritis following lateral unicompartmental knee replacement. *Knee* 2006;13(5):374-377.

    Thirty-two lateral unicompartmental arthroplasties were assessed after 5 years. There was a significant increase in radiographic OA at 5 years compared to that seen on the immediate postoperative radiograph. Six patients required revision for progression of OA in the retained compartments.

28. El-Yussif E, Engh GA: A technique for lateral unicompartmental arthroplasty: A road less traveled. *Semin Arthroplasty* 2009;20:6-10.

    The important aspects of the lateral UKA include using a figure-of-4 leg position, downsizing the femoral component to avoid patellofemoral impingement, avoiding tibial component external rotation, and lateralizing the femoral component.

29. Chang CB, Seong SC, Kim TK: Evaluations of radiographic joint space: Do they adequately predict cartilage conditions in the patellofemoral joint of the patients undergoing total knee arthroplasty for advanced knee osteoarthritis? *Osteoarthritis Cartilage* 2008; 16(10):1160-1166.

    Radiographic joint space height and intraoperative cartilage loss were assessed in 151 TKAs. The prediction of cartilage loss in the patellofemoral joint based on radiographs was found to be inaccurate.

30. Robinson BJ, Rees JL, Price AJ, et al: Dislocation of the bearing of the Oxford lateral unicompartmental arthroplasty: A radiological assessment. *J Bone Joint Surg Br* 2002;84(5):653-657.

31. Gunther TV, Murray DW, Miller R, et al: Lateral unicompartmental arthroplasty with the Oxford meniscal knee. *Knee* 1996;3:33-39.

32. Davies AP, Vince AS, Shepstone L, Donell ST, Glasgow MM: The radiologic prevalence of patellofemoral osteoarthritis. *Clin Orthop Relat Res* 2002;402(402): 206-212.

33. McAlindon TE, Snow S, Cooper C, Dieppe PA: Radiographic patterns of osteoarthritis of the knee joint in

the community: The importance of the patellofemoral joint. *Ann Rheum Dis* 1992;51(7):844-849.

34. Leadbetter WB, Seyler TM, Ragland PS, Mont MA: Indications, contraindications, and pitfalls of patellofemoral arthroplasty. *J Bone Joint Surg Am* 2006;88(Suppl 4):122-137.

   This review article analyzed trends in the literature of patellofemoral arthroplasty to identify critical factors contributing to the success or failure of these operations. A review of clinical experience of the Avon Patellofemoral arthroplasty (Stryker Orthopaedics, Mahwah, NJ) is presented, including indications, contraindications, pitfalls, and midterm follow-up.

35. Lonner JH: Patellofemoral arthroplasty. *J Am Acad Orthop Surg* 2007;15(8):495-506.

   This review article presents the latest published data concerning patellofemoral joint arthroplasty to include indications, patient evaluation, surgical and postoperative management, and clinical results.

36. Lonner JH, Mehta S, Booth RE Jr: Ipsilateral patellofemoral arthroplasty and autogenous osteochondral femoral condylar transplantation. *J Arthroplasty* 2007;22(8):1130-1136.

   This study reports the short-term results of ipsilateral patellofemoral arthroplasty and autologous osteochondral transplantation in four patients, with an average age of 40 years, who had patellofemoral arthritis and focal full-thickness chondral defects of the femoral condyles. At a mean of 2.7 years after surgery, the mean Knee Society function score improved from 49 to 93 and the clinical score improved from 47 to 95.

37. Hendrix MR, Ackroyd CE, Lonner JH: Revision patellofemoral arthroplasty: Three- to seven-year follow-up. *J Arthroplasty* 2008;23(7):977-983.

   This study showed that significant improvement in patellar tracking can be obtained when revising an inlay-style patellofemoral arthroplasty to an onlay design with a more accommodating implant design, provided there is no tibiofemoral arthritis.

38. Australian Orthopaedic Association National Joint Replacement Registry: http://www.dmac.adelaide.edu.au/aoanjrr/publications.jsp. Accessed March 29, 2011.

   The tendency for revision after patellofemoral arthroplasty differs significantly depending on whether an inlay or onlay-style trochlear component is used. For instance in that series, the cumulative 5-year revision rate was 21.8% with the LCS prosthesis (DePuy, Warsaw, IN) and 9.9% with the Avon implant. Data on newer systems are not yet available in that registry.

39. Lonner JH: Patellofemoral arthroplasty: The impact of design on outcomes. *Orthop Clin North Am* 2008;39(3):347-354, vi.

   This review highlights the impact of trochlear design features on outcomes and patellar tracking after patellofemoral arthroplasty.

40. Cartier P, Sanouiller J-L, Khefacha A: Long-term results with the first patellofemoral prosthesis. *Clin Orthop Relat Res* 2005;436(436):47-54.

   The authors report on the long-term results of 70 patients (79 knees) undergoing patellofemoral arthroplasty from 1975 to 1991 with average follow-up of 10 years and 75% survival at a minimum of 6 years.

41. Kooijman HJ, Driessen AP, van Horn JR: Long term results of patellofemoral arthroplasty: A report of 56 arthroplasties with 17 years of follow-up. *J Bone Joint Surg Br* 2003;85(6):836-840.

42. Ackroyd CE, Newman JH, Evans R, Eldridge JD, Joslin CC: The Avon patellofemoral arthroplasty: Five-year survivorship and functional results. *J Bone Joint Surg Br* 2007;89(3):310-315.

   A review of 109 patellofemoral replacements in 85 patients with minimum follow-up of 5 years is presented. The survival rate was 95.8% with no cases of loosening. Success was based on the Bristol Pain Score and reported at 80%. Twenty-five patients (28%) had implant failure due to progression of tibiofemoral arthritis.

43. Argenson JN, Flecher X, Parratte S, Aubaniac JM: Patellofemoral arthroplasty: An update. *Clin Orthop Relat Res* 2005;440:50-53.

   Sixty-six knees underwent patellofemoral arthroplasty and were followed for an average of 16.2 years. Twenty-nine of the 66 knees required conversion to TKA at latest follow-up, 11 due to trochlear loosening and 14 due to progression of tibiofemoral joint disease.

44. Lonner JH, Jasko JG, Booth RE Jr: Revision of a failed patellofemoral arthroplasty to a total knee arthroplasty. *J Bone Joint Surg Am* 2006;88(11):2337-2342.

   Twelve failed patellofemoral arthroplasties were revised to posterior stabilized TKAs for isolated progressive tibiofemoral arthritis, isolated patellofemoral catching and maltracking, or a combination of both. No stems, augments, or structural bone graft were necessary. At a mean follow-up of 3.1 years, there was significant improvement in Knee Society scores (p < 0.001). Mean Knee Society clinical and functional scores increased from 57 to 96 and 51 to 91, respectively. At most recent follow-up, there is no clinical or radiographic evidence of patellofemoral maltracking, loosening, or wear.

45. Noble PC, Gordon MJ, Weiss JM, Reddix RN, Conditt MA, Mathis KB: Does total knee replacement restore normal knee function? *Clin Orthop Relat Res* 2005;431:157-165.

   Two hundred forty-three TKA patients and 257 individuals without knee disorders were surveyed. Activities that were biomechanically more demanding such as squatting, dancing, carrying heavy objects, kneeling, turning, and cutting were avoided by TKA patients.

46. Dennis DA, Komistek RD, Mahfouz MR, Haas BD, Stiehl JB: Multicenter determination of in vivo kine-

2: Knee

matics after total knee arthroplasty. *Clin Orthop Relat Res* 2003;416(416):37-57.

47. Argenson JN, Komistek RD, Aubaniac JM, et al: In vivo determination of knee kinematics for subjects implanted with a unicompartmental arthroplasty. *J Arthroplasty* 2002;17(8):1049-1054.

48. Akizuki S, Mueller JK, Horiuchi H, Matsunaga D, Shibakawa A, Komistek RD: In vivo determination of kinematics for subjects having a Zimmer Unicompartmental High Flex Knee System. *J Arthroplasty* 2009; 24(6):963-971.

    Thirty medial UKAs in 18 patients were studied with in vivo fluoroscopy. On average, the implant experienced posterior femoral rollback and normal axial rotation during flexion.

49. Argenson JA, Parratte S, Bertani A, et al: The new arthritic patient and arthroplasty treatment options. *J Bone Joint Surg Am* 2009;91 (Suppl 5):43-48.

    Early outcomes of 17 patients with two-piece non-linked bicompartmental (medial or lateral tibiofemoral and patellofemoral) arthroplasty were reviewed. All patients had mild or no pain, could rise unassisted, and were able to ascend stairs leg over leg.

50. Wang H, Dugan E, Frame J, Rolston L: Gait analysis after bi-compartmental knee replacement. *Clin Biomech (Bristol, Avon)* 2009;24(9):751-754.

    Gait and knee extension strength were evaluated in 10 healthy control subjects and 8 bicompartmental knee arthroplasty patients. Bicompartmental patients exhibited good frontal plane knee mechanics and were able to produce a knee extensor moment equivalent to healthy control limbs.

51. Rolston L, Siewert K: Assessment of knee alignment after bicompartmental knee arthroplasty. *J Arthoplasty* 2009;24(7):1111-1114.

    Mechanical axis alignment was assessed in 137 bicompartmental knee arthroplasties. Preoperatively, 77 knees (56%) had a mechanical axis passing medial to the center of the knee. Postoperatively, 130 knees (95%) had a mechanical axis passing through the center of the knee.

52. Tria AJ Jr: Bicompartmental arthroplasty of the knee. *Instr Course Lect* 2010;59:61-73.

    Forty patients (42 knees) underwent bicompartmental knee arthroplasty. Ten patients had persistent anterior knee pain, three patients had "global" knee pain, and two knees were revised. One tibial tray fractured, and one collapsed anteriorly.

Chapter 10

New Technology for Knee Arthroplasty

Michael P. Bolognesi, MD   Andrew D. Pearle, MD   Jeremy M. Oryhon, MD   Ryan M. Nunley, MD

Computer-Assisted Total Knee Arthroplasty
Michael P. Bolognesi, MD

Computer-assisted total knee navigation systems allow the surgeon to plan and perform the femoral and tibial bone cuts in a very precise fashion, and have been supported by numerous reports in the literature.[1-8] All systems rely on some type of signaling technology that allows surgical instrumentation to be positioned in the desired position for bone resection. The signaling options that exist include, but are not limited to, infrared and electromagnetic signaling. Some systems require three-dimensional preoperative imaging such as CT; others use intraoperative imaging (fluoroscopy), and some are imageless. Despite all of these various options, the guiding principles behind a navigated technique remain very simple. The system needs to be "educated" about where the limb and knee joint are in space. This is achieved by registering the required anatomic points in such a fashion that the system knows the location of the center of the hip joint, and resection landmarks in the knee and the center of the ankle joint at all times. Trackers must be placed on the femur and tibia to allow this information to remain constant and accurate while the leg is moved during the surgical procedure. These trackers can be passive or active and must be secured rigidly to the respective bone with stable fixation. If they are not rigidly fixed

or they lose fixation, the accuracy of the registration is affected and the surgeon might have to consider switching to a standard technique. When tracker placement is done correctly, the surgeon is afforded a continuous and real-time depiction of the deformity of the limb before resections are performed and documentation of the correction of these deformities as bone resections and ligament releases are made.

Computer navigation systems can have image-based or imageless platforms. One technique requires a preoperative CT scan. The surgeon can use the three-dimensional anatomic data provided by the CT scan to plan the idealized intraoperative component positioning. In the operating room the surgeon must register actual anatomic points in the surgical field to allow the procedure to be performed. This registration lets the surgeon then make bone resections in idealized planes on the CT scan. There has been some concern expressed over the radiation dose associated with a CT scan as well as the additional cost of the study. There have been studies performed that confirm the accuracy that can be obtained with a CT-based technique.[9,10]

Another technique uses intraoperative fluoroscopic imaging. Most platforms require that two or more images be obtained and then the procedure can be performed while navigating on these images. This avoids the expense of the preoperative CT scan but does require fluoroscopy in the operating room. Some surgeons have expressed concern about the potential increased risk of infection with extra personnel in the room, as well as the radiation exposure to the members of the surgical team as disadvantages of this technique. This technique has also provided a high accuracy of coronal component position.[11]

The imageless navigation technique for total knee arthroplasty (TKA) requires the surgeon to register all of the appropriate anatomic points in the operating room. This navigation system then creates a "virtual" image of the limb and the knee joint. This technique requires that the trackers on the femur and the tibia remain fixed throughout the procedure. The surgeon can use instrumentation specific to the navigation system to position resection blocks or use reference arrays that can be positioned within cutting slots in standard instrumentation to perform navigated bone preparation. This

Dr. Bolognesi or an immediate family member is a member of a speakers' bureau or has made paid presentations on behalf of Zimmer; serves as a paid consultant to or is an employee of Biomet, Zimmer, and Amedica; has received research or institutional support from Zimmer, Wright Medical Technology, DePuy, and Biomet; and owns stock or stock options in Amedica. Dr. Pearle or an immediate family member has received research or institutional support from Brainlab, Praxim, Medvision, and MAKO Surgical. Dr. Nunley or an immediate family member serves as a paid consultant for or is an employee of Smith & Nephew, Wright Medical Technology, and Salient Surgical and has received research or institutional support from Biomet, Wright Medical Technology, Stryker, Smith & Nephew, Biospace, and Mobile Compression Systems. Neither Dr. Oryhon nor any immediate family member has received anything of value from or owns stock in a commercial company or institution related directly or indirectly to the subject of this chapter.

2: Knee

technique has tended to be the most frequently used because no preoperative or intraoperative imaging is required. Imageless systems are available from many vendors and most have universal software applications that avoid the need to use a specific implant. These systems have continued to evolve with a decrease in size in the operating room. With some systems, the computer is completely ceiling mounted and can be contained within a single overhead boom (**Figure 1**). The software applications have also improved with time to allow for improved screen outputs and more facile interfacing for the surgeon with the navigated approach (**Figure 2**). The actual trackers and the associated instruments have also improved with the systems (**Figure 3**).

Tracking Technologies

A large number of computer navigation systems use infrared tracking, in which the computer hardware is linked to a camera that can detect the position of the trackers and any instrument that has a tracker array affixed to it. Other systems use an electromagnetic ap-

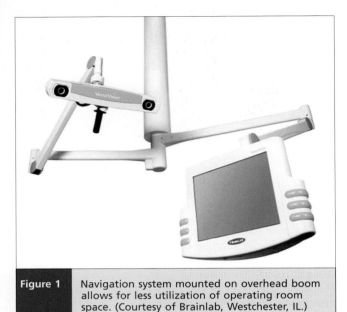

Figure 1 Navigation system mounted on overhead boom allows for less utilization of operating room space. (Courtesy of Brainlab, Westchester, IL.)

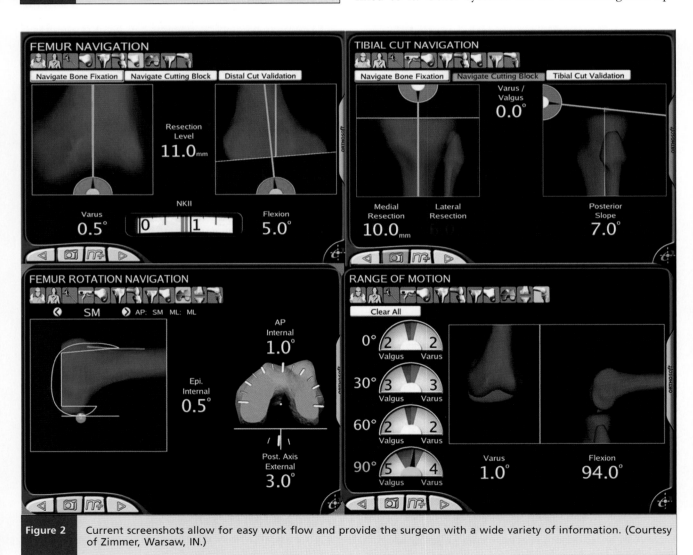

Figure 2 Current screenshots allow for easy work flow and provide the surgeon with a wide variety of information. (Courtesy of Zimmer, Warsaw, IN.)

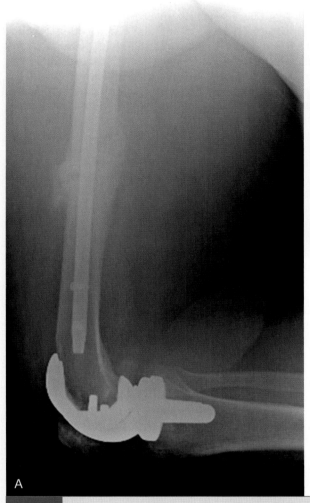

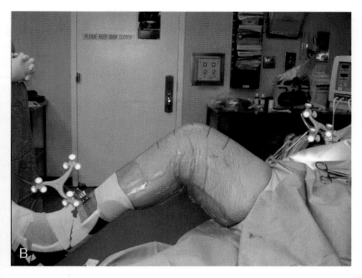

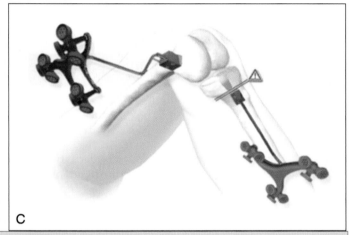

Figure 5 **A**, Radiograph showing femur fracture after tracker placement treated with a trochanteric start point intramedullary nail. Avoiding tracker placement in the midshaft of the femur (**B**) and using a distal metaphyseal placement (**C**) might be safer. (Panel C courtesy of Zimmer, Warsaw, IN.)

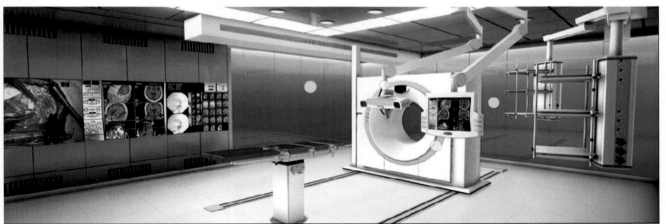

Cranial   Spine   Hip   ☺

Figure 6 The ability to perform intraoperative imaging in the "operating rooms of the future" will likely facilitate navigated surgical techniques and allow for streamlined registration. (Courtesy of Brainlab, Westchester, IL.)

2: Knee

cost savings could be obtained with navigation if the additional cost was contained to $629.[35] Another study suggested that navigation could be cost-effective in large-volume total joint centers.[36] It is hoped that in the future the additional costs will decrease relative to other costs associated with the procedure.

The tracker pin sites on the femur and the tibia can be sites of complications, including fracture and infection.[37-39] One study reported 980 consecutive primary knee arthroplasties performed with navigation and no fractures.[40] However, this study reported tibial tracker pin site infections requiring antibiotic treatment. As tracking technology improves, these complications may be avoided based on changes in the method and need for fixation. With the current systems that rely on rigid pin fixation to the femur and tibia, the surgeon must be aware of these potential complications (**Figure 5**). Intraoperative imaging in the operating room of the future will allow for easier registration and navigated surgical techniques (**Figure 6**).

Robot-Assisted Knee Surgery
Andrew L. Pearle, MD

The increase in demand for minimally invasive orthopaedic procedures over the past two decades has been met with a surge in the production of "smart tools" to adequately adapt to the smaller size of the surgical field. Innovations in computer-assisted surgery have led to improvements in the precision of orthopaedic procedures. By combining advanced imaging technologies (such as CT) with registration algorithms, computer navigation systems can accurately reproduce the individual anatomy of the patient and convert it into an interactive virtual model on the computer screen. This technology allows the surgeon to create an accurate surgical plan and to reproduce it in the operating room.

Surgical precision, however, still has limitations. Available conventional tools have inherent limitations that may introduce errors into the surgical procedure. The skill of the surgeon also directly influences the outcome of the procedure, especially considering the steep learning curve required for certain manual procedures. Robotic technology was developed to improve the surgeon's abilities and precision, to improve outcomes and recovery times for the patient, and to reduce the number of mechanical instruments required in the operating room. Robots may potentially provide standardization of conventional surgical procedures.

In joint arthroplasty surgery, alignment of the components directly influences the longevity of the prosthesis and the clinical outcome of the procedure. Malalignment can lead to reduced life of the prosthesis, suboptimal mechanical function, and arthrosis in other joints. Good clinical outcomes in TKAs are associated with postoperative leg alignment of 3° or less.[41] During conventional procedures, the surgeon must estimate the alignment of the cutting tools and the prosthetic com-

ponents, leading to variable results. Computer assistance has improved limb-alignment outcomes in comparison with unassisted surgical techniques; however, reports indicate that inadequate limb alignment still occurs in 20% to 30% of patients.[1,42] Robots have been introduced specifically to reduce positioning and execution errors during surgery. Imprecise bone sawing has been suggested as one of the main factors contributing to joint malalignment. Because robots can saw a stiff object very precisely, there have been numerous attempts at developing reliable and functional robotic devices for use in orthopaedic surgery.

Classification
Robots may be classified as passive, active, and semiactive, according to their level of involvement in performing a procedure. An active robot autonomously performs part of the surgical procedure, based on information provided to the robotic system. The surgeon observes the procedure being performed by the robot and may intervene at any time to stop the procedure and may then continue the surgery using the conventional technique. When using semiactive robots, the surgeon moves the cutting tool while the robot restricts its motion based on boundaries set in the preoperative plan. Passive robots, such as navigation systems, do not actively perform any part of the surgical procedure, but provide information to the surgeon regarding the position of the instruments relative to the anatomy of the patient and the surgical plan.

Based on their role in the surgical procedure, robots may be categorized as either positioning tools for placing surgical instruments or implants or as execution tools for performing a step of the operation, such as bone cutting. Robots may also be described as floor-mounted, table-mounted, or bone-mounted devices.

Advantages and Disadvantages
It has been suggested that robots are effective tools for minimally invasive orthopaedic procedures. Their high accuracy has increased the precision of bone-cutting techniques for prosthesis implantation, leading to improvements in implant positioning, fit, placement, and alignment. This improved alignment may lead to a reduced risk of implant loosening. When used appropriately, robots provide consistent performance, reducing the percentage of alignment outliers. Robots may also decrease the learning curve for surgeons, allowing a high level of proficiency in a shorter period of time.

Important disadvantages remain in the use of surgical robots. The high initial acquisition costs of robotic arm units make them economically prohibitive for low- and mid-volume surgical centers. Although robots may decrease surgical time in some instances, this decrease is the exception rather than the norm. Because robotics is a relatively new and continuously evolving technology, long-term follow-up on the impact of robots in surgical orthopaedic outcomes cannot be readily evaluated.

History and Development

Several orthopaedic robotic technologies have been developed over the past decade (**Tables 1** and **2**). A chronologic listing along with a description of the features of the main robotic systems is presented in this section.

ROBODOC System

The ROBODOC system (Curexo Technology, Fremont, CA) was developed in 1986 in a joint collaboration between IBM Research and the University of California, Davis. Commercialized by Integrated Surgical Systems in 1992, ROBODOC became the first active robot used for surgery on humans.[43,44] It was introduced in Germany in 1994 and has since been used mainly in primary and revision hip arthroplasty.[43]

The system was developed to improve implant selection, implant sizing, positioning of the implant within the bone, and accurate preparation of the bone cavity that accepts the implant. ROBODOC uses a preoperative planning computer workstation (ORTHODOC) and a five-axis robotic arm with a high-speed milling device. Three-dimensional preoperative planning is performed by the computer workstation based on data obtained from CT scans. Data and the optimized plan are transferred to ROBODOC, which mills the bone cavity as determined by the plan after registration of the femur. For registration, three titanium screw fiducials are necessary.[43] One of the disadvantages of the system is the need for a separate preliminary surgery for placing the fiducials.[45]

Studies evaluating the ROBODOC system show conflicting results. Two studies, one with 97 patients and another with 65 patients, reported equal outcomes with the robotic and manual techniques.[43,44] The fit and positioning of the femoral component, varus-valgus orientation of the stem, and limb-length similarity were significantly better on postoperative radiographs of patients treated with the robotic technique.[45,46] Using ROBODOC, there was a significant reduction in the occurrence of intraoperative femoral fractures.[43,45] At longer follow-ups of 6 and 12 months, the group treated with robotic implantation had better clinical scores. However, by the 24-month follow-up, there was no detectable difference between the groups with regard to the Mayo clinical scores and the Harris hip scores.[46]

Among the disadvantages of the ROBODOC were the high number of technical complications and system failures, directly or indirectly related to the robot, which reportedly occurred in 9% to 18% of implantations.[44,46] The durations of the robotic procedures were longer than those of the manual procedures, and slightly more heterotopic ossification was reported in the ROBODOC group. The most serious complication was hip dislocation. Recurrent dislocation and pronounced limping were indications for revision surgery in patients treated with robotic implantation. No patients in the control group had indications for revision

surgery. The ROBODOC system also required soft-tissue cutting. Rupture of the gluteus medius tendon was observed during all of the revisions in the robotic group and was believed to be responsible for the higher dislocation rate. Nerve injury was unacceptably high at 7%. The sciatic nerve may have been injured by the femoral fixator clamp or the decreased blood supply to the nerve.[46] Following widespread reports of gluteus medius damage and the subsequent lawsuits, ROBODOC use in Germany was ended by 2003. ROBODOC is not approved by the FDA for use in the United States.

Acrobot Sculptor System

The Acrobot Sculptor system (Acrobot, London, England) was designed for use in TKA and then adapted for use in unicompartmental knee arthroplasty. This system provides the surgeon with an accurate tool with real-time computer visualization capabilities.[47] Preoperative virtual planning is performed using the Acrobot Modeller and Planner software packages that incorporate three-dimensional CT data and allow bone segmentation and calculation of the volume of bone that needs to be removed before implant placement. This information is then uploaded to the Sculptor robotic system.

The robot works through a hands-on integrated system for accurately machining the bone, with the surgeon controlling the position of the milling tool using a handle instrumented with a force sensor.[48] The Acrobot Sculptor is a semiactive robot that consists of two devices: (1) a high-speed cutter that provides the active constraints and (2) a robotic positioning device on which the cutter is mounted. The robot assists the surgeon in milling bone about the knee and prevents the surgeon from cutting bone away from outside the areas determined by the preoperative plan, based on three-dimensional CT models of the leg.[49] The surgeon remains in charge of the operation by retaining full control of the system at all times.[47] No fiducial markers are needed with the Acrobot system; however, bone clamps are used, which result in four extra stab wounds in addition to the surgical cuts.[49,50]

When first built, the Acrobot system was believed to achieve a more consistent angular alignment of the prosthesis and of the corresponding tibiofemoral alignment in the coronal plane than conventional instrumentation.[49] In several studies, the Acrobot system showed a significant improvement in the accuracy of implant placement in relationship to the planned placement compared with the accuracy achieved with the conventional method.[47,49,50] However, the duration of the robotic procedure was significantly longer.[49]

The Acrobot system has been successfully used to accurately register and cut the knee bones in knee arthroplasty. This device demonstrates the great potential of a hands-on robot for improving accuracy and increasing patient safety.[48]

Table 1

The Main Robotic Systems Used in Orthopaedic Surgery

Classification	Name	Manufacturer	Year of Introduction	Surgery
Active	ROBODOC	Curex Technology	1992	Hip and knee
Semiactive	MAKO Tactile Guidance System	MAKO Surgical Corporation	2006	Knee
Semiactive	Acrobot Sculptor	Acrobot	1999; first trials 2002	Knee
Semiactive	PiGalileo	Smith and Nephew	2004	Hip and knee
Semiactive	iBlock	Praxim	2004	Knee

Table 2

Study Results of Robotics Literature

Author	Procedure/System	No. of Patients	Surgical Time (min)	Follow-up Time
Lonner et al[56]	UKA/MAKO	31	N/A	3 months
Pearle et al[54]	UKA/MAKO	10	132 (mean, 118 to 152)	6 weeks
Sinha[57]	UKA/MAKO	20	N/A	N/A
Cobb et al[49]	UKA/Acrobot	13 patients, 13 knees	104 ± 16.6	18 weeks

RMSE = root mean square error; UKA = unicompartmental knee arthroplasty

PiGalileo System

The PiGalileo system (Smith and Nephew, London, England) was first introduced by PLUS Endoprothetik AG (Rotkreuz, Switzerland) in 2004 as a practical navigation system with an integrated bone-mounted robot that serves as a cutting block. An integrated ligament tensioning device measures and applies the correct tension. The navigation is performed by an infrared optical system (Polaris; NDI, Waterloo, Canada). After registration of the bone landmarks and the mechanical axis through kinematic analysis and direct palpation, the computer can move the cutting block in precalculated positions. To alter the tension of the ligaments, it is possible to move the cutting block in 0.5-mm steps in the cranial-caudal and ventral-dorsal directions as directed by the force sensors.

Clinical results for 69 consecutive implantations found a mean deviation of only 1° from the ideal femoral axis.[51] An analysis of blood loss, the length of hospitalization, range of motion on discharge, and complications showed no significant differences when compared with conventional surgery.

MAKO Tactile Guidance System

The MAKO Tactile Guidance System (MAKO Surgical Corporation, Ft. Lauderdale, FL) is the only minimally invasive robotic system currently in use for knee surgery. It is a semiactive system used for unicompartmental knee arthroplasty. The first study of patients treated using the MAKO robot was published in 2010.[52]

Customized CT-based planning is performed before surgery. Bone surfaces are segmented by the software package to produce patient-specific three-dimensional models that allow the virtual positioning of implants for preoperative planning. Once optimal parameters are defined by the surgeon, bone resection areas and boundaries for cutting are established in the robotic system to prevent incorrect cutting. This preliminary plan may be modified intraoperatively according to gap measurements throughout flexion and dynamic lower limb alignment values.

The system consists of a robotic arm and a standard optical infrared camera (**Figure 7**). During the actual surgical procedure, the surgeon moves the robotic arm by guiding the force-controlled tip within the pre-

Table 1

The Main Robotic Systems Used in Orthopaedic Surgery (continued)

Technique	Current Status	Imaging Used
Milling device	Rarely used after first introduction	Fluoroscopic
Burring tool	Currently used in unicompartmental knee arthroplasty	CT-based
Cutting tool	Currently used	Fluoroscopic CT-based
Cutting guide	Currently used	Image-free
Cutting guide	FDA approval pending	CT-based

Table 2

Study Results of Robotics Literature (continued)

Tibial Component Posterior Slope	Tibial Component Coronal Slope	Alignment Outliers	Complications
RMSE = 1.9°	0.2° ± 1.8°	0	One case of tibial subsidence at 3 months
N/A	N/A	0	0
4.29° ± 3.24°	4.60° ± 1.76°	0 flexion outliers; 19% tibial slope outliers (versus 25% preoperative)	N/A
N/A	1.5° ± 1.4°	0	Three mild adverse events (nonserious; swelling, skin blister), one intermediate adverse event (serious; urinary retention)

RMSE = root mean square error; UKA = unicompartmental knee arthroplasty

defined boundaries. The active feedback mechanism (haptic and audio) of the robot ensures cutting only in the previously specified areas (Figure 8). If the surgeon attempts to move the cutting burr past the predefined volume while the cutting burr is set to the burring mode, the robotic arm applies a force simulating contact with a rigid wall, thereby confining the tip to the correct region in space. The system permits intraoperative tissue balancing and controls the preparation of osseous surfaces directly through tactile guidance of the cutting burr. With the augmented surgical control of the haptic robotic system and bone-sparing implants, a limited surgical exposure can be used.[53-55]

A report on the first 10 patients successfully treated using the MAKO robot showed a difference between the planned and intraoperative femoral angles of only 1°, and a postoperative long-leg mechanical axis within 1.6°.[52] One advantage of the MAKO robot is that the system does not depend on any permanent or rigid fixation to the patient, thereby reducing complications caused by the weight and movement of the robot. The robot is very accurate in burring the exact cavity required for the implant.

A study of 31 patients treated with unilateral medial unicompartmental knee arthroplasty with the MAKO robot arm showed a reduction in both error and variance of the alignment of the tibial component in the coronal and sagittal planes.[56] Results were similar to those of conventional unicompartmental knee arthroplasty with regard to complications, patient function, and the surgeon's learning curve.

Limitations of the MAKO Tactile Guidance System include the initially longer surgical time when compared with conventional methods; learning curve issues, which usually occur with new techniques; and the cost of the robotic arm base unit.[52,57] Given the recent adoption of this technology, no long-term follow-up studies are available in the literature. Further follow-up is necessary to determine if the reduction in error and variance of alignment observed with the MAKO system will influence implant function or survival after unicompartmental knee arthroplasty.[52,57]

iBlock
Development of iBlock (Praxim, Grenoble, France), a semiautomatic cutting guide (formerly referred to as

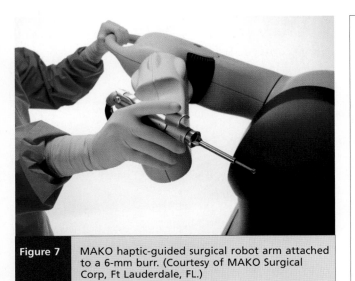

Figure 7 | MAKO haptic-guided surgical robot arm attached to a 6-mm burr. (Courtesy of MAKO Surgical Corp, Ft Lauderdale, FL.)

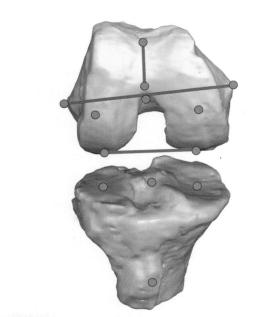

Figure 9 | Computer modeling software creates a three-dimensional model of the distal femur and proximal tibia to analyze the bony topography to help calculate component size, alignment, and rotation of the implants.

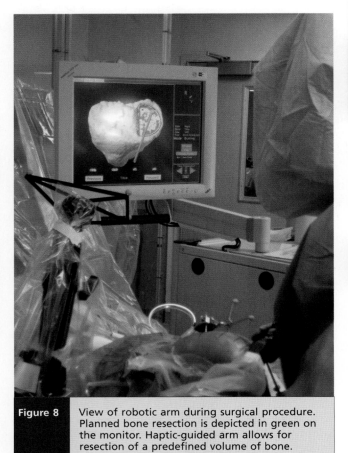

Figure 8 | View of robotic arm during surgical procedure. Planned bone resection is depicted in green on the monitor. Haptic-guided arm allows for resection of a predefined volume of bone.

different planes to guide the cuts for the femoral component.[58]

Ongoing cadaver testing has shown the iBlock to have easy setup, reduced surgical time, and more precise cuts. No clinical results are yet available.

Patient-Specific Cutting Guides
Jeremy M. Oryhon, MD
Ryan M. Nunley, MD

Over the past several years, computer-assisted technology has evolved to include patient-specific custom cutting guides, which have the benefits of computer-aided accuracy and the potential for more efficient intraoperative resource and time management, without the need for costly investments in capital equipment.

Technology
Traditional computer-navigated TKA is completely intraoperative; these intraoperative navigation systems recognize the position of carefully arranged tracking arrays mounted on pins placed into the tibia and femur. The surgeon must manually register certain bony landmarks to calculate the optimal bony resections and implant position. Conversely, patient-specific cutting guide technology removes the intraoperative variability and time requirements by shifting the bony landmark registration and implant positioning to the preoperative setting. Preoperative CT or MRI is required to con-

Praxiteles) commenced in 2004. iBlock is a semiactive, bone-mounted, robotic cutting jig that integrates with the Praxim navigation system by attachment to the medial femoral condyle with a navigation array. After all calculations have been done using the navigation software, two motors allow the iBlock jig to move in five

2: Knee

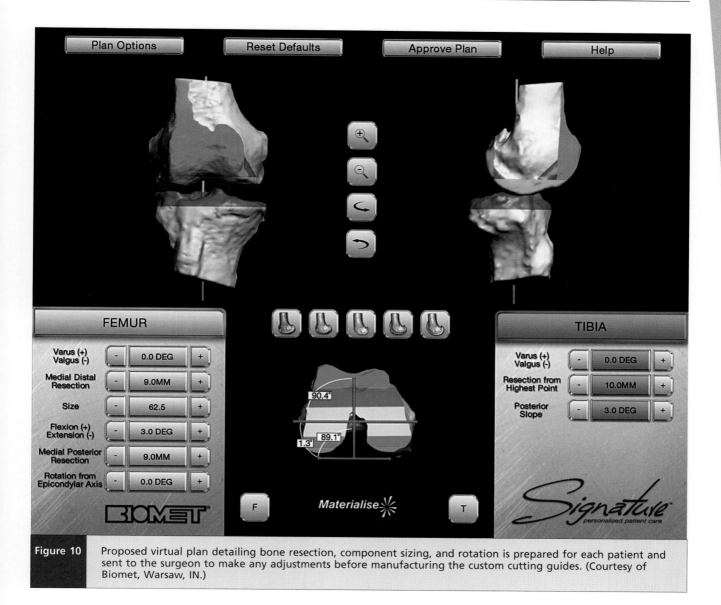

Figure 10 Proposed virtual plan detailing bone resection, component sizing, and rotation is prepared for each patient and sent to the surgeon to make any adjustments before manufacturing the custom cutting guides. (Courtesy of Biomet, Warsaw, IN.)

struct a virtual three-dimensional model of the knee. Images through the hip and ankle are obtained from either a scout CT scan, an MRI with selected cuts at the hip and ankle, or from a long cassette radiograph. These images are then used to determine the mechanical alignment of the lower extremity. Computer modeling software analyzes the bony topography to create a virtual knee model (**Figure 9**) that is used to calculate the proper size femoral and tibial components, and the ideal component alignment and rotation for stock (noncustom) components. Default implant sizing and proposed alignment targets are predetermined by the individual surgeon and mapped onto the virtual knee images, which are then sent to the surgeon for review (**Figure 10**). The surgeon may modify the proposed virtual plan to incorporate any patient-specific clinical findings, such as flexion contractures or ligament deficiencies, before the actual manufacturing of the custom cutting guides.

Once the preoperative plan is finalized, the exact bone resections are designed into the patient-specific cutting blocks to match the virtual knee specifications for component sizing, alignment, and rotation.

Using a process of rapid prototyping, the approved virtual three-dimensional models are converted into disposable patient-specific cutting guides that use the patient's existing osteophytes and unique bony topography to lock onto the distal femur and proximal tibia (**Figures 11 and 12**). Once the custom guides are accurately positioned they are secured to the bone with pins. Some of the custom guides are designed with the cutting slots already incorporated into the custom guide. Other systems use the custom guides to establish the accurate placement of the fixation pins, and then the custom guides are replaced with conventional cutting jigs.

The custom femoral guide determines the rotation, distal resection (axial alignment and extension gap), AP

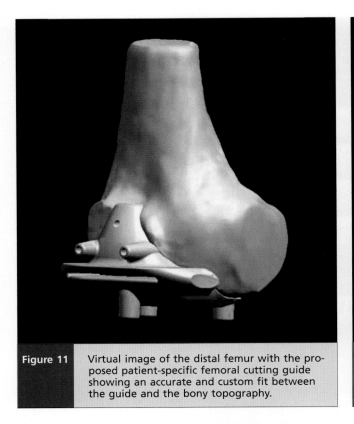

Figure 11   Virtual image of the distal femur with the proposed patient-specific femoral cutting guide showing an accurate and custom fit between the guide and the bony topography.

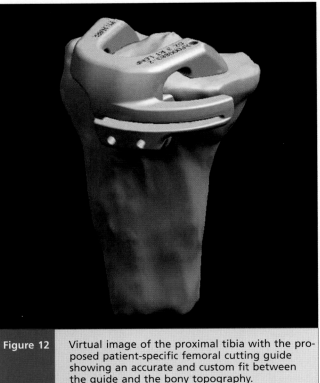

Figure 12   Virtual image of the proximal tibia with the proposed patient-specific femoral cutting guide showing an accurate and custom fit between the guide and the bony topography.

resections (component size and flexion gap), and flexion-extension of the femoral component. The custom tibial guide determines the thickness of the tibial resection, axial alignment, posterior tibial slope, tibial component size, and polyethylene liner thickness. Most commercially available patient-specific cutting guides are designed to obtain the same rotational and axial alignment goals as would be expected with conventional instrumentation.

There is a second type of patient-specific cutting guide technology commercially available called the OtisKnee (OtisMed, Alameda, CA) that uses similar three-dimensional knee modeling technology but is designed to restore the knee to its prearthritic state, which may not necessarily restore the mechanical axis of the lower extremity. With this system, a preoperative MRI of the knee is analyzed with proprietary software and cartilage wear in the medial and lateral aspects of the knee joint is calculated. A virtual model can be generated with the goal of only restoring the knee to its prearthritic alignment. Thereafter, the process is essentially the same with the manufacturing of the patient-specific custom guides and the utilization of stock implants to replicate the shape-matched restored knee. The OtisKnee system operates on a different philosophy that is based on kinematic alignment rather than mechanical alignment. There has been some controversy regarding this system's apparent disregard for restoring the mechanical axis, which has been a fundamental tenet of TKA surgery for several decades. A

limited amount of short-term data are available to assess both of these new technologies.

Advantages and Disadvantages

Early reports indicated that there is some improvement in component positioning using intraoperative computer assistance, but alignment outliers still occur. There is a tendency for surgeons to override the computer system, and long-term functional data are lacking. One of the anticipated benefits of patient-specific cutting guides is the potential to more accurately and reliably place the TKA implants with fewer outliers, which may improve patient outcomes, satisfaction, and implant durability.

One of the criticisms of intraoperative computer navigation is the additional time required during surgery to use this technology, even for proficient surgeons. Patient-specific cutting blocks have the unique advantage of moving the navigational component outside of the operating room and reducing the number of intraoperative steps required to perform the procedure. The steps that are avoided or significantly reduced include reduced soft-tissue exposure, avoidance of intramedullary and extramedullary instruments, time required to secure multiple cutting/alignment jigs in place, and avoidance of femoral and tibial sizing and resection devices. Avoiding these steps is potentially advantageous for the surgeon, the patient, and the hospital. The surgeon might benefit from more efficient surgery, improved implant sizing/alignment, decreased intraoperative decision making (which may reduce surgeon stress), and the potential to perform more surgical procedures due to the time saved.[59] The patient might benefit from decreased surgical time, with potentially decreased anesthetic complications; shorter tourniquet time (which might decrease postoperative pain, deep venous thrombosis risk, and muscle ischemia); and less blood loss and possible arthrofibrosis due to avoidance of instrumenting the intramedullary canal. The hospital may benefit from faster surgery with the potential to perform more surgical cases; fewer instruments and trays are required to perform the surgery so there is less to clean and sterilize; surgical technicians are not overwhelmed with all the trays and instrumentation; and inventory may be reduced because fewer trays are needed to perform the case and, with known sizing of the implants, fewer carts of implants are necessary.

High start-up capital equipment costs may deter an otherwise promising technology from being implemented, even if it may lead to long-term cost savings by direct price reduction, increases in efficiency, alternative revenue flows, decreases in complications (and the cost associated with them) or a combination thereof.[60,61] Unlike computer-assisted surgery, patient-specific cutting guides do not require any capital equipment expenditures by the hospital or surgeon; therefore, the start-up costs for this new technology are minimal. However, there is the additional cost of CT or MRI that must be obtained preoperatively (in patients who normally would not require such radiographic imaging for TKA); these costs usually are billed to the patient's health insurance. There is also a charge associated with the analysis of the MRI and the production of the patient-specific cutting guides; the implant company bills the hospital for these costs in addition to the cost of the stock TKA components. To date, there have been no published studies reporting the cost-benefit analysis for patient-specific cutting guides used in TKA.

Compared to computer-assisted surgery, patient-specific cutting guides have a minimal intraoperative learning curve. There is a learning curve that involves working with the company engineers preoperatively to refine the custom blocks prior to manufacture. Although it has been shown that minimally invasive TKA might account for a higher percentage of overall revisions and earlier time to revision,[62] patient-specific cutting blocks may have a role in allowing the surgeon to safely and more accurately perform TKA surgery through smaller incisions.

Results

There are only a few studies of the results of TKA using patient-specific custom cutting guide technology. A cadaver study with CT-based guides showed accuracy in bone cuts, implant sizing, and implant positioning with a mean error for alignment and bone resection within 1.7°/mm and maximum error less than 2.3°/mm.[63] Another study reported on 44 TKAs with MRI-based custom cutting guides.[64] All components were found to be accurately sized and implanted in satisfactory alignment (4° to 8° valgus), with no instability and no reoperations at 6 weeks after surgery.

A report on the OtisKnee system involving 48 knees showed no adverse events and an average surgical time of 53 minutes (range, 39 to 71 minutes).[65] It was reported that the custom cutting guides fit well, but 3% of the femoral guides and 3% of the tibial guides did not conform well to the distal femur or proximal tibia. These problems were attributed to the MRI techniques. Long-leg CT alignment averaged −1.4° ± 2.8° valgus. At 3 months postoperatively, 35% of patients reported their knee felt "normal" and 60% reported that the knee felt "nearly normal." There was a mean of 114° (range, 92° to 134°) of active flexion, with an average Knee Society score of 171 (range, 130 to 200). The OtisKnee has been reported to have minimal prevalence of adduction/lateral lift-off and reverse axial rotation, which are undesirable consequences and are reported to be higher with traditional TKA techniques.[66] Another report on the OtisKnee found the recommended cuts were more than 3° off the mechanical axis and the authors raised the concern that the malalignment with this system might place the implant at high risk for early failure.[67]

Future Directions

Computer navigation for TKA must continue to evolve so that the advantages inherent to the technique can outweigh current limitations and reported complications. The technique must become so simple that the surgery time is not affected. The technique should deviate minimally from a standard, nonnavigated approach. The work flow between the navigation system and the surgeon's instruments has to be seamless. Cost for the hardware, software, and instrumentation must not be prohibitive. The technique must avoid introducing new complications not associated with a standard approach. It is likely that these systems will become integrated in the operating rooms of the future. Surgical suites can now be married to a CT scanner or MRI scanner, which can be used with the patient positioned on the surgical table. The surgeon can then perform the required registration in the surgical field and immediately navigate in reference to the imaging study just obtained. This process avoids the need for obtaining the study in an outpatient setting before the patient goes to the operating room.

This type of integration may occur for both the three-dimensional imaging navigation platforms and imageless platforms. The ideal scenario would be an approach that allows the surgeon to perform the procedure in a way that closely resembles a standard approach, but provides the surgeon with the information associated with the navigated approach. These data would be available to the surgeon in real time.

Because all navigated systems are composed of computer hardware and software, it is understood that the

2: Knee

process will evolve. Computer navigation may be considered routinely for complicated cases and it may be adapted for widespread use in the future. To make an assumption on the role of navigation in the future based solely on the status and the performance of the current systems that are available would be shortsighted.

Robots increase the precision and accuracy of the bone-cutting techniques used in joint reconstruction surgery, as well as the positioning and alignment of the prosthetic implants. They may also decrease the surgeon's learning curve associated with certain conventional procedures, helping to achieving a more consistent performance.

Possibly increased surgical times, conflicting clinical outcome reports, and a high cost-benefit ratio remain as limitations of robotic implementation in orthopaedic surgery. As the number of TKAs increase annually, future developments in smart tool technology should resolve current safety concerns and could result in measurable benefits.

Patient-specific cutting guides for TKA are an emerging technology that may offer some potential advantages over both traditional instrumentation and intraoperative computer navigation. There have been few studies validating its use and no studies on the cost-benefit ratio of implementing this technology. Future research and longer follow-up is necessary to determine the accuracy, durability, and time efficiency of patient-specific cutting guides in TKA surgery.

Annotated References

1. Bäthis H, Perlick L, Tingart M, Lüring C, Zurakowski D, Grifka J: Alignment in total knee arthroplasty: A comparison of computer-assisted surgery with the conventional technique. *J Bone Joint Surg Br* 2004;86(5): 682-687.

2. Bohling U, Schamberger H, Grittner U, Scholz J: Computerized and technical navigation in total knee-arthroplasty. *J Orthop Traumatol* 2005;5:69.

   The authors concluded that computerized navigation improved precision during TKA, with possible reduction of aseptic loosening.

3. Chauhan SK, Scott RG, Breidahl W, Beaver RJ: Computer-assisted knee arthroplasty versus a conventional jig-based technique: A randomised, prospective trial. *J Bone Joint Surg Br* 2004;86(3):372-377.

4. Chin PL, Yang KY, Yeo SJ, Lo NN: Randomized control trial comparing radiographic total knee arthroplasty implant placement using computer navigation versus conventional technique. *J Arthroplasty* 2005; 20(5):618-626.

   The authors compared the radiologic outcome of conventional techniques with computer-navigated surgery for TKA and found that computer-navigated TKA helps increase accuracy and reduce outliers for implant placement.

5. Oberst M, Bertsch C, Würstlin S, Holz U: CT analysis of leg alignment after conventional vs. navigated knee prosthesis implantation: Initial results of a controlled, prospective and randomized study. *Unfallchirurg* 2003;106(11):941-948.

6. Saragaglia D, Picard F, Chaussard C, Montbarbon E, Leitner F, Cinquin P: Computer-assisted knee arthroplasty: Comparison with a conventional procedure. Results of 50 cases in a prospective, randomized study. *Rev Chir Orthop Reparatrice Appar Mot* 2001;87(1): 18-28.

7. Sparmann M, Wolke B, Czupalla H, Banzer D, Zink A: Positioning of total knee arthroplasty with and without navigation support: A prospective, randomised study. *J Bone Joint Surg Br* 2003;85(6):830-835.

8. Stulberg DS, Picard F, Saragaglia D: Computerassisted total knee replacement arthroplasty. *Oper Tech Orthop* 2000;10:25.

9. Bäthis H, Perlick L, Tingart M, Lüring C, Perlick C, Grifka J: Radiological results of image-based and non-image-based computer-assisted total knee arthroplasty. *Int Orthop* 2004;28(2):87-90.

10. Mizu-uchi H, Matsuda S, Miura H, Okazaki K, Akasaki Y, Iwamoto Y: The evaluation of post-operative alignment in total knee replacement using a CT-based navigation system. *J Bone Joint Surg Br* 2008;90(8): 1025-1031.

    Thirty-nine TKAs implanted using a conventional alignment guide system were compared with 37 implanted using a CT-based navigation system. The ideal angles of all alignments (using full-length weight-bearing AP radiographs, lateral radiographs, and CT scans) in the navigated group were obtained at significantly higher rates than in the conventional group.

11. Victor J, Hoste D: Image-based computer-assisted total knee arthroplasty leads to lower variability in coronal alignment. *Clin Orthop Relat Res* 2004;428:131-139.

12. Kilian P, Plaskos C, Parratte S, et al: New visualization tools: Computer vision and ultrasound for MIS navigation. *Int J Med Robot* 2008;4(1):23-31.

    Echo surgetics, a new image acquisition method used for minimally invasive computer-assisted surgical procedures, was found to have significantly improved results over conventional digitization.

13. Song EK, Seon JK, Park SJ, Yoon TR: Accuracy of navigation: A comparative study of infrared optical and electromagnetic navigation. *Orthopedics* 2008; 31(10, Suppl 1).

    The authors studied the accuracy of infrared optical and electromagnetic navigation systems in measuring the mechanical axis of patients having TKA and in a bone model. Accuracy of both systems was affected by erroneous registration, with the optical system more reproducible than the electromagnetic system.

14. Tigani D, Busacca M, Moio A, Rimondi E, Del Piccolo N, Sabbioni G: Preliminary experience with electromagnetic navigation system in TKA. *Knee* 2009;16(1): 33-38.

    This report analyzes the postoperative radiologic results of 32 knees treated using an electromagnetic system and found an ideal alignment for the mechanical axis (180°± 3°) in 30 of 32 cases. All patients achieved a value of 90°± 3° for both femoral and tibial frontal component angles. An apparently overcorrected implant position for the sagittal femoral component was reported, with a mean value of 11.2°± 3.6°.

15. Lionberger DR, Weise J, Ho DM, Haddad JL: How does electromagnetic navigation stack up against infrared navigation in minimally invasive total knee arthroplasties? *J Arthroplasty* 2008;23(4):573-580.

    Forty-six primary TKAs were performed using either an electromagnetic (EM) or infrared (IR) navigation system. Mechanical alignment was ideal in 92.9% of EM and 90.0% of IR cases based on spiral CT imaging and 100% of EM and 95% of IR cases based on radiographs. Individual measurements of component varus/valgus and sagittal measurements showed EM to be equivalent to IR.

16. Graydon AJ, Malak S, Anderson IA, Pitto RP: Evaluation of accuracy of an electromagnetic computer-assisted navigation system in total knee arthroplasty. *Int Orthop* 2009;33(4):975-979.

    The authors assessed the accuracy of an electromagnetic computer navigation system for TKA in a limb with normal or abnormal mechanical alignment and found that deformity did not affect accuracy.

17. Alan RK, Shin MS, Tria AJ Jr: Initial experience with electromagnetic navigation in total knee arthroplasty: A radiographic comparative study. *J Knee Surg* 2007; 20(2):152-157.

    Electromagnetic navigation in TKA is studied.

18. Mason JB, Fehring TK, Estok R, Banel D, Fahrbach K: Meta-analysis of alignment outcomes in computer-assisted total knee arthroplasty surgery. *J Arthroplasty* 2007;22(8):1097-1106.

    This study identified 29 studies of computer-assisted surgery in comparison with conventional TKA and determined that mechanical axis malalignment of greater than 3° occurred in 9.0% of patients in the computer-assisted group compared with 31.8% of conventional TKA patients. Tibial and femoral slope both showed statistical significance in favor of computer-assisted surgery at greater than 2° malalignment. This meta-analysis demonstrated significant improvement in component orientation and limb alignment when computer-assisted surgery was used.

19. Alden KJ, Pagnano MW: The consequences of malalignment: Are there any? *Orthopedics* 2008;31(9): 947-948.

    The authors discuss the possible consequences of malalignment.

20. Del Gaizo D, Soileau ES, Lachiewicz PF: Value of preoperative templating for primary total knee arthroplasty. *J Knee Surg* 2009;22(4):284-293.

    In this study, tibial and femoral resections were templated in 200 primary TKAs. Postoperative tibiofemoral alignment was within 3° of the goal alignment in 189 (94.5%) knees. Postoperative femoral and tibial component coronal alignment was within 3° of the goal alignment in 190 (95%) and 199 (99.5%) knees, respectively. This study demonstrated a very low incidence of outliers using a conventional technique.

21. Kamat YD, Aurakzai KM, Adhikari AR, Matthews D, Kalairajah Y, Field RE: Does computer navigation in total knee arthroplasty improve patient outcome at midterm follow-up? *Int Orthop* 2009;33(6):1567-1570.

    The outcome of computer-navigated and conventional TKA was compared, and radiologically malaligned knees were analyzed.

22. Molfetta L, Caldo D: Computer navigation versus conventional implantation for varus knee total arthroplasty: A case-control study at 5 years follow-up. *Knee* 2008;15(2):75-79.

    The authors compared computer-assisted and conventional TKA in patients with varus knee osteoarthritis. No significant clinical difference between the two groups was found 5 years after surgery.

23. van Strien T, van der Linden-van der Zwaag E, Kaptein B, van Erkel A, Valstar E, Nelissen R: Computer assisted versus conventional cemented total knee prostheses alignment accuracy and micromotion of the tibial component. *Int Orthop* 2009;33(5):1255-1261.

    The authors compared conventional TKA with CT-free and CT-based computer-assisted surgery and evaluated TKA alignment and micromotion. No clinically significant difference in alignment was found. There was a significant difference for micromotion in subsidence between the three groups.

24. Fehring TK, Mason JB, Moskal J, Pollock DC, Mann J, Williams VJ: When computer-assisted knee replacement is the best alternative. *Clin Orthop Relat Res* 2006;452:132-136.

    Sixteen patients (18 knees) with posttraumatic femoral deformity, retained femoral hardware, a history of osteomyelitis, or severe cardiopulmonary disease were managed with a computer-assisted surgical technique. The mechanical axis of the limb using computer-assisted surgery was acceptable in 16 of the 17 knees that were successfully navigated. Computer-assisted surgery was helpful in these difficult cases where the use of traditional instrumentation was not ideal.

25. Klein GR, Austin MS, Smith EB, Hozack WJ: Total knee arthroplasty using computer-assisted navigation in patients with deformities of the femur and tibia. *J Arthroplasty* 2006;21(2):284-288.

    Five patients with extra-articular femoral and/or tibial deformity, retained hardware, or intramedullary implants underwent TKA using a computer navigation system. In all cases the navigation system proved to be

2: Knee

an effective tool for restoration of limb alignment and provided an alternative approach to the traditional intramedullary instrumentation for treating these patients in an effective manner.

26. Mullaji A, Shetty GM: Computer-assisted total knee arthroplasty for arthritis with extra-articular deformity. *J Arthroplasty* 2009;24(8):1164-1169, e1.

Forty extra-articular deformities (22 femoral and 18 tibial) in 34 patients were managed with a computer-assisted surgical technique. The mean postoperative limb alignment was 179.1°. Computer-assisted surgery was an effective means of managing these complex cases.

27. Bottros J, Klika AK, Lee HH, Polousky J, Barsoum WK: The use of navigation in total knee arthroplasty for patients with extra-articular deformity. *J Arthroplasty* 2008;23(1):74-78.

Computer-assisted navigation was found to be as effective as high technology instrumentation in improving and restoring the lower limb mechanical axis in patients with deformity.

28. Church JS, Scadden JE, Gupta RR, Cokis C, Williams KA, Janes GC: Embolic phenomena during computer-assisted and conventional total knee replacement. *J Bone Joint Surg Br* 2007;89(4):481-485.

The authors conducted a double-blind, randomized study to compare the cardiac embolic load sustained during computer-assisted and conventional, intramedullary-aligned, total knee replacement, as measured by transoesophageal echocardiography. There were 26 consecutive procedures performed by a single surgeon at a single hospital. The results demonstrated a highly significant increase (P = 0.004) in embolic load in the conventional group.

29. Kalairajah Y, Cossey AJ, Verrall GM, Ludbrook G, Spriggins AJ: Are systemic emboli reduced in computer-assisted knee surgery? A prospective, randomised, clinical trial. *J Bone Joint Surg Br* 2006; 88(2):198-202.

This study compared noninvasive Doppler signals in 14 patients undergoing TKA with a computer-assisted technique to 9 patients treated with standard instrumentation. The difference between the two groups was highly significant using the Wilcoxon nonparametric test (P = 0.0003). The findings show that computer-assisted TKA, when compared with conventional jig-based surgery, significantly reduces systemic emboli as detected by transcranial Doppler ultrasonography.

30. Kim YH, Kim JS, Hong KS, Kim YJ, Kim JH: Prevalence of fat embolism after total knee arthroplasty performed with or without computer navigation. *J Bone Joint Surg Am* 2008;90(1):123-128.

Two hundred ten primary TKAs performed with navigation were compared with 210 cases done without navigation. The prevalence of fat and/or bone-marrow-cell embolization was not significantly different between the patients who underwent TKA with navigation and those who underwent it without navigation.

31. O'Connor MI, Brodersen MP, Feinglass NG, Leone BJ, Crook JE, Switzer BE: Fat emboli in total knee arthroplasty: A prospective randomized study of computer-assisted navigation vs standard surgical technique. *J Arthroplasty* 2010;25(7):1034-1040.

The authors studied fat emboli in patients undergoing TKA who were randomly assigned to surgery with computer-assisted navigation or the standard surgical technique and concluded that any difference in the extent of emboli between the two groups is not likely to be clinically significant.

32. Kalairajah Y, Simpson D, Cossey AJ, Verrall GM, Spriggins AJ: Blood loss after total knee replacement: Effects of computer-assisted surgery. *J Bone Joint Surg Br* 2005;87(11):1480-1482.

The authors evaluated blood loss in 60 patients who underwent TKA; 30 patients underwent a computer-assisted procedure and 30 had a standard surgical procedure. The reduction of blood drainage and the calculated hemoglobin loss between the two groups was highly significant. In patients in whom blood products are not acceptable, computer-assisted surgery may be useful.

33. Browne JA, Cook C, Hofmann AA, Bolognesi MP: Postoperative morbidity and mortality following total knee arthroplasty with computer navigation. *Knee* 2010;17(3):152-156.

The authors identified 101,596 patients who underwent TKA; 1,156 of these patients had a computer-assisted procedure. Computer navigation was associated with a lower rate of postoperative cardiac complications, a shorter length of hospital stay, and fewer hematomas.

34. Jenny JY, Miehlke RK, Giurea A: Learning curve in navigated total knee replacement: A multi-centre study comparing experienced and beginner centres. *Knee* 2008;15(2):80-84.

This observational study was performed at 13 European orthopaedic centers. Navigated techniques initially took an additional 10 to 20 minutes, but were reduced to 7 minutes after a 30-procedure learning period.

35. Novak EJ, Silverstein MD, Bozic KJ: The cost-effectiveness of computer-assisted navigation in total knee arthroplasty. *J Bone Joint Surg Am* 2007;89(11): 2389-2397.

A decision-analysis model was used to estimate the cost-effectiveness of computer-assisted surgery in TKA. The model assumes computer-assisted surgery to be both more effective and more expensive than mechanical alignment systems. This model indicates that cost savings could be achieved if the added cost of computer-assisted surgery was $629 or less per operation.

36. Slover JD, Tosteson AN, Bozic KJ, Rubash HE, Malchau H: Impact of hospital volume on the economic value of computer navigation for total knee replacement. *J Bone Joint Surg Am* 2008;90(7):1492-1500.

A Markov decision model was used to evaluate the impact of hospital volume on the cost-effectiveness of computer-assisted knee arthroplasty in a theoretic cohort of patients. Computer navigation was less likely to be a cost-effective investment in health care improvement in centers with a low volume of joint arthroplasties. This model suggests that it may be a cost-effective technology for centers with a higher volume of joint arthroplasties.

37. Wysocki RW, Sheinkop MB, Virkus WW, Della Valle CJ: Femoral fracture through a previous pin site after computer-assisted total knee arthroplasty. *J Arthroplasty* 2008;23(3):462-465.

   The authors discuss two instances of femoral fracture via a previous pin site, a complication that has not previously been reported in the literature.

38. Manzotti A, Confalonieri N, Pullen C: Intra-operative tibial fracture during computer assisted total knee replacement: A case report. *Knee Surg Sports Traumatol Arthrosc* 2008;16(5):493-496.

   The authors discuss the case of an elderly man with an intraoperative tibial fracture at the site of insertion of a navigation tracker during computer-assisted TKA.

39. Li CH, Chen TH, Su YP, Shao PC, Lee KS, Chen WM: Periprosthetic femoral supracondylar fracture after total knee arthroplasty with navigation system. *J Arthroplasty* 2008;23(2):304-307.

   The authors report on a patient who sustained a supracondylar periprosthetic fracture 1 month after computer-assisted TKA; pinhole fracture is a possible complication.

40. Owens RF Jr, Swank ML: Low incidence of postoperative complications due to pin placement in computer-navigated total knee arthroplasty. *J Arthroplasty* 2009. Epub ahead of print.

   Postoperative complications after primary TKA (n = 984) were studied; 17 patients had minor pin-related complications and 12 had a superficial infection near the tibial pin site that was treated with antibiotics.

41. Rand JA, Coventry MB: Ten-year evaluation of geometric total knee arthroplasty. *Clin Orthop Relat Res* 1988;232:168-173.

42. Victor J, Hoste D: Image-based computer-assisted total knee arthroplasty leads to lower variability in coronal alignment. *Clin Orthop Relat Res* 2004;Nov(428): 131-139.

43. Bargar WL, Bauer A, Börner M: Primary and revision total hip replacement using the Robodoc system. *Clin Orthop Relat Res* 1998;354:82-91.

44. Schulz AP, Seide K, Queitsch C, et al: Results of total hip replacement using the Robodoc surgical assistant system: Clinical outcome and evaluation of complications for 97 procedures. *Int J Med Robot* 2007;3(4): 301-306.

   The authors report on 97 total hip arthroplasties performed using the ROBODOC system. ROBODOC ap-peared to achieve equal clinical outcomes compared with manual technique; however, it had a 9.3% rate of technical complications.

45. Nishihara S, Sugano N, Nishii T, et al: Clinical accuracy evaluation of femoral canal preparation using the ROBODOC system. *J Orthop Sci* 2004;9(5):452-461.

46. Honl M, Dierk O, Gauck C, et al: Comparison of robotic-assisted and manual implantation of a primary total hip replacement: A prospective study. *J Bone Joint Surg Am* 2003;85-A(8):1470-1478.

47. Barrett AR, Davies BL, Gomes MP, et al: Computer-assisted hip resurfacing surgery using the acrobot navigation system. *Proc Inst Mech Eng H* 2007;221(7): 773-785.

   An overview of the Acrobot system for unicompartmental knee arthroplasty is presented. Preoperative and intraoperative processes are described.

48. Jakopec M, Harris SJ, Rodriguez y Baena F, Gomes P, Cobb J, Davies BL: The first clinical application of a "hands-on" robotic knee surgery system. *Comput Aided Surg* 2001;6(6):329-339.

49. Cobb J, Henckel J, Gomes P, et al: Hands-on robotic unicompartmental knee replacement: A prospective, randomised controlled study of the acrobot system. *J Bone Joint Surg Br* 2006;88(2):188-197.

   The authors present the results of a prospective randomized controlled trial of 28 knees, comparing the performance of the Acrobot system with conventional surgery in unicompartmental knee arthroplasty. Tibiofemoral alignment and other parameters were measured. The Acrobot group appeared to have a favorable alignment in all knees, compared with only 40% of knees in the conventional group. Surgical time was longer with the Acrobot system.

50. Rodriguez F, Harris S, Jakopec M, et al : Robotic clinical trials of uni-condylar arthroplasty. *Int J Med Robot* 2005;1(4):20-28.

   The results of a randomized controlled clinical trial comparing the Acrobot system (13 patients) with the conventional technique (15 patients) are presented. Preoperative CT-based plans were compared with postoperative CT scans. The Acrobot system showed a significant improvement in execution accuracy.

51. Ritschl P Jr, Machacek F, Fuiko R, Zettl R, Kotten B: The Galileo System for implantation of total knee arthroplasty: An integrated solution comprising navigation, robotics and robot-assisted ligament balancing, in Stiehl JB, Konermann WH, Haaker RG, eds: *Navigation and Robotics in Total Joint and Spine Surgery*. New York, NY, Springer, 2004, pp 281-361.

52. Pearle AD, O'Loughlin PF, Kendoff DO: Robot-assisted unicompartmental knee arthroplasty. *J Arthroplasty* 2010;25(2):230-237.

   The authors describe the preoperative, intraoperative, and postoperative management of patients treated with unicompartmental knee arthroplasty with both conventional and robotic techniques.

53. Conditt MA, Roche MW: Minimally invasive robotic-arm-guided unicompartmental knee arthroplasty. *J Bone Joint Surg Am* 2009;91(Suppl 1):63-68.

   The first description of a new robotic technology (MAKO Tactile Guidance System) for minimally invasive unicompartmental knee arthroplasty is presented.

54. Pearle AD, Kendoff D, Stueber V, Musahl V, Repicci JA: Perioperative management of unicompartmental knee arthroplasty using the MAKO robotic arm system (MAKOplasty). *Am J Orthop* 2009;38(2, Suppl)16-19.

   The authors report on the first clinical series of 10 patients treated with unicompartmental knee arthroplasty using the MAKO Tactile Guidance System, a semiactive robotic system for unicondylar knee arthroplasty. A detailed description of the robotic system and surgical time are presented. The robotic system showed promising results in preoperative, perioperative, and postoperative alignment.

55. Roche M, O'Loughlin PF, Kendoff D, Musahl V, Pearle AD: Robotic arm-assisted unicompartmental knee arthroplasty: Preoperative planning and surgical technique. *Am J Orthop* 2009;38(2, Suppl)10-15.

   The authors describe a new semiactive robotic system that has potential to improve alignment in unicompartmental knee arthroplasty. Details are given about the preoperative planning and the intraoperative technique of the MAKO system.

56. Lonner JH, John TK, Conditt MA: Robotic arm-assisted UKA improves tibial component alignment: A pilot study. *Clin Orthop Relat Res* 2010;468(1):141-146.

   This study showed similar outcomes with robotic and manual techniques, but better component alignment was achieved using the MAKO robot.

57. Sinha RK: Outcomes of robotic arm-assisted unicompartmental knee arthroplasty. *Am J Orthop* 2009;38(2, Suppl):20-22.

   The author reports on early outcomes of unicompartmental knee arthroplasty performed with the MAKO system. The results were promising in regard to accuracy and component positioning.

58. Plaskos C, Cinquin P, Lavallée S, Hodgson AJ: Praxiteles: A miniature bone-mounted robot for minimal access total knee arthroplasty. *Int J Med Robot* 2005;1(4):67-79.

   The authors developed a new bone-mounted robot (Praxiteles) for minimally invasive total knee arthroplasty. The robot, prototypes, and techniques are described.

59. Radermacher K, Portheine F, Anton M, et al: Computer assisted orthopaedic surgery with image based individual templates. *Clin Orthop Relat Res* 1998;354(354):28-38.

60. Slover JD, Tosteson AN, Bozic KJ, Rubash HE, Malchau H: Impact of hospital volume on the economic value of computer navigation for total knee replacement. *J Bone Joint Surg Am* 2008;90(7):1492-1500.

   With a Markov decision model, computer-assisted TKA was less likely to be cost effective at low-volume surgery centers than at high-volume centers.

61. Novak EJ, Silverstein MD, Bozic KJ: The cost-effectiveness of computer-assisted navigation in total knee arthroplasty. *J Bone Joint Surg Am* 2007;89(11):2389-2397.

   A decision-analysis model was used to determine the cost-effectiveness of computer-assisted TKA. Cost savings is realized if the added cost is less than $629 per operation. Computer-assisted TKA is potentially cost-effective but many variables must be accounted for.

62. Barrack RL, Barnes CL, Burnett RS, Miller D, Clohisy JC, Maloney WJ: Minimal incision surgery as a risk factor for early failure of total knee arthroplasty. *J Arthroplasty* 2009;24(4):489-498.

   A consecutive series of revision TKA from three centers and five surgeons was analyzed after excluding revisions and infections. Minimal incision surgery primary TKA accounted for a high percentage of overall revisions, and time to revision of less than 24 months was significantly higher for the minimal incision group.

63. Hafez MA, Chelule KL, Seedhom BB, Sherman KP: Computer-assisted total knee arthroplasty using patient-specific templating. *Clin Orthop Relat Res* 2006;444:184-192.

   Forty-five TKAs were performed on 16 cadaver knees and 29 plastic knees using CT-based custom cutting blocks. Bone cuts were accomplished in a mean time of 9 minutes with an assistant and 11 minutes without. Mean bone cut errors for alignment and bone resection were 1.7° and 0.8 mm (max 2.3° and 1.2 mm), respectively.

64. Lombardi AV Jr, Berend KR, Adams JB: Patient-specific approach in total knee arthroplasty. *Orthopedics* 2008;31(9):927-930.

   Fifty-four TKAs were performed with MRI-based alignment and custom jigs. Surgical time averaged 81.5 minutes overall, reflecting time intraoperatively for validation of cuts with traditional instrumentation on the first 26 knees. Surgical time averaged 10 minutes less for the second 26 knees. At 6 weeks after surgery, alignment was between 4° and 8° of valgus, there was no instability, and Knee Society pain, clinical, and functional scores were improved.

65. Howell SM, Kuznik K, Hull ML, Siston RA: Results of an initial experience with custom-fit positioning total knee arthroplasty in a series of 48 patients. *Orthopedics* 2008;31(9):857-863.

   Forty-eight TKAs were performed using the OtisKnee system. Follow-up was 3 months. Alignment averaged −1.4° ± 2.8° valgus. At 3 months after surgery, 35% of patients reported their knee "normal" and 60% "nearly normal" with average active flexion of 114°

2: Knee

(92° to 134°) and average Knee Society Score of 171 (130-200).

66. Howell SM, Hodapp EE, Kuznik K, Hull ML: In vivo adduction and reverse axial rotation (external) of the tibial component can be minimized. *Orthopedics* 2009;32(5):319.

Thirty-five TKAs implanted with the shape-matching OtisKnee system were analyzed by radiographic image-matching technique to determine contact kinematics during standing and while kneeling. There was a minimal prevalence of adduction/lateral lift-off (3%) and reverse axial rotation (8.5%), which are undesirable consequences reported in other studies and at much higher prevalence using traditional TKA techniques.

67. Klatt BA, Goyal N, Austin MS, Hozack WJ: Custom-fit total knee arthroplasty (OtisKnee) results in malalignment. *J Arthroplasty* 2008;23(1):26-29.

Four TKAs were performed with the OtisKnee system. The recommended cuts by the system resulted in alignment more than 3° off the mechanical axis. It was concluded that this system has the potential for component malalignment and therefore may result in early mechanical failure of the TKAs.

2: Knee

Chapter 11

Mini-Incision Total Knee Arthroplasty: New Data

Erik P. Severson, MD   Mark W. Pagnano, MD

Introduction

Minimally invasive surgery (MIS) techniques related to total knee arthroplasty (TKA) have gained popularity in recent years. Although some of the initial enthusiasm has waned as it has become clear that MIS techniques are not for all patients or for all surgeons, MIS techniques are unlikely to disappear from the armamentarium of contemporary total knee surgeons. MIS surgical techniques have been developed with the intention of reducing perioperative morbidity, shortening recovery times, and allowing a more rapid return to function. As MIS has evolved, new instrumentation and implant designs have emerged and techniques have subsequently been developed to facilitate a variety of surgical approaches. The MIS approaches for TKA included the mini-subvastus, the mini-midvastus, the mini-medial parapatellar, the direct lateral, and the so-called quadriceps-sparing approach.[1] In the past 5 years a clearer picture has emerged regarding the technical obstacles associated with each of these approaches and those will be reviewed. Additionally, the most recent scientific data pertaining to minimally invasive surgical techniques in TKA will be presented, including associated levels of evidence.

Principles of Minimally Invasive TKA

It is important to understand that the benefits of minimally invasive TKA are dependent on excellent perioperative anesthesia and coordinated postoperative analgesia. It should be noted that the introduction of MIS TKA has been accompanied by substantial advancements in the efficacy of perioperative anesthetic tech-

Dr. Pagnano or an immediate family member has received royalties from DePuy and has received research or institutional support from DePuy, Musculoskeletal Transplant Foundation, National Institutes of Health, Stryker, and Zimmer. Neither Dr. Severson nor any immediate family member has received anything of value from or owns stock in a commercial company or institution related directly or indirectly to the subject of this chapter.

niques.[2] Although the definition of MIS TKA remains debatable, the tenets typically associated with that term include a shorter skin incision, avoiding patellar eversion, limiting the degree of surgical dissection in the suprapatellar pouch, and limiting the extent of cutting into the quadriceps tendon. Ten evolutionary features of minimally invasive TKA have previously been proposed and are shown in Table 1.

The evolution of MIS TKA has taken place since the early 1990s and was actually first described in the setting of unicompartmental arthroplasty in 1999.[3] Specific techniques for MIS TKA have been reported in the literature;[4,5] the idea that MIS techniques could be translated from the unicompartmental knee to the total knee was popularized.

Proposed Advantages of MIS TKA

The primary impetus that continues to support MIS TKA stems from studies citing a shorter hospital stay, improved knee range of motion, and the use of less pain medicine when compared with traditional TKA techniques.[6-9] Recently, some evidence of improved functional recovery has emerged, particularly in regard to quadriceps recovery after MIS TKA.[9] In a prospective study of 50 patients who underwent the mini-subvastus technique, isokinetic muscle testing was performed to objectively evaluate the recovery of quadriceps and hamstring muscle strength after such a procedure. The testing was performed before surgery and then at 6 weeks, 3 months, 6 months, and 1 year. Quadriceps muscle strength returned to preoperative levels by 3 months postoperatively and was 17% stronger at 6 months and 30% stronger at 1 year than preoperative levels ($P < 0.05$).[9] These findings can be contrasted with strength testing studies after traditional TKA, which show quadriceps strength deficit in the operated knee that is persistent at 1 year after surgery.[10] After traditional TKA, according to one study, there was a 24% deficit in quadriceps strength of the operated knee compared with the uninvolved knee at 1 year after surgery, and at 2 years, this deficit was still 20%.[10] There have been several strength studies performed on patients undergoing TKA where use of the uninvolved knee serves as a control. After TKA with a

Table 1

Ten Evolutionary Features of Minimally Invasive TKA

Decreases the skin incision length

Controls the flexion and extension of the leg to gain more exposure

Uses retractors symbiotically to achieve a mobile skin window

Uses quadriceps-sparing approaches

Uses inferior and superior patellar releases to mobilize the patella

Avoids patellar eversion

In situ bone cuts are performed to avoid joint dislocation

Uses downsized instrumentation

Uses bone platforms to complete bone cuts

Possible use of the suspended leg approach to optimize exposure with gravity as an aid

Reproduced from Bonutti PM: Minimally invasive total knee arthroplasty, in Barrack RL, Booth RE Jr, Lonner JH, McCarthy JC, Mont MA, Rubash HE, eds: *Orthopaedic Knowledge Update Hip and Knee Reconstruction 3.* Rosemont, IL, American Academy of Orthopaedic Surgeons, 2006, pp 81-91.

standard medial parapatellar arthrotomy, these strength studies have shown persistent weakness of the operated knee compared with the uninvolved knee.[10-12]

Disadvantages of MIS TKA

Although some evidence suggests that MIS TKA approaches result in an accelerated recovery and decreased hospital stay, this must be weighed against a potentially higher revision rate due to aseptic loosening or component malalignment as well as a higher overall reoperation rate.[13]

The authors of one study reviewed reoperations undertaken after 221 unicompartmental arthroplasties were performed using a minimally invasive technique. Although this was a report on unicompartmental arthroplasty, it is relevant to the discussion because it facilitated a comparison with a traditional, open approach and highlighted the potential errors encountered when less exposure is available. The 221 unicompartmental arthroplasties were compared to 514 standard unicompartmental arthroplasties that underwent standard arthrotomy and patellar eversion. The rate of revision due to aseptic loosening was 3.7% in the MIS group compared to 1.0% in the standard group. The overall reoperation rate in the MIS group was 11.3% compared to 8.6% in the standard group.[13]

In addition, MIS TKA has been shown to increase the risk of component malalignment. In a recent study that compared 30 patients who underwent MIS TKA to a group of 30 patients who underwent standard TKA, varus malalignment was seen more frequently on the tibial component in the MIS group.[14]

Indications/Contraindications

To properly interpret the literature regarding outcomes comparing the various approaches, it is important to understand the differing elements of each MIS approach as well as accompanying indications and contraindications. The indications for MIS TKA are essentially the same as for a standard TKA: disabling pain that is accompanied by advanced degenerative joint disease.

Relative contraindications include surgeon inexperience with the approach or instrumentation. Most surgeons should consider additional specific training that includes both the surgical approach and the instrumentation. Seemingly small details involving placement of the skin incision, choice of retractors, and positioning of the limb during surgery can make substantial differences in the technical difficulty of these procedures. Most surgeons would avoid MIS approaches in patients with substantial patella baja or marked knee stiffness. It can be difficult to translate the patella laterally in those situations that compromise visualization of both the proximal tibia and distal femur, and efforts to improve that visualization place the patellar tendon at risk of avulsion. In addition, patients with compromised skin or medical comorbidities contributing to impaired wound healing (poorly controlled diabetes, peripheral vascular disease, or chronic steroid use) are not ideal candidates for the MIS approach because substantially more tension is placed on the skin edges. Other variables such as obesity or muscle mass are not absolute contraindications but do increase technical difficulty. A final consideration is the quality of the bone, which may impact the surgeon's ability to retract appropriately during an MIS approach.

Approaches

Mini-subvastus

The subvastus exposure has been shown to be a reliable, safe, and reproducible approach to the knee.[8,15] It is the only approach that maintains the integrity of the entire extensor mechanism. In an anatomic study, it was found that the vastus medialis obliquus (VMO) inserts at a 50° angle relative to the long axis of the femur and that the distalmost attachment is at the midpole of the patella on the medial side.[16] In an examination of 150 knees (100 knees intraoperatively at the time of TKA, 45 cadaver specimens and MRIs of 5 normal knees) the medial anatomy of the extensor mechanism was consistent. The inferior edge of the VMO was inserted at, or near, the midpole of the patella in each case.[16] The authors of that study concluded that any medial arthrotomy that extends more proximal than the midpole of the patella detaches a portion of the quadriceps tendon. Therefore, the term "quadriceps sparing" should not be applied to any surgical approach with a capsular incision that extends more proximal than the midpole of the patella.[16]

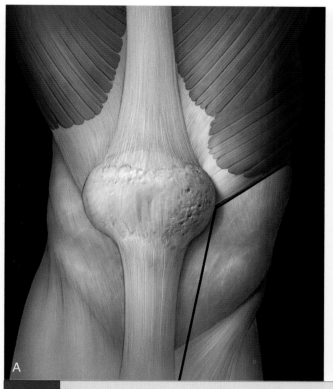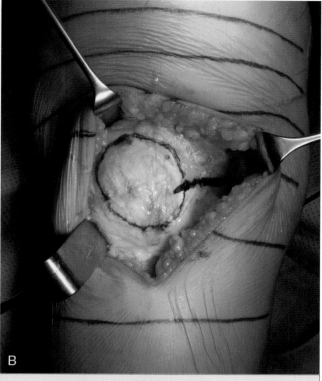

Figure 1 **A,** Schematic drawing depicting the anatomy of the mini-subvastus approach. The dark line indicates the length and direction of the deep capsular incision (or arthrotomy). **B,** Intraoperative photograph displaying the anatomy of the VMO. Insertion of the VMO at approximately the midpole of the patella is seen. (Panel A reproduced with permission from the Mayo Foundation for Medical Education and Research, Rochester, MN.)

With the mini-subvastus approach, a straight, midline, or medially based incision is made starting at the superior pole of the patella and extending distally to the top of the tibial tubercle. A medial full-thickness skin flap is raised to clearly identify the distal border and insertion of the VMO, while preserving its overlying fascia (**Figure 1**). It is helpful to establish a plane between the undersurface of the VMO and capsule before making the arthrotomy. This can be accomplished by incising the overlying fascia of the VMO and bluntly freeing the muscle belly from the underlying synovial layer (**Figure 2**) to preserve a myofascial band of tissue at the inferior border of the VMO, where the retractor will rest against later. If the tendon is not preserved, the retractor will move proximally and tear or macerate the VMO muscle fibers, causing unwanted damage and bleeding. The arthrotomy is then made and starts along the inferior border of the VMO, extends laterally to the midpole of the patella, and then turns distally to parallel the medial border of the patellar tendon to the level of the tibial tubercle.

After sufficient patellar mobility is ensured, a 90° bent Hohmann retractor is placed in the lateral gutter and rests against the tendon edge of the VMO that was carefully preserved during the exposure. The patella is subluxated (not everted) into the lateral gutter with relatively little tension on the VMO.

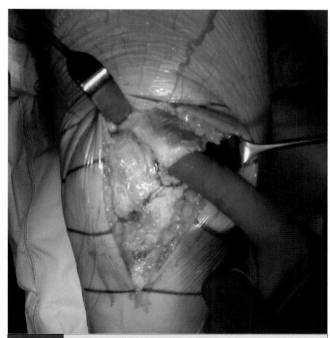

Figure 2 Intraoperative photograph showing development of the plane between the undersurface of the VMO muscle belly and the synovium. At this point, the surgeon's finger is still extracapsular.

2: Knee

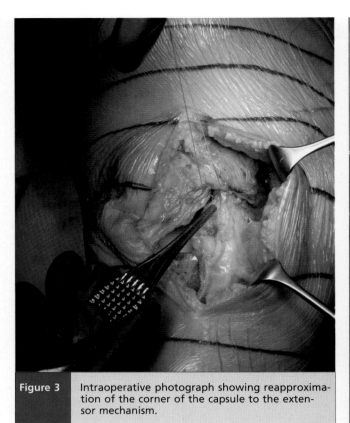

Figure 3   Intraoperative photograph showing reapproximation of the corner of the capsule to the extensor mechanism.

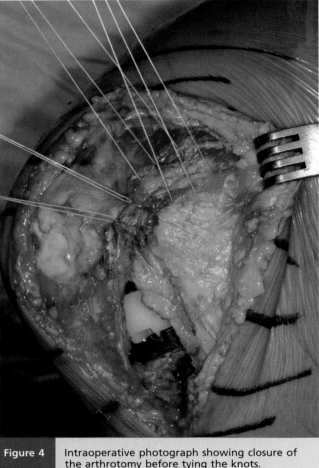

Figure 4   Intraoperative photograph showing closure of the arthrotomy before tying the knots.

Two key maneuvers can aid in visualization of the distal femur during critical steps such as placing the intramedullary guide, femoral sizing, anterior resection, and cementation. The first is bringing the knee into more extension, which decreases tension on the extensor mechanism and allows more of the distal femur to be seen. The second is to place a small knee retractor to slightly elevate the extensor mechanism from the distal femur. With subluxation of the patella into the lateral gutter, the patellar tendon tends to push the tibial proximal resection block medially. As a result, it is critical to keep the distal guide toward the medial malleolus to compensate for this position and avoid a varus resection of the tibia.

The arthrotomy closure begins at the midpole of the patella, reapproximating the corner of the capsule to the extensor mechanism (Figure 3). Next, interrupted Vicryl sutures are placed deep to the VMO muscle belly (not in the muscle belly itself) in the myofascial sleeve defined at the time of exposure and reapproximated to the medial retinacular tissue. The distal vertical limb is closed by suturing the medial retinacular tissue to the medial edge of the patellar tendon (Figure 4).

The complication unique to the mini-subvastus approach is a subvastus hematoma, which occurs when the blood vessels that course through the adductor canal and branch through the VMO are torn with excessive retraction. The possibility of subvastus hematoma is minimized by translation (not eversion) of the patella

to decrease the tension on this area. The medial skin flap must be elevated far enough to clearly identify the inferior border of the VMO. The arthrotomy should never extend proximal to the midpole of the patella, because this will cause the VMO muscle fibers to tear, split, or macerate during the remainder of the operation. After making the arthrotomy, the surgeon must make certain the patella is mobile by translating the patella into the lateral gutter while the knee is extended. If difficulty is encountered, release of the medial patellofemoral ligament and any soft-tissue attachments overlying the quadriceps should be ensured to assist with patellar mobility.

Mini-midvastus

The mini-midvastus approach has no definite contraindications, but the procedure is contraindicated in the significantly obese patient and those with large quadriceps muscle mass, patella baja, and deformity.[17] A midline incision is made from the superior pole of the patella to the midpoint of the tibial tubercle distally (Figure 5). A medial arthrotomy is begun distally 5 mm medial to the tibial tubercle and extended proximally just medial to the patellar border. At the superomedial

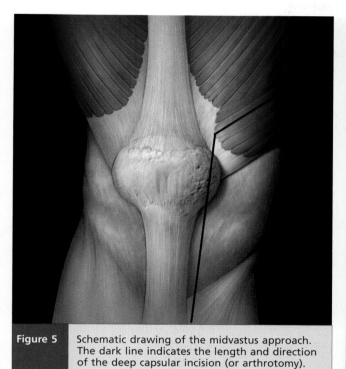

Figure 5 | Schematic drawing of the midvastus approach. The dark line indicates the length and direction of the deep capsular incision (or arthrotomy).

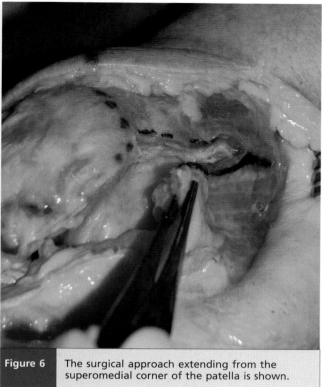

Figure 6 | The surgical approach extending from the superomedial corner of the patella is shown.

corner of the patella, the arthrotomy is turned proximally-medially and a 2-cm split is made in line with the muscle fibers of the VMO (**Figure 6**). The patella is subluxated laterally (but not everted in an attempt to prevent proximal tearing of the VMO) with a bent Hohmann retractor around the margin of the lateral femoral condyle. The distal femoral resection is easier if the knee is in 70° of flexion.

It is important to remember that the VMO is dually innervated by the terminal branches of the femoral and saphenous nerves and can be safely dissected 4.5 cm from the patellar insertion without risk of denervating the muscle distally.

Mini-medial Parapatellar

The mini-medial parapatellar approach is the most popular minimally invasive TKA approach because of its familiarity and simplicity. It can be converted into a standard medial parapatellar approach at any time. The indications are similar to the other MIS TKA approaches, and this approach is beneficial because of the limited damage to knee structures, not necessarily a shortened incision length.[18] The approach is performed through a midline or slightly medially based incision that extends from the superior pole of the patella to the top of the tibial tubercle (**Figure 7**). Because of the elasticity of the skin, the incision can stretch and allows for the use of "mobile windows." The medial parapatellar arthrotomy is performed in a manner similar to that of the standard medial parapatellar approach, except that the proximal extent of the quadriceps tendon incision is only 2 to 4 cm. The success of the procedure will depend on extending the arthrotomy more proximally.

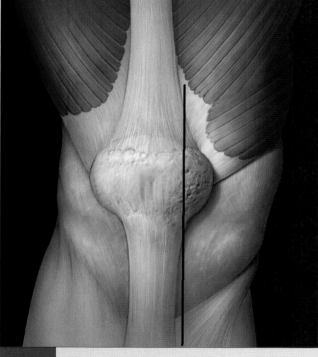

Figure 7 | Schematic drawing of the mini-medial parapatellar approach. The dark line indicates the length and direction of the deep capsular incision (or arthrotomy). (Reproduced with permission from the Mayo Foundation for Medical Education and Research, Rochester, MN.)

2: Knee

Table 2

Results of Minimally Invasive Total Knee Arthroplasty

Authors/Year	Study Design	Number of Knees	Approach
Aglietti et al[27] 2006	Prospective randomized	60 total (30 subvastus and 30 quadriceps sparing)	Subvastus versus quadriceps sparing
Chin et al[25] 2007	Prospective randomized	90	Midvastus versus side-cutting versus standard
Karachalios et al[19] 2008	Prospective randomized	100	Midvastus versus standard
Jackson et al[26] 2008	Prospective cohort	209	Mini parapatellar
Huang et al[24] 2007	Prospective cohort	67 (32 MIS vs 35 standard)	Quadriceps sparing versus medial parapatellar
Han et al[23] 2008	Prospective	30 (15 MIS vs 15 standard)	Mini-medial parapatellar versus standard parapatellar
Boerger et al[20] 2005	Prospective	120	Subvastus versus medial parapatellar
Dalury and Dennis[14] 2005	Retrospective	60	Mini-incision (midvastus) vs standard medial parapatellar
Pagnano and Meneghini[8] 2006	Descriptive and retrospective	103	Subvastus
Haas et al[6] 2004	Retrospective	40	Midvastus
Schroer et al[21] 2008	Matched retrospective	300	Subvastus versus medial parapatellar
Laskin et al[17] 2004	Matched retrospective	58	Midvastus versus medial parapatellar

Patients with large femurs are difficult to treat with this approach because a wide femur necessitates more exposure to implant a large femoral component. In addition, patients with deformity greater than 15° of varus or valgus or a flexion contracture greater than 10° will require more extensive soft-tissue dissection to correct the deformity. As in all other MIS approaches, a shortened patellar tendon will make it more difficult to subluxate the patella laterally and will require a longer incision.[18]

Quadriceps Sparing

The quadriceps-sparing TKA has an even more limited medial parapatellar exposure than the mini-medial parapatellar approach, with the arthrotomy stopping at the superior pole of the patella. Although this approach is actually similar to the open medial meniscectomy approach, it offers the poorest visualization of any of the minimally invasive TKA approaches. Whether this approach is truly quadriceps sparing is controversial. As stated earlier, the medial VMO insertion goes distally to the midpole of the patella; therefore, the approach does involve detachment of the VMO along the upper half of the medial border of the patella.[16]

The skin incision can be curved around the medial aspect of the patella or a straight incision that is just medial to the patella. The arthrotomy is from the superior pole of the patella to 2 cm below the tibial joint line, just medial to the tibial tubercle (Figure 8). Because of poor visualization of the area to be operated, the procedure must be performed with instruments that cut from medial to lateral and demands partial bone cuts through resection guides followed by freehand finishing cuts. This approach would be extremely difficult to perform in the more muscular male with a low inserting VMO as well as the patient with patella baja. Because this approach requires custom instruments, it is important for the operating surgeon to become familiar with them to avoid inaccurate cuts.

Outcomes

There are few published studies reporting long-term data on minimally invasive TKA. In recent years, however, multiple short-term studies have emerged (Table 2). To summarize the available literature, the primary advantages shown in minimally invasive TKA include earlier improvements in flexion, reduced blood loss, and a shortened length of hospital stay.[6,8,19-23] Disadvantages found in the literature include increases in operating room time, component malalignment, and lon-

2: Knee

Table 2

Results of Minimally Invasive Total Knee Arthroplasty (continued)

Mean Follow-up	Results	Level of Evidence
3 mo	Subvastus showed earlier straight leg raise and had better flexion at 10 and 30 days	Level I
N/A	Side cutting technique negatively affects accuracy of implant placement	Level I
23 mo	MIS group with earlier flexion and better early functional outcomes. No difference at final follow-up.	Level I
6 mo	Markedly increased complication rate in the first 100 knees	Level II
24 mo	MIS group with quicker return of quadriceps strength. Longer operating room time and more malalignment in MIS group	Level II
28 mo	Bilateral MIS group had quicker functional recovery vs standard bilateral group	Level II
90 days	MIS group with less blood loss, better early flexion, faster straight leg raise	Level II
3 mo	Varus malalignment more common in mini-midvastus knees	Level III
1 yr	Excellent early functional results with comparable alignment to standard	Level III
1 yr	Midvastus approach achieved motion faster and maintained better motion at 1 year compared with historic standard control	Level III
2 yrs	Subvastus had earlier straight leg raise, shorter hospital stay, and better flexion	Level III
3 mo	Passive flexion better in MIS group, MIS group had lower visual analog score and more rapid increase in Knee Society score	Level III

ger tourniquet times, as well as a higher rate of intraoperative ligament ruptures and unintended retention of cement.[14,19,24-26]

Level I Evidence

There are four level I studies that report on minimally invasive TKA.[19,25,27,28] A recent prospective randomized clinical trial compared a mini-midvastus surgical approach to a standard medial parapatellar approach. There were 50 patients in each arm with a mean follow-up of 2 years. In the mid-vastus group, a statistically better amount of flexion was seen early; however, at final follow-up there was no difference. In addition, the MIS group showed better Oxford Knee Scores, which related to function, up to 9 months after surgery. This study reported a higher rate of technical errors, however, as 12% of patients in the MIS group demonstrated varus malposition of the tibial component on postoperative radiographs and a longer duration of surgery. It should also be noted that 6 of the 56 patients originally randomized to the MIS group in this study had to be converted to the standard group because of partial patellar tendon avulsion in 2 patients, an inability to displace the patella in 2 other patients,

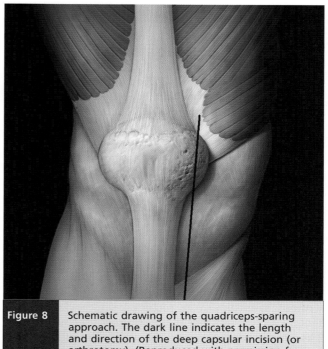

Figure 8 Schematic drawing of the quadriceps-sparing approach. The dark line indicates the length and direction of the deep capsular incision (or arthrotomy). (Reproduced with permission from the Mayo Foundation for Medical Education and Research, Rochester, MN.)

2: Knee

and overall bad exposure in the remaining 2 patients. This prospective, randomized trial concluded that MIS is safe for use in a select patient population, although the authors did not specify which patient population would be ideal.[19]

Another level I study compared only the radiologic outcomes of TKA using the conventional technique versus MIS techniques. Results were found to be comparable radiologically with the midvastus approach and the standard medial parapatellar approach; however, the MIS side-cutting group demonstrated significantly poorer postoperative limb alignment and showed improper femoral component position when compared to the midvastus and standard groups.[25]

The third available level I evidence study was a prospective, randomized, double-blind study comparing the early results of the quadriceps-sparing approach versus the mini-subvastus approach.[27] There was no significant difference between the two groups with regard to tourniquet time, blood loss, and postoperative pain. Active straight leg raising was achieved faster in the mini-subvastus group by one half day. Range of motion also was similar between the two groups.[27]

In a prospective, randomized study, the results of primary TKA using a quadriceps-sparing technique versus standard arthroplasty were compared in 120 patients. All patients had bilateral TKA under the same anesthetic. This study found significantly longer surgery times and tourniquet use as well as an increased complication rate in the quadriceps-sparing group.[28]

Level II Evidence

One single-surgeon study reported on 120 consecutive patients who had undergone minimally invasive TKA with a mini-subvastus approach and who were compared with a cohort of patients for whom a medial parapatellar approach was used.[20] The mini-subvastus group showed better flexion at 30, 60, and 90 days, reaching statistical significance ($P < 0.02$). The MIS group also demonstrated 100 mL less blood loss. It should be noted, however, that the MIS group had, on average, 15 more minutes in tourniquet time.[20]

Another study investigated whether bilateral minimally invasive TKA was advantageous over conventional TKA with respect to faster functional recovery.[23] Thirty patients undergoing bilateral TKA were prospectively randomized into a mini-medial parapatellar approach or a conventional medial parapatellar approach. There were 15 patients in each group. Range of motion and time required to regain the ability to walk without assistance were recorded. In the MIS group blood loss was less, but the tourniquet time was longer. The time needed to regain the ability to walk without assistance was significantly faster in the MIS group ($P = 0.043$). In addition, the gain of range of motion was faster in the MIS group ($P = 0.002$).[23]

Authors of one report compared 32 minimally invasive quadriceps-sparing TKAs to 35 standard TKAs and followed them prospectively for 24 months. The usual MIS benefits of a quicker recovery and faster ability to regain quadriceps strength was seen; however, some significant negative consequences to the MIS approach were highlighted.[24] There were more bony injuries and more patients with postoperative malalignment in the MIS group. In addition, there was a 17% higher operating room cost because of an average 122-minute tourniquet time compared to 55 minutes in the standard group ($P < 0.001$).[24]

The potential disadvantages of MIS TKA were reported prospectively in 209 patients who underwent quadriceps-sparing TKA through a mini-medial parapatellar approach.[26] Surgical complications were frequent and included two patellar tendon avulsions, two lateral collateral ligament ruptures, and one medial collateral ligament rupture. Arthrofibrosis occurred in 10% of MIS patients requiring manipulation, and there was an unacceptably high rate of wound complications (11%). This study highlighted the importance of the difficult learning curve as the second 100 patients in the MIS group had a complication rate similar to standard TKA. Complications were more common in patients with peripheral vascular disease, a body mass index greater than 33, and valgus deformity greater than 10°.[26]

Level III Evidence

In a retrospective review of the mini-subvastus approach, one study reported a significant decrease in duration of hospital stay ($P = 0.00013$).[21] This study was unique in that the learning curve was taken into account. The authors compared their first 150 MIS TKAs with to their last 150 patients who underwent a standard medial parapatellar approach. At 1-year follow-up, the MIS group showed persistently significantly better flexion ($P = 0.0001$). In addition, fewer patients in the MIS group were transferred to extended care facilities upon hospital discharge.[21]

Another retrospective review reported on patients demonstrating a lower average visual analog pain score at 6 week-follow-up.[22] This study reported on the midvastus approach and generally reported favorable outcomes, especially better flexion.[22]

One surgeon reported on 40 MIS knees that underwent a midvastus approach during which the patella was not everted and hyperflexion was minimized during surgery.[6] It was theorized that those modifications would lead to less stretching of the patellar tendon as well as less spreading of the VMO, minimizing the risk of denervation. This retrospective review showed no difference in radiographic appearance when compared to standard techniques, and the MIS approach allowed for improved early functional results; improved motion continued at 1-year follow-up.[6]

Another single-surgeon study described an optimized subvastus approach and highlighted the importance of the MIS tenets of TKA: smaller skin incision, no eversion of the patella, minimal disruption of the suprapatellar pouch to prevent scarring, and minimal disruption of the quadriceps tendon. In all 103 TKAs, the procedure was completed without extending the skin incision beyond 3.5 inches. In 102 cases, the mechanical axis passed through the central third of the knee; the mechanical axis passed through the lateral third of the knee in 1 case. Every tibial component, except one, was placed 90° +/− 2° with the other one being placed at 3° of valgus relative to 90°. According to Knee Society criteria, every knee had acceptable varus-valgus and anteroposterior stability at final follow-up. Longer surgery times were seen in larger patients requiring larger components.[8]

A concerning finding in a recent study was that minimally invasive TKA can increase the risk of component malalignment. In a comparison of 30 patients who had MIS TKA and 30 patients who had a standard TKA, varus malalignment of the tibia was seen in the MIS group. This report concluded that although MIS TKA provides some early functional advantages, the approach can impede a surgeon's vision and may lead to component malalignment resulting in the potential for long-term problems.[14]

The Learning Curve

One study identified the learning phase as approximately 10 months, or 21 knee replacements, using the MIS technique.[29] According to another study, it takes 25 minimally invasive TKAs before the surgery time equals that of the open technique.[30] Another study reported that the first 100 cases were associated with a significantly higher complication rate but that the second 100 patients had complication rates equivalent to that of standard TKA.[26] Increased surgical time is a frequent finding in MIS TKA even after the learning curve has been experienced. The literature indicates that minimally invasive TKA is, in general, more difficult to perform than standard TKA, with difficulty in obtaining adequate radiologic outcome during the learning curve.[31]

Summary

Minimally invasive techniques related to TKA introduced in recent years appear to have a role in contemporary knee surgery but they have not supplanted traditional TKA techniques. The available evidence suggests that there is some advantage to minimally invasive TKA in regard to quicker recovery, better early motion, and a shorter hospital stay, but those advantages come at the cost of a longer time for surgery, a higher risk of component malposition, and a greater risk of early reoperation.

Annotated References

1. Scuderi GR, Tenholder M, Capeci C: Surgical approaches in mini-incision total knee arthroplasty. *Clin Orthop Relat Res* 2004;428:61-67.

2. Horlocker TT, Kopp SL, Pagnano MW, Hebl JR: Analgesia for total hip and knee arthroplasty: A multimodal pathway featuring peripheral nerve block. *J Am Acad Orthop Surg* 2006;14(3):126-135.

   This article talks about peripheral nerve blockade of the lumbosacral plexus emerging as an alternative analgesic approach to the traditional intravenous patient-controlled analgesia or epidural analgesia for patients undergoing total hip and knee arthroplasty. Peripheral nerve block techniques may be the optimal analgesic method following total joint arthroplasty.

3. Repicci JA, Eberle RW: Minimally invasive surgical technique for unicondylar knee arthroplasty. *J South Orthop Assoc* 1999;8(1):20-27, discussion 27.

4. Bonutti PM, Mont MA, Kester MA: Minimally invasive total knee arthroplasty: A 10-feature evolutionary approach. *Orthop Clin North Am* 2004;35(2):217-226.

5. Tria AJ Jr, Coon TM: Minimal incision total knee arthroplasty: Early experience. *Clin Orthop Relat Res* 2003;416:185-190.

6. Haas SB, Cook S, Beksac B: Minimally invasive total knee replacement through a mini midvastus approach: A comparative study. *Clin Orthop Relat Res* 2004;428: 68-73.

7. Laskin RS: New techniques and concepts in total knee replacement. *Clin Orthop Relat Res* 2003;416:151-153.

8. Pagnano MW, Meneghini RM: Minimally invasive total knee arthroplasty with an optimized subvastus approach. *J Arthroplasty* 2006;21(4, Suppl 1):22-26.

   The authors of this study describe the subvastus approach and communicate outcomes on more than 100 patients. The minimally invasive subvastus approach provides very good exposure through a small incision, preserves all four attachments of the quadriceps to the patella, does not require patella eversion, minimizes disruption in the suprapatellar pouch, and allows rapid and reliable closure to the knee. When coupled with instruments designed specifically for small incision surgery, the modified subvastus approach is reliable, reproducible, and safe.

9. Schroer WC, Diesfeld PJ, Reedy ME, Lemarr AR: Isokinetic strength testing of minimally invasive total knee arthroplasty recovery. *J Arthroplasty* 2010;25(2): 274-279.

   This prospective study demonstrated that the minisubvastus TKA technique led to a more rapid and more complete recovery of muscle strength than has

2: Knee

been previously demonstrated after TKA with a medial parapatellar arthrotomy.

10. Berman AT, Bosacco SJ, Israelite C: Evaluation of total knee arthroplasty using isokinetic testing. *Clin Orthop Relat Res* 1991;271:106-113.

11. Rossi MD, Brown LE, Whitehurst M: Knee extensor and flexor torque characteristics before and after unilateral total knee arthroplasty. *Am J Phys Med Rehabil* 2006;85(9):737-746.

    In this article, the authors show that 1 year after unilateral TKA, there continues to be knee extensor and flexor strength asymmetry between limbs. Moreover, within the first month after surgery, the knee extensors and flexors are at the weakest point compared with before surgery and 60 days and 1 year after surgery. Isokinetic testing is a useful tool to document torque production before and in the early time after unilateral TKA.

12. Chang CH, Chen KH, Yang RS, Liu TK: Muscle torques in total knee arthroplasty with subvastus and parapatellar approaches. *Clin Orthop Relat Res* 2002; 398:189-195.

13. Hamilton WG, Collier MB, Tarabee E, McAuley JP, Engh CA Jr, Engh GA: Incidence and reasons for reoperation after minimally invasive unicompartmental knee arthroplasty. *J Arthroplasty* 2006;21(6, Suppl 2)98-107.

    This report reviewed reoperations undertaken on the initial 221 unicompartmental arthroplasties performed using a minimally invasive technique. A comparison was then performed between these cases and the previous 514 open medial unicompartmental arthroplasties performed at the authors' institution. Despite an accelerated recovery and decreased hospital stay in the minimally invasive unicompartmental arthroplasties, the rate of revision due to aseptic loosening and the overall reoperation rate compare unfavorably with those performed with an open technique.

14. Dalury DF, Dennis DA: Mini-incision total knee arthroplasty can increase risk of component malalignment. *Clin Orthop Relat Res* 2005;440:77-81.

    This study compared 30 patients who had TKA with a mini-incision to a similar group of 30 patients who had TKA with a standard length incision. Although TKA performed using a minimal incision may provide some early advantages, minimal incisions can impede a surgeon's vision and may influence component alignment and possibly compromise long-term outcome.

15. Hofmann AA, Plaster RL, Murdock LE: Subvastus (Southern) approach for primary total knee arthroplasty. *Clin Orthop Relat Res* 1991;269(269):70-77.

16. Pagnano MW, Meneghini RM, Trousdale RT: Anatomy of the extensor mechanism in reference to quadriceps-sparing TKA. *Clin Orthop Relat Res* 2006; 452: 102-105.

    The authors demonstrate that any medial arthrotomy that extends more proximal than the midpole of the patella detaches a portion of the quadriceps tendon. From an anatomic perspective, the term "quadriceps sparing" should not be applied to any surgical approach with a capsular incision that extends more proximal than the midpole of the patella.

17. Laskin RS, Beksac B, Phongjunakorn A, et al: Minimally invasive total knee replacement through a mini-midvastus incision: An outcome study. *Clin Orthop Relat Res* 2004;428:74-81.

18. Scuderi GR: Minimally invasive total knee arthroplasty with a limited medial parapatellar arthrotomy. *Oper Tech Orthop* 2006;16:145-152.

    The surgical techniques associated with the variety of MIS approaches for TKA, including the limited parapatellar, midvastus, and subvastus approaches, and the quadriceps-sparing approach, are reviewed. The extensibility of these approaches allows surgeons to adapt and modify the procedure should intra-operative difficulties arise.

19. Karachalios T, Giotikas D, Roidis N, Poultsides L, Bargiotas K, Malizos KN: Total knee replacement performed with either a mini-midvastus or a standard approach: A prospective randomised clinical and radiological trial. *J Bone Joint Surg Br* 2008;90(5):584-591.

    The authors report the clinical and radiologic results of a three-year prospective randomized study that was designed to compare a MIS technique with a standard technique in total knee replacement and was undertaken between January 2004 and May 2007. Based on the results, the authors currently use MIS techniques in total knee replacement in selected cases only.

20. Boerger TO, Aglietti P, Mondanelli N, Sensi L: Mini-subvastus versus medial parapatellar approach in total knee arthroplasty. *Clin Orthop Relat Res* 2005;440: 82-87.

    The authors compared short-term clinical results of the mini-subvastus approach with the standard parapatellar approach for TKA. The mini-subvastus approach offers early but short-lived benefits for patients at the expense of a longer operation and a higher risk of complications.

21. Schroer WC, Diesfeld PJ, Reedy ME, LeMarr AR: Mini-subvastus approach for total knee arthroplasty. *J Arthroplasty* 2008;23(1):19-25.

    This study compares the authors' first 150 MIS TKA patients to their previous 150 traditional TKA patients. Comparison between the MIS and traditional techniques demonstrated no increase in the number or severity of complications and no difference in operating room time.

22. Laskin RS: Surgical exposure for total knee arthroplasty: for everything there is a season. *J Arthroplasty* 2007;22(4, Suppl 1)12-14.

    The author has used a mini-midvastus lesser-invasive knee approach for 5 years for patients undergoing a primary TKA. The approach involves a modified capsular and muscular incision, displacement but not eversion of the patella, and avoidance of anterior dislocation of the tibia before bony resections. This has resulted in a more rapid return of flexion and functional ability with a lesser amount of postoperative pain as compared with previous larger median parapatellar approaches with patellar eversion.

23. Han I, Seong SC, Lee S, Yoo JH, Lee MC: Simultaneous bilateral MIS-TKA results in faster functional recovery. *Clin Orthop Relat Res* 2008;466(6):1449-1453.

 The authors asked whether bilateral MIS-TKA had advantages over conventional TKA with respect to faster functional recovery. Functional recovery in the MIS group was faster in rehabilitation milestones of walking without assistance and gain in range of motion. Minimally invasive TKA may benefit patients undergoing simultaneous bilateral procedures with faster functional recovery.

24. Huang HT, Su JY, Chang JK, Chen CH, Wang GJ: The early clinical outcome of minimally invasive quadriceps-sparing total knee arthroplasty: Report of a 2-year follow-up. *J Arthroplasty* 2007;22(7):1007-1012.

 The results of 32 minimally invasive quadriceps-sparing TKAs were compared with those of a matched group of 35 standard TKAs. The quadriceps-sparing technique showed better and faster recovery, but there were more outliers and bone injuries during surgery, and this, coupled with length of tourniquet time, were the major disadvantages in early studies.

25. Chin PL, Foo LS, Yang KY, Yeo SJ, Lo NN: Randomized controlled trial comparing the radiologic outcomes of conventional and minimally invasive techniques for total knee arthroplasty. *J Arthroplasty* 2007;22(6):800-806.

 The objective of this study was to compare the radiologic outcomes of TKA using the conventional technique with those using MIS techniques. Ninety patients were randomized to undergo conventional (control), MIS mini-incision midvastus (mini), or MIS side-cutting techniques for their TKAs. The side-cutting technique appears to affect the accuracy of implant placement.

26. Jackson G, Waldman BJ, Schaftel EA: Complications following quadriceps-sparing total knee arthroplasty. *Orthopedics* 2008;31(6):547.

 This study examined whether quadriceps-sparing TKA through a minimal medical incision could be performed without an increased risk of complications. This quadriceps-sparing technique required a progressive learning curve and has not yet proven to be superior to standard approaches. However, complication rates after extensive experience were not significantly increased.

27. Aglietti P, Baldini A, Sensi L: Quadriceps-sparing versus mini-subvastus approach in total knee arthroplasty. *Clin Orthop Relat Res* 2006;452:106-111.

 In this prospective randomized double-blind study, the authors compared the postoperative recovery and early results of two groups of 30 patients having TKA with MIS techniques using either a mini-subvastus or a modified quadriceps-sparing approach. They believe there was no difference between the mini-subvastus and quadriceps-sparing approach in relation to short-term recovery or early results.

28. Kim YH, Kim JS, Kim DY: Clinical outcome and rate of complications after primary total knee replacement performed with quadriceps-sparing or standard arthrotomy. *J Bone Joint Surg Br* 2007;89(4):467-470.

 This is a prospective randomized study of 120 patients who underwent bilateral TKA under the same anesthetic. They found significantly longer surgery times and tourniquet use in addition to an increased rate of complications in the quadriceps-sparing group.

29. Kashyap SN, Van Ommeren JW, Shankar S: Minimally invasive surgical technique in total knee arthroplasty: A learning curve. *Surg Innov* 2009;16(1):55-62.

 Clinical experience of learning a new technique of MIS for TKA is presented. Close monitoring of the technique, pitfalls, learning tips, and tricks are discussed. There was no incidence of increased complications during the learning phase. Functional results such as stair climbing, walking distance, and walking with aids was significantly better after minimally invasive technique than after standard technique.

30. King J, Stamper DL, Schaad DC, Leopold SS: Minimally invasive total knee arthroplasty compared with traditional total knee arthroplasty: Assessment of the learning curve and the postoperative recuperation period . *J Bone Joint Surg Am* 2007;89(7):1497-1503.

 This study compared to each other the first 100 MIS knee procedures by a high-volume surgeon and then compared them to 50 TKAs done through the traditional approach. The learning curve was that 25 knees had a surgery time equal to that of the traditional approach. The MIS group had better clinical outcomes with regard to hospital stay, need for inpatient rehabilitation, narcotic usage at 2 and 6 weeks after surgery, and the need for assistive devices at 2 weeks. The authors cautioned that the learning curve may be unacceptably long for a low-volume arthroplasty surgeon.

31. Chen HF, Alan RK, Redziniak OE, Tria AJ Jr: Quadriceps-sparing total knee replacement: The initial experience with results at two to four years. *J Bone Joint Surg Br* 2006;88(11):1448-1453.

 This retrospective review compared results in patients with quadriceps-sparing TKA versus standard TKA. Fifty-seven patients were available for follow-up. There was no difference in complications and in Knee Society scores at final follow-up. Radiologic outcomes, however, were inferior in the quadriceps-sparing group.

Chapter 12

The Results of Contemporary Total Knee Arthroplasty

James Benjamin, MD

Introduction

Refinements in prosthetic design and surgical technique have made total knee arthroplasty (TKA) a reliable and reproducible procedure for relieving pain associated with arthritis and restoring function to the knee. The results of second-generation implant designs using modular tibial components have demonstrated survival rates of 90% to 99% at 10 to 23 years of follow-up.[1-7]

Outcomes after TKA can be measured in several ways. Patient satisfaction can be measured using established tools such as the Western Ontario and McMaster Universities Arthritis Index (WOMAC) and the Medical Outcomes Study 36-Item Short Form (SF-36) scoring systems. The WOMAC scale is a validated questionnaire that measures the patient's impression of his or her pain, disability, and joint stiffness after hip or knee arthroplasty. The SF-36 is also a validated patient questionnaire that profiles functional health and well-being as well as the patient's perception of his or her own physical and mental health. The Knee Society Clinical Rating System (KSS), introduced in 1989, is probably the most commonly used scoring system to evaluate the outcome of knee arthroplasty.[8] It consists of a knee/prosthesis score and a patient function score. The knee score evaluates three parameters: pain, stability, and range of motion (ROM) with deductions for flexion contracture, extension lag, and malalignment. The function score evaluates walking distance and stair climbing with deductions for the use of walking aids. Both the knee score and the function score have a maximum of 100 points. Although the knee score does not appear to deteriorate significantly with time, the functional score is probably more valid in the early to intermediate follow-up period, as it has been demonstrated to decline as a patient's age and comorbidities limit his or her activity. As a result, the functional score of the

KSS may not be as useful as the knee score in long-term follow-up studies to evaluate the results of knee arthroplasty.[9]

Survivorship (the length of time a prosthesis remains in service without the need for any type of revision surgery) is another measure of success. Survivorship is commonly used in large joint registries as well as institutional series and has the power to identify early problems with individual prostheses or surgical technique because of the large numbers of patients included. Although survivorship is a useful measurement of an implant's success, it does not provide significant information regarding the function of an individual prosthesis or the level of patient satisfaction.

When evaluating the success of a specific implant, it is important to recognize the causes of both early and late failure of TKA. Many studies document that more than 50% of revisions after TKA occur within 5 years of the index procedure.[10-12] The reasons for early failure are infection, instability, loosening, and patellofemoral problems. Infection, as a cause of failure, is unrelated to the implant. Instability and patellofemoral problems after TKA are the result of errors in surgical technique and are not related to the implant selection. Of the complications resulting in early revision, only loosening can be related to implant selection but may also be caused by poor surgical technique. Late causes of failure, specifically polyethylene wear and osteolysis, can be multifactorial in etiology.[10-14]

The results obtained in centers of surgeon-designers who characteristically perform many surgical procedures and publish many reports on the outcomes of individual prosthetic designs probably represent the best-case scenarios. The use of a specific prosthetic design is no guarantee that the results obtained by the individual surgeon will necessarily be equivalent. Another unfortunate problem with evaluating the outcomes of knee designs is that often by the time long-term results are published, the specific prosthesis is no longer in production or has been "updated or improved." Changes in design or manufacturing do not always guarantee an improved result from that of the original prosthesis.

2: Knee

Fixed-Bearing TKA

Fixed-bearing TKA designs currently represent the predominant style of knee prostheses being implanted in North America, and account for more than 85% of implants sold. With fixed-bearing designs, the femoral and tibial components are anchored to the host with all of the joint motion occurring at the prosthetic bearing surface. These designs attempt to re-create the rolling and gliding motion seen at the articular surface in the normal knee. Fixed-bearing knees have had excellent results in both improvement of function and survivorship. These knees fall into two broad categories, posterior cruciate retaining (CR), which maintains a slight lead in sales at approximately 54%, and posterior cruciate substituting (PS) knee designs. CR designs attempt to retain the function of the posterior cruciate ligament (PCL) during the arthroplasty. This is based on biomechanical studies that demonstrate the importance of the PCL in facilitating femoral rollback that is critical to achieving deep flexion in the normal knee. Whether or not this can be routinely achieved in TKA is a hotly debated issue. Fluoroscopic studies of "successful" well-functioning TKAs demonstrate that, regardless of design, prosthetic knees do not duplicate normal knee kinematics. Proponents of posterior stabilized designs think that by the time a knee has reached the point of requiring a TKA, the PCL is dysfunctional and that it is an impediment to achieving a balanced and well-functioning knee. Posterior stabilized knees require excision of the PCL and use a cam and post design in the prosthesis to control and direct the kinematics in flexion.

The reported results with both designs are equivalent. Selection of one style of prosthesis over another is mainly based on surgeon experience and preferred surgical technique. A 2008 study reported on 8-year follow-up of the Press Fit Condylar–Sigma CR knee design (PFC-Sigma CR, DePuy, Warsaw, IN) in 284 patients with a 99% survival rate.[15] The mean KSS prosthesis score was 94 and the mean ROM at last follow-up was 123°. In a multicenter study of 1,970 knees, using the same prosthesis in both CR and PS designs, there was a reported 97.2% 10-year survival rate and a mean ROM of 116 for the PS knees and 114° for the CR knees.[16]

In a short-term follow-up using the Triathalon design (Stryker, Mahwah, NJ), in a consecutive series of 2,035 knees, a mean postoperative prosthesis score of 96 and a mean ROM of 126° were reported.[17] A single-surgeon series on the NexGen CR prosthesis (Zimmer, Warsaw, IN), with 7-year follow-up, reported a mean ROM of 123° and mean knee score of 97. There was a 98% survivorship in this intermediate follow-up series.[18] In a report on the Genesis prosthesis (Smith & Nephew, Memphis, TN) in both CR and PS design, one surgeon reported a 98% survival at 10 years and prosthesis scores of 89 for the CR design and 92 for the PS design.[19] The ROM also varied slightly between the two designs, 117° for the CR and 114° for the PS.

The biggest difference between contemporary TKA designs and the previous generation is an increase in postoperative ROM. Second-generation modular TKA designs had reported mean ROM of 100° to 113° versus current designs that routinely obtain more than 120° of flexion postoperatively.[1-7] Although it would be easy to attribute this finding solely to improvement in prosthesis design, it may be more related to advances in surgical technique, including minimally invasive surgical approaches, modern perioperative pain control regimens, and aggressive rehabilitation protocols.

There are some potential drawbacks to each style of fixed-bearing prosthesis that should be recognized to avoid complications. Not all knees can be reconstructed leaving the native PCL intact. In some knees the PCL is contracted and if left in situ can result in excessive tightness in flexion. This is manifested in restricted flexion or excessive rollback of the femoral component that can lead to early polyethylene wear or failure. In these cases, the surgeon is often required to perform a PCL recession or segmental lengthening procedure to restore balance in flexion. If the PCL is rendered incompetent or if PCL failure occurs after surgery, symptomatic PCL insufficiency may result. Patients with a PCL-insufficient CR TKA often experience anterior knee pain, recurrent effusions, and clinical instability that require revision to a PS TKA to resolve.[20] This has prompted some surgeons to recommend that CR knee designs are contraindicated in patients with combined fixed coronal and sagittal deformities of greater than 15° who require extensive soft-tissue releases to obtain alignment.[21] CR prostheses may also be ill advised in patients with patellectomy, in whom the extensor mechanism is already compromised and in whom posterior subluxation of the tibia further exacerbates the quadriceps weakness (Figure 1).

Resection of the PCL during surgery preferentially increases the flexion gap, a condition that can lead to flexion instability of PS knee designs. As a result, the use of a PS knee often dictates the use of surgical techniques that balance the flexion and extension gaps to achieve stability in both positions. PS designs often result in an elevation of the joint line, because additional distal femoral resection is required to compensate for the increase in flexion gap created by the PCL resection. This elevation of the joint line of up to 1 cm does not appear to have any deleterious effects on outcomes or longevity of these designs.[22,23]

Patellar clunk is another complication that is unique to PS designs. This phenomenon, associated mainly with first-generation PS knee designs, resulted from the entrapment of a hyperplastic retropatellar nodule in the intercondylar notch of the femoral component during active knee extension. This condition would often result in painful catching that frequently required surgical intervention.[24] The incidence of this complication ranged from 3% to 7% with early PS TKA designs. Al-

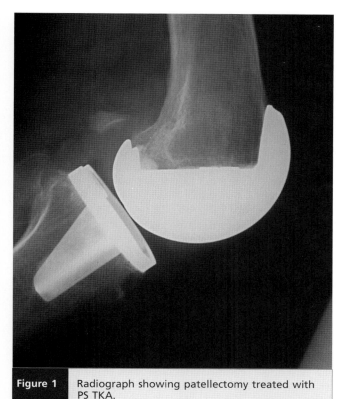

though the etiology of this complication is multifactorial, femoral component design has been identified as one of the leading causes. Recent studies, with current generation posterior stabilized knees, have reported a significant reduction and even elimination of patellar clunk,[25,26] but patellar crepitus appears to remain an issue with these designs. One study reported a 3.3% incidence of patellar crepitus in a series of 60 PS knees.[27] In a review of 428 patients with PS knees of two different designs, 1 in 4 patients reported patellar crepitus after knee replacement.[28]

Current fixed-bearing TKA designs provide excellent clinical outcomes and midterm survivorship with increased ROM compared to the previous generation of knee designs. The choice of CR or PS designs is mainly based on surgeon preference, and results have not demonstrated any clear advantage between the two designs.

Mobile-Bearing TKA

Mobile-bearing knees represent a departure from "standard" fixed-bearing prosthetic designs. Mobile-bearing knees attempt to separate the rolling and gliding motions of the knee, allowing these motions to occur at different interfaces. The original mobile-bearing knee, introduced in 1977, used a meniscal-bearing design. Although meniscal-bearing knees are still in production, most current mobile-bearing prostheses use variations of a rotating platform to achieve this design philosophy. In these designs there is increased congruency between the femoral component and the tibial polyethylene that essentially limits the motion at this interface to flexion and eliminates the sliding or gliding motion. The gliding/rotational motion of the knee takes place between the polyethylene and a polished tibial tray. The increase in contact area and congruency of these designs has the benefit of decreasing the strain seen at the polyethylene interface; by separating the motions into two different locations, the shear forces on the polyethylene can also be significantly decreased. The theoretic benefit of these designs is a potential decrease in polyethylene wear by decreasing stress and shear at the polyethylene interface.

There are several long-term follow-up studies that document the success of mobile-bearing knee designs. One surgeon reported on a 20-year follow-up for the Low Contact Stress Rotating Platform (LCS RP, DePuy) knee in 233 patients using cement and cementless fixation. The rate of survivorship was 97.7% at both 10 and 20 years. The mean ROM was 107° in the cemented group and 110° in the cementless group.[29] In another report of 598 patients undergoing LCS meniscal-bearing and rotating platform knee replacement, the follow-up ranged from 10 to 15 years, with a survival rate of 92% for the rotating platform design. The mean ROM in the study was 105°.[30] Another study reported on 371 knees using the same prosthesis with a mean follow-up of 8.1 years. Using the New Jersey knee scoring system, 99.7% of patients had good to excellent results. The mean ROM in this series was 112° and the survivorship was 89.5%.[31] A fourth study also reported an excellent 10-year survival rate (99%) with the LCS prosthesis, but the mean ROM was only 100°.[32]

The use of mobile-bearing knee designs requires significant attention to ligament balancing and mandates the use of a gap balancing technique to avoid flexion-extension imbalance. Leaving the knee with tightness in flexion, especially an asymmetric flexion space, can lead to dislocation or spinout of the polyethylene. The incidence of polyethylene-bearing dislocation ranges from 0% to 9% depending on the series.[33-35] It is a more frequent occurrence with meniscal-bearing designs and is related to surgical technique. Increased experience with the prosthesis and surgical technique can minimize this complication.

Despite the excellent long-term survival, mobile-bearing knees have not been shown to provide clinical results superior to those of fixed-bearing knees. In a prospective randomized study of mobile-bearing versus fixed-bearing knees using the same femoral component, the authors failed to demonstrate any difference in ROM, Knee Society scores, WOMAC scores, or SF-36 scores between the two groups.[36] In a study of 174 patients undergoing bilateral TKA with a mobile-bearing implant (Press Fit Condylar–Rotating Platform [PFC-RP], DePuy) on one side and a fixed-bearing implant (Press Fit Condylar–Cruciate Retaining PFC-CR) on

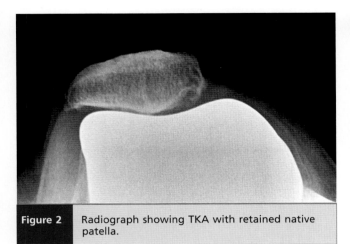

Figure 2 Radiograph showing TKA with retained native patella.

the other, there was no difference in pain scores, function scores, or ROM between the two knee designs at 5.6-year mean follow-up.[37] Another bilateral TKA series using the NexGen CR and Rotaglide prostheses (Zimmer) reported similar results.[38] In a series of 213 knees randomized to receive a fixed-bearing or mobile-bearing tibial component, there was no difference in postoperative ROM. The two groups also did not show any significant change between their preoperative ROM and ROM at a minimum follow-up of 2 years.[39] In a prospective randomized trial of 312 patients comparing a Sigma Rotating Platform-Postenor Stabilized implant (Sigma RP-PS) (DePuy) to a fixed-bearing PFC with an all-polyethylene PS tibia, there was no difference in ROM, KSS, or WOMAC scores at 42-month follow-up. The increase in cost for the mobile-bearing knee was $1,100.[40]

Although mobile-bearing knee designs offer the theoretic advantage of decreasing articular stresses at the polyethylene interface, they do not eliminate wear or osteolysis. Studies have demonstrated comparable rates of polyethylene wear and osteolysis to those seen in fixed-bearing designs.[41-43] These knee designs have not been proven to decrease lateral release rates or provide clinical outcomes that are superior to fixed-bearing designs.[44] Finally, regardless of design, mobile-bearing knees, like their fixed-bearing counterparts, do not recreate "normal" knee kinematics when evaluated in vivo.[45-47] Compared to fixed-bearing prostheses, mobile-bearing designs carry a significant increase in cost that may be difficult to justify on a routine basis.

New designs of mobile-bearing knees have recently appeared globally and, to a lesser extent, in the North American market. Some of these designs allow both gliding and rotation at the polyethylene-tibial interface, a philosophy that may defeat the purpose of avoiding shear forces on the polyethylene. Long-term clinical trials will be required to determine if these newer prostheses yield the same results as the existing designs.

Patellar Resurfacing During TKA

Patellar resurfacing is commonly performed during TKA because many patients undergoing arthroplasty have tricompartmental disease. Although this is standard procedure for most surgeons in North America, patellar arthroplasty during TKA remains a controversial subject in the global community. The incidence of patellar resurfacing during TKA ranges from a high of 70% in the Danish arthroplasty registry to 5% in the Norwegian total joint registry. As a compromise to the "all or none" approach, there are authors who recommend selective resurfacing based on the status of the patella at the time of arthroplasty and host factors such as age, weight, and disease process.

Opponents of routine patellar resurfacing cite problems with patellar fracture, osteonecrosis, extensor mechanism injury, and patellar clunk as reasons to retain the native patella during TKA. The high failure rate of early metal-backed patellar designs also added support to this argument. In contrast to first- and second-generation femoral components, contemporary femoral designs have trochlear articulations with unconstrained surfaces that have been described as patellar "friendly." Biomechanical studies of native patella's articulation against prosthetic femoral components have demonstrated larger contact areas and lower stresses than are seen with polyethylene patellar prostheses[48] (Figure 2).

There are clinical studies that demonstrate excellent results with retention of the native patella during TKA. In a randomized prospective study of 100 knees, there was no difference in KSS, the incidence of anterior knee pain, or radiographic findings at 10-year follow-up.[49] However, the overall rate of revision was higher in the knees without resurfacing. The status of the patellar articular surface at the time of surgery was not a predictor of outcome, which would argue against selective resurfacing. In a 30-second stair-climbing trial, the patients with nonresurfaced knees were able to ascend more stairs than patients who had undergone patellar resurfacing. In a second study of patients undergoing bilateral TKA, with and without patellar resurfacing, findings were similar.[50]

Despite the concerns regarding patellar resurfacing, the evidence provided by large total joint registries would support its routine use. In the Australian joint registry, failure to resurface the patella increased the risk of needing a revision procedure by 30%.[51] In the Swedish registry, the risk of required revision surgery increased by 20% when the patella was not resurfaced, and in the Norwegian registry, revision surgery for anterior knee pain increased 5.7 times when the patella was not resurfaced.[14]

In a meta-analysis of 14 prospective randomized trials, a statistically significant reduction in anterior knee pain was noted in patients who underwent resurfacing. Although the analysis demonstrated that there was no significant difference in the rate of revision surgery between the native and resurfaced groups, it did show that patients with native patellae had an 8.7% incidence of secondary resurfacing.[52] Another meta-analysis of 1,223 knees in 10 prospective randomized trials concluded that resurfacing the patella reduced the risk of reoperation by 4.6% and the risk of anterior knee pain by 13.8%.[53] In a meta-analysis of 1,490 knees, an increased incidence of revision for patellofemoral complications was noted in unresurfaced patellae, 6.5% versus a rate of 2.3% for patellae that had been resurfaced at the time of the index arthroplasty. An increased incidence of anterior knee pain was noted in unresurfaced knees; 22.3% versus 7.6% in knees that had patellar resurfacing.[54] Despite there being no measurable clinical difference in patients with and without patellar resurfacing, another study reported a 15% revision rate in the nonresurfaced knees and a 5% revision rate in knees implanted with a patellar prosthesis. This difference was not found to be statistically significant.[49]

Retention of the native patella during TKA does not result in any apparent decrease in clinical function after TKA. Because there is a subset of patients who have persistent anterior knee pain following TKA, even with patellar resurfacing, it is often difficult to identify the exact etiology of this problem. Despite these findings, meta-analysis of numerous series as well as the findings from national joint registries demonstrate a significant incidence of secondary reoperation for patellofemoral problems in patients with a retained native patella during TKA.

Cemented Versus Cementless Fixation

Although the same technology used successfully in total hip arthroplasty for cementless fixation has been applied to TKA, it has not met with the same success. Cementless TKA currently represents 5% to 6% of knees implanted in North America, whereas hybrid TKA, a cemented tibial component and cementless femur, comprises 9% of knees implanted.

Cementless knees that do survive have a good track record, and the fixation has been shown to be durable with a very low incidence of late loosening. In a single-surgeon report of 176 cementless knees with 12 years follow-up, a 93.4% survivorship was reported when revisions for infection and polyethylene liner exchanges were excluded.[55] In another single-surgeon series using a different implant, a 98.6% survival rate was reported at 15 to 18 years, with loosening as the endpoint.[56] According to a 2010 study, there was a 97% 20-year survivorship of the cementless anatomic graduated component (AGC, Biomet, Warsaw, IN) prosthesis in a multisurgeon series. There were two early failures of tibial component fixation in this series but no femoral component failures.[57] Cementless TKA is a more demanding procedure requiring precise bone cuts to maximize implant-host contact and initial implant stability.

The excellent results with cementless designs using sintered porous-coated implants are from single-surgeon series, and these results have not always carried over to their general use.

The success of cementless fixation varies by component. Early cementless patellae had high failure rates that were attributed to design problems and poor patellofemoral kinematics created by femoral component designs with constrained trochlear articulations and a lack of understanding of the importance of femoral component rotation. These early designs failed mainly because of wear or dissociation of the thin polyethylene from the metal baseplate. A 16.4% failure rate of metal-backed patellae was reported at less than 10 years follow-up.[57] More recent cementless patellar designs using inset designs have had better survival rates. Femoral components, because of the ability to obtain an initial stable interference fit, have demonstrated success rates equivalent to cemented fixation with a very low incidence of failure of fixation. Cementless tibial components have not met with the same success, and failure of fixation of this component is the most commonly cited reason leading to revision in cementless TKA.

Examination of large joint registries can provide some insight into the outcomes of cementless TKA in a broader setting. The Norwegian joint registry did not demonstrate any difference in implant survival based on the type of fixation, although cementless fixation was used in only 2% of knees and hybrid fixation in 10% of knees contained in the registry. Because the hybrid fixation was no better than cemented fixation, the authors did not believe that the increase in cost of cementless technology justified its routine use.[58]

The Kaiser Permanente US joint registry reported on 30,815 knee replacements and documented a threefold increase in revision for loosening with cementless TKAs when compared to cemented or hybrid fixation.[59] These findings implicate the failure of tibial fixation as the main cause of failure in these patients. In a review of 11,606 TKAs from the Mayo Clinic, a significant difference in survivorship between cemented and cementless TKAs at 10 years was reported: 92% versus 61%.[60] In a meta-analysis of 15 published studies evaluating the method of fixation, no difference in KSS was demonstrated between cemented and cementless TKAs but there was a 4.2-fold greater risk for revision due to loosening with knees implanted without cement.[61] The Swedish knee arthroplasty registry reported on 41,223 knees implanted between 1988 and 1997 and found that knees implanted with a cementless tibia had a 1.4-fold risk of revision for loosening. There was no difference in revision risk when a cementless femur or patella was implanted. It is important to note that patellar resurfacing was only performed in 30% of knees during the study period.[14]

Recently, trabecular metal technology has been introduced into cementless knee designs and has met with early success. Radiostereophotogrammetric studies with a trabecular metal cementless knee design (Nex-

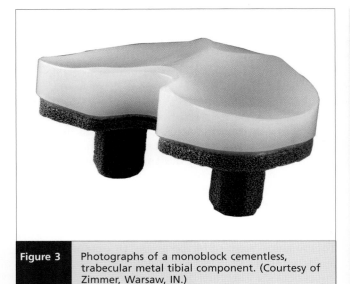

Figure 3 Photographs of a monoblock cementless, trabecular metal tibial component. (Courtesy of Zimmer, Warsaw, IN.)

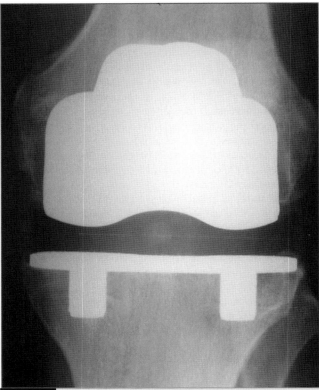

Figure 4 Radiograph of a cementless trabecular metal tibial component. (Courtesy of Zimmer, Warsaw, IN.)

Gen) did not show any difference in magnitude and pattern of migration at 2 years when compared to the same knee implanted with cement.[62] A similar study with NexGen trabecular metal tibial components showed migration during the first 3 months of implantation with subsequent stabilization. Motion was mainly subsidence and was different than that seen in other cementless tibial designs that routinely migrate by tilting.[63] These results are encouraging and clinical studies are needed to determine if these newer designs can eliminate the problem of early loosening of previous cementless tibial designs (Figures 3 and 4).

Although cementless fixation can provide durable fixation and excellent long-term results, the use of this technology introduces a significant risk of early tibial component failure not seen with cemented fixation. Cementless technology also introduces a significant increase in the cost of the implant without any improvement in clinical outcomes as measured by existing patient evaluation tools. Newer technology may improve the ability to obtain reliable early fixation but this remains to be documented in clinical studies.

Cross-linked Polyethylene in TKA

Cross-linked polyethylene has enjoyed great success in total hip arthroplasty with numerous in vitro, radiostereophotogrammetric, and retrieval studies that demonstrate a significant decrease in linear and volumetric wear. Although it would appear logical that these findings would also be applicable in TKA, the transition has not been as dramatic. Increased cross-linking is routinely obtained with ionizing radiation, and the polyethylene is subsequently treated by annealing (heating to a temperature below melting) or melting to remove free radicals created by the irradiation. The free radicals, when present, can lead to oxidation and deterioration of the polyethylene. Although melting is more effective at eliminating free radicals, it has been demonstrated to produce a larger reduction in the ultimate tensile strength and a decrease in elongation to failure that is related to increased cross-linking.

The hip, with its constrained interface and linear wear mechanisms, appears to be an ideal application of this technology. The kinematics in the knee, which demonstrate linear as well as multidirectional wear patterns, represent a significantly different environment. In this setting the shear at the polyethylene interface can potentially expose the weakened mechanical properties of ultra-high-molecular-weight polyethylene, especially if thinner metal-backed inserts are used.

There are certainly no short-term clinical benefits that have been demonstrated with the use of cross-linked polyethylene in the knee.[64] The potential long-term benefits of this material would be decreased wear and hopefully a decrease in the incidence of osteolysis. Whether the increased cost of this material is justified for most patients undergoing TKA is uncertain.

High-Flexion Knee Designs

In response to the perception that high-demand patients require increased flexion routinely in their daily activities, manufacturers have modified existing knee designs to allow increased femoral-tibial contact in deep flexion. Essentially all of these designs accomplish this by increasing the amount of bone resected from the posterior condyles of the femur and replacing it with the prosthesis. This modification decreases edge loading in extremes of flexion (130°) by increasing the prosthetic contact area and subsequently decreasing the stress on the polyethylene.

There are some studies that would support the concept of increasing flexion through modification of prosthetic design. One series of 218 knees reported a mean flexion of 140° using a high-flexion, mobile-bearing knee design.[65] In a 3.8-year follow-up study of 259 fixed-bearing high-flexion knee prostheses, a mean ROM of 135° was reported, a significant improvement over the preoperative ROM of 117°.[66]

Other studies have failed to demonstrate any significant increase in ROM resulting from the use of high-flexion TKA designs. In a prospective study evaluating a high-flexion tibial polyethylene insert articulating with the same femoral component, no difference in ROM was seen at 2-year follow-up. There were also no differences in clinical evaluation scores.[67] In a fluoroscopic study of patients with standard and high-flexion knee inserts of the same design, there was also no difference in ROM.[68] In a randomized study using a standard and high-flexion modification of a single implant system, there was no difference between the two designs although both groups had a significant increase in ROM from preoperative measurements.[69] In another prospective randomized study, no difference in clinical outcomes or ROM was noted between a standard or high-flexion modification of the same knee design.[70]

There is one report of complications with the use of a high-flexion knee design. A 38% incidence of loosening of the femoral component at a mean of 32 months follow-up was reported.[71] The components routinely migrated into flexion, a finding that may implicate loss of posterior bone support and/or some substantial difference in surgical technique leading to this problem.

It has been reported that high flexion is rarely used in most patients during activities of daily living. The authors of a 2009 study monitored 21 patients with high-flexion TKA designs with a digital goniometer 2 years postoperatively and found that knee flexion exceeded 90° only 1.2% of the time. Flexion was more than 120° in only eight patients, on average 2.2 minutes in a 36-hour period.[72] It is important to remember that the best determinant of the amount of postoperative ROM is the preoperative ROM. TKA allows the opportunity to increase flexion in patients with arthritis, but use of a high-flexion design is not a guarantee that increased flexion will be achieved. The reality is that surgical technique, patient motivation, and postoperative rehabilitation are as influential as prosthetic design in determining ROM. In a patient with preoperative flexion greater than 120°, in whom high-flexion activities can be predicted postoperatively, a high-flexion design may be warranted but the increased cost realistically does not make it practical for global use.

Sex–Specific Knee Prostheses

There has recently been a significant amount of attention directed toward sex differences in the osseous anatomy of the distal femur. There are variations in distal femoral anatomy related to sex, race, and the disease process affecting the joint, with female knees tending to be smaller than male knees. The aspect ratio, defined as the mediolateral dimension of the femur divided by the anteroposterior dimension, has been the focus of the controversy as it relates to sex-specific prosthetic design.

In a study of 200 knees undergoing TKA, the aspect ratio measured at the time of surgery was 122 in women and 127 in men.[73] This finding was confirmed in a study of measurement of the distal femurs of 1,000 patients undergoing TKA.[74] A large percentage, 98%, of the smallest knees in the series were those of women, and there was significant variability between narrow and wide mediolateral dimensions in this group of patients. In the knees that were intermediate in size, the knees of females were narrower than those of males. The femoral dimensions were also related to body habitus; both male and female patients with a short and wide morphotype (endomorphs) had wider femurs. In contrast, patients with long, narrow morphotypes (ectomorphs) had narrower knees.[74]

Claims of improved clinical outcomes with the use of sex-specific knee designs have not been substantiated. In a prospective study using a sex-neutral TKA design, there was no sex bias in clinical outcome scores and the use of sex-specific implants could not be supported.[75] In a literature review of 19 studies evaluating patients with sex-neutral femoral prostheses, the clinical results in women were as good if not better than those in men.[76] Based on these findings, the need for sex-specific implants was not supported.

Regardless of the range of prostheses sizes provided by a manufacturer, there will always be knees for which the surgeon will have to make minor compromises in sizing. It is important to remember that matching anteroposterior sizing is most critical to restoring knee kinematics. Overhang of the femoral or tibial component in the mediolateral plane should be avoided to reduce the incidence of soft-tissue impingement and irritation. Current standard TKA designs are designed to accommodate the variations in distal femoral anatomy encountered in most patients. Standard TKAs have aspect ratios that range from 107 to 119 in the smallest sizes to 105 to 109 in the largest sizes. These ratios fall well under the aspect ratios that have been demonstrated for both male and female femurs and would allow reconstruction of the anteroposterior dimensions without mediolateral overhang of the prosthesis in most patients, whether male or female, undergoing TKA.

2: Knee

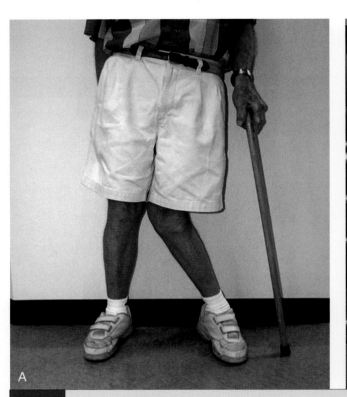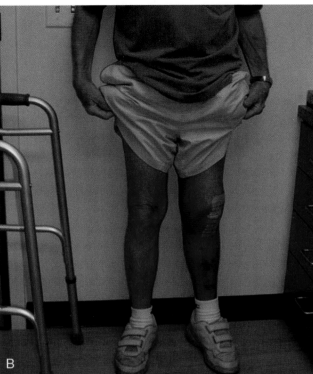

Figure 5   **A,** Photograph of a patient with severe valgus deformity and an incompetent medial collateral ligament. **B,** Photograph of the patient 2 weeks after primary TKA with a constrained prosthesis.

Constrained Implants for Primary TKA

Most arthritic knees can be managed with standard, minimally constrained implant designs and ligament balancing to yield a stable reconstruction. Revision implants usually use a constrained condylar design using a deeper femoral box and larger tibial keel that limits varus-valgus and rotational motion to less than 5°. In severe valgus knees with an incompetent medial collateral ligament, constrained implant designs have been used successfully in the primary setting (**Figure 5**).

The authors of one study reported on 44 primary knee replacements treated with the Constrained Condylar Knee (CCK) prosthesis (Zimmer).[77] The mean valgus deformity in the series was 17.6°, and 28 patients had follow-up of 7.8 years. The mean age of the patients in the series was 73 years. The KSS prosthesis scores improved from 27 to 95 and the functional scores improved from 32 to 67. There were no peroneal nerve palsies or cases of loosening or prosthesis failure. Although stem extensions were routinely used in this series, they were noncemented and implanted in a "loose press-fit manner." It was the authors' contention that the stems would allow some motion at the diaphyseal interface permitting load sharing.

A series of 54 knees treated with two different constrained condylar designs were reported in another study.[78] Although most of the knees had severe valgus deformity with an incompetent medial collateral liga-

ment, approximately 20% of the knees had severe preoperative flexion contracture for which the author could not obtain satisfactory balance at the time of surgery. Ten of the knees were treated with a nonmodular Total Condylar III prosthesis (Zimmer) that had fixed cemented stems on both the femoral and tibial component. A modular Insall-Burstein II prosthesis (Zimmer) was used to treat the remainder of the knees. In this group, stem extensions were used in six femoral and seven tibial components. Two knees were revised for loosening, and the 10-year survival rate with loosening as an endpoint in the 42 knees with follow-up was 96%. There were no tibial post fractures or peroneal nerve palsies in this series.

A third study reported on a series of 55 severe valgus knees treated with a nonmodular CCK design (Exactech, Gainesville, FL) placed without stem extensions.[79] The mean follow-up was 44.5 months (range, 2 to 6 years) and the mean age at the time of surgery was 73 years. The KSS prosthesis scores improved from 34 to 93 points and the functional score improved from 40 to 74 points. There were no peroneal nerve palsies and no cases of postoperative instability. There was one case of implant loosening and one tibial post fracture, both occurring in young, active patients.

The use of constrained condylar implant designs in patients with severe valgus deformities (> 15°) and compromise of the medial collateral ligament is supported in multiple studies. The use of stem extensions does not appear to be necessary on a routine basis and a successful outcome can be achieved without reconstruction of the medial collateral ligament. Implant loosening and tibial post fracture remain valid concerns in younger active patients.

Summary

The biggest difference in the results obtained with contemporary TKA designs over the previous generation is an increase in ROM, with most series routinely reporting more than 120° of postoperative flexion.[15,17] To attribute this finding solely to changes in implant design may be erroneous because changes in surgical technique, pain management, and rehabilitation protocols may have more to do with the increase in ROM than prosthetic modifications. Long-term follow-up will be needed to determine if the current designs of TKA can match the excellent survival rate of the previous generation.

The incidence of lateral retinacular release performed in conjunction with TKA also has decreased significantly in the past decade. Historically, reported lateral release rates were routinely greater than 50% and currently are well below 10% in most published series.[44] As with increased ROM, this is the result of multiple factors that may be unrelated to prosthetic design. The importance of femoral component rotation, and the effect of the tourniquet on patellar tracking, are several issues that are currently recognized as having an impact on this issue.[80] Surgeons have also become more tolerant of slight patellar tilt at the time of arthroplasty without strict reliance on the "rule of no thumb" (evaluating patellar tracking at the time of surgery with no manual pressure on the patella or capsular closure) that previously was the dominant factor in determining lateral release.[81,82]

There have been significant improvements over the past decade in implant materials and manufacturing. The understanding of the deleterious effects of gamma irradiation in air on polyethylene and extended shelf life on the integrity of this material has led to manufacturing and sterilization changes that have eliminated early catastrophic polyethylene failures. The effect of highly cross-linked polyethylene in TKA, however, remains to be demonstrated. Backside wear has been addressed with improvements in modular locking mechanisms and the use of polished tibial components. The effect of other modifications in prosthesis design, and sex-specific and high-flexion femoral components, have not been conclusively shown to improve the outcome of TKA.

With the current high quality of implant design and manufacturing, long-term success of TKA may be less associated with a specific implant and more related to avoiding infection, achieving durable fixation, and obtaining good soft-tissue stability. Despite the media emphasis on demands for high-performance arthroplasty, surgeons need to recognize that, in most series, the mean age of patients receiving TKA is still the sixth and seventh decades of life. It is also important to realize that the mortality following TKA is approximately 3% per year. This means that at 10 years, 30% of patients will be deceased and at 15 years only 50% of the patients will be alive. Surgeons should critically weigh the impact of newer high-performance knee designs with regard to their potential benefits against their significant increase in cost before adopting their use on a routine basis.

Annotated References

1. Pavone V, Boettner F, Fickert S, Sculco TP: Total condylar knee arthroplasty: A long-term followup. *Clin Orthop Relat Res* 2001;388:18-25.

2. Rand JA, Ilstrup DM: Survivorship analysis of total knee arthroplasty: Cumulative rates of survival of 9200 total knee arthroplasties. *J Bone Joint Surg Am* 1991;73(3):397-409.

3. Ritter MA, Herbst SA, Keating EM, Faris PM, Meding JB: Long-term survival analysis of a posterior cruciate-retaining total condylar total knee arthroplasty. *Clin Orthop Relat Res* 1994;309:136-145.

4. Ritter MA, Worland R, Saliski J, et al: Flat-on-flat, nonconstrained, compression molded polyethylene total knee replacement. *Clin Orthop Relat Res* 1995;321:79-85.

5. Schai PA, Thornhill TS, Scott RD: Total knee arthroplasty with the PFC system: Results at a minimum of ten years and survivorship analysis. *J Bone Joint Surg Br* 1998;80(5):850-858.

6. Ranawat CS, Flynn WF Jr, Saddler S, Hansraj KK, Maynard MJ: Long-term results of the total condylar knee arthroplasty: A 15-year survivorship study. *Clin Orthop Relat Res* 1993;286:94-102.

7. Ritter MA, Berend ME, Meding JB, Keating EM, Faris PM, Crites BM: Long-term followup of anatomic graduated components posterior cruciate-retaining total knee replacement. *Clin Orthop Relat Res* 2001;388:51-57.

8. Insall JN, Dorr LD, Scott RD, Scott WN: Rationale of the Knee Society clinical rating system. *Clin Orthop Relat Res* 1989;248:13-14.

9. Benjamin J, Johnson R, Porter S: Knee scores change with length of follow-up after total knee arthroplasty. *J Arthroplasty* 2003;18(7):867-871.

10. Sharkey PF, Hozack WJ, Rothman RH, Shastri S, Jacoby SM: Insall Award paper: Why are total knee arthroplasties failing today? *Clin Orthop Relat Res* 2002;404:7-13.

2: Knee

11. Gioe TJ, Killeen KK, Grimm K, Mehle S, Scheltema K: Why are total knee replacements revised? Analysis of early revision in a community knee implant registry. *Clin Orthop Relat Res* 2004;428:100-106.

12. Hofmann S, Graf R: Why do prosthesis fail early: Analysis of 100 consecutive revision surgeries in TKA. 2009 *Annual Meeting Proceedings*. Rosemont, IL, American Academy of Orthopaedic Surgeons, 2009, p 528.

    A consecutive single-surgeon series of revisions demonstrated that 78% were performed within 5 years of the index procedure. Malrotation of components was the reason for revision in 54%, followed by malalignment (41%), instability (36%), and infection (19%).

13. Fehring TK, Odum S, Griffin WL, Mason JB, Nadaud M: Early failures in total knee arthroplasty. *Clin Orthop Relat Res* 2001;392:315-318.

14. Lidgren L, Robertsson O: *Annual Report 2008: The Swedish Knee Arthroplasty Register.* Lund, Sweden, Wallin & Dalholm, 2008.

    Fifty percent of revisions were done within 4 years of the index procedure, with loosening being the most common reason for revision (44%). Polyethylene wear/lysis (12.4%) and infection (9.9%) were the other leading causes of revision.

15. Dalury DF, Gonzales RA, Adams MJ, Gruen TA, Trier K: Midterm results with the PFC Sigma total knee arthroplasty system. *J Arthroplasty* 2008;23(2):175-181.

    The authors present a prospective study on 284 knees with 8-year survival rate of 99%. Mean postoperative knee scores were 93.8 and mean ROM was 123°.

16. Dalury DF, Barrett WP, Mason JB, Goldstein WM, Murphy JA, Roche MW: Midterm survival of a contemporary modular total knee replacement: A multicentre study of 1970 knees. *J Bone Joint Surg Br* 2008; 90(12):1594-1596.

    The authors present a multicenter study of 1970 PFC CR and PS knees with a mean follow-up of 7.3 years. ROM was 115.9 in PS knees versus 114.4° in CR knees. The 10-year survival rate was 97.2%.

17. Harwin SF, Greene KA, Hitt K: Triathlon total knee arthroplasty: 4-year outcomes with a high-performance implant. *J Knee Surg* 2008;21(4):320-326.

    Short-term follow-up on 2,035 consecutive knees with knee scores of 96 and mean ROM of 126° at 21 months is discussed.

18. Bertin KC: Cruciate-retaining total knee arthroplasty at 5 to 7 years followup. *Clin Orthop Relat Res* 2005; 436: 177-183.

    Intermediate follow-up on 198 NexGen CR knees with mean ROM of 123° and 98% survival is discussed. Mean knee scores were 97 at follow-up.

19. Laskin RS: The Genesis total knee prosthesis: A 10-year followup study. *Clin Orthop Relat Res* 2001;388: 95-102.

20. Waslewski GL, Marson BM, Benjamin JB: Early, incapacitating instability of posterior cruciate ligament-retaining total knee arthroplasty. *J Arthroplasty* 1998; 13(7):763-767.

21. Laskin RS: The Insall Award: Total knee replacement with posterior cruciate ligament retention in patients with a fixed varus deformity. *Clin Orthop Relat Res* 1996;331:29-34.

22. Partington PF, Sawhney J, Rorabeck CH, Barrack RL, Moore J: Joint line restoration after revision total knee arthroplasty. *Clin Orthop Relat Res* 1999;367:165-171.

23. Figgie HE III, Goldberg VM, Heiple KG, Moller HS III, Gordon NH: The influence of tibial-patellofemoral location on function of the knee in patients with the posterior stabilized condylar knee prosthesis. *J Bone Joint Surg Am* 1986;68(7):1035-1040.

24. Hozack WJ, Rothman RH, Booth RE Jr, Balderston RA: The patellar clunk syndrome: A complication of posterior stabilized total knee arthroplasty. *Clin Orthop Relat Res* 1989;241:203-208.

25. Lonner JH, Jasko JG, Bezwada HP, Nazarian DG, Booth RE Jr: Incidence of patellar clunk with a modern posterior-stabilized knee design. *Am J Orthop* 2007;36(10):550-553.

    The authors report elimination of patellar clunk using the NexGen PS TKA system versus 4% incidence with Insall-Bernstein II prosthesis.

26. Clarke HD, Fuchs R, Scuderi GR, Mills EL, Scott WN, Insall JN: The influence of femoral component design in the elimination of patellar clunk in posterior-stabilized total knee arthroplasty. *J Arthroplasty* 2006; 21(2):167-171.

    After minimum 2-year follow-up on 238 NexGen PS TKAs, there was no incidence of patellar clunk or revision for patellofemoral problems.

27. Ip D, Wu WC, Tsang WL: Early results of posterior-stabilized NexGen Legacy total knee arthroplasty. *J Orthop Surg* 2003;11(1):38-42.

    The authors discuss follow-up on 60 knees at 21 months with a 3.3% incidence of patellar crepitus.

28. Pagnano M, Trousdale R: Clunk is solved but patellar crepitus persists: Prevalence, severity and natural history in two contemporary posterior stabilized knee designs. *25th Annual Interim Meeting Proceedings*. Rosemont, IL, Knee Society, 2008, p 69.

    A total of 428 patients with PS TKAs were followed for 3.9 years and 24% reported some patellar crepitus. Only 6% of patients believed the condition was painful, audible, or a source of dissatisfaction. This is a report on patient follow-up in 428 TKAs using PFC PS or NexGen PS prostheses. On a patient questionnaire, 25% reported patellar crepitus.

29. Buechel FF Sr, Buechel FF Jr, Pappas MJ, D'Alessio J:

Twenty-year evaluation of meniscal bearing and rotating platform knee replacements. *Clin Orthop Relat Res* 2001;388:41-50.

30. Huang CH, Ma HM, Lee YM, Ho FY: Long-term results of low contact stress mobile-bearing total knee replacements. *Clin Orthop Relat Res* 2003;416:265-270.

31. Sorrells RB, Voorhorst PE, Murphy JA, Bauschka MP, Greenwald AS: Uncemented rotating-platform total knee replacement: A five to twelve-year follow-up study. *J Bone Joint Surg Am* 2004;86-A(10):2156-2162.

32. Ali MS, Mangaleshkar SR: Uncemented rotating-platform total knee arthroplasty: A 4-year to 12-year follow-up. *J Arthroplasty* 2006;21(1):80-84.

This is a follow-up on 109 LCS-RP knees with a 10-year survival rate of 99%. The mean ROM in this series was 100°.

33. Sorrells RB: The rotating platform mobile bearing TKA. *Orthopedics* 1996;19(9):793-796.

34. Bert JM: Dislocation/subluxation of meniscal bearing elements after New Jersey low-contact stress total knee arthroplasty. *Clin Orthop Relat Res* 1990;254(254):211-215.

35. Callaghan JJ, O'Rourke MR, Iossi MF, et al: Cemented rotating-platform total knee replacement: A concise follow-up, at a minimum of fifteen years, of a previous report. *J Bone Joint Surg Am* 2005;87(9):1995-1998.

The authors report on 37 surviving patients from the original series. There were no bearing dislocations or implant loosening. The mean ROM was 105° and three patients demonstrated osteolysis.

36. Harrington MA, Hopkinson WJ, Hsu P, Manion L: Fixed- vs mobile-bearing total knee arthroplasty: Does it make a difference? A prospective randomized study. *J Arthroplasty* 2009;24(6, Suppl)24-27.

No difference in clinical outcome measurements or ROM between the two designs at 2-year follow-up was noted.

37. Kim YH, Kim DY, Kim JS: Simultaneous mobile- and fixed-bearing total knee replacement in the same patients: A prospective comparison of mid-term outcomes using a similar design of prosthesis. *J Bone Joint Surg Br* 2007;89(7):904-910.

The authors present a prospective study on patients undergoing bilateral TKA with PFC-RP and PFC-CR. At 5.6 years there was no difference in KSS pain scores, function scores, or ROM.

38. Watanabe T, Tomita T, Fuji M, Hashimoto J, Sugamoto K, Yoshikawa H: Comparison between mobile-bearing and fixed-bearing knees in bilateral total knee replacements. *Int Orthop* 2005;29(3):179-181.

This is a report on 22 patients with NexGen CR and Rotaglide prostheses. No difference in KSS or ROM was noted. Five patients favored the mobile-bearing knee and 16 had no preference.

39. Evans MC, Parsons EM, Scott RD, Thornhill TS, Zurakowski D: Comparative flexion after rotating-platform vs fixed-bearing total knee arthroplasty. *J Arthroplasty* 2006;21(7):985-991.

A retrospective review of 113 PFC-RP and 100 PFC-CR knees is presented. No difference in postoperative ROM or complications between the two groups was noted.

40. Gioe TJ, Glynn J, Sembrano J, Suthers K, Santos ER, Singh J: Mobile and fixed-bearing (all-polyethylene tibial component) total knee arthroplasty designs: A prospective randomized trial. *J Bone Joint Surg Am* 2009;91(9):2104-2112.

The authors present a randomized prospective study using identical PS femoral component (PFC PS) with RP or FB all-polyethylene tibial components. No difference in postoperative KSS, WOMAC, or ROM was noted.

41. Kim YH, Kim JS: Prevalence of osteolysis after simultaneous bilateral fixed- and mobile-bearing total knee arthroplasties in young patients. *J Arthroplasty* 2009;24(6):932-940.

The authors discuss follow-up on 61 patients with Anatomic Modular Knee (AMK, DePuy) and LCS TKA at 10.8 years. No difference in clinical outcomes, revision rates, or incidence of osteolysis was noted.

42. Wright T, Fu R, Kelly N, Padgett D: Retrieval analysis of mobile bearing total knee prosthesis. *26th Annual Interim Meeting Proceedings*. Rosemont, IL, Knee Society, 2009, p 34.

Forty-eight mobile-bearing retrievals were evaluated for articular and backside wear. The mean length of implantation was 3.2 years and revisions were for lysis, stiffness, instability, and infection. Articular wear was comparable to that of fixed-bearing designs, and backside wear showed wear from third-body interposition.

43. Huang CH, Ma HM, Lee YM, Ho FY: Long-term results of low contact stress mobile-bearing total knee replacements. *Clin Orthop Relat Res* 2003;416:265-270.

44. Pagnano MW, Trousdale RT, Stuart MJ, Hanssen AD, Jacofsky DJ: Rotating platform knees did not improve patellar tracking: A prospective, randomized study of 240 primary total knee arthroplasties. *Clin Orthop Relat Res* 2004;428:221-227.

45. D'Lima DD, Trice M, Urquhart AG, Colwell CW Jr: Comparison between the kinematics of fixed and rotating bearing knee prostheses. *Clin Orthop Relat Res* 2000;380:151-157.

46. Insall J, Aglietti P, Baldini A, Easley M: Meniscal-

bearing knee replacement, in Insall J, Scott W, eds: *Surgery of the Knee*, ed 3. New York, NY, Churchill Livingstone, 2001, pp 1717-1738.

47. Stiehl JB, Dennis DA, Komistek RD, Keblish PA: In vivo kinematic analysis of a mobile bearing total knee prosthesis. *Clin Orthop Relat Res* 1997;345:60-66.

48. Benjamin JB, Szivek JA, Hammond AS, Kubchandhani Z, Matthews AI Jr, Anderson P: Contact areas and pressures between native patellas and prosthetic femoral components. *J Arthroplasty* 1998;13(6):693-698.

49. Burnett RS, Haydon CM, Rorabeck CH, Bourne RB: Patella resurfacing versus nonresurfacing in total knee arthroplasty: Results of a randomized controlled clinical trial at a minimum of 10 years' followup. *Clin Orthop Relat Res* 2004;428:12-25.

50. Burnett RS, Boone JL, McCarthy KP, Rosenzweig S, Barrack RL: A prospective randomized clinical trial of patellar resurfacing and nonresurfacing in bilateral TKA. *Clin Orthop Relat Res* 2007;464:65-72.

    Ten-year follow-up demonstrated no difference in ROM, KSS, revision rates, or incidence of anterior knee pain.

51. Graves S, Davidson D, de Steiger R, Tomkins A: *Australian Orthopaedic Association National Joint Replacement Registry: Annual Report.* Adelaide, Australia, Australian Orthopaedic Association, 2008, p 152.

    The risk of revision, for any reason, at 5 years was 30% higher in patients who did not have patellar resurfacing.

52. Parvizi J, Rapuri VR, Saleh KJ, Kuskowski MA, Sharkey PF, Mont MA: Failure to resurface the patella during total knee arthroplasty may result in more knee pain and secondary surgery. *Clin Orthop Relat Res* 2005;438:191-196.

    A meta-analysis of 14 prospective randomized studies showed a lower risk of anterior knee pain with patellar resurfacing.

53. Pakos EE, Ntzani EE, Trikalinos TA: Patellar resurfacing in total knee arthroplasty: A meta-analysis. *J Bone Joint Surg Am* 2005;87(7):1438-1445.

    A meta-analysis of 10 prospective randomized studies reported lower incidence of reoperation and anterior knee pain with patellar resurfacing.

54. Nizard RS, Biau D, Porcher R, et al: A meta-analysis of patellar replacement in total knee arthroplasty. *Clin Orthop Relat Res* 2005;432:196-203.

    A meta-analysis of 12 prospective randomized studies reported a lower risk of reoperation for patellofemoral problems and decreased risk of anterior knee pain with patellar resurfacing.

55. Hofmann AA, Evanich JD, Ferguson RP, Camargo MP: Ten- to 14-year clinical followup of the cementless Natural Knee system. *Clin Orthop Relat Res* 2001;388:85-94.

56. Whiteside LA: Long-term followup of the bone-ingrowth Ortholoc knee system without a metal-backed patella. *Clin Orthop Relat Res* 2001;388:77-84.

57. Ritter M, Meneghini R: Twenty-year survivorship of cement-less anatomic graduated component total knee arthroplasty. *J Arthroplasty* 2010;25(4):507-513.

    The authors report minimum 10-year follow-up on 73 cementless anatomic graduated component TKAs with 97.4% tibial component survivorship and no femoral failures. The patellar failure rate was 16.4%.

58. Furnes O, Espehaug B, Lie SA, Vollset SE, Engesaeter LB, Havelin LI: Early failures among 7,174 primary total knee replacements: A follow-up study from the Norwegian Arthroplasty Register 1994-2000. *Acta Orthop Scand* 2002;73(2):117-129.

59. Paxton E, Inacio M, Slipchenko T, Fithian D: The Kaiser Permanente national total joint replacement registry. *The Pemanente Journal* 2008;12(3):12-16.

    This is a follow-up study of more than 30,000 TKAs, demonstrating main causes of revision due to infection, loosening, and ligament instability. Noncemented TKAs had a threefold incidence of loosening.

60. Rand JA, Trousdale RT, Ilstrup DM, Harmsen WS: Factors affecting the durability of primary total knee prostheses. *J Bone Joint Surg Am* 2003;85-A(2):259-265.

61. Gandhi R, Tsvetkov D, Davey JR, Mahomed NN: Survival and clinical function of cemented and uncemented prostheses in total knee replacement: A meta-analysis. *J Bone Joint Surg Br* 2009;91(7):889-895.

    In this review of 15 studies, there was no difference in KSS, but revision for loosening was 4.2 times greater in cementless prostheses.

62. Gao F, Henricson A, Nilsson KG: Cemented versus uncemented fixation of the femoral component of the NexGen CR total knee replacement in patients younger than 60 years: A prospective randomised controlled RSA study. *Knee* 2009;16(3):200-206.

    Radiostereogrammetric studies of 41 patients demonstrated no difference in magnitude or pattern of migration between cemented or uncemented femoral components.

63. Henricson A, Linder L, Nilsson KG: A trabecular metal tibial component in total knee replacement in patients younger than 60 years: A two-year radiostereophotogrammetric analysis. *J Bone Joint Surg Br* 2008;90(12):1585-1593.

    The authors report on a radiostereogrammetric analysis of monoblock trabecular metal tibial components and cemented tibial components demonstrating stabilization of cementless tibial tray migration at 3 months.

64. Minoda Y, Aihara M, Sakawa A, et al: Comparison between highly cross-linked and conventional polyethylene in total knee arthroplasty. *Knee* 2009;16(5):348-

351.

No difference in ROM or KSS was reported between patients with cross-linked or standard polyethylene in the same CR knee system.

65. Tarabichi S, Tarabichi Y, Hawari M: Achieving deep flexion after primary total knee arthroplasty. *J Arthroplasty* 2010;25(2):219-224.

Five year follow-up on 218 mobile-bearing, high-flexion knees with a mean ROM of 140° was studied.

66. Kim TH, Lee DH, Bin SI: The NexGen LPS-flex to the knee prosthesis at a minimum of three years. *J Bone Joint Surg Br* 2008;90(10):1304-1310.

A prospective series of a mobile-bearing high-flexion TKA with a mean postoperative ROM of 135° is presented. The mean preoperative ROM in this series was 117°.

67. McCalden RW, MacDonald SJ, Bourne RB, Marr JT: A randomized controlled trial comparing "high-flex" vs "standard" posterior cruciate substituting polyethylene tibial inserts in total knee arthroplasty. *J Arthroplasty* 2009;24(6, Suppl):33-38.

A high flexion tibial insert was compared to a standard tibial polyethylene insert, with no difference in clinical measures or ROM.

68. Suggs JF, Kwon YM, Durbhakula SM, Hanson GR, Li G: In vivo flexion and kinematics of the knee after TKA: Comparison of a conventional and a high flexion cruciate-retaining TKA design. *Knee Surg Sports Traumatol Arthrosc* 2009;17(2):150-156.

A fluoroscopic study of knees with and without a high-flexion tibial insert performing weight-bearing flexion is presented. No difference in ROM between the two designs was noted.

69. Nutton RW, van der Linden ML, Rowe PJ, Gaston P, Wade FA: A prospective randomised double-blind study of functional outcome and range of flexion following total knee replacement with the NexGen standard and high flexion components. *J Bone Joint Surg Br* 2008;90(1):37-42.

A randomized study of 56 patients receiving either a standard or high-flexion TKA implant is presented. Both groups had significant improvement in ROM, but there was no difference between the two designs.

70. Kim YH, Choi Y, Kim JS: Range of motion of standard and high-flexion posterior cruciate-retaining total knee prostheses a prospective randomized study. *J Bone Joint Surg Am* 2009;91(8):1874-1881.

No difference in weight bearing or non–weight-bearing ROM between the two designs was noted.

71. Han HS, Kang SB, Yoon KS: High incidence of loosening of the femoral component in legacy posterior stabilised-flex total knee replacement. *J Bone Joint Surg Br* 2007;89(11):1457-1461.

A significant incidence of early femoral loosening, 38%, at a mean of 32 months was reported. Knees with loosening had higher flexion than stable femurs: 136° versus 125°.

72. Huddleston JI, Scarborough DM, Goldvasser D, Freiberg AA, Malchau H: 2009 Marshall Urist Young Investigator Award: How often do patients with high-flex total knee arthroplasty use high flexion? *Clin Orthop Relat Res* 2009;467(7):1898-1906.

Twenty-one patients with high-flexion prosthetic designs were monitored for 36 hours. Knees were flexed greater than 90° 0.5% of the time, and only eight knees were flexed more than 120° for 0.1% of the testing period.

73. Chin KR, Dalury DF, Zurakowski D, Scott RD: Intraoperative measurements of male and female distal femurs during primary total knee arthroplasty. *J Knee Surg* 2002;15(4):213-217.

74. Bellemans J, Carprentier K, Vandenneucker H, Vanlauwe J, Victor J: The John Insall Award: Both morphotype and gender influence the shape of the knee in patients undergoing TKA. *Clin Orthop Relat Res* 2010;466(1):29-36.

Femurs of 1,000 patients were measured at the time of TKA. Significant anteroposterior/mediolateral ratio variations were found with femur size, sex, and body habitus.

75. MacDonald SJ, Charron KD, Bourne RB, Naudie DD, McCalden RW, Rorabeck CH: The John Insall Award: Gender-specific total knee replacement. Prospectively collected clinical outcomes. *Clin Orthop Relat Res* 2008;466(11):2612-2616.

No sex bias in outcome scores using generic implants was noted in a prospective study of 5,279 TKAs. Results did not support the premise of using sex-specific implants.

76. Merchant AC, Arendt EA, Dye SF, et al: The female knee: Anatomic variations and the female-specific total knee design. *Clin Orthop Relat Res* 2008;466(12):3059-3065.

A literature review of 19 studies of TKA with sex-neutral prosthesis is presented. Results in females were equivalent to those of males, which did not support the need for a sex-specific implant.

77. Easley M, Insall J, Scuderi G, Bullek D: Primary constrained condylar knee arthroplasty for the arthritic valgus knee. *Clin Orthop Relat Res* 2000;380:58-64.

78. Lachiewicz P, Soileau E: Ten-year survival and clinical results of constrained components in primary total knee arthroplasty. *J Arthroplasty* 2006;21:803-808.

The authors studied 44 primary constrained TKAs with a 10-year survival rate and loosening rate of 96%. There were no peroneal nerve injuries or tibial post fractures.

79. Anderson J, Baldini A, MacDonald J, Pellicci P, Sculco T: Primary constrained condylar knee arthroplasty without stem extensions for the valgus knee. *Clin Or-*

2: Knee

thop Relat Res 2006;422:199-203.

Fifty-five nonstemmed constrained primary TKAs were followed for 44 months. There was one tibial post fracture and one patellar dislocation, but no nerve injuries.

80. Marson BM, Tokish JT: The effect of a tourniquet on intraoperative patellofemoral tracking during total knee arthroplasty. *J Arthroplasty* 1999;14(2):197-199.

81. Benjamin J, Chilvers M: Correcting lateral patellar tilt at the time of total knee arthroplasty can result in overuse of lateral release. *J Arthroplasty* 2006;21(6, Suppl 2)121-126.

Ninety-nine consecutive patients without lateral release at time of TKA were studied. There were no patellar subluxations/dislocations. Patellar tilt and congruence were improved postoperatively.

82. Scott RD: Prosthetic replacement of the patellofemoral joint. *Orthop Clin North Am* 1979;10(1):129-137.

2: Knee

Chapter 13

Revision Total Knee Arthroplasty

R. Michael Meneghini, MD

Introduction

With annual rates of primary total knee arthroplasty (TKA) on the rise, the current and projected incidence of revision TKA procedures is expected to increase dramatically. One study reported projections that the number of knee revision procedures in the United States will double from the year 2005 to 2015 and increase 601% by the year 2030.[1] Compared with primary TKA, revision procedures are more technically demanding and generally have higher risks of complications. Therefore, it is critical that surgeons understand the principles of the evaluation, etiologies of failure, surgical reconstruction, and clinical outcomes associated with revision TKA.

Evaluation of the Painful TKA

Because the etiologies of dysfunction and pain after TKA can be numerous,[2-4] it is important to approach the diagnosis in a systematic fashion. A logical approach includes a thorough history, physical examination, and radiographic modalities while being aware of the differential diagnosis of the painful TKA. The etiologies can be grouped into two large categories: intrinsic or intra-articular (**Table 1**) and extrinsic or extra-articular (**Table 2**).

Systematic Approach

The history and physical examination are critical and have the ability to identify and/or eliminate most extrinsic etiologies. The final requisite test is a plain radiograph, which can identify many of the intrinsic causes of pain, particularly if serial examinations are available. In most patients with a painful TKA, basic laboratory testing that includes an assessment of complete blood count (CBC), erythrocyte sedimentation rate (ESR), and C-reactive protein (CRP) level can identify the possibility of occult infection. If the etiology of

Dr. Meneghini or an immediate family member is a paid consultant for or is an employee of Stryker; has received research or institutional support from Stryker; and has received nonincome support (such as equipment or services), commercially derived honoraria, or other non-research–related funding (such as paid travel) from Stryker.

pain has not been conclusively determined after the above-mentioned efforts, advanced radiographic imaging such as CT, a nuclear bone scan, or MRI may be advantageous. A diagnostic injection of lidocaine into the knee may also provide further confirmatory evidence of a suspected etiology for pain.

History

A thorough patient history is requisite to determining the etiology of pain after TKA. Pain that is constant and does not abate with rest or activity modification should alert the surgeon to the strong possibility of infection. Pain that is related to activity and is relieved with rest may indicate noninfectious causes of mechanical pain, as is associated with instability or loosening. Associated symptoms such as stiffness or instability are also important indicators of the potential etiology of pain.

The onset and duration of the symptoms is also critical and help narrow the differential diagnosis. Pain that is persistent throughout the first few months of the early postoperative period is more likely to represent infection, instability, or soft-tissue conditions such as impingement. When infection is suspected, it is essential to assess the status of the wound early after surgery and determine if problems such as persistent drainage or treatment with oral antibiotics occurred. If so, a detailed workup to evaluate the TKA for infection is mandatory. An additional consideration in patients who have early postoperative pain that is similar in those with preoperative pain is whether the TKA was performed for the correct diagnosis. Rarely, knee pain can be referred from the spine or hip, which must be investigated in detail if suspected clinically. Pain that presents late, such as years after the procedure, is typically indicative of mechanical problems such as aseptic loosening, polyethylene wear, or osteolysis. If there is an acute and dramatic onset of pain years later in a well-functioning and pain-free knee, hematogenous infection should be suspected.

Physical Examination

The workup of a painful TKA must include a thorough, systematic, and detailed physical examination performed with an emphasis on the differential diagnosis. Each patient should be examined for any gait disturbance such as antalgia or varus-valgus thrust. A

Table 1

Intrinsic or Intra-articular Etiologies

1. Infection
2. Instability
   a. Axial
   b. Flexion
3. Malalignment
   a. Axial
   b. Flexion
4. Aseptic loosening
5. Polyethylene wear
6. Osteolysis
7. Implant fracture
8. Arthrofibrosis
9. Soft-tissue impingement
10. Patellar clunk
11. Popliteus tendon impingement
12. Component overhang/excess cement
13. Extensor mechanism dysfunction
    a. Patellar instability
    b. Patellar fracture
    c. Patellar pain
       i. Unresurfaced patella
       ii. Lateral facet impingement
       iii. Patella baja
       iv. Excessive composite thickness
    d. Quadriceps / patellar tendon rupture

Table 2

Extrinsic or Extra-articular Etiologies

1. Hip pathology
2. Lumbar spine
   a. Stenosis
   b. Radiculopathy
3. Neuroma
4. Complex regional pain syndrome
5. Vascular claudication
6. Soft-tissue inflammation
   a. Pes bursitis
   b. Patellar tendinitis
   c. Quadriceps tendinitis
7. Periprosthetic fractures
   a. Tibial stress fracture
   b. Patellar stress fracture
   c. Traumatic fractures

careful visual examination should note all incisions around the knee. The knee is palpated to determine the presence of effusion and to note any specific areas of tenderness. The stability of the knee to varus-valgus stress should be assessed in full extension, midflexion, and at 90° of flexion. The assessment in midflexion is critical to isolate the medial and lateral collateral ligaments via relaxation of the posterior capsule, which can act as a stabilizer in full extension. Equally important is the examination of the knee at 90° to ascertain if any flexion instability exists. In combination with symptoms that include pain while ascending or descending stairs, while squatting, or during knee flexion, tenderness over the anterior knee particularly in the pes anserine region or exaggerated anterior tibial translation at 90° on physical examination strongly suggest a diagnosis of flexion instability.

The surgeon should carefully evaluate patellar tracking through the entire range of motion with special attention on the stability and position of the patella relative to the trochlear groove of the femoral component. Patellar clunk syndrome is typically observed near 30° to 45° as the knee extends from the flexed position and is manifested as a palpable and even audible "clunk" of

the patella.[5] It is also important to evaluate the strength and integrity of the extensor mechanism through passive and active motion assessment. This allows the surgeon to ascertain whether a limitation of full extension is from a flexion contracture or an extensor lag, which is critical in determining the etiology of extensor mechanism dysfunction. In addition, the strength of the quadriceps muscle should be assessed; in cases of patellar instability, the vastus medialis obliquus should be examined specifically.

A thorough neurovascular examination, including assessment of lower extremity pulses, is mandatory. Every patient with a painful TKA should have the ipsilateral hip examined to avoid missing hip osteoarthritis that may present as knee pain. A lumbar spine and lower extremity neurologic examination may also be warranted.

Radiographic Evaluation

Plain radiographs should include weight-bearing AP, lateral, and axial views of the patella. The standing AP view provides the alignment and interfaces of the implants in the coronal plane. The lateral view should be examined for osteolysis, which is most commonly observed in the posterior condyles. The lateral view also can reveal the relationship of the patella relative to the femoral condyle, tibial tubercle, and joint line to determine patella alta or baja. The lateral view can also be evaluated to determine the femoral component size, posterior condylar offset, and tibial slope. The axial view of the patella helps determine patellar maltracking or instability, as well as loosening or osteolysis. All plain radiographs should be closely examined for radiolucent lines at either the bone-cement or cement-prosthesis interface. If a cementless device is being examined, visualization of the prosthesis-bone interface is critical and requires persistence in technique to obtain a true AP view of the tibial component and a true lateral view of the femoral and tibial components without view-obscuring angulation. Fluoroscopy may be helpful to clearly evaluate the interfaces "in plane" to more accurately assess the implant fixation. If possible, the patient's preoperative radiographs should be obtained to assess the degree of osteoarthritis present before TKA. Rare instances of relatively normal-looking preoperative radiographs can be an indication that persistent pain after TKA may be caused by other pathologic conditions such as hip osteoarthritis, soft-tissue inflammation, or psychosomatic issues. Serial radiographs are valuable and required to ascertain any change in component position or progression of radiolucent lines over time that may be suggestive of loosening.

Additional Radiographic Studies

If the diagnosis of the painful TKA is uncertain, nuclear imaging studies may be helpful in the diagnosis of aseptic loosening, infection, complex regional pain syndrome, and periprosthetic stress fractures. However, caution must be exercised when using this diagnostic modality, because a three-phase technetium bone scan may show increased uptake in TKA indefinitely. Increased uptake of approximately 89% tibial and 63% femoral implants have been demonstrated more than 1 year after the index TKA surgery. Unfortunately, this persistent uptake limits the usefulness of the study when performed alone. An indium-labeled leukocyte scan has an accuracy of 78% when used alone for the diagnosis of infection; however, when combined with a technetium-99 sulfur-colloid marrow scan, the accuracy improves to 88% to 95%.[6]

CT may be helpful to more accurately define the extent of osteolytic lesions, which are typically underestimated on plain radiographs. Recently, MRI techniques have been shown to potentially offer advantages with metal artifact suppression when assessing TKA for osteolysis.[7] CT is also helpful to assess femoral and tibial component malrotation in the case of patellofemoral instability. Internal rotation of the femoral component is associated with patellar instability and lateral flexion laxity, which are both associated with poorer clinical function.[8]

Laboratory Analysis

Infection was recently reported to be the leading etiology for revision TKA in the United States based on newly developed ICD-9 codes.[9] ESR and CRP are the most commonly used laboratory tests in the evaluation of the painful TKA. It has recently been shown that if the ESR is less than 30 mm/h and the CRP is less than 10 mg/dL, infection is very unlikely.[10,11] However, intra-articular joint fluid aspiration is required if there is a high clinical suspicion of sepsis, such as with clinical presentation or with a high-risk patients who may be immunocompromised. Joint aspiration is suggested if

either the CRP or ESR is elevated, regardless of the clinical presentation. Newly reported criteria for chronic periprosthetic sepsis state that when fluid analysis shows a synovial leukocyte count of greater than 1,100 cells/cm^3 and differential greater than 64% in the face of elevated CRP and ESR, sepsis is very likely (98.6%).[10] Recently, it has been established that aspiration of a suspected early postoperative TKA infection is essential to accurately determine whether sepsis is confirmed. With a cutoff of 27,800 cells/μL, synovial white blood cell count predicted infection within 6 weeks after primary TKA with a positive predicted value of 94% and a negative predictive value of 98%.[12]

Establish Etiology Prior to Revision TKA

An intra-articular lidocaine injection can be a useful adjunct to confirm intra-articular and extra-articular pathology, particularly aseptic loosening, soft-tissue impingement, and pes anserine bursitis. It can also be a useful diagnostic modality to differentiate psychosomatic issues from true pathology in certain patients. However, if the etiology for pain after TKA cannot be determined, it is not advisable to perform revision TKA. A very low probability of success has been reported with revision TKA for unexplained pain. Additional caution is warranted before isolated patella revision[13] or tibial polyethylene exchange,[14] because poor results are likely the result of failure to address the underlying failure mechanism, which is likely multifactorial and related to component malposition.

Surgical Technique and Principles

The goals of revision TKA include proper axial limb alignment, accurate positioning and adequate fixation of prosthetic components, symmetric ligament balance in flexion and extension, satisfactory patellofemoral mechanics, and an acceptable knee range of motion. These goals, particularly proper ligamentous balance and prosthetic fixation, are highly dependent on the management of bone loss. The magnitude of bone loss has significant implications for decisions regarding the use of bone graft or prosthetic augmentation, choice of prosthesis sizing, selection of prosthetic articular constraint, and need for supplemental stem fixation.[15]

Preoperative Planning

If a lateral radiograph of the knee obtained before the original arthroplasty is unavailable, it is helpful to obtain a lateral radiograph of the opposite knee to determine the appropriate anteroposterior dimension of the knee. The optimal joint line position is roughly 2 cm below the origin of the medial collateral ligament and 2.5 cm below the prominence of the lateral epicondyle. It is also helpful to anticipate the bone loss that might be encountered and the supplemental stem fixation required, which is typical in revision TKA. It is advantageous to anticipate the level of articular constraint that

2: Knee

might be required to ensure that the various options are available in the operating room during the procedure.

Surgical Technique

Revision TKA typically is performed in a stepwise sequence. The initial step is to perform the surgical incision and exposure of the knee joint. If multiple longitudinal incisions are present about the knee, the surgeon should use the most lateral incision through which adequate exposure can be obtained. Because the superficial blood supply to the knee originates medially, medially based incisions may create the possibility of detrimental skin necrosis and subsequent infection. Care should be taken to create minimal flaps, which should be full thickness at the level of the patella retinaculum. Surgical exposure of the knee joint is most commonly performed via a medial parapatellar approach. Occasionally, more extensile approaches, such as a rectus snip or tibial tubercle osteotomy, may be necessary based on the specific location identified as limiting adequate exposure of the knee joint. Recently, a "banana peel" technique has been recommended as a safe method of exposure. This involves peeling the patella tendon as a sleeve off the tibia, leaving the extensor mechanism intact with a lateral hinge of soft tissue.[16] Authors of a 2007 study retrospectively reviewed the use of this technique in conjunction with a proximal quadriceps snip in 102 consecutive patients undergoing revision TKA.[16] At a minimum 2-year follow-up, no patient reported disruption of the extensor mechanism or decreased ability to extend the surgically treated knee.

After exposure of the knee, removal of the implants is performed with specific attention to preservation of viable remaining bone. This is typically accomplished with a combination of osteotomes, a reciprocating saw, a Gigli saw, and offset impactors. Once the implants are removed, all remaining synovial tissue is débrided, bone deficiencies are exposed, fibrous tissue is cleaned away, and reconstruction strategies are assessed. Four main procedural steps are essential and should occur in the following sequence: tibial platform reconstruction, establishment of the flexion space, balance of the extension space, and patellofemoral reconstruction.

Tibial Platform Reconstruction

The initial reconstructive step in revision TKA is to establish the tibial platform. A minimal "freshening" cut is made perpendicular to the mechanical axis of the tibia using intramedullary alignment or extramedullary alignment jigs. The proximal tibial plateau frequently has significant bone deficiency and requires supplemental fixation into the tibial diaphysis with a prosthetic stem extension.[15] Additional mechanical support of the tibial platform on deficient bone may require reconstruction with cement and screws, modular metal augments, morcellized or bulk allograft, or newer strategies such as porous tantalum cones. Although reconstitution of the joint line is desirable, a mechani-

cally stable and well-fixed tibial platform is of paramount importance to achieve a stable and well-balanced knee arthroplasty. Knees with severe bone deficiency may have severe ligament attenuation or conversely have severe scarring or contracture, and, therefore, strict anatomic replication of the bone architecture is likely not practical.

Femoral Reconstruction

Once the stable tibial platform is established, the flexion space is assessed and established. It is often valuable to check both the flexion and extension space to determine whether the flexion space is greater, as is frequently seen with posterior femoral osteolysis or flexion instability. It is advisable to start by reestablishing or maximizing replacement of posterior femoral bone deficiency and then adjusting the distal femoral reconstruction to obtain final ligamentous balance via the distal resection or buildup as required. Reconstruction of the posterior femoral deficiency is most commonly addressed with modular metal augments. It may be necessary to "upsize" the femoral component and use even larger augments in cases of flexion instability. Excessive stretching or contracture of the collateral ligaments and posterior capsular structures often requires considerable judgment and adjustment to the reconstruction of bone defects. Once the flexion space has been established, equalization of the extension space can be performed and freshening cuts made to facilitate stable implant opposition and bone contact. If the knee is too tight in extension, additional resection of the distal femur can be performed. More commonly, modular distal augments can be used to balance the knee in extension space to minimize the overall polyethylene insert thickness when possible. Finally, the knee must be stable to varus and valgus stress in full extension, mid-flexion, and at 90° of flexion. Frequently with the revision TKA, scarring of the medial and posterior soft tissues creates a significant challenge in balancing the knee in the mediolateral plane with traditional techniques. If the knee remains unbalanced despite release of contracted tissues, it is advisable to use a tibiofemoral articulation with more intrinsic constraint than the typical cruciate retaining or posterior substituting designs. This use of semiconstrained tibiofemoral articulation typically requires the use of supplemental stem fixation for the implants.

Patellofemoral Reconstruction

In all revision TKA procedures, but particularly revision for patellar instability, careful attention is paid to ensure the proper femoral and tibial rotation. Femoral component rotation is aligned with the epicondylar axis when available. Tibial component rotation should be aligned so that the implant is in line with the medial third of the tibial tubercle. Because of distorted and damaged anatomy frequently seen in revision TKA, the normal bony landmarks may not be available and a reduction with trial implants is advised to assess patellar tracking and determine the optimal rotational position of the components.[17]

The decision of whether to retain a well-fixed patella without bone loss at the time of revision TKA depends largely on the type of patella that currently exists. If the particular patella design has a successful long-term history, is free of any visual delamination, polyethylene damage, or wear and is tracking adequately in the femoral trochlea, it may be retained with expected good outcomes.[18,19] However, if the patella is composed of polyethylene that was gamma-sterilized in air, it is advisable to revise the patella to a modern polyethylene patella that will resist oxidation and long-term wear.[19] If the patella is malpositioned, is mechanically loose, or has visible damage, a patellar component revision is recommended. Various reconstructive methods are available and are detailed in the following sections.

Reconstruction for Bone Loss

Bone Loss Assessment
The critical step in revision TKA is to determine the amount and location of the bone loss.[15] After component removal, it is important to determine whether the defects are contained or uncontained (segmental). The location of supportive bone that surrounds the bone loss is essential, and will dictate the type and size of the augmentation that is required. Smaller contained defects can be treated with either cement fill with screw augmentation or morcellized allograft fill, particularly in older patients. However, larger uncontained defects typically require larger reconstructive measures such as modular block augments, bulk allograft, or highly porous metal metaphyseal cones.

Cement and Screws
The use of cement as a reconstructive augment has the benefits of being simple, inexpensive, and efficient, because the revision TKA is already using the material for fixation in most instances. This reconstruction method is typically used for smaller contained defects less than 5 mm in depth,[20] although some authors have advocated its use in larger defects.[21] When cement is used for defects, augmentation with bone screws are typically recommended to enhance the biomechanical properties of the construct. However, if the patient is young and active, it may be more advantageous to use morcellized allograft to restore bone stock in these types of defects.

Satisfactory midterm results have been reported with the use of screws and cement for bone defects in TKA. In one study, 125 TKAs that used screws and cement to fill large medial tibial defects secondary to severe varus deformities were reported at a mean follow-up of 7.9 years.[21] The authors reported two failures that occurred due to medial tibial collapse at 5 and 10 years, but no other failures or loosening were observed. However, this was a series of primary TKAs without the typical stem extensions used in revision TKA to augment fixation and prevent medial collapse in the setting of bone deficiency and suboptimal bone quality.

Morcellized Allograft
Bone loss in revision TKA has been successfully treated with morcellized cancellous allograft.[22-24] This method is typically reserved for contained defects and is particularly attractive for younger patients in whom restoration of deficient bone stock is a priority. Biologically, morcellized cancellous allograft appears to incorporate similarly to cancellous autograft, albeit at a much slower rate. It is beneficial to have a well-vascularized recipient bed to facilitate incorporation of the allograft bone. If a highly sclerotic defect is encountered, it may be beneficial to either burr away the sclerotic bone to underlying cancellous and vascular bone or conversely use another reconstruction method such as a block augment. If the defect is large and segmental, reconstruction with more robust structural augments such as metal blocks, bulk allograft, or metaphyseal porous metal cones will typically produce more biomechanically stable constructs; however, some authors have reported adequate results with impaction allografting.[23,24]

Midterm results are available for the technique of impaction allograft reconstruction in revision TKA. The midterm results of 48 consecutive revision TKAs with bone loss treated with impaction allografting were prospectively studied.[24] At an average follow-up of 3.8 years, no mechanical failures of the revisions were reported and all radiographs demonstrated incorporation and remodeling of the bone graft. The technique is time-consuming and technically demanding.[24]

Structural Allograft
Bulk structural allograft has frequently been used to reconstruct large bone defects with the intention of providing mechanical support and reconstituting bone. Bulk allograft is typically indicated for defects that are larger than 1.5 cm in depth and exceed the dimensions of typical metal block augments. The advantage of bulk allograft is the potential for bone reconstitution, particularly important in young patients. The disadvantages are the potential for graft resorption, collapse, and graft-host nonunion. Patient factors, including health status, physiologic age, bone quality, and activity level must be considered when contemplating using this reconstructive technique.

The authors of a 2007 study reported 46 revision TKAs with reconstruction of massive tibial defects using bulk allograft.[25] Only four failures were reported, including two for infection, at a mean of 95 months follow-up, without evidence of graft collapse.[25] Resorption and collapse of bulk allograft has been a concern for others.[17] In a study of 52 revisions with bulk allograft followed prospectively, it was reported that 13 knee replacements failed, yielding a 75% success rate at 97 months follow-up.[26] Five knees had graft resorption with implant loosening and two knees had nonunion

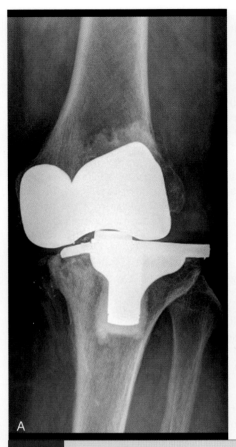
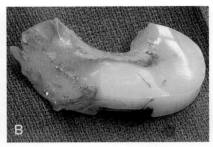
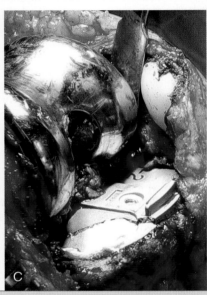
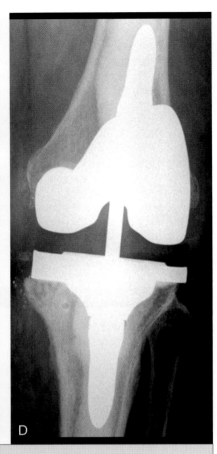

Figure 1 AP radiograph (**A**) and intraoperative photographs (**B** and **C**) of failed TKA due to medial tibial collapse and a broken tibial tray. **D**, Revision TKA radiograph showing reconstruction with a modular medial tibial augment and cemented stem fixation.

between the host bone and the allograft. The survival rate of the allografts was 72% at 10 years.[26] In a retrospective study from the Mayo Clinic, 65 knees with bulk allograft had a 10-year revision-free survivorship of only 76%. Sixteen patients (22.8%) had failed reconstructions and underwent additional surgery, with 8 of 16 revisions caused by allograft failure and 3 caused by failure of a component unsupported by allograft.[27]

Reconstruction With Modular Blocks or Wedges

Modular blocks and wedges are indicated in small to moderate segmental tibial and femoral defects (Figure 1). Modular metal blocks have the advantages of being versatile, efficient, technically straightforward, and not requiring osseointegration. They are particularly useful in older and less active patients, but have the disadvantage of failing to restore bone stock. Most revision total knee systems have numerous shapes and sizes of augments for both the tibia and femur, which facilitates restoration of the joint line and proper balancing of the knee.

Several studies have reported successful midterm results with modular metal augments in revision knee ar-

throplasty. One study reported the postoperative 5- to 10-year results of 102 revision knee arthroplasties in patients with type 2 defects treated with augments and stems.[28] The average follow-up was 7 years. Nonprogressive radiolucent lines were observed around the augment in 14% of knees, but were not associated with increased failure of the implants. The overall survivorship of the components was 92% at 11 years.[28]

Reconstruction With Porous Metal Metaphyseal Cones

Highly porous metal metaphyseal cones have recently been developed and used for large tibial and femoral defects and were designed to avoid nonunion and resorption associated with bulk allograft reconstructions. Highly porous metals, particularly porous tantalum, are biomaterials that offer several potential advantages over traditional materials, including low stiffness, high porosity, and high coefficient of friction. The design intent for these porous tantalum metaphyseal cones is to address the variable patterns of severe bone loss encountered during revision TKA, in addition to providing mechanical support with biologic integration. Short-term evidence now exists that supports the use of

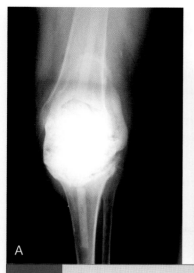
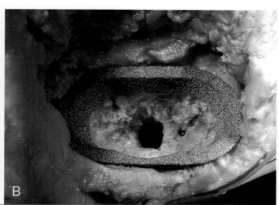
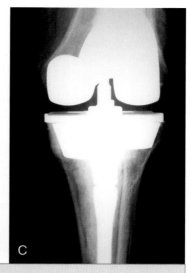

Figure 2 **A,** Radiograph showing failed revision TKA secondary to infection with a static antibiotic cement tibiofemoral spacer in place. **B,** Intraoperative view of tibial porous tantalum metaphyseal cone in place with stable interference fit. **C,** Radiograph showing revision TKA tibial reconstruction with tibial porous tantalum metaphyseal cone and cemented stem supplemental fixation.

these implants in the reconstruction of large tibial defects in revision TKA.[29-32]

The indications for the use of the highly porous metaphyseal cones are similar to those traditionally used for bulk allograft and include large contained (Anderson Orthopaedic Research Institute [AORI] type 2B) or uncontained (AORI type 3) tibial or femoral bony defects (AORI type 3) in a failed TKA. The size of the defect is typically larger than is appropriately reconstructed with traditional modular blocks or wedges. The defects can be classified and characterized by moderate to severe cancellous and/or cortical defects (Figure 2). The surgeon should keep in mind, however, that contained defects with a substantial supportive cortical rim may be more appropriate for impaction grafting, particularly in younger patients, and small uncontained defects that are less than 5 to 10 mm in depth and isolated to one tibial plateau will likely be more amenable to standard metal blocks. Alternatively, reconstruction of large tibial or femoral defects in young patients may be more appropriately performed with bulk allograft in an attempt to reconstitute bone stock for future revision surgery. Furthermore, large defects in patients with insufficient bone support or decreased potential for osseointegration may be amenable to reconstruction with custom prostheses or tumor megaprostheses.

Surgical Technique

The most common tibial scenario appropriate for the porous metaphyseal cones is typically a severe contained or uncontained medial tibial plateau bony defect with varying amounts of lateral tibial plateau remaining for structural support. The most common femoral defect appropriate for porous metal cones is a severe medial and lateral condyle cancellous bone deficiency with intact, yet minimally supportive, cortical rim. Visual inspection of the metaphyseal region and associated defect is performed with respect to the fit of the porous metal cone trial, and a high-speed burr is used to contour the metaphyseal bone to accommodate the implant trial with the maximal bone contact and stability possible (Figure 2, B). The final implant is impacted in the tibial or femoral metaphysis carefully and the frictional coefficient of the actual porous tantalum implant will create significant resistance to insertion and subsequent stability. Once the porous metal cone is in its final and stable position, any areas or voids between the periphery of the porous tantalum cone and the adjacent bone of the proximal tibia are filled with morcellized cancellous bone or putty to prevent any egress of bone cement between the cone and host bone during cementation of the stemmed component.

The tibial and/or femoral revision prosthetic component is inserted through the cone using either cementless or cemented stem extensions. With either type of stem fixation, polymethylmethacrylate is placed between the porous cone and the tray and the proximal keel of the tibial component and/or between the box and augments of the femoral component.

Clinical Results

The early outcomes with highly porous metaphyseal cones for use in large tibial defects for revision TKA have been reported in two studies.[29,31] Fifteen revision knee arthroplasties performed with a porous metal metaphyseal tibial cone were followed for a minimum of 2 years. All tibial cones were found to be osseointegrated radiographically and clinically at final follow-up with no reported failures in this initial series.[29] In a series of 16 revision TKAs with severe tibial defects, good results were reported with osseointegration of the porous tantalum cone in 14 of 16 cases at a minimum 2-year follow-up. Two metaphyseal cones required removal for recurrent sepsis and were found to be well fixed at surgery.[31] These early results appear equivalent to those obtained with bulk allograft, custom implants, or large modular metal augments at the same time interval. Further clinical and radiographic follow-up will provide insight into the long-term durability of these highly porous augments.

Patellar Reconstruction

Severe patellar loss, which precludes adequate fixation of another patellar implant, may be treated by patellectomy, retention of the remaining patellar bony shell (resection arthroplasty), a porous tantalum patellar implant, or patellar bone grafting.[33] The results of patellectomy performed as a portion of a revision TKA have been associated with poorer functional results, extensor mechanism weakness, or delayed extensor mechanism disruption. The patellar resection arthroplasty has been associated with poorer clinical results due to lower knee scores, retropatellar pain, patellar maltracking, difficulty ascending or descending stairs, and delayed patellar fragmentation.

As an alternative to resection arthroplasty, a recent study reported on a series of 12 patellar reconstructions using a gull-wing osteotomy technique.[34] The technique involves longitudinally bisecting the residual patellar cortical shell, allowing the apex of the osteotomy to reside in the depth of the trochlear groove. At follow-up, radiographs revealed successful healing of the osteotomy in all patients with central tracking of the patella in the trochlear groove. The authors reported no patellar fractures or significant patellar malalignment and concluded that it is a viable method of patellar salvage reserved for the most advanced cases of patellar bone stock compromise.[34]

Another reconstructive method is the use of a porous tantalum patella, which may be used in the setting of deficient patellar bone stock.[35-37] It has been reported that 50% or greater of the porous tantalum surface of the implant must be in contact with host bone.[37] In a comparative study of revision TKA with deficient patellae, it was reported that with less than 50% residual bone stock, the porous metal implant loosened in all cases. In 10 of 11 knees with at least 50% host bone contact, the metal implant remained well fixed and stable at early follow-up.[37] Patellar bone grafting provided the potential for restoration of deficient patellar bone.[33] The technique involves using a tissue flap created from one of several sources, including peripatellar fibrotic tissue, or a free tissue flap obtained from either the suprapatellar pouch or fascia lata from the lateral gutter of the knee joint. The tissue flap is sewn to the peripheral patellar rim and the patellar defect filled with cancellous autograft harvested from the metaphyseal portion of the central femur during preparation of the femur for the revision implant. It should be emphasized that the initial success of this procedure is likely due in part to the use of an anatomic femoral trochlea and the correct rotational positioning of the femoral and tibial components. Use of this procedure as an isolated patellar reconstruction, particularly if there have been patellar maltracking difficulties leading to the patellar failure, is likely to be unsuccessful.

Cemented or Cementless Stems

When revision TKA occurs in the setting of bone deficiency, stem augmentation is generally required to supplement the fixation of the implant via bypassing the deficient bone and achieving fixation in the viable metaphyseal or diaphyseal bone. When additional tibiofemoral constraint (constrained condylar or rotating hinge prosthesis) is used, stem supplementation is necessary to help resist the articular forces transmitted from the constraint to the implant fixation interface. Adequate long-term results have been reported with both cemented and press-fit cementless stem fixation in revision TKA, with greater than 90% survivorship at 10 years with both fixation types.[38-40] However, because of the lack of comparative studies, the choice of cemented versus cementless stems remains a choice based on personal philosophy, past experience, and intraoperative judgment. Regardless of fixation type, close attention should be paid to cement technique to ensure adequate implant stability. If supplemental press-fit cementless stem fixation is used, however, it is advisable to ensure adequate tibial or femoral prosthesis cementation into the metaphyseal region while achieving intimate endosteal contact and interference fit of the uncemented stem into the metadiaphyseal region.[39,40]

Clinical Outcomes

Outcomes of revision TKAs have shown midterm results of greater than 90% survivorship free of aseptic loosening at 10 years.[38,40] However, reoperation and re-revision occur at greater frequency than after primary TKA. A recent study identified the variables and mechanisms associated with failure after revision TKA.[41] Five hundred sixty-six index revision TKAs were studied. Twelve percent failed at an average of 40.1 months and demonstrated an overall survivorship of 82% at 12 years. The predominant failure mechanisms included infection (46%), aseptic loosening (19%), and instability (13%). Revision TKA is more likely to fail in younger patients and in those who underwent polyethylene exchanges. Revision TKA performed for infection is four times more likely to fail than that performed for aseptic loosening.[41] Other authors have reported that reoperations after revision TKA are frequent and occur in approximately 20% of patients in a large series, with a higher risk of reoperation in revisions performed for infection, loosening, and instability.[42]

Summary

Revision TKA remains challenging and is associated with higher complication rates requiring reoperation, particularly periprosthetic sepsis. Thorough preoperative evaluation and accurate diagnosis of failure etiology is critical, and meticulous surgical technique with appropriate mechanical reconstruction and careful attention to prevention of complications is essential to optimize outcomes.

Annotated References

1. Kurtz S, Ong K, Lau E, Mowat F, Halpern M: Projections of primary and revision hip and knee arthroplasty in the United States from 2005 to 2030. *J Bone Joint Surg Am* 2007;89(4):780-785.

   The Nationwide Inpatient Sample (1990 to 2003) was used in conjunction with US Census Bureau data to quantify primary and revision arthroplasty rates. The authors found the demand for hip revision procedures is projected to double by the year 2026, while the demand for knee revisions is expected to double by 2015.

2. Fehring TK, Odum S, Griffin WL, Mason JB, Nadaud M: Early failures in total knee arthroplasty. *Clin Orthop Relat Res* 2001;392:315-318.

3. Mulhall KJ, Ghomrawi HM, Scully S, Callaghan JJ, Saleh KJ: Current etiologies and modes of failure in total knee arthroplasty revision. *Clin Orthop Relat Res* 2006;446:45-50.

   A multicenter prospective observational cohort study of 318 consecutive patients investigated the etiologies of revision TKA failure. Infection, instability, loosening and wear were determined to be the leading causes of failure in revision TKA. Level of evidence: II.

4. Sharkey PF, Hozack WJ, Rothman RH, Shastri S, Jacoby SM: Insall Award paper: Why are total knee arthroplasties failing today? *Clin Orthop Relat Res* 2002;404:7-13.

5. Clarke HD, Fuchs R, Scuderi GR, Mills EL, Scott WN, Insall JN: The influence of femoral component design in the elimination of patellar clunk in posterior-stabilized total knee arthroplasty. *J Arthroplasty* 2006; 21(2):167-171.

   A retrospective review of 238 TKAs was done to determine the incidence of patellar clunk with an optimized third-generation, posterior-stabilized prosthesis. Conclusions support that femoral component design is a predictor of the occurrence of patellar clunk.

6. Scher DM, Pak K, Lonner JH, Finkel JE, Zuckerman JD, Di Cesare PE: The predictive value of indium-111 leukocyte scans in the diagnosis of infected total hip, knee, or resection arthroplasties. *J Arthroplasty* 2000; 15(3):295-300.

7. Vessely MB, Frick MA, Oakes D, Wenger DE, Berry DJ: Magnetic resonance imaging with metal suppression for evaluation of periprosthetic osteolysis after total knee arthroplasty. *J Arthroplasty* 2006;21(6):826-831.

   A retrospective review of 11 patients with suspected periprosthetic osteolysis who underwent MRI is presented. Radiographic and MRI findings and findings at revision arthroplasty were correlated. Osteolysis was confirmed in 10 patients by MRI, and in 9 of 11 patients, the extent of osteolysis was greater on MRI than estimated radiographically.

8. Romero J, Stähelin T, Binkert C, Pfirrmann C, Hodler J, Kessler O: The clinical consequences of flexion gap asymmetry in total knee arthroplasty. *J Arthroplasty* 2007;22(2):235-240.

   A retrospective review of 18 knees with lateral flexion instability after TKA is presented. The study demonstrated that increased lateral flexion laxity is associated with increased internal femoral component rotation and a less favorable clinical outcome.

9. Bozic KJ, Kurtz SM, Lau E, et al: The epidemiology of revision total knee arthroplasty in the United States. *Clin Orthop Relat Res* 2010;468(1):45-51.

   Causes of failure of revision TKA performed in the United States were assessed using ICD-9-CM diagnosis and procedure codes from the Nationwide Inpatient Sample database. Clinical, demographic, and economic data were reviewed and analyzed from 60,355 revision TKA procedures performed in the United States between October 1, 2005, and December 31, 2006. Level of evidence: II.

10. Ghanem E, Parvizi J, Burnett RS, et al: Cell count and differential of aspirated fluid in the diagnosis of infection at the site of total knee arthroplasty. *J Bone Joint Surg Am* 2008;90(8):1637-1643.

    Synovial fluid that had been aspirated preoperatively from 429 knees that had undergone revision arthroplasty at three different institutions was analyzed. The cutoff values for optimal accuracy in the diagnosis of infection were more than 1,100 cells/10^{-3} cm^3 for the fluid leukocyte count and more than 64% for the neutrophil differential.

11. Schinsky MF, Della Valle CJ, Sporer SM, Paprosky WG: Perioperative testing for joint infection in patients undergoing revision total hip arthroplasty. *J Bone Joint Surg Am* 2008;90(9):1869-1875.

    Two hundred thirty-five consecutive total hip arthroplasties were evaluated using a consistent algorithm to identify infection. A synovial fluid cell count of more than 3,000 white blood cells/mL was the most predictive perioperative testing modality for determining the presence of periprosthetic infection when combined with an elevated ESR and CRP level.

12. Bedair H, Ting N, Jacovides C, et al: The Mark Coventry Award: Diagnosis of early postoperative TKA infection using synovial fluid analysis. *Clin Orthop Relat Res* 2011;469(1):34-40.

2: Knee

A review of more than 11,000 TKAs was undertaken to evaluate the accuracy of laboratory and synovial fluid cell counts for predictors of periprosthetic sepsis. Investigators found that a cutoff of 27,800 cells/µL in synovial white blood cell count predicted infection within 6 weeks after primary TKA. Level of evidence: II.

13. Leopold SS, Silverton CD, Barden RM, Rosenberg AG: Isolated revision of the patellar component in total knee arthroplasty. *J Bone Joint Surg Am* 2003;85-A(1): 41-47.

14. Babis GC, Trousdale RT, Pagnano MW, Morrey BF: Poor outcomes of isolated tibial insert exchange and arthrolysis for the management of stiffness following total knee arthroplasty. *J Bone Joint Surg Am* 2001; 83-A(10):1534-1536.

15. Engh GA, Ammeen DJ: Bone loss with revision total knee arthroplasty: Defect classification and alternatives for reconstruction. *Instr Course Lect* 1999;48: 167-175.

16. Lahav A, Hofmann AA: The "banana peel" exposure method in revision total knee arthroplasty. *Am J Orthop (Belle Mead NJ)* 2007;36(10):526-529.

A retrospective review of 102 consecutive patients who underwent revision TKA with an exposure technique involves peeling the patella tendon as a sleeve off the tibia, leaving the extensor mechanism intact with a lateral hinge of soft tissue. The authors state it is a safe method that can be used along with a proximal quadriceps snip and does not violate the extensor mechanism.

17. Chin KR, Bae DS, Lonner JH, Scott RD: Revision surgery for patellar dislocation after primary total knee arthroplasty. *J Arthroplasty* 2004;19(8):956-961.

The authors studied risk factors for patellar dislocation following primary TKA. Functional outcomes were significantly improved.

18. Barrack RL, Rorabeck C, Partington P, Sawhney J, Engh G: The results of retaining a well-fixed patellar component in revision total knee arthroplasty. *J Arthroplasty* 2000;15(4):413-417.

19. Lonner JH, Mont MA, Sharkey PF, Siliski JM, Rajadhyaksha AD, Lotke PA: Fate of the unrevised all-polyethylene patellar component in revision total knee arthroplasty. *J Bone Joint Surg Am* 2003;85-A(1):56-59.

20. Aleto TJ, Berend ME, Ritter MA, Faris PM, Meneghini RM: Early failure of unicompartmental knee arthroplasty leading to revision. *J Arthroplasty* 2008; 23(2):159-163.

Thirty-two consecutive revisions from unicompartmental knee arthroplasty to TKA were retrospectively reviewed. The predominant mode of failure was medial tibial collapse, most of which were all-polyethylene tibial components and required more complex reconstruction with stems, augments, and screws and cement.

21. Ritter MA, Harty LD: Medial screws and cement: A possible mechanical augmentation in total knee arthroplasty. *J Arthroplasty* 2004;19(5):587-589.

The authors found that screws placed beneath the medial tibial plateau to fill large defects after TKA helps prevent collapse of the medial tibia.

22. Bradley GW: Revision total knee arthroplasty by impaction bone grafting. *Clin Orthop Relat Res* 2000; 371: 113-118.

23. Lonner JH, Lotke PA, Kim J, Nelson C: Impaction grafting and wire mesh for uncontained defects in revision knee arthroplasty. *Clin Orthop Relat Res* 2002; 404:145-151.

24. Lotke PA, Carolan GF, Puri N: Impaction grafting for bone defects in revision total knee arthroplasty. *Clin Orthop Relat Res* 2006;446:99-103.

The authors present a prospective study of the midterm results of 48 consecutive revision TKAs with substantial bone loss treated with impaction allograft. No mechanical failures were reported and all radiographs demonstrated graft incorporation and remodeling. Level of evidence: IV.

25. Engh GA, Ammeen DJ: Use of structural allograft in revision total knee arthroplasty in knees with severe tibial bone loss. *J Bone Joint Surg Am* 2007;89(12): 2640-2647.

The authors present a retrospective review of the clinical and radiographic outcomes of 49 revision TKAs in which structural allograft was used for severe tibial bone defects. The authors found no instance of graft collapse or aseptic loosening associated with the structural allograft.

26. Clatworthy MG, Ballance J, Brick GW, Chandler HP, Gross AE: The use of structural allograft for uncontained defects in revision total knee arthroplasty: A minimum five-year review. *J Bone Joint Surg Am* 2001;83-A(3):404-411.

27. Bauman RD, Lewallen DG, Hanssen AD: Limitations of structural allograft in revision total knee arthroplasty. *Clin Orthop Relat Res* 2009;467(3):818-824.

A retrospective review of 79 revision TKAs with structural allografts for major bone defects is discussed. Revision-free survival of 76% at 10 years was reported, which supports the selective use of structural allograft for large cavitary defects. Level of evidence: IV.

28. Patel JV, Masonis JL, Guerin J, Bourne RB, Rorabeck CH: The fate of augments to treat type-2 bone defects in revision knee arthroplasty. *J Bone Joint Surg Br* 2004;86(2):195-199.

29. Meneghini RM, Lewallen DG, Hanssen AD: Use of porous tantalum metaphyseal cones for severe tibial bone loss during revision total knee replacement.

J Bone Joint Surg Am 2008;90(1):78-84.

The authors discuss a retrospective review of 15 revision TKAs using novel highly porous tantalum metaphyseal cones for large tibial defects at minimum 2 year follow-up. All metaphyseal cones showed evidence of osseointegration with no evidence of loosening or migration.

30. Meneghini RM, Lewallen DG, Hanssen AD: Use of porous tantalum metaphyseal cones for severe tibial bone loss during revision total knee replacement: Surgical technique. *J Bone Joint Surg Am* 2009;91(Suppl 2 Pt 1): 131-138.

The authors discuss a surgical technique detailing the implantation and procedural rationale for highly porous tantalum metaphyseal tibial cones for use in the reconstruction of large tibial bone defects in revision total knee replacement.

31. Long WJ, Scuderi GR: Porous tantalum cones for large metaphyseal tibial defects in revision total knee arthroplasty: A minimum 2-year follow-up. *J Arthroplasty* 2009;24(7):1086-1092.

The authors present a retrospective review of 16 revision total knee replacements using highly porous tantalum metaphyseal cones for reconstruction of severe tibial bone defects. Good results were obtained with no evidence of aseptic loosening or mechanical failure observed at short-term follow-up.

32. Radnay CS, Scuderi GR: Management of bone loss: Augments, cones, offset stems. *Clin Orthop Relat Res* 2006;446:83-92.

A retrospective review of 10 revision total knee replacements using highly porous tantalum metaphyseal cones for reconstruction of severe tibial bone defects is presented. No evidence of aseptic loosening or mechanical failure observed at short-term follow-up. Level of evidence: V.

33. Hanssen AD: Bone-grafting for severe patellar bone loss during revision knee arthroplasty. *J Bone Joint Surg Am* 2001;83-A(2):171-176.

34. Klein GR, Levine HB, Ambrose JF, Lamothe HC, Hartzband MA: Gull-wing osteotomy for the treatment of the deficient patella in revision total knee arthroplasty. *J Arthroplasty* 2010;25(2):249-253.

In a retrospective review, 12 patients with unresurfaceable patella at the time of revision TKA were treated with a technique of gull-wing osteotomy. Successful healing of the osteotomy occurred in all patients with central tracking of the patella.

35. Tigani D, Trentani P, Trentani F, Andreoli I, Sabbioni G, Del Piccolo N: Trabecular metal patella in total knee arthroplasty with patella bone deficiency. *Knee* 2009;16(1):46-49.

A retrospective review is presented of 10 porous tantalum patellar components used in the setting of patellar bone deficiency or prior patellectomy. At short-term follow-up, the only failure occurred in the lone case of prior patellectomy.

36. Nelson CL, Lonner JH, Lahiji A, Kim J, Lotke PA: Use of a trabecular metal patella for marked patella bone loss during revision total knee arthroplasty. *J Arthroplasty* 2003;18(7, Suppl 1)37-41.

37. Ries MD, Cabalo A, Bozic KJ, Anderson M: Porous tantalum patellar augmentation: The importance of residual bone stock. *Clin Orthop Relat Res* 2006;452:166-170.

The authors present a retrospective review of 18 revision TKAs with severe patellar bone loss using trabecular metal patellar reconstruction with short-term follow-up. The results suggest stable fixation of a trabecular metal patellar component can be achieved when residual bone is present for implant fixation.

38. Mabry TM, Vessely MB, Schleck CD, Harmsen WS, Berry DJ: Revision total knee arthroplasty with modular cemented stems: Long-term follow-up. *J Arthroplasty* 2007;22(6, Suppl 2):100-105.

In a retrospective review, 73 revision TKAs used a posterior stabilized implant with modular, fully cemented femoral and tibial stems. Five- and 10-year implant survivorship free of revision for aseptic failure was 98% and 92%, respectively.

39. Peters CL, Erickson JA, Gililland JM: Clinical and radiographic results of 184 consecutive revision total knee arthroplasties placed with modular cementless stems. *J Arthroplasty* 2009;24(6, Suppl):48-53.

Fifty consecutive revision TKAs placed with metaphyseal cemented femoral and tibial components with press-fit cementless stems were retrospectively reviewed. Short-term outcomes were acceptable and were not associated with significant thigh and leg pain.

40. Wood GC, Naudie DD, MacDonald SJ, McCalden RW, Bourne RB: Results of press-fit stems in revision knee arthroplasties. *Clin Orthop Relat Res* 2009;467(3):810-817.

One hundred thirty-five knees underwent revision TKA using a press-fit technique (press-fit diaphyseal fixation and cemented metaphyseal fixation) and were retrospectively reviewed. Kaplan-Meier survivorship analysis revealed a probability of survival free of revision for aseptic loosening of 98% at 12 years.

41. Suarez J, Griffin W, Springer B, Fehring T, Mason JB, Odum S: Why do revision knee arthroplasties fail? *J Arthroplasty* 2008;23(6, Suppl 1):99-103.

Five hundred sixty-six index revision knee arthroplasties were retrospectively reviewed to determine the etiology of failure. Predominant revision failure modes included infection, aseptic loosening, and instability. The survivorship for the entire cohort, with revision for any reason as an end point, was 82% at 12 years.

42. Sierra RJ, Cooney WP IV, Pagnano MW, Trousdale RT, Rand JA: Reoperations after 3200 revision TKAs: Rates, etiology, and lessons learned. *Clin Orthop Relat Res* 2004;425:200-206.

2: Knee

Chapter 14

Complications After Total Knee Arthroplasty

Michael P. Nett, MD   Fred D. Cushner, MD

Introduction

The results after total knee arthroplasty (TKA) are generally excellent, with greater than 90% survivorship at 20 years. With the new Surgical Care Improvement Project (SCIP) initiative, renewed emphasis has been placed on avoiding preventable complications during the perioperative period, including treatment of such complications.

Medical Complications

Prior to TKA, the patient should be evaluated by his or her primary care physician for preoperative optimization of medical comorbidities. A recent review of more than four million discharges reported on in-hospital complications, including mortality, after unilateral, bilateral, and revision TKA.[1] In this series, in-hospital mortality was highest for patients with bilateral TKA (0.5%) compared to a 0.3% mortality rate for those with unicompartmental TKA. Patients with revision TKAs also had a mortality rate of 0.3%. Although the overall complication rate during hospitalization was higher for bilateral TKAs at 12.2%, the rates for in-hospital complications following unicompartmental TKAs was still 8.2%.

Some elements of the patient's medical history should alert the orthopaedic surgeon to proceed with caution. A patient with a cardiac stent may require a more intensive preoperative cardiac evaluation. Antiplatelet medications are usually withheld at least 1 week before surgery and reinitiated during the postoperative period, once hemostasis is obtained. Changes in a surgeon's postoperative thromboembolism prophy-

laxis protocol may be required. Preoperative consultation with a cardiologist and neurologist is generally recommended.

Several studies have demonstrated success in bilateral procedures, but with a higher risk of complications.[2] However, patients approximately 65 years old or younger and in good health may tolerate a bilateral procedure with little increased risk.[2] Increased medical complications can be seen in physiologic older patients, obese patients, and those with numerous medical problems. Bilateral TKAs seem to have a higher complication and mortality rate than unilateral procedures. Postoperative telemetry should be considered after bilateral TKAs.

Fewer medical complications occur when the patient's postoperative hemoglobin levels are maximized. A patient-specific approach is favored. The patient's hemoglobin level is evaluated prior to scheduling surgery. Patients with a hemoglobin level less than 13 g/dL received 40,000 units of erythropoietin alpha with iron supplements at 3 weeks, 2 weeks, and 1 week before the surgery. With this approach, there is a decreased transfusion rate and higher levels of hemoglobin and hematocrit when the patient is discharged from the hospital.[3] Preautologous donations are no longer advocated because they have been demonstrated to increase the patient's need for allogeneic blood and lead to lower postoperative blood levels.[4]

The SCIP project has also made recommendations regarding the use of beta blockers. The current emphasis on dosing beta blockers on the day of surgery has been stressed. Recent studies suggest that the beta blockers should not be stopped after the first dose on the day of surgery. A recent study looked at 5,158 patients undergoing hip or knee arthroplasty; 992 received beta blockers on the day of surgery only and 252 had the beta blocker continued during the hospital stay.[5] Fewer myocardial infarctions occurred in those in whom beta blocker dosing was continued.

Patients with diabetes mellitus have been shown to have higher complication rates, including deep venous thrombosis (DVT) and infection.[6,7] Several studies have shown that normalization of the hemoglobin A1C level can decrease morbidity in the postoperative period. One recent study evaluated the impact of glycemic control and diabetes on perioperative outcomes after TKA.[8] This study analyzed a nationwide patient sample with more than one million patients, comparing those with controlled and uncontrolled diabetes. The risk of stroke, urinary tract infection, ileus, and death was decreased with better glycemic control during the preoperative period. The American Association of Clinical Endocrinologists recommends that patients with type 2 diabetes maintain a hemoglobin A1C level less than 6.5% to decrease the incidence of postoperative morbidity.[8]

Hematoma

The symptoms of postoperative hematoma include intense palpable hemarthrosis, skin discoloration, bruising, increased pain, decreased range of motion, and wound drainage.

An increased rate of infection occurs with prolonged wound drainage. A recent study demonstrated that an increase in the initial postoperative drainage in the recovery room was most indicative of further drainage on days 2 through 5.[9] Better control of blood loss and wound drainage in the immediate postoperative period leads to less wound drainage on subsequent hospitalization days. Limiting blood loss in the recovery room begins in the operating room, with plugging of the intramedullary canal and electrocautery of geniculate vessels and the posterior capsule. Intraoperative tourniquet deflation has not been shown to decrease blood loss, and a meta-analysis showed an increase in blood loss when this is done.[10]

Other intraoperative methods of decreasing the prevalence of wound hemarthrosis include fibrin sprays, cautery devices, and tranexamic acid. Tranexamic acid works as an antifibrinolytic agent to help stop the breakdown of fibrin.[11,12] A 10 mg/kg dose before the incision and at the time of tourniquet deflation for high-risk patients can be considered. Other doses include a 15 mg/kg one-time dose.[13] In one study of tranexamic acid use in TKA patients, a 1-g bolus was given at the time of anesthesia induction, and there was a significant decrease in early postoperative blood loss, total blood loss, and transfusion rates.[14] There was no increase in thrombosis. Another randomized, double-blind study in 100 TKA patients with a 15 mg/kg dose of tranexamic acid demonstrated less blood loss without an increase in thromboembolisms.[15] A meta-analysis of 20 available prospective studies in orthopaedic surgery concluded that patients receiving tranexamic acid demonstrated a reduced transfusion need, reduced blood loss, and no increase in DVT.[12] Tranexamic acid may decrease the occurrence of postoperative hemarthrosis, hematoma, and wound drainage after TKA.

Although no difference in transfusion rates has been noted, some studies have shown a decrease in overall blood loss after injection of bupivacaine and epineph-

rine. However, one study showed no benefit when the epinephrine lavage was used in total joint arthroplasty.[16] Another method to decrease the occurrence of hemarthrosis has been the use of bipolar cautery. High-risk areas for bleeding can be coagulated to obtain hemostasis, with reports of less tissue damage. These high-risk areas include exposed surface of the bone, the posterolateral corner, and the posterior capsule. Bipolar technology may decrease intraoperative total blood loss while minimizing tissue damage when compared to conventional electrocautery, but no prospective randomized trials exist.

Topical fibrin sealants and autologous platelet gels have also been recommended for management of intraoperative blood loss. One study compared three groups in a randomized trial of 150 patients undergoing TKA.[17] One group received a topical fibrin spray applied intraoperatively, one group received tranexamic acid, and the third group received both treatments. Both tranexamic acid and the topical spray were effective in decreasing blood loss compared to the control. There was no difference between the groups receiving tranexamic acid or the fibrin spray. Another study used an autologous platelet gel and fibrin sealant in 85 unilateral TKA patients, with 80 other unilateral TKA patients serving as a control group.[18] The hemoglobin level following discharge was 11.3 g/dL with the platelet gel, versus 8.9 g/dL for the control group. This study demonstrated a decrease in the rate of allogenic transfusions, fewer wound complications, and a 1.4% decrease in the length of hospital stay.

A watertight closure of the capsule is of utmost importance in preventing wound drainage. This closure should include a good seal at the arthrotomy site, with special care at the distal medial aspect of the tibia. If excessive wound drainage occurs in the recovery room, knee flexion and clamping of the drain can be performed. Stopping the continuous passive motion (CPM) machine at 60° of flexion is recommended to allow for hemostasis and clamping the drain for a 4-hour period. Immediate CPM in the recovery room is no longer recommended. The leg is maintained in full extension to help facilitate hemostasis before initiation of range of motion on the first postoperative day.

If a large hematoma occurs, use of the CPM machine and anticoagulation therapy should be stopped, but use of pneumatic compression devices for DVT prophylaxis is continued. If symptoms do not resolve with this treatment, hematoma evacuation may be considered, with a complete irrigation and débridement with antibiotic solution performed and cultures obtained. A recent study reviewed the Mayo Clinic experience of the outcomes of 59 TKAs following early irrigation and débridement for wound complication following TKA.[19] The study demonstrated a 7% incidence of chronic deep infection and a 5.3% rate of major reoperation following early irrigation and débridement. In an earlier series at the same institution, outcomes of 42 knees that underwent irrigation and débridement of a postop-

Table 1

Factors Affecting Wound Complication After TKA

Systemic Factors	Local Factors	Surgical Technique	Postoperative Factors
Diabetes mellitus	Previous incisions	Length of incisions	Postoperative hematoma
Vascular disease	Significant deformity (varus/rotational)	Minimally invasive surgical technique with excessive wound tension	Overaggressive anticoagulation
Rheumatoid arthritis or prolonged steroid use	Local irradiation	Large, thin subcutaneous flaps	Excessive knee flexion (> 40°) with high-risk wounds
Tobacco use	Local burns or trauma	Failure to preserve subcutaneous fascial layer	Use of O_2 via nasal cannula to increase O_2 tension
Albumin level < 3.5 g/dL	Dense adherent scar tissue	Lateral release	Excessive CPM machine use with postoperative hematoma
Total lymphocyte count < 1,500 mm^3	Local blood supply	Large medial release	Prolonged wound drainage
Obesity	Use of tissue expanders preoperatively	Meticulous wound closure	Early postoperative fall and wound dehiscence

erative hematoma within 30 days of the index arthroplasty were reviewed.[20] In this series, the 2-year cumulative probability of undergoing subsequent major surgery or the development of deep infection was 12.3% and 10.5%, respectively. These series stress the importance of avoiding early postoperative wound complication and hematoma.

Avoiding Other Wound Complications

Preoperative planning, intraoperative technique, and postoperative management are critical to avoid wound complications, especially in high-risk patients and including those with prior incisions (Table 1). Consultation with a plastic surgeon may be appropriate in some situations.

Preoperative evaluation of TKA should include an evaluation of the skin. Systemic concerns include vascular compromise, obesity, malnutrition, prolonged steroid or nonsteroidal anti-inflammatory drug use, diabetes, an immunocompromised state, or a history of smoking. Local factors that may play a role in wound healing could include the inability to incorporate a previous incision into the planned incision, a small skin bridge between the previous incision and the planned incision, local irradiation or burns, or dense adherent scar tissue. The correction of severe varus and rotational deformity may make subsequent closure difficult. As the deformity is corrected, there may not be enough skin to close the inferior aspect of the wound over the subcutaneous surface of the tibia. Previous trauma may play a role because of previously placed skin incisions, scarring, and loss of skin mobility.

Terminal branches of the peripatellar anastomotic ring of arteries are responsible for most of the blood supply to the anterior skin and subcutaneous tissues. The blood supply to the skin arises through a subdermal plexus supplied by arterioles in the subcutaneous fascia. Flap formation over the anterior aspect of the knee should be limited and performed deep to the subcutaneous fascia. A midline skin incision remains the optimal approach if possible, because this reduces the dimensions of the lateral skin flap where lower skin oxygen tension is noted. Previous longitudinal incisions can be safely used. Some degree of modification is often performed to incorporate previous paramedian incisions. If multiple parallel longitudinal incisions exist, the most lateral incision is chosen because the predominant blood supply enters medially.

Transverse skin incisions, such as those from previous patella surgery or osteotomy, can be safely approached at a 90° angle. Short, oblique incisions such as previous meniscectomies can often be ignored. However, when there are long, oblique incisions or oblique incisions that cross the midline, crossing these incisions may result in a narrow point of intersection. When the planned surgical incision and prior incision create an angle of less than 60°, alternative techniques should be considered.

If skin conditions are extremely poor, the preferred technique is soft-tissue expansion, which is indicated when insufficient or inadequate soft tissue is present for wound healing. Inadequate soft tissue may result after multiple crossing and combined incisions, previous skin grafts or flaps, severe preoperative deformity, or when expanded soft-tissue coverage is required. The completion of soft-tissue expansion takes 8 to 10 weeks. The most recent review included 64 knees.[21] One major wound complication occurred in a patient with previ-

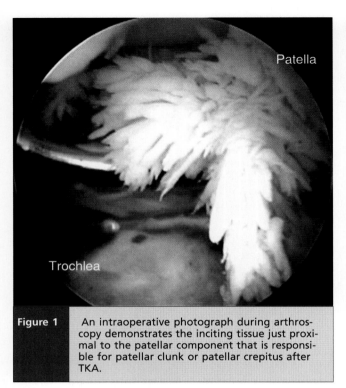

Patella

Trochlea

Figure 1 An intraoperative photograph during arthroscopy demonstrates the inciting tissue just proximal to the patellar component that is responsible for patellar clunk or patellar crepitus after TKA.

ously irradiated skin, necessitating abandonment of the planned arthroplasty. Fourteen minor complications (22%) were noted during the expansion phase and responded to local treatment. Six major complications (9%) were encountered, requiring reoperation. Contraindications for soft-tissue expansion would include active infection, previous local irradiation, or skin graft that is directly adherent to underlying bone or fascia.[21]

A prearthroplasty soft-tissue flap may be considered in patients with prior skin graft, local irradiation, or densely adherent scar tissue. The choice of flap depends on the location of the lesion, the extent of coverage required, and the status of the limb. Most lesions can be covered adequately with a medial or lateral gastrocnemius muscle or myocutaneous flap. Lesions proximal to the superior pole of the patella may require a free flap. If large areas of superficial skin loss have occurred, split-thickness skin grafting is an option. Recently, vacuum-assisted wound closure has prepared the knee before the tissue graft procedure is performed. A bed of healthy granulation tissue provides the best environment for skin graft healing. For large defects, anterolateral thigh fasciocutaneous flaps are frequently available for coverage in the area of the knee. However, their use should be limited to small, superficial defects without evidence of infection.[22] Large areas of soft-tissue breakdown and exposed tendon or bone require greater coverage than the local fasciocutaneous flap. The workhorse for local coverage about the knee is a gastrocnemius muscle. The two heads are divided by a median raphe and the blood supply is usually a separate, individual artery, which

provides the pedicle about which they are rotated. The medial head is larger and longer and thus can be used in most cases. In far lateral wounds, the lateral head may be used, but care must be taken to avoid the peroneal nerve as it passes around the proximal fibula. Specific complications of flaps involve injury to the nearby neurovascular structures, including the sural nerve and short and long saphenous veins. Other complications include hematoma formation in the calf because of failure to achieve hemostasis, graft strangulation secondary to an insufficiently wide subcutaneous tunnel, and damage to the vascular pedicle from excessive stretch. Cosmetic concerns include a decrease in calf girth and the excessive soft-tissue mass on the anterior aspect of the knee. One study reported the results on 12 TKA patients who underwent medial gastrocnemius coverage.[23] Limb salvage and prosthetic survival occurred in all but one patient (92%), but with a 25% incidence of major reoperation.[23] Poor results have been demonstrated in the face of chronic infection and delayed soft-tissue coverage. Complication rates increase with attempted coverage of more proximal lesions over the patellar or quadriceps tendon. Free flaps around the knee are indicated when local flaps are insufficient because of the location or size of the defect, or the compromised status of the traditional gastrocnemius flap.

Patella Complications

Patella complications can range from 1% to 10% and can be a cause for reoperation.[24-27] Patella pain following TKA can be related to prosthetic design, surgical technique, or not resurfacing the patella at the time of the initial procedure.

The symptoms of patellar clunk syndrome include pain and an audible clunk when extending the knee from 60° to 30° of flexion. The inciting tissue forms just proximal to the patella and catches on the femoral flange as the knee extends (**Figure 1**). The etiology is not clear but appears to be related to prosthetic design. Recent prosthetic modifications, such as elongation of the trochlea and a more anatomic femoral component, as well as increased attention to the removal of superficial patella synovium, have led to a decrease in this complication. One study evaluated two posterior-stabilized prostheses to define the incidence of patellar clunk.[26] One prosthesis had a 4% incidence of patellar clunk, but the complication was eliminated with the other prosthesis.

Arthroscopic débridement is effective treatment for refractory patellar clunk syndrome. A recent retrospective review of 25 patients undergoing arthroscopic débridement for patellofemoral clunk or synovial hyperplasia demonstrated improvement in pain, crepitus, and knee scores, but range of motion was unchanged.[27]

Extensor Mechanism Disruption

Quadriceps Tendon Rupture

Extensor mechanism disruption after TKA has been reported as high as 1.1%; a recent report identified 24 knees from the Mayo Clinic joint registry (0.1% incidence).[28] Although patient-specific factors and traumatic events may play a role in the incidence of quadriceps rupture, the main preventable cause involves surgical technique. Overaggressive resection of the patella can weaken the quadriceps insertion and predispose patients to rupture. The quadriceps snip technique has been described as an oblique extension of the standard medial arthrotomy to aid in difficult exposure. Although a correctly performed snip does not predispose patients to quadriceps tendon ruptures, poor technique can damage the integrity of the tendon.

If a partial injury occurs, treatment should be nonsurgical. One study reported good results in those treated with partial injuries, whereas 7 of the 11 patients with complete tears who underwent surgical reconstruction experienced poor outcomes and a high complication rate.[28] Another study described 14 patients with chronic extensor mechanism rupture who underwent allograft reconstruction. Preoperatively, all patients had full passive motion, an extensor lag, and averaged 7 months from rupture to surgery.[29] At follow-up, all patients were ambulators, nearly 50% required the use of a cane, and all demonstrated a rather persistent extensor lag despite improvement in their functional status. A study of extensor mechanism allograft reconstructions concluded that loosely tensioned allografts resulted in persistent extensor lag and clinical failure, but allografts that were tightly tensioned in full extension could restore active knee extension.[30] Another study reviewed extensor allografts with a nearly 5-year follow-up; only one patient required a cane and overall successful reconstruction was noted.[31] If allograft reconstruction is performed, an extended period of immobilization is needed to allow for allograft incorporation. Newer graft jacket devices may aid in the improvement of vascularization of the allograft tissue. Suture anchors and transpatellar or transtubercular placement of polyethylene surgical tape can facilitate and protect the repair while healing progresses. The allograft is tensioned in full extension and the knee is not flexed intraoperatively.[32] Most often an unresurfaced allograft patella is used and the knee is left in extension for 6 weeks.

Patellar Tendon Ruptures

Patellar tendon ruptures are more common than quadriceps tendon ruptures, occurring in 1.7% to 2.0% of TKA patients. With the advent of minimally invasive surgery there has been an emphasis on avoiding eversion of the patella. Tension on the tendon of insertion should be observed intraoperatively to avoid inadvertent rupture (**Figure 2**).

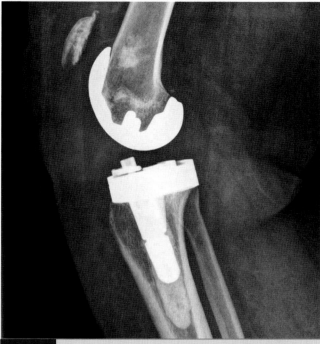

Figure 2 A postoperative radiograph of the knee of a revision TKA patient demonstrates significant patellar alta consistent with patellar tendon rupture.

In patients with rheumatoid arthritis, the patellar tendon may peel off the tubercle. This issue should be identified early, the arthrotomy lengthened to decrease the tension, and a Kirschner wire or fixation pin placed in the area of the tendon insertion to decrease continuation of patellar peel. Hyperflexion of the knee without attention to patellar tendon tensioning can lead to an avulsion-type injury.

Primary repair of a patellar tendon rupture alone has been unsuccessful. Various augmentation techniques, including autologous tissue, allografts, and synthetic materials, have been developed to improve the outcomes when primary repair is attempted. Allograft augmentation as described above in the discussion of quadriceps tendon ruptures is recommended. The procedure involves keying the allograft bone into the tibial tubercle with bicortical fixation achieved. An allograft extensor mechanism with the patella can be used, or an Achilles tendon can be used if only the patellar tendon is to be reconstructed. These types of repairs can be reinforced with the use of polyethylene surgical tape. It is preferable to create a transverse drill hole through the tubercle for placement of the polyethylene surgical tape. A transverse hole can be made through the patella or the quadriceps tendon and then tightened both medial and lateral to the patella. This helps to facilitate the tension at the repair site and takes the tension off the graft. If an allograft patella is used, it remains controversial whether the patella needs to be resurfaced.

2: Knee

Table 2

New Classification for Periprosthetic Femoral Fractures

Type	Fracture Reducible	Bone Stock in Distal Segment	Component Well Fixed and Well Aligned
IA	Yes	Good	Yes
IB	No	Good	Yes
II	Yes/No	Good	No
III	Yes/No	Poor	No

Adapted with permission from Berry DJ: Epidemiology: Hip and knee. *Orthop Clin North Am* 1999;30:183-190.

Periprosthetic Fracture

The incidence of periprosthetic fracture is increasing.[33,34] Most patients sustaining periprosthetic fractures are elderly with osteopenia and multiple medical comorbidities. Many fractures are related to loose implants or extensive osteolysis, often requiring component revision and fracture fixation. Often with a well-fixed implant, the prosthesis interferes with traditional methods of fracture fixation. Involvement of the ligamentous structures about the knee may result in implant instability requiring increased constraint at the time of reconstruction.

The exact incidence of periprosthetic fracture following TKA remains unknown. Studies from the total joint registry at the Mayo Clinic report a 2% overall incidence in periprosthetic fracture after TKA, a 0.39% incidence of intraoperative fracture during primary TKA, a 0.1% and 0.4% incidence of tibial periprosthetic fracture during and after TKA, respectively, and supracondylar femur fracture from 0.3 to 2.5% after primary TKA.[33,34]

A recent study proposed a new classification for supracondylar periprosthetic fracture that provides more information and aids in management.[34] This system is based on the quality of bone in the distal segment, the status of the implant with regard to fixation and position, and the reducibility of the fracture (Table 2).

Periprosthetic Fracture of the Tibia

A type I fracture is frequently associated with a loose first-generation prosthesis. These situations require revision arthroplasty with a stemmed implant to bypass the defect, and management of the bony defect with cement, bone graft, or augmentation as indicated. If a type I fracture occurs intraoperatively (type IC), it can usually be treated with cancellous screw fixation and a stemmed component to bypass the fracture. A type II fracture occurs at the metaphyseal-diaphyseal junction adjacent to the stem of the tibial prosthesis. With a well-fixed component and a minimally displaced fracture, patients can be treated successfully with rigid immobilization; otherwise, fracture fixation is required with traditional techniques.[33,34] A type IIB fracture typ-

Table 3

Classification of Tibial Periprosthetic Fractures

Major Anatomic Pattern	Subtype
I: Tibial plateau	A. Radiographically well-fixed prosthesis
II: Adjacent to component stem	B. Radiographically loose prosthesis
III: Distal to prosthesis	C. Intraoperative fracture
IV: Tibial tubercle	

ically occurs around a loose, stemmed component. These patients require revision arthroplasty to a long-stemmed design with structural bone graft or impaction grafting to fill the ectatic canal. Type III injuries are diaphyseal fractures, and most occur with a well-fixed prosthesis (IIIA). The fracture should be treated according to typical principles with regard to the management of tibial shaft fractures. If the fracture occurred as a result of a stress fracture related to malalignment, revision arthroplasty should be considered. Type IV fractures involve the tibial tubercle. Most occur following a fall and are associated with a well-fixed prosthesis. If the fracture is nondisplaced, immobilization in extension is adequate; otherwise, open reduction versus extensor mechanism reconstruction is necessary. The classification of tibial periprosthetic fractures is summarized in Table 3.

Periprosthetic Fracture of the Femur

Postoperative periprosthetic fracture of the femur is the most common periprosthetic fracture following TKA. Nonsurgical treatment should be considered for stable fractures with minimal displacement, a well-fixed and well-aligned prosthesis, and good bone stock (type 1A fracture).[33] Type IB fractures are irreducible and require open reduction and internal fixation. Some controversy still exists regarding the use of supracondylar retrograde nails versus locked periarticular plates for these fractures.[35-37] With improved options for the distal placement of locking screws in supracondylar in-

Table 4	

Classification of Periprosthetic Fracture of the Patella

Type	Description
I	Implant intact/extensor mechanism intact
II	Implant intact/extensor mechanism disrupted
III	Implant loose IIIA: Good bone stock IIIB: Poor bone stock

tramedullary nails, there has been a resurgence of interest in load-sharing intramedullary nail fixation. In 29 case series including 415 fractures, the nonunion rate was 9%, the failure rate was 4%, the infection rate was 3%, and the revision surgery rate was 13%.[35] Retrograde nails demonstrated a statistically significant relative risk reduction of 87% for nonunion and 70% for requiring revision surgery compared to traditional nonlocking plates. Locking plates had a nonsignificant relative risk reduction of 57% for nonunion and 43% for revision surgery compared to nonlocking plates.[35] Another study reviewed the treatment of 14 supracondylar periprosthetic femur fractures treated with a retrograde nail and had a 100% union rate with a low complication rate.[36] However, in a recent review of 50 patients with supracondylar fracture, locked condylar plating resulted in less blood loss, better alignment, and a lower complication rate compared to nonlocked plating or retrograde intramedullary nailing. All seven patients treated with intramedullary nailing in this series went on to nonunion or malunion.[37] Additional randomized prospective studies are needed to compare these modern implants.

Patients with type II fractures have a loose or poorly aligned prosthesis and good bone stock, and are best managed with revision arthroplasty using a stemmed prosthesis and fracture fixation. Although results are variable, there is little controversy that this treatment will provide the best outcome for most patients.[34] In elderly patients with limited mobility or suboptimal health, a hinged-type distal femoral replacement could be considered. In a younger or more active patient, a type III fracture presents a difficult dilemma. The surgeon could proceed with resection arthroplasty, fracture fixation, and bone grafting. This treatment is then followed by delayed reimplantation. Another option with shorter convalescence is revision arthroplasty with an allograft-prosthetic composite.

Periprosthetic Fracture of the Patella
Type I fractures are the most common and by definition have a well-fixed patellar component and an intact extensor mechanism. These patients should be treated nonsurgically. Type II fractures are associated with dis-

ruption of the extensor mechanism. These patients can be treated with open reduction and internal fixation, or partial patellectomy and extensor mechanism advancement to bone. Type III fractures are associated with a loose patellar component. If the patient is sufficiently symptomatic, surgical treatment is warranted. Type IIIA fractures are best treated with patelloplasty and component revision or resection arthroplasty. Type IIIB fractures are often treated with component removal and patelloplasty or complete patellectomy. Other modern salvage options could include allograft reconstruction, the use of a trabecular metal revision component, or impaction grafting. The classification of periprosthetic fractures of the patella is summarized in Table 4.

Arthrofibrosis
The etiology of arthrofibrosis often is unclear. A recent review discussed factors linked with poor postoperative motion. Patient diagnosis, preoperative range of motion, prosthetic geometry, surgical technique, intraoperative range of motion, capsular closure, postoperative rehabilitation, and wound healing factors all play a role in the development of a stiff knee.[38] Ipsilateral hip arthritis can also inhibit postoperative recovery, leading to stiffness.

One study looked at the preoperative and postoperative range of motion for a contralateral TKA in patients with a history of knee stiffness after TKA.[39] The range of motion was not significantly different than that of a control group at 2-year follow-up, but the rate of manipulation was 26.7% in the study group compared to 8% in the control group.

If the knee stiffness fails to resolve after adjustments in pain medication and physical therapy, manipulation may be considered at 6 weeks, when adequate wound healing has occurred. Manipulation tends to be more successful for improving flexion, but mild improvement can be made in extension. A recent study of 1,188 TKAs showed the prevalence of stiffness to be 5.3%.[40] When manipulation was performed, the average pre-manipulation range of motion was 67° and improved to 117°. Better results were seen in patients undergoing early manipulation (within 8 weeks after surgery). Another recent study of stiffness after TKA reported a prevalence of 1.3%.[41] In this study stiffness was associated with knees having a preoperative flexion contracture of 15°, or less than 75° of flexion. In the most recent review of manipulation following TKA, 37 of 800 TKAs (4.6%) were manipulated. The range of motion improved from 68° to 109°.[42]

When manipulation is unsuccessful or if it is too late to consider manipulation, further intervention may be warranted. Arthroscopic lysis of adhesions within the first 6 months following arthroplasty has been reported. In this procedure, retinacular releases are performed both medially and laterally, and patella mobil-

2: Knee

ity must be restored. Regional anesthesia may be continued postarthroscopy to allow for intensive mobilization and early range of motion. The role of isolated arthrolysis and polyethylene component downsizing in patients with a stiff arthroplasty and well-fixed, well-aligned components remains unclear. Poor results with a high complication rate and no significant improvement in range of motion or pain have been demonstrated in the literature. Revision of both components is usually necessary and likely to provide improved results, but improvement in range of motion and pain is modest.[43]

Instability

Instability accounts for 10% to 22% of TKA failures requiring revision.[44,45] The direction of instability at the tibiofemoral articulation can occur in the coronal (varus-valgus) plane, the sagittal (anteroposterior) plane, or as a combination of planes. Instability following TKA is best divided into three categories: extension instability, flexion instability, and global instability with genu recurvatum.

Extension Instability

Symmetric extension instability occurs when the extension space is not filled by the thickness of the components. This condition can be caused by overresection of the tibia or the distal femur. Although overresection of the tibia results in equally large flexion and extension gaps, excessive resection from the distal femur results in asymmetric flexion and extension gaps. If overresection of the tibia is recognized intraoperatively, it can be easily managed by increasing the size of the polyethylene insert. Overresection of the distal femur creates a much different scenario because the joint line is elevated, which creates a larger extension gap compared to the flexion gap. By simply increasing the size of the tibial insert, the result will be a knee that is too tight in flexion. The elevated joint line will also affect patellar tracking, limit flexion, and may result in "midflexion" instability. It is best in this situation to restore the joint line by adding distal femoral augmentation.[45]

An asymmetric extension gap with appropriate bony resection is most often caused by inadequate correction of the preoperative soft-tissue deformity.[45] Extension instability can also be caused by iatrogenic injury of the collateral ligaments, which requires repair, reconstruction, or increased constraint. A recent retrospective study of 15 TKAs reported successful treatment for intraoperative iatrogenic detachment of the medial collateral ligament (MCL) from the tibia.[46] No increased constraint, bracing, or ligament reconstruction was performed. No significant difference was seen between MCL-intact TKAs and the knees with iatrogenic MCL injury at a minimum 2-year follow-up.[46]

Flexion Instability

Flexion instability results from inadequate filling of the flexion gap or attenuation of the posterior cruciate ligament following placement of cruciate-retaining prostheses. Early flexion instability is likely secondary to gap imbalance with or without laxity of a collateral ligament.[45] This instability can be caused by overresection of the posterior femoral condyles and a reduction in femoral offset. Alternatively, the creation of excessive tibial slope can result in a knee that is well balanced in extension but remains loose in flexion. Late flexion instability can occur in both cruciate-retaining and posterior-stabilized TKAs, but the etiology is different. In patients with cruciate-retaining knees, it is not uncommon for the posterior cruciate ligament to elongate or attenuate. Late flexion instability in posterior-stabilized knees may result from significant wear or fracture of the tibial polyethylene post.[45] Symptoms can range from a vague sense of instability and recurrent effusions to dislocation. Flexion instability is best assessed with the knee in 90° of flexion while the patient sits on the end of the examination table. In a review of 1,370 revision TKAs, 10 revisions were performed for flexion instability.[47] Eight (80%) had successful outcomes after revision of both components and appropriate balancing of the flexion and extension gaps. The excessively large flexion gap was frequently managed by upsizing the femoral component following posterior femoral augmentation.[47] Treatment of cruciate-retaining knees with flexion instability most often involves revision arthroplasty to a posterior-stabilized design.[45] At the time of revision, a larger femoral component is frequently used following posterior femoral augmentation. This improves posterior femoral offset and reduces the size of the flexion gap. If excessive posterior slope is present preoperatively, revision of the tibial resection is performed. Careful balancing of the flexion and extension gaps is then performed.

Global Instability With Genu Recurvatum

Because genu recurvatum is known to recur in patients with certain neuromuscular disorders, the etiology of the hyperextension deformity must be elucidated thoroughly before surgery. In the absence of neuromuscular disease, hyperextension deformities tend not to recur after TKA.[48] Patients with quadriceps weakness secondary to neuromuscular disease rely on hyperextension of the knee to prevent limb collapse during the stance phase of gait. In the absence of neuromuscular disease, recurvatum may develop in patients with a fixed valgus deformity associated with a contracted iliotibial band or in patients with rheumatoid arthritis.[47]

Several options have been described to prevent the recurrence of recurvatum when performing a TKA in a patient with preoperative recurvatum. One option is to use a rotating-hinged component with an extension stop, which traditionally has been recommended in patients with poliomyelitis with less-than-antigravity quadriceps strength. However, a recent study demonstrated 95% good to excellent results in 16 TKAs performed in patients with poliomyelitis using a posterior-stabilized or constrained condylar design.[49] Anteroposterior stability was restored in all patients. Only one patient required a hinged implant for reconstruction. However, caution is advised when treating patients with less-than-antigravity quadriceps function.

A second alternative for patients with preoperative recurvatum is to underresect the distal femur, creating a relatively smaller extension gap. By filling the flexion gap with the largest polyethylene insert possible, the knee will have a slight flexion contracture, preventing hyperextension.

Persistent Pain and Dissatisfaction

Persistent anterior knee pain after TKA is a relatively frequent complaint. A recent review found that despite substantial advances in primary knee arthroplasty, most studies still report only 80% to 90% good to excellent results.[50] In this series of 1,700 primary knees, approximately 19% of patients were not satisfied with the outcome; pain relief varied from 70% to 80% and was frequently associated with activities of daily living. In another review of 112 patients, preoperative expectations with regard to time to full recovery, pain, and limitations in everyday activities were examined.[51] Patients significantly underestimated the time for full recovery (expected 4.7 ± 2.8 months, recalled actual time, 6.1 ± 3.7 months; $P = 0.005$). They were also overly optimistic about the likelihood of being pain-free (85% expected it, 43% were; $P < 0.05$) and of not being limited in usual activities (52% expected it, 20% were; $P < 0.05$). Despite these findings, global outcomes were good to excellent in 87.5% of patients. A study of TKA in Asian patients reported severe functional disabilities with kneeling, squatting, sitting with legs crossed, sexual activity, and recreational activities.[52] In this series, 23 patients (20%) were dissatisfied with their TKA. This group had more functional disabilities than the patients who were satisfied with their outcome. Those who were dissatisfied tended to perceive functional disability in high flexion-type activities. Patient expectations can affect overall satisfaction. Preoperatively, patient education must provide realistic expectations with regard to time to recovery, pain relief, and postoperative functional limitations. Appropriate preoperative consultation must address unrealistic expectations to reduce the risk of dissatisfaction.

Summary

The results after TKA are generally excellent, with more than 90% implant survivorship at 20 years. Unfortunately, medical and surgical complications following TKA remain. Emphasis must be placed on prevention because these complications often lead to a significant increase in patient morbidity.

Annotated References

1. Memtsoudis SG, Ma Y, González Della Valle A, et al: Perioperative outcomes after unilateral and bilateral total knee arthroplasty. *Anesthesiology* 2009;111(6):1206-1216.

   Procedure-related complications and in-hospital mortality were more frequent after bilateral TKA than unilateral TKA (9.45% versus 7.07% and 0.30% versus 0.14%; $P < 0.0001$ each). With regard to bilateral TKA, an increased rate of complications was associated with a staged (same hospitalization) versus simultaneous approach with no difference in mortality (10.30% versus 9.15%; $P < 0.0001$ and 0.29% versus 0.26%; $P = 0.2875$).

2. Cushner FD, Scott WN, Scuderi G, Hill K, Insall JN: Blood loss and transfusion rates in bilateral total knee arthroplasty. *J Knee Surg* 2005;18(2):102-107.

   The authors present a review of blood management during 170 bilateral TKAs. Blood management included preoperative autologous donation, symptom-based transfusion, and autoreinfusion devices. The perioperative allogeneic transfusion rate for patients who donated two units of blood was 0.00%. Preoperative autologous donation greater than two units resulted in lower preoperative hemoglobin levels. Therefore, for bilateral TKA, a protocol of two preoperative autologous donation units was recommended.

3. Cushner FD, Lee GC, Scuderi GR, Arsht SJ, Scott WN: Blood loss management in high-risk patients undergoing total knee arthroplasty: A comparison of two techniques. *J Knee Surg* 2006;19(4):249-253.

   The authors present a comparison of preoperative autologous donation with preoperative administration of epoetin alfa in high-risk patients undergoing TKA. Although both preoperative autologous donation and epoetin alfa were successful in decreasing the need for allogeneic blood transfusions, epoetin alfa was more effective in maximizing perioperative hemoglobin levels.

4. Cushner FD, Hawes T, Kessler D, Hill K, Scuderi GR: Orthopaedic-induced anemia: The fallacy of autologous donation programs. *Clin Orthop Relat Res* 2005;431(431):145-149.

   In 148 unilateral primary TKA patients, a preoperative autologous donation program resulted in increased preoperative anemia. Whereas only 26.2% of patients were in the high transfusion-risk group (hemoglobin > 10 g/dL and ≤ 13 g/dL) before surgery, 55.7% of patients were in this high-risk category after preoperative autologous donation.

5. van Klei WA, Bryson GL, Yang H, Forster AJ: Effect of beta-blocker prescription on the incidence of postoperative myocardial infarction after hip and knee arthroplasty. *Anesthesiology* 2009;111(4):717-724.

   Nine hundred ninety-two arthroplasty patients were treated with beta blockers on the day of surgery. Discontinuation of the beta blocker prescription during the hospital stay was significantly associated with a

2: Knee

higher rate of myocardial infarction (odds ratio 2.0; 95% CI 1.1 to 3.9) and death (odds ratio 2.0; 95% CI 1.0 to 3.9).

6. Dowsey MM, Choong PF: Obese diabetic patients are at substantial risk for deep infection after primary TKA. *Clin Orthop Relat Res* 2009;467(6):1577-1581.

A review of 1,214 consecutive primary TKAs demonstrated that the odds for a deep prosthetic infection were greater in patients with morbid obesity (odds ratio [OR], 8.96) and diabetes (OR, 6.87).

7. Bolognesi MP, Marchant MH Jr, Viens NA, Cook C, Pietrobon R, Vail TP: The impact of diabetes on perioperative patient outcomes after total hip and total knee arthroplasty in the United States. *J Arthroplasty* 2008;23(6, Suppl 1)92-98.

The authors present a review of 751,340 primary or revision total hip arthroplasty (THA) or TKA patients. Patients with diabetes had fewer routine discharges and higher inflation-adjusted hospital charges for all procedures. These patients also had significantly increased odds of pneumonia, stroke, and transfusion ($P < 0.001$) after primary arthroplasty.

8. Marchant MH Jr, Viens NA, Cook C, Vail TP, Bolognesi MP: The impact of glycemic control and diabetes mellitus on perioperative outcomes after total joint arthroplasty. *J Bone Joint Surg Am* 2009;91(7):1621-1629.

In a nationwide inpatient sample of more than 1 million patients who underwent joint arthroplasty surgery, in comparison with patients with controlled diabetes mellitus, patients with uncontrolled diabetes mellitus had a significantly increased odds of stroke, urinary tract infection, ileus, postoperative hemorrhage, transfusion, wound infection, and death. In addition, length of hospital stay was significantly longer.

9. Patel VP, Walsh M, Sehgal B, Preston C, DeWal H, Di Cesare PE: Factors associated with prolonged wound drainage after primary total hip and knee arthroplasty. *J Bone Joint Surg Am* 2007;89(1):33-38.

A retrospective study of 1,226 primary TKAs is presented. An increased volume of drain output was the only independent risk factor for prolonged wound drainage in TKA. Each day of prolonged wound drainage increased the risk of wound infection by 29% following TKA.

10. Rama KR, Apsingi S, Poovali S, Jetti A: Timing of tourniquet release in knee arthroplasty: Meta-analysis of randomized, controlled trials. *J Bone Joint Surg Am* 2007;89(4):699-705.

A meta-analysis of 11 studies involving 893 primary knee arthroplasties is presented. Early release of the tourniquet increased the total measured blood loss and increased blood loss as calculated on the basis of the maximum decrease in hemoglobin concentration. However, the risk difference of reoperations due to postoperative complications was 3% higher without early tourniquet release.

11. Camarasa MA, Ollé G, Serra-Prat M, et al: Efficacy of aminocaproic, tranexamic acids in the control of bleeding during total knee replacement: A randomized clinical trial. *Br J Anaesth* 2006;96(5):576-582.

The authors studied 127 TKA patients. Total blood loss was 1,099 mL in the group that received antifibrinolytic agents and 1,784 mL in the control group ($P < 0.001$). Five patients (7.5%) in the study group and 23 (38.3%) in the control group ($P < 0.001$) received blood transfusions. Mean reduction in hemoglobin levels between preoperative and fifth day postoperative readings was 2.5 (0.9) in the study group and 3.4 (1.2) in the control group ($P < 0.001$).)

12. Kagoma YK, Crowther MA, Douketis J, Bhandari M, Eikelboom J, Lim W: Use of antifibrinolytic therapy to reduce transfusion in patients undergoing orthopedic surgery: A systematic review of randomized trials. *Thromb Res* 2009;123(5):687-696.

A meta-analysis of 29 studies including 1,981 patients is presented. Patients receiving antifibrinolytic agents had reduced transfusion needs, reduced blood loss, and no increase in the risk of venous thromboembolism.

13. Orpen NM, Little C, Walker G, Crawfurd EJ: Tranexamic acid reduces early post-operative blood loss after total knee arthroplasty: A prospective randomised controlled trial of 29 patients. *Knee* 2006; 13(2):106-110.

A statistically significant ($P = 0.006$) decrease in blood loss was seen with tranexamic acid use. There was no significant difference in total blood loss ($P = 0.55$) or transfusion requirements. There was no evidence of DVT in either group.

14. Rajesparan K, Biant LC, Ahmad M, Field RE: The effect of an intravenous bolus of tranexamic acid on blood loss in total hip replacement. *J Bone Joint Surg Br* 2009;91(6):776-783.

In 73 THAs, tranexamic acid reduced the rate of early postoperative blood loss and total blood loss, but not intraoperative blood loss. The tranexamic acid group required fewer transfusions and had no increased incidence of DVT.

15. Johansson T, Pettersson LG, Lisander B: Tranexamic acid in total hip arthroplasty saves blood and money: A randomized, double-blind study in 100 patients. *Acta Orthop* 2005;76(3):314-319.

One hundred THA patients received tranexamic acid (15 mg/kg) or placebo intravenously. Blood loss averaged 0.97 L in the THA group and 1.3 L in the placebo group ($P < 0.001$). There was a significant reduction in transfusion rates with THA ($P = 0.009$). No thromboembolic complications occurred.

16. Malone KJ, Matuszak S, Mayo D, Greene P: The effect of intra-articular epinephrine lavage on blood loss following total knee arthroplasty. *Orthopedics* 2009; 32(2):100.

Of 189 TKAs, 82 procedures were performed without epinephrine and 107 procedures were performed with lavage. No significant differences were found in blood loss among the patients in the two groups. Intra-articular epinephrine lavage does not affect blood loss after TKA.

17. Molloy DO, Archbold HA, Ogonda L, McConway J, Wilson RK, Beverland DE: Comparison of topical fibrin spray and transexamic acid on blood loss after total knee replacement: A prospective randomized controlled trial. *J Bone Joint Surg Br* 2007;89(3):306-309.

The authors studied 150 TKA patients with a preoperative level of hemoglobin of 13.0 g/dL. Fifty patients were treated with topical fibrin spray, 50 received tranexamic acid, and 50 patients in the control group received no intervention. There was a significant reduction in the total calculated blood loss for those in the topical fibrin spray group and tranexamic acid group compared with the control group.

18. Everts PA, Devilee RJ, Oosterbos CJ, et al: Autologous platelet gel and fibrin sealant enhance the efficacy of total knee arthroplasty: Improved range of motion, decreased length of stay and a reduced incidence of arthrofibrosis. *Knee Surg Sports Traumatol Arthrosc* 2007;15(7):888-894.

Of a total 165 TKA patients, 85 were treated with autologous platelet gel and fibrin sealant and 80 served as the control group. The treatment group had a smaller decrease in hemoglobin, superior postoperative range of motion, and a lower incidence of arthrofibrosis and subsequent forced manipulation.

19. Galat DD, McGovern SC, Larson DR, Harrington JR, Hanssen AD, Clarke HD: Surgical treatment of early wound complications following primary total knee arthroplasty. *J Bone Joint Surg Am* 2009;91(1):48-54.

A review of 59 TKAs requiring early irrigation and débridement for wound complication following TKA is presented. There was a 7% incidence of chronic deep infection and a 5.3% major reoperation rate following early irrigation and débridement.

20. Galat DD, McGovern SC, Hanssen AD, Larson DR, Harrington JR, Clarke HD: Early return to surgery for evacuation of a postoperative hematoma after primary total knee arthroplasty. *J Bone Joint Surg Am* 2008; 90(11):2331-2336.

Forty-two of 17,784 TKAs (incidence: 0.24%) required return to the operating room for evacuation of an early hematoma within 30 days from initial surgery. In patients requiring hematoma evacuation, the 2-year cumulative probability of undergoing subsequent major surgery or developing deep infection was 12.3% and 10.5%, respectively.

21. Manifold SG, Cushner FD, Craig-Scott S, Scott WN: Long-term results of total knee arthroplasty after the use of soft tissue expanders. *Clin Orthop Relat Res* 2000;380(380):133-139.

22. Wei FC, Jain V, Celik N, Chen HC, Chuang DC, Lin CH: Have we found an ideal soft-tissue flap? An experience with 672 anterolateral thigh flaps. *Plast Reconstr Surg* 2002;109(7):2219-2230.

23. Ries MD, Bozic KJ: Medial gastrocnemius flap coverage for treatment of skin necrosis after total knee arthroplasty. *Clin Orthop Relat Res* 2006;446:186-192.

Twelve patients were treated with a medial gastrocnemius flap after TKA. A functioning TKA was salvaged in 11 patients (92%). Defects that extended more proximally over the patella or quadriceps tendon were more likely to require additional procedures to achieve adequate soft-tissue coverage.

24. Kelly MA: Extensor mechanism complications in total knee arthroplasty. *Instr Course Lect* 2004;53:193-199.

25. Schoderbek RJ Jr, Brown TE, Mulhall KJ, et al: Extensor mechanism disruption after total knee arthroplasty. *Clin Orthop Relat Res* 2006;446:176-185.

A systematic review of the different types of treatment options available for extensor mechanism rupture after TKA that are supported by the literature is presented. The second part of the study looks at the results following 290 revision TKAs. Six of the 290 revision patients had extensor mechanism disruption as a cause of TKA failure, and this group of patients had overall worse functional outcomes.

26. Lonner JH, Jasko JG, Bezwada HP, Nazarian DG, Booth RE Jr: Incidence of patellar clunk with a modern posterior-stabilized knee design. *Am J Orthop (Belle Mead NJ)* 2007;36(10):550-553.

This series compares the incidence of patellar clunk with two different knee prostheses, the Insall-Burstein II (IB) and the NexGen Legacy PS (NG), both manufactured by Zimmer (Warsaw, IN). There were 150 NG TKAs in each group. The incidence of patellar clunk was reduced from 4% with the IB design to 0% with the NG design.

27. Dajani KA, Stuart MJ, Dahm DL, Levy BA: Arthroscopic treatment of patellar clunk and synovial hyperplasia after total knee arthroplasty. *J Arthroplasty* 2010;25(1):97-103.

A retrospective review is presented of 25 patients who underwent arthroscopic débridement after primary TKA to treat the patellar clunk syndrome (15 knees) or patellofemoral synovial hyperplasia (10 knees). Knee pain and crepitus as well as Knee Society knee and function scores improved in both groups, but postoperative knee range of motion remained unchanged.

28. Dobbs RE, Hanssen AD, Lewallen DG, Pagnano MW: Quadriceps tendon rupture after total knee arthroplasty: Prevalence, complications, and outcomes. *J Bone Joint Surg Am* 2005;87(1):37-45.

29. Barrack RL, Stanley T, Allen Butler R: Treating extensor mechanism disruption after total knee arthroplasty. *Clin Orthop Relat Res* 2003;416:98-104.

30. Burnett RS, Berger RA, Della Valle CJ, et al: Extensor mechanism allograft reconstruction after total knee arthroplasty. *J Bone Joint Surg Am* 2005;87(Pt 2, Suppl 1):175-194.

2: Knee

31. Prada SA, Griffin FM, Nelson CL, Garvin KL: Allograft reconstruction for extensor mechanism rupture after total knee arthroplasty: 4.8-year follow-up. *Orthopedics* 2003;26(12):1205-1208.

32. Burnett RS, Butler RA, Barrack RL: Extensor mechanism allograft reconstruction in TKA at a mean of 56 months. *Clin Orthop Relat Res* 2006;452:159-165.

    Nineteen patients with extensor mechanism disruption after TKA were studied. All patients underwent reconstruction with either quadriceps tendon-patella-patellar tendon-tibial tubercle allograft, or Achilles tendon allograft. At a mean follow-up of 56 months, all patients were community ambulators. There was no loss of knee flexion. The mean postoperative extensor lag was 14°. Fifteen patients had an extensor lag of less than 10°.

33. Berry DJ: Epidemiology: Hip and knee. *Orthop Clin North Am* 1999;30(2):183-190.

34. Kim KI, Egol KA, Hozack WJ, Parvizi J: Periprosthetic fractures after total knee arthroplasties. *Clin Orthop Relat Res* 2006;446:167-175.

    A review of the general concepts, treatment algorithms, and the overall treatment outcomes of femoral and tibial periprosthetic fractures after TKA is presented. A new classification system for periprosthetic femoral fractures is proposed that takes into account the status of the prosthesis, the quality of distal bone stock, and the reducibility of the fracture.

35. Herrera DA, Kregor PJ, Cole PA, Levy BA, Jönsson A, Zlowodzki M: Treatment of acute distal femur fractures above a total knee arthroplasty: Systematic review of 415 cases (1981-2006). *Acta Orthop* 2008; 79(1):22-27.

    Twenty-nine series containing 415 fractures were studied. There was an overall nonunion rate of 9%, fixation failure rate of 4%, infection rate of 3%, and revision surgery rate of 13%. Retrograde nailing was associated with relative risk reduction of 87% for nonunion and 70% revision surgery compared to traditional plating methods. Risk reductions for locking plates were not statistically significant (57% for nonunion, $P = 0.2$; 43% for revision surgery, $P = 0.23$).

36. Chettiar K, Jackson MP, Brewin J, Dass D, Butler-Manuel PA: Supracondylar periprosthetic femoral fractures following total knee arthroplasty: Treatment with a retrograde intramedullary nail. *Int Orthop* 2009;33(4):981-985.

    A retrospective review of 14 fractures treated by retrograde intramedullary supracondylar nailing demonstrates good functional outcomes, low complication rates, and 100% fracture union.

37. Large TM, Kellam JF, Bosse MJ, Sims SH, Althausen P, Masonis JL: Locked plating of supracondylar periprosthetic femur fractures. *J Arthroplasty* 2008; 23(6, Suppl 1):115-120.

    Fifty periprosthetic supracondylar femur fractures were reviewed. Fractures were treated with locked condylar plating, nonlocked plating systems, or intramedullary fixation. Patients treated with locked plates had less blood loss during surgery, healed with better knee alignment, and had greater knee motion. All seven patients treated with a retrograde intramedullary nail developed a malunion or nonunion.

38. Scott RD: Stiffness associated with total knee arthroplasty. *Orthopedics* 2009;32(9).

    A review of the etiology and treatment of arthrofibrosis following TKA is presented.

39. Lang JE, Guevara CJ, Aitken GS, Pietrobon R, Vail TP: Results of contralateral total knee arthroplasty in patients with a history of stiff total knee arthroplasty. *J Arthroplasty* 2008;23(1):30-32.

    This study evaluated the clinical outcomes of a second primary TKA in patients whose initial (contralateral) primary TKA was complicated by stiffness. There was no significant difference in final postoperative range of motion or Knee Society scores compared to control subjects. However, there was a statistically significant higher rate of closed manipulation.

40. Yercan HS, Sugun TS, Bussiere C, Ait Si Selmi T, Davies A, Neyret P: Stiffness after total knee arthroplasty: Prevalence, management and outcomes. *Knee* 2006; 13(2):111-117.

    The authors reviewed 1,188 posterior-stabilized TKAs. The prevalence of stiffness was 5.3%. The patients were treated with manipulation or secondary surgery. In the manipulation group (n = 46), the mean range of motion improved from 67° before manipulation to 117° afterward. Motion at final follow-up was better for those manipulated early to those done later. In the secondary surgery group (n = 10), the mean gain in motion was 49° at final follow-up.

41. Kim J, Nelson CL, Lotke PA: Stiffness after total knee arthroplasty: Prevalence of the complication and outcomes of revision. *J Bone Joint Surg Am* 2004;86-A(7):1479-1484.

42. Rubinstein RA Jr, DeHaan A: The incidence and results of manipulation after primary total knee arthroplasty. *Knee* 2010;17(1):29-32.

    Thirty-seven of 800 TKAs were manipulated (4.6% incidence). The pre-TKA stiff group included 16 knees and was defined as less than 110° total arc of motion. Patients with pre-TKA stiffness improved from a total arc of motion of 94 to 109 ($P < 0.001$) whereas patients without pre-TKA stiffness changed from 121 to 118 ($P = 0.169$).

43. Haidukewych GJ, Jacofsky DJ, Pagnano MW, Trousdale RT: Functional results after revision of well-fixed components for stiffness after primary total knee arthroplasty. *J Arthroplasty* 2005;20(2):133-138.

    Sixteen TKAs were revised in 15 patients for stiffness. Of 15 patients, 10 (66%) were satisfied with the results of the procedure. The mean Knee Society pain score improved from 28 to 65 points, and the mean functional score improved from 45 to 58 points. The mean arc of motion improved from 40° preoperatively to 73° postoperatively. Recurrent stiffness required additional intervention in four knees (3 patients, 25%).

44. Vince KG, Abdeen A, Sugimori T: The unstable total knee arthroplasty: Causes and cures. *J Arthroplasty* 2006;21(4, Suppl 1):44-49.

   A review of TKA etiology and treatment is presented.

45. Parratte S, Pagnano MW: Instability after total knee arthroplasty. *J Bone Joint Surg Am* 2008;90(1):184-194.

   A review of TKA etiology and treatment is presented.

46. Koo MH, Choi CH: Conservative treatment for the intraoperative detachment of medial collateral ligament from the tibial attachment site during primary total knee arthroplasty. *J Arthroplasty* 2009;24(8):1249-1253.

   Fifteen primary TKAs complicated with intraoperative complete detachment of the MCL from the tibial attachment site were all treated with nonsurgical conservative treatment without a brace. Compared to the MCL-intact contralateral knees, there was no significant difference in terms of clinical and radiologic outcome at a minimum of 2 years after surgery. There were no cases of instability.

47. Schwab JH, Haidukewych GJ, Hanssen AD, Jacofsky DJ, Pagnano MW: Flexion instability without dislocation after posterior stabilized total knees. *Clin Orthop Relat Res* 2005;440:96-100.

   Ten patients had revision of a posterior stabilized TKA for isolated symptomatic flexion instability. Revision TKA was reliable in alleviating pain (mean Knee Society pain scores improved from 68 points preoperatively to 89 points postoperatively), improving stability (nine of 10 patients had < 5 mm anterior tibial translation postoperatively) and improving patient satisfaction (9 of 10 patients were satisfied).

48. Meding JB, Keating EM, Ritter MA, Faris PM, Berend ME: Genu recurvatum in total knee replacement. *Clin Orthop Relat Res* 2003;416(416):64-67.

49. Jordan L, Kligman M, Sculco TP: Total knee arthroplasty in patients with poliomyelitis. *J Arthroplasty* 2007;22(4):543-548.

   Seventeen TKAs were performed in 15 patients with limbs affected by poliomyelitis. Eight patients had a constrained condylar knee design, eight a posterior stabilized design, and one a hinged design. Knee stability was obtained in all patients, including four patients with less-than-antigravity quadriceps strength.

50. Bourne RB, Chesworth BM, Davis AM, Mahomed NN, Charron KD: Patient satisfaction after total knee arthroplasty: Who is satisfied and who is not? *Clin Orthop Relat Res* 2010;468(1):57-63.

   A study of 1,703 primary TKAs is presented. One in five primary TKA patients was not satisfied with the outcome. The strongest predictors of patient dissatisfaction after primary TKA were expectations not met (10.7x greater risk), a low 1-year Western Ontario and McMaster Universities osteoarthritis index (2.5x greater risk), preoperative pain at rest (2.4x greater risk) and a postoperative complication requiring hospital readmission (1.9x greater risk).

51. Mannion AF, Kämpfen S, Munzinger U, Kramers-de Quervain I: The role of patient expectations in predicting outcome after total knee arthroplasty. *Arthritis Res Ther* 2009;11(5):R139.

   One hundred twelve patients completed a questionnaire about their expectations regarding months until full recovery, pain, and limitations in everyday activities after TKA surgery. Two years postoperatively, they were asked what the reality was for each of these domains, and rated the global outcome and satisfaction with surgery. Patients significantly underestimated the time for full recovery, were overly optimistic about the likelihood of being pain-free and of not being limited in usual activities. Global outcomes were 46.2% excellent, 41.3% good, 10.6% fair, and 1.9% poor.

52. Kim TK, Kwon SK, Kang YG, Chang CB, Seong SC: Functional disabilities and satisfaction after total knee arthroplasty in female Asian patients. *J Arthroplasty* 2009;25(3):458-464.e2.

   Two hundred sixty-one TKA patients completed questionnaires. The top five severe functional disabilities were difficulties in kneeling, squatting, sitting with legs crossed, sexual activity, and recreational activities. The top five in order of perceived importance were difficulties in walking, using a bathtub, working, recreational activities, and climbing stairs. The 23 patients (8.8%) dissatisfied with their replaced knees had more severe functional disabilities than the patients who reported satisfaction with most activities. The dissatisfied patients tended to perceive functional disabilities in high-flexion activities to be more important than did the satisfied patients did.

Chapter 15

Polyethylene Wear and Osteolysis in Total Knee Arthroplasty

William L. Griffin, MD

Introduction

Polyethylene wear and the subsequent development of periprosthetic osteolysis can initiate a variety of failure mechanisms, including aseptic loosening, periprosthetic fracture, component fracture, catastrophic polyethylene failure, or recurrent painful effusions, all of which may be indications for revision surgery.[1-5] Up to 25% of total knee revisions are performed for polyethylene wear and osteolysis.[6,7] Therefore, wear and osteolysis remain a critical area of continued research and review.

Etiology and Factors Affecting Wear

Bone loss secondary to osteolysis is caused by a complex inflammatory response that is influenced by the size, shape, type, and number of particles generated and shows individual variability due to genetic predisposition.[8] The particle-induced inflammatory response triggers osteoclastic activity, leading to progressive bone loss[8] (Figure 1). Because of the combination of rolling, sliding, and rotational motions of the knee and the less congruent nature of the articular surfaces, total knee articulations are a more severe environment for polyethylene components than the more congruent total hip articulation.[9]

Historically, the wear debris generated from total knee polyethylene inserts has occurred in the form of pitting and delamination at the articular surface, secondary to polyethylene fatigue failure from high-contact stresses and oxidation of gamma radiation in air-sterilized polyethylene[9,10] (Figure 2). When pitting and delamination occur, the wear debris generated

Dr. Griffin or an immediate family member has received royalties from DePuy; is a member of a speakers' bureau or has made paid presentations on behalf of DePuy; serves as a paid consultant for or is an employee of DePuy; owns stock or stock options in DePuy; has received research or institutional support from DePuy, Zimmer, Biomet, Wright Medical Technology, and Stryker; and is a board member, owner, officer, or committee member of the American Association of Hip and Knee Surgeons and the Knee Society.

tends to be larger and, therefore, not as bioactive or as likely to incite an osteolytic reaction as the submicron particles produced as a result of the microadhesion and microabrasion that occurs with total hip articulations.[11]

With the introduction of modular tibial trays, however, came the potential for abrasive wear of the polyethylene liner's backside caused by micromotion between the insert and the tibial tray.[12-14] Patterns of backside wear are distinctly different from the types of polyethylene wear observed at the articular surface, with burnishing being the most common mode of backside wear.[15] Moreover, the amount of debris released from the backside articulation has been estimated to be up to 100 times greater than the debris generated from the articular surface.[16] This increase in the amount of particles coupled with the submicron size of the debris has led to an increase in osteolysis as a common cause of failure in total knees. Factors that determine the amount of debris generated from backside wear include the extent of micromotion, the surface roughness of the tibial base plate, and the resistance of the polyethylene insert to abrasive wear[13,14,17] (Figure 3).

A host of other factors also influence the generation of particulate wear debris and the subsequent development of osteolysis in total knee arthroplasty (TKA), including patient variables, surgical technique, design of the femoral and tibial components, type of polyethylene and its fabrication method, and method of sterilization.[10,14,18-22] In a review of 1,287 press-fit condylar total knee replacements, age and sex were patient factors that had a substantial effect on the rate of osteolysis.[22] A 5% decrease in wear-related failure was documented for every 1-year increase in patient age, and men were 2.8 times more likely than women to have wear-related failure.[22] These data suggest that patient size and activity increase the risk of polyethylene wear.

Surgical techniques that lead to malalignment or poor ligamentous balance can also increase the risk of osteolysis. Malalignment can lead to medial or lateral compartment overload, increasing the stress on the polyethylene, whereas an unstable TKA increases the shear stresses on the polyethylene, both of which lead to increased wear.[23] Surgical strategies to encourage uniform loading of the polyethylene component include

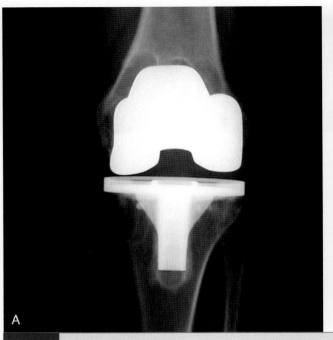
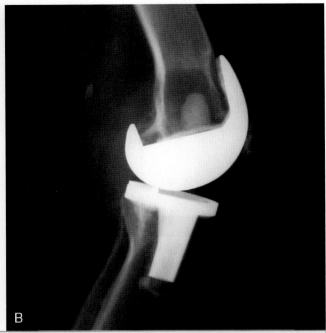

Figure 1 **A,** AP radiographic view of extensive femoral and tibial osteolysis. **B,** Lateral radiographic view of femoral osteolysis.

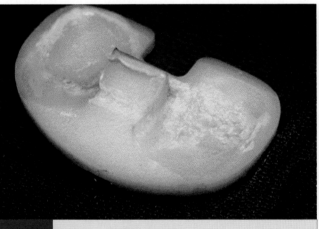

Figure 2 Pitting and delamination of a polyethylene insert is shown. (Reproduced from Griffin WL: Revision total knee arthroplasty: Management of osteolysis, in Lieberman JR, Barry DJ, Azar FM, eds: *Advanced Reconstruction Knee*. Rosemont, IL, American Academy of Orthopaedic Surgeons, 2011, pp 373-378.)

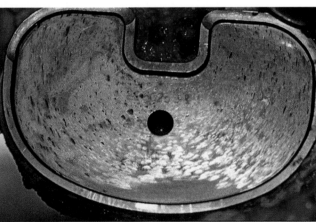

Figure 3 Tibial tray burnishing due to backside micromotion and wear. (Reproduced from Griffin WL: Revision total knee arthroplasty: Management of osteolysis, in Lieberman JR, Barry DJ, Azar FM, eds: *Advanced Reconstruction Knee*. Rosemont, IL, American Academy of Orthopaedic Surgeons, 2011, pp 373-378.)

precise ligament balancing, reproducing anatomic extremity alignment, restoring the proper joint line level, and ensuring symmetry and balance of the flexion and extension gaps.

Component design, in particular the congruency of the articular components, also plays a major role in the generation of polyethylene wear.[9,10,24] The stress experienced by the polyethylene insert is inversely proportional to the contact area of the articulating surfaces. The more conforming the surfaces, the less contact stress on the polyethylene, and the better the wear environment. However, as the articular surface becomes increasingly conforming, more stress is transferred to the tibial tray locking mechanism and to the component-bone interface, which may lead to increased micromotion and backside polyethylene wear or increased fixation interface stress. To address this dilemma, rotating platform mobile-bearing components have been developed.[25] Rotating platform designs provide a very congruent articular surface with a polished

2: Knee

cobalt-chromium tibial tray intended for backside motion. This design accomplishes two goals. First, with its congruent surfaces, it decreases stress on the articular side of the polyethylene. Second, with the ability of the polyethylene insert to rotate on the tibial tray, it eliminates the cross-shear stress on the polyethylene resulting from femoral component rotation on a fixed liner during gait. The reduction in cross-shear inherent in the design of the rotating platform mobile-bearing knee has been documented to reduce wear by 50% compared with a standard fixed-bearing knee under normal kinematic conditions.[10] A recent meta-analysis of 19 studies encompassing 3,506 TKAs has documented that these components perform well, and reports a 96.4% survivorship of rotating platform designs at 15 years.[26] One drawback related to these components, however, is that there are two surfaces generating wear.

The materials used in a TKA, particularly the type of polyethylene and its fabrication method, also have a great impact on wear. First, the quality of polyethylene used to manufacture components can differ among vendors. A study of 2,091 press-fit condylar implants comparing the rate of wear-related failure from different vendors showed that polyethylene from one vendor was 36 times more likely to have wear-related failure than polyethylene from another vendor.[22] Second, the method of manufacture may affect wear behavior. Some have hypothesized that machining components from extruded polyethylene stock may create subsurface material cracking that can increase in vivo delamination, resulting in greater articular wear than occurs with compression-molded components.[27,28] This has been demonstrated clinically in an analysis of 39 tibial inserts where direct compression-molded polyethylene was found superior to molded machined polyethylene in reducing backside wear regardless of time in vivo.[15]

The type of polyethylene sterilization has a strong and well-documented association with wear and may have the greatest impact on the potential for osteolysis. Historically, most polyethylenes used in TKA were sterilized by gamma irradiation and the components were packaged and stored in air. Gamma irradiation produces free radicals in the polyethylene that allows oxidation to occur when the component is exposed to an oxygenated environment. This oxidation reduces the polyethylene's strength and elongation properties and significantly decreases the resistance of polyethylene bearings to fatigue.[29] Gamma irradiation in air, especially when coupled with a long shelf life, has been associated with wear-related failure of polyethylene components.[30] Implant manufacturers have subsequently changed sterilization techniques to ethylene oxide gas or gamma irradiation in an oxygen-free environment. This has resulted in clinically decreased wear-related failures as indicated by one study, which reported a significant decrease in failure between 1,287 first-generation press-fit condylar modular knees with inserts sterilized by gamma irradiation in air and 1,183 second-generation press-fit condylar prostheses having

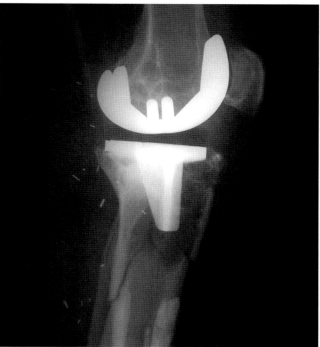

Figure 4 Radiograph showing periprosthetic fracture secondary to osteolysis. (Reproduced from Griffin WL: Revision total knee arthroplasty: Management of osteolysis, in Lieberman JR, Barry DJ, Azar FM, eds: *Advanced Reconstruction Knee.* Rosemont, IL, American Academy of Orthopaedic Surgeons, 2011, pp 373-378.)

inserts packaged and sterilized in an oxygen-free environment. The wear-related failure rate for the components with gamma irradiation in an oxygen-free environment was 1.1% and 10-year survivorship was 97.0%, compared with 8.3% failure and 87.7% 10-year survival for the components with gamma irradiation in air.[18]

Diagnosis

Clinically, patients with osteolysis around a TKA can present with a variety of symptoms. These patients may be completely asymptomatic, have painless effusions, or present with pain secondary to inflammation, loosening, or periprosthetic fracture (**Figure 4**). Osteolysis may be difficult to detect on plain radiographs, and the amount of bone loss is usually underestimated because a more than 30% loss of bone mineral is necessary before a change can be detected radiographically.[31] Reliable assessment of osteolysis and its progression, therefore, require analysis of a temporal series of follow-up radiographs.[32] Routine follow-up radiographs should include good-quality AP and lateral views. If osteolysis is suspected, oblique views can be obtained to better evaluate the posterior aspects of the medial and lateral femoral condyles (**Figure 5**).

2: Knee

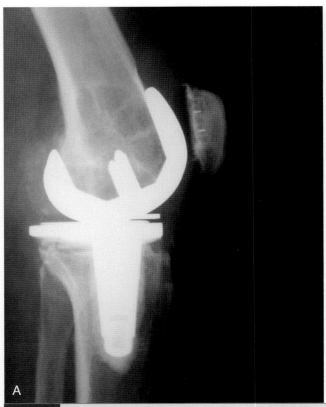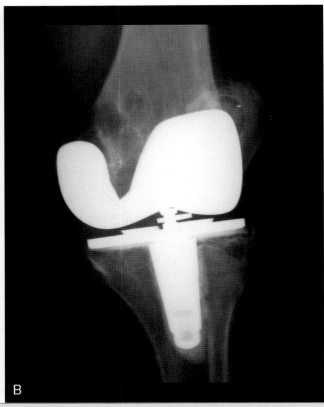

Figure 5 A, Lateral radiographic view of medial femoral condyle osteolysis. B, Oblique radiographic view of medial femoral condyle osteolysis and lack of femoral bony support. (Reproduced from Griffin WL: Revision total knee arthroplasty: Management of osteolysis, in Lieberman JR, Barry DJ, Azar FM, eds: *Advanced Reconstruction Knee*. Rosemont, IL, American Academy of Orthopaedic Surgeons, 2011, pp 373-378.)

In some patients with severe osteolysis, preoperative CT with metal subtraction techniques can be used to quantify the amount of bone loss and help determine appropriate preoperative plans. Although CT can be used to assess the extent of osteolysis, a recent study suggests that MRI is a more sensitive method of detecting osteolysis. According to one study, the sensitivity of detecting lesions by MRI was 95.4%, compared with 74.7% with CT and 51.7% with plain radiography.[33]

Treatment and Results

There is general agreement that treating accelerated wear, the timing of the treatment, and the ability to arrest the osteolytic process with bone preservation and the least morbid methods are paramount to preventing more severe wear-related complications from occurring. Despite this, a general consensus as to the management of osteolytic lesions does not exist and the timing of surgical intervention for osteolysis remains controversial.

For patients with small asymptomatic lesions that do not jeopardize the stability of the implants, for older patients who are less active, or for patients who are poor surgical candidates because of medical comorbidities, treatment can be limited to periodic serial radiographic evaluation and intervention only when the patient becomes symptomatic.

If the patient is symptomatic or the osteolysis is progressive, then surgical intervention can be considered. When surgical intervention is deemed appropriate, the best treatment options are dictated by the extent of osteolytic bone loss, the fixation of the components, and the track record of the TKA design.

For those patients with well-aligned, stable implants that have good locking mechanisms and for which a modern replacement polyethylene insert is available, modular polyethylene insert exchange should be considered. Insert exchange with component retention may result in a quicker recovery, decreased blood loss, decreased cost, and bone stock preservation compared with a complete revision. Early studies on modular polyethylene tibial insert exchange for osteolysis have been unfavorable, reporting a considerable recurrent early failure rate—greater than 27% within 5 years—if the polyethylene exchange is performed because of advanced wear.[30,34] More recent studies, however, using polyethylene not sterilized by gamma irradiation in air have reported more favorable results, documenting failure rates below 16% at midterm follow-up[1,35,36] (Table 1). These studies also demonstrated no significant progression of osteolysis-induced bone loss when defects

Table 1

Failure Rates for Polyethylene Insert Exchange and Full Component Revision for Osteolysis

Authors (Year)	Procedure	Mean Age (Years; Range)	No. of TKAs	Mean F/U (Months)	Revision Rate (%)
Engh et al[30] (2000)	Polyethylene exchange	68 (43-90)	22	90	27
Babis et al[34] (2002)	Polyethylene exchange	66 (35-83)	24	54	33
Griffin et al[1] (2007)	Polyethylene exchange	68 (41-85)	68	44	16
Callaghan et al[36] (2010)	Polyethylene exchange	N/A	22	40	0
Suarez et al[6] (2008)	Full revision	65.7	122	35	11
Burnett et al[37] (2009)	Full revision	N/A	26	48	14

F/U = follow-up; N/A = not available.

were treated with either bone grafting or cement fillers. Of note, femoral components were more susceptible to loosening after isolated insert exchange than tibial components. It seems as though the stem on the tibial component provides some additional protection because osteolysis rarely extended down to the tip of the tibial stem. Moreover, isolated insert exchange should not be performed when there is accelerated wear of the insert with delamination or severe backside wear because these variables have been associated with poor outcomes.[30,34]

When there is impending or definite loosening, component fracture, poor alignment, or a poorly functioning total knee component, full component revision is indicated. There is little information in the literature regarding full component revision specifically for osteolysis and wear. In a series of 122 patients who underwent full component revision for osteolysis, there was an 11% failure rate at an average follow-up of 3 years.[6] In a comparable study with 4-year follow-up, revision surgery for osteolysis failed in 14% of the 26 knees.[37] The primary pitfall encountered with revision surgery for osteolysis is the preoperative underestimation of bone loss present at the time of surgery.

Attempting an isolated polyethylene insert exchange in patients with inadequate bone support of the components can lead to early failure. In addition, not having the appropriate equipment to deal with unexpected large structural bone defects will also lead to poor results. Preparing for worst-case scenarios is particularly important when revising total knees for polyethylene wear and osteolysis.

Technique of Revision for Polyethylene Wear

The knee should be exposed through the previous knee incision with a standard medial parapatellar arthrotomy. If additional previous incisions exist, the most lateral one should be used to preserve blood supply to the anterior skin flaps. Minimal incisions with limited ex-

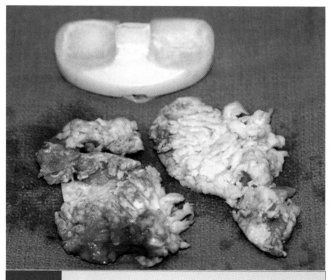

Figure 6 Polyethylene insert with broken locking tab and hypertrophic synovitis is shown. (Reproduced from Griffin WL: Revision total knee arthroplasty: Management of osteolysis, in Lieberman JR, Barry DJ, Azar FM, eds: *Advanced Reconstruction Knee*. Rosemont, IL, American Academy of Orthopaedic Surgeons, 2011, pp 373-378.)

posure are strongly discouraged. Revision surgery for osteolysis with potential significant bone loss requires excellent visualization to inspect and test the components for secure fixation, and inspect the bone for osteolytic defects. Adequate exposure also avoids excessive retraction force, which can cause fractures of the weakened epicondyles or tibial tubercle.

The first step in the revision procedure is to remove the polyethylene insert to create more space and take the extensor mechanism tension off of the tibial tubercle. The next step is a complete synovectomy to decrease the particulate burden within the knee and provide improved exposure (**Figure 6**).

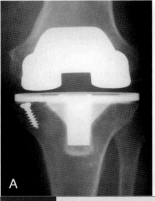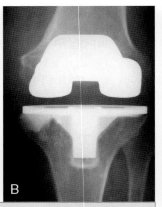

Figure 7 **A,** Preoperative AP radiographic view of medial tibial plateau osteolysis in a well-fixed, well-aligned TKA. **B,** Postoperative radiograph of the new polyethylene insert and the cement augmentation of the osteolytic defect. (Reproduced from Griffin WL: Revision total knee arthroplasty: Management of osteolysis, in Lieberman JR, Barry DJ, Azar FM, eds: *Advanced Reconstruction Knee*. Rosemont, IL, American Academy of Orthopaedic Surgeons, 2011, pp 373-378.)

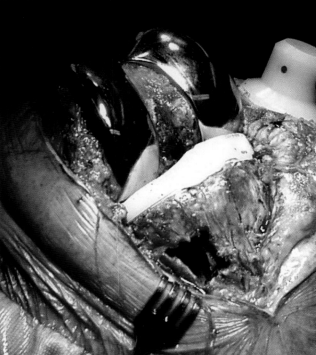

Figure 8 Clinical photograph of the osteolytic lesion exposed through a window in the medial tibial plateau. (Reproduced from Griffin WL: Revision total knee arthroplasty: Management of osteolysis, in Lieberman JR, Barry DJ, Azar FM, eds: *Advanced Reconstruction Knee*. Rosemont, IL, American Academy of Orthopaedic Surgeons, 2011, pp 373-378.)

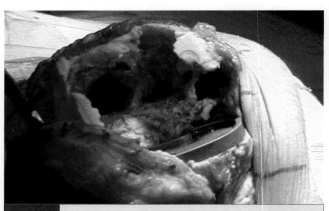

Figure 9 Extensive bone loss secondary to osteolysis is shown. (Reproduced from Griffin WL: Revision total knee arthroplasty: Management of osteolysis, in Lieberman JR, Barry DJ, Azar FM, eds: *Advanced Reconstruction Knee*. Rosemont, IL, American Academy of Orthopaedic Surgeons, 2011, pp 373-378.)

Using a hemostat as a probe and preoperative radiographs for guidance, the periprosthetic bone is then palpated to check for bone defects behind the components. In particular, the posterior femoral condyles should be assessed for bone loss because this is an important area of support for the femoral component. The components are then stressed to determine if they remain solidly fixed to the bone. Rather than impacting the components with a mallet, a torque force should be applied and the bone/cement/prosthesis interface inspected for motion and extrusion of blood. If any motion is detected, the component should be revised.

If the components remain well fixed and have adequate bony support, an isolated polyethylene insert exchange can be considered. However, components should be revised if significant ligamentous instability exists, either with a mismatch between the flexion and extension gaps, an incompetent posterior cruciate ligament with a posterior cruciate-retaining design, or varus/valgus instability requiring additional constraint. Trial inserts are used to assess the ligamentous balance of the knee. Usually an insert one to two sizes thicker than the original polyethylene is required to achieve stability.

Accessible bone defects should be débrided and packed with morcellized bone graft or filled with doughy cement using a large-bore syringe (**Figures 7** and **8**). There are no definitive data available to guide the surgeon regarding the use of cement augmentation or morcellized bone graft to treat osteolytic lesions. For younger patients who are more likely to require repeat revision surgeries in the future, it seems reasonable to use bone graft in an attempt to restore bone stock. In elderly, more sedentary patients who are less likely to require a revision, cement augmentation of osteolytic defects provides immediate stability and eliminates concerns about bone graft resorption.

Another consideration is whether the osteolytic defect is contained or uncontained. With an uncontained bone defect it is difficult to keep the morcellized bone graft within the lesion. Bone particles dislodged from the defect can create an abrasive slurry, potentially accelerating wear. For this reason, cement augmentation may be the better option for uncontained bone defects, particularly in older patients. Both techniques have performed well with limited follow-up.

If full component revision is required due to loosening, impending failure, or instability, extensive bone loss should be expected (**Figure 9**). Preoperative plain radiographs consistently underestimate the amount of bone loss in patients with osteolysis. A full range of revision instruments is required for component removal and reconstruction.

Bone defects can be treated in several ways. Small, contained defects can be treated with morcellized allograft or metal component augments. Larger, uncontained defects can be treated with metal augments, cones or sleeves, or structural allografts. The degree of implant constraint should be tailored on an individual basis. In revisions for osteolysis, the implants used should be at least posterior cruciate substituting and have the ability to provide varus/valgus support for an incompetent collateral ligament or to act as an internal splint for a weakened epicondyle. Stems should be used to bypass stress risers and to provide additional support for more constrained constructs.

Future Directions/Improvements

The incidence of polyethylene-induced osteolysis is decreasing[38] because of continued research and improvements in the three main areas that affect the generation of polyethylene debris. These areas are:

(1) Reducing backside wear. Newer-generation component designs that incorporate better polyethylene locking mechanisms, monoblock tibial tray designs, and polished cobalt-chromium tibial baseplates are three changes that have helped reduce the amount of backside wear due to micromotion between the polyethylene insert and the tibial tray.

(2) Making the polyethylene more resistant to wear. This has occurred as a result of changes in sterilization techniques as well as the development of moderately cross-linked polyethylenes. Implant manufacturers have used gamma irradiation to create improved polyethylene structure by cross-linking and eliminating the free radicals via thermal stabilization. In simulator studies, the cross-linked polyethylenes now available for TKA are substantially more resistant to abrasive backside and topside wear and offer more hope for further decreasing the incidence of osteolysis.[39]

(3) Exploring alternative bearing materials. Ceramic femoral components have some theoretic advantages over metal components that make them more attractive for use as a bearing material. These advantages include chemical inertness, low coefficient of friction, and high resistance to third-body wear damage. Recent improvements in ceramic quality have allowed more complex implants, such as femoral and tibial components for TKA, to be manufactured. Knee simulator studies of these ceramics have demonstrated encouraging improvements in topside wear.[20,21]

Continued research in these areas is imperative to continue a decrease in polyethylene wear and eliminate osteolysis.

Annotated References

1. Griffin WL, Scott RD, Dalury DF, Mahoney OM, Chiavetta JB, Odum SM: Modular insert exchange in knee arthroplasty for treatment of wear and osteolysis. *Clin Orthop Relat Res* 2007;464:132-137.

   This study evaluated the results of isolated polyethylene exchange for wear and/or osteolysis in 68 press-fit condylar TKAs. At a mean of 44 months, there were 11 failures (16.2%). Radiographic review demonstrated no progression of osteolytic lesions in 97% of knees. Level of evidence: IV, therapeutic study.

2. Amstutz HC, Campbell P, Kossovsky N, Clarke IC: Mechanism and clinical significance of wear debris-induced osteolysis. *Clin Orthop Relat Res* 1992;276:7-18.

3. Benevenia J, Lee FY, Buechel F, Parsons JR: Pathologic supracondylar fracture due to osteolytic pseudotumor of knee following cementless total knee replacement. *J Biomed Mater Res* 1998;43(4):473-477.

4. Huang CH, Yang CY, Cheng CK: Fracture of the femoral component associated with polyethylene wear and osteolysis after total knee arthroplasty. *J Arthroplasty* 1999;14(3):375-379.

5. Niki Y, Matsumoto H, Otani T, Yoshimine F, Inokuchi W, Morisue H: Gigantic popliteal synovial cyst caused by wear particles after total knee arthroplasty. *J Arthroplasty* 2003;18(8):1071-1075.

6. Suarez J, Griffin W, Springer B, Fehring T, Mason JB, Odum S: Why do revision knee arthroplasties fail? *J Arthroplasty* 2008;23(6, Suppl 1):99-103.

   This study identified the mechanisms of failure in 566 index revision TKAs. Of index revisions, 12% failed at an average of 40.1 months. Predominant revision failure modes included infection (46%), aseptic loosening (19%), and instability (13%).

7. Sharkey PF, Hozack WJ, Rothman RH, Shastri S, Jacoby SM: Insall Award paper: Why are total knee arthroplasties failing today? *Clin Orthop Relat Res* 2002;404:7-13.

8. Jacobs JJ, Roebuck KA, Archibeck M, Hallab NJ, Glant TT: Osteolysis: Basic science. *Clin Orthop Relat Res* 2001;393:71-77.

2: Knee

9. Bartel DL, Rawlinson JJ, Burstein AH, Ranawat CS, Flynn WF Jr: Stresses in polyethylene components of contemporary total knee replacements. *Clin Orthop Relat Res* 1995;317:76-82.

10. Fisher J, Jennings LM, Galvin AL, Jin ZM, Stone MH, Ingham E: 2009 Knee Society Presidential Guest Lecture: Polyethylene wear in total knees. *Clin Orthop Relat Res* 2010;468(1):12-18.

   Two low-wearing tribologic TKA design solutions are discussed: a rotating platform with reduced cross-shear provides reduced wear with conformity and intrinsic stability; and a low-conformity fixed bearing with reduced surface area and reduced wear but less intrinsic stability that requires good soft-tissue function.

11. McKellop HA, Campbell P, Park SH, et al: The origin of submicron polyethylene wear debris in total hip arthroplasty. *Clin Orthop Relat Res* 1995;311:3-20.

12. Wasielewski RC, Parks N, Williams I, Surprenant H, Collier JP, Engh G: Tibial insert undersurface as a contributing source of polyethylene wear debris. *Clin Orthop Relat Res* 1997;345(345):53-59.

13. Parks NL, Engh GA, Topoleski LD, Emperado J: The Coventry Award: Modular tibial insert micromotion: A concern with contemporary knee implants. *Clin Orthop Relat Res* 1998;356:10-15.

14. Galvin A, Jennings LM, McEwen HM, Fisher J: The influence of tibial tray design on the wear of fixed-bearing total knee replacements. *Proc Inst Mech Eng H* 2008;222(8):1289-1293.

   A new fixed-bearing cobalt-chromium tibial tray design with an improved locking mechanism significantly reduced polyethylene wear compared with a previous titanium alloy tray. The decrease in wear was suggested to be due to a reduction in backside wear.

15. Lombardi AV Jr, Ellison BS, Berend KR: Polyethylene wear is influenced by manufacturing technique in modular TKA. *Clin Orthop Relat Res* 2008;466(11): 2798-2805.

   Results from analysis of 39 tibial inserts demonstrate that direct compression-molded polyethylene is superior to nondirect compression-molded machined polyethylene in reducing backside wear regardless of time in vivo.

16. Rao AR, Engh GA, Collier MB, Lounici S: Tibial interface wear in retrieved total knee components and correlations with modular insert motion. *J Bone Joint Surg Am* 2002;84(10):1849-1855.

17. Azzam MG, Roy ME, Whiteside LA: Second-generation locking mechanisms and ethylene oxide sterilization reduce tibial insert backside damage in total knee arthroplasty. *J Arthroplasty* 2011;26(4):523-530.

   Peripheral capture locking mechanisms, when combined with polyethylene sterilized by ethylene oxide gas instead of gamma radiation, is effective in preventing major backside damage to the polyethylene insert, irrespective of patient factors associated with increased activity.

18. Griffin WL, Fehring TK, Pomeroy DL, Gruen TA, Murphy JA: Sterilization and wear-related failure in first- and second-generation press-fit condylar total knee arthroplasty. *Clin Orthop Relat Res* 2007;464: 16-20.

   The 5-year wear-related failure rate for 1,183 second-generation TKAs having inserts sterilized in an oxygen-free environment was 1.1%; 10-year survivorship was 97.0%. The 1,287 first-generation TKAs with inserts gamma irradiated in air experienced 8.3% failure and 87.7% 10-year survival. Level of evidence: III, therapeutic study.

19. Utzschneider S, Paulus A, Datz JC, et al: Influence of design and bearing material on polyethylene wear particle generation in total knee replacement. *Acta Biomater* 2009;5(7):2495-2502.

   This study analyzed the impact of knee designs combined with cross-linked polyethylenes on the amount, size, and shape of particles. For all six material combinations tested, wear size and shape were similar. The number of particles, however, was related to TKA design.

20. Tsukamoto R, Williams PA, Clarke IC, et al: Y-TZP zirconia run against highly crosslinked UHMWPE tibial inserts: Knee simulator wear and phase-transformation studies. *J Biomed Mater Res B Appl Biomater* 2008;86(1):145-153.

   The wear of yttria-stabilized zirconia (YZr) femoral condyles on 7-Mrad tibial inserts was compared with cobalt-chromium bearings on 3.5-Mrad inserts. At 10 Mc the cobalt-chromium/3.5-Mrad bearing wear averaged 4.5 mm(3)/Mc and the condyles' roughness increased substantially; the YZr/7-Mrad bearing wear was unmeasurable and the condyles remained pristine.

21. Oonishi H, Ueno M, Kim SC, Oonishi H, Iwamoto M, Kyomoto M: Ceramic versus cobalt-chrome femoral components; wear of polyethylene insert in total knee prosthesis. *J Arthroplasty* 2009;24(3):374-382.

   Simulator tests revealed that ultra-high molecular weight polyethylene inserts had remarkably lower wear against ceramic femoral components than against cobalt-chromium components. However, the retrieval study revealed no significant difference between ceramic and cobalt-chromium.

22. Fehring TK, Murphy JA, Hayes TD, Roberts DW, Pomeroy DL, Griffin WL: Factors influencing wear and osteolysis in press-fit condylar modular total knee replacements. *Clin Orthop Relat Res* 2004;428(428): 40-50.

23. Callaghan JJ, O'rourke MR, Saleh KJ: Why knees fail: Lessons learned. *J Arthroplasty* 2004;19(4, Suppl 1): 31-34.

24. Galvin AL, Kang L, Udofia I, et al: Effect of conformity and contact stress on wear in fixed-bearing total knee prostheses. *J Biomech* 2009;42(12):1898-1902.

    This study showed that a low-conforming, high–contact stress knee with a low-medium level of cross-shear resulted in significantly lower wear rates in comparison to a standard cruciate-sacrificing, fixed-bearing knee.

25. Dennis DA, Komistek RD: Mobile-bearing total knee arthroplasty: Design factors in minimizing wear. *Clin Orthop Relat Res* 2006;452:70-77.

    The clinical and basic science studies of factors affecting polyethylene wear are reviewed. Emphasis is placed on mobile-bearing designs with features that should lessen polyethylene wear.

26. Carothers JT, Kim RH, Dennis DA, Southworth C: Mobile-bearing total knee arthroplasty a meta-analysis. *J Arthroplasty* 2011;26(4):537-542.

    A meta-analysis of 19 studies encompassing 3,506 TKAs has documented that these components perform well, and reports a 96.4% survivorship of rotating platform designs at 15 years.

27. Won CH, Rohatgi S, Kraay MJ, Goldberg VM, Rimnac CM: Effect of resin type and manufacturing method on wear of polyethylene tibial components. *Clin Orthop Relat Res* 2000;376:161-171.

28. Berzins A, Jacobs JJ, Berger R, et al: Surface damage in machined ram-extruded and net-shape molded retrieved polyethylene tibial inserts of total knee replacements. *J Bone Joint Surg Am* 2002;84-A(9):1534-1540.

29. Collier JP, Sperling DK, Currier JH, Sutula LC, Saum KA, Mayor MB: Impact of gamma sterilization on clinical performance of polyethylene in the knee. *J Arthroplasty* 1996;11(4):377-389.

30. Engh GA, Koralewicz LM, Pereles TR: Clinical results of modular polyethylene insert exchange with retention of total knee arthroplasty components. *J Bone Joint Surg Am* 2000;82(4):516-523.

31. Engh CA Jr, McAuley JP, Sychterz CJ, Sacco ME, Engh CA Sr: The accuracy and reproducibility of radiographic assessment of stress-shielding: A postmortem analysis. *J Bone Joint Surg Am* 2000;82(10):1414-1420.

32. Engh CA Jr, Sychterz CJ, Young AM, Pollock DC, Toomey SD, Engh CA Sr: Interobserver and intraobserver variability in radiographic assessment of osteolysis. *J Arthroplasty* 2002;17(6):752-759.

33. Weiland DE, Walde TA, Leung SB, et al: Magnetic resonance imaging in the evaluation of periprosthetic acetabular osteolysis: A cadaveric study. *J Orthop Res* 2005;23(4):713-719.

    This study compared MRI to plain film analysis in assessing periacetabular bone loss. MRI was 95% sensitive in the detection of lesions, specificity was 98%, and accuracy was 96%. Using conventional radiographs, the overall sensitivity of lesion detection was 52%, and the specificity was 96%.

34. Babis GC, Trousdale RT, Morrey BF: The effectiveness of isolated tibial insert exchange in revision total knee arthroplasty. *J Bone Joint Surg Am* 2002;84(1):64-68.

35. Whiteside LA, Katerberg B: Revision of the polyethylene component for wear in TKA. *Clin Orthop Relat Res* 2006;452:193-199.

    This study assessed isolated liner exchange for wear in 49 TKAs. In 36 knees, a locking mechanism was fabricated with a carbide bit and acrylic cement. Overall, isolated polyethylene component exchange was successful. Fabricating a locking mechanism proved effective in laboratory testing and clinical application.

36. Callaghan JJ, Reynolds ER, Ting NT, Goetz DD, Clohisy JC, Maloney WJ: Liner exchange and bone grafting: Rare option to treat wear and lysis of stable TKAs. *Clin Orthop Relat Res* 2011;469(1):154-159.

    In this review of 25 revision TKAs in knees with extensive osteolysis around well-fixed components, liner exchange and bone grafting provided durable results. At a mean of 59 months, 84.6% and 70% of femoral and tibial osteolytic lesions, respectively, showed evidence of complete or near complete graft incorporation. Level of evidence: IV, therapeutic study.

37. Burnett RS, Keeney JA, Maloney WJ, Clohisy JC: Revision total knee arthroplasty for major osteolysis. *Iowa Orthop J* 2009;29:28-37.

    Results from 28 knees revised for major osteolytic defects demonstrated that both morcellized and structural bone grafting, in combination with stemmed components, was successful in managing this condition. At a mean of 48 months, 96% of knees demonstrated clinical and functional improvement.

38. Marshall A, Ries MD, Paprosky W, Implant Wear Symposium 2007 Clinical Work Group: How prevalent are implant wear and osteolysis, and how has the scope of osteolysis changed since 2000? *J Am Acad Orthop Surg* 2008;16(1, Suppl 1):S1-S6.

    Clinical experience before 2000 included wear rates and osteolysis from 10% to 70% at 7- to 14-year follow-up. With recent advances in polyethylene manufacturing, alternative bearing surfaces, implant design, and revision techniques, early clinical results demonstrate 50% to 81% decreases in radiographic wear rates.

39. Fisher J, McEwen HM, Tipper JL, et al: Wear, debris, and biologic activity of cross-linked polyethylene in the knee: Benefits and potential concerns. *Clin Orthop Relat Res* 2004;428:114-119.

2: Knee

Chapter 16

Infection in Total Knee Arthroplasty

Jeffrey A. Krempec, MD   John L. Masonis, MD   Thomas K. Fehring, MD

Introduction

The diagnosis of infection must always be considered when evaluating the patient with a painful total knee arthroplasty (TKA). Diagnosis and management of prosthetic joint infection have evolved in recent years in response to improvements in detection methods and the growing prevalence of antibiotic-resistant organisms, with effective treatment of both acute and chronic infections. With a predicted exponential increase in TKAs and a stable infection rate, prevention and appropriate treatment of prosthetic TKA infections is paramount.

Incidence and Risk Factors

The incidence of prosthetic knee infection is typically less than 1% in the general population for primary arthroplasty[1,2] and up to 5.6% for revision arthroplasty.[3] Multiple studies have shown an increased risk in certain patient populations (**Table 1**).

Diabetes is an independent risk factor for deep infection, with older studies reporting infection rates as high as 5.5% to 6%.[4,5] A larger, more recent study has shown a lower risk of infection. One study reported a 1.9% incidence of infection in patients with diabetes in a prospective series of 1,509 consecutive TKAs over a 5-year follow-up period.[6]

Obesity has been considered a risk factor for prosthetic knee infection. A 2005 study reported on 1,813 TKA patients comparing outcomes in highly obese, obese, and nonobese patients.[7] The highly obese TKA

Dr. Masonis or an immediate family member has received royalties from Smith & Nephew; serves as a paid consultant to or is an employee of Smith & Nephew; serves as an unpaid consultant for Stryker; and has received research or institutional support from DePuy, Smith & Nephew, and Zimmer. Dr. Fehring or an immediate family member has received royalties from DePuy; serves as a paid consultant to or is an employee of DePuy; and has received research or institutional support from DePuy. Neither Dr. Krempec nor any immediate family member has received anything of value from or owns stock in a commercial company or institution related directly or indirectly to the subject of this chapter.

patients (body mass index [BMI] ≥ 35) had a significantly higher rate of postoperative infection (1.1%) than the obese group (BMI < 35) (0.3%). The odds ratio was 6.7 times higher for risk of infection in highly obese TKA patients. However, several smaller recent studies have not demonstrated an increased rate of infection in obese patients.[8-10]

In a review of more than 43,000 knees in the Finnish Arthroplasty Registry, patients with seropositive rheumatoid arthritis with a 2.29 risk ratio had twice the rate of infection compared with those with primary osteoarthritis (1.32% and 0.66%, respectively).[1] Other systemic illnesses such as HIV infection, sickle cell disease, and hemophilia are associated with higher rates of infection.[11] Additional associations with increased rates of infection are prior open surgery, poor nutrition, hypokalemia, pharmacologic immunosuppression, psoriatic skin lesions, and current infection at a remote site.[12]

Bacteremia from a variety of sources can cause hematogenous seeding of bacteria into the prosthetic knee joint, both in the early postoperative period and for the life of the implant. Bacteremia associated with acute infection in the oral cavity or skin, and respiratory, gastrointestinal, and urogenital systems and/or other sites can cause late implant infection. Patients with joint arthroplasties who undergo invasive procedures such as dental extraction, cystoscopy, and colonoscopy or who have other infections are at increased risk for hematogenous seeding of their prosthesis. In 2009, the American Academy of Orthopaedic Surgeons (AAOS) issued an information statement regarding antibiotic prophylaxis for bacteremia in patients with joint arthroplasties.[13] It was recommended that antibiotic prophylaxis be considered for all total joint arthroplasty patients before performing any invasive procedure that may cause bacteremia. This is particularly important for those patients with one or more certain risk factors (**Table 1**).

Etiology

Coagulase-negative staphylococcus and *Staphylococcus aureus* continue to be the most common infecting organisms of TKA, accounting for 36% and 25% of in-

2: Knee

Table 1

Conditions Placing Patients at Potential Increased Risk for Hematogenous Total Joint Infection

Immunocompromised/immunosuppressed state

Inflammatory arthropathies (rheumatoid arthritis, systemic lupus erythematosus)

Drug-induced immunosuppression

Radiation-induced immunosuppression

Comorbidities (diabetes, obesity, HIV, smoking history)

Previous prosthetic joint infections

Malnourishment

Hemophilia

HIV infection

Type I diabetes

Malignancy

Megaprostheses

fections, respectively, in a series of 4,788 TKAs.[2] Some common but less frequent organisms include *Streptococcus* species, enterococci, *Escherichia coli, Pseudomonas,* and *Klebsiella.*

Fungal infection is a rare complication of TKA. *Candida albicans* is the most frequent infecting fungal organism, with other species of *Candida, Aspergillus,* and others less frequent. Risk factors predisposing patients to prosthetic fungal infections include intravenous catheters, prolonged use of antibiotics, intensive care unit stays, steroid use, and immunocompromised hosts. Systemic antifungal agents (amphotericin B) are used for prolonged courses because of the difficulty in eradicating fungal infection. Delayed diagnosis is common because of the lack of systemic symptoms, and outcomes are less favorable than for bacterial infections. In a recent multiinstitutional study, fungal infections of TKA more often required resection arthroplasty, fusion, and amputation.[14]

In a retrospective study of 2,116 episodes of periprosthetic joint infection over a period of 22 years, only 7 (0.3%) were caused by mycobacterium.[15] The risk of reactivation of tuberculosis in patients undergoing total hip arthroplasty (THA) or TKA for quiescent tuberculosis native septic arthritis varies between 0% and 31%. The risk is higher for patients receiving TKA (27%) than those with THA (6%). The diagnosis of tuberculosis prosthetic joint infection is often delayed because of a low level of clinical suspicion and its unusual clinical presentation in patients at risk. Joint effusion may be bloody and have minimally elevated inflammatory markers, histology of synovium showing lack of acute inflammation, and granulomatous inflammation with giant cells, histiocytes, and necrosis. The optimal therapy for tuberculosis prosthetic joint infection is still

unclear. Patients with unsuspected tuberculosis septic arthritis discovered at the time of implantation or in the early postoperative period can be successfully treated with antituberculosis drugs for 12 to 18 months. With late onset of tuberculosis prosthetic joint infection, medical treatment alone is usually unsuccessful and two-stage exchange is often required.[15]

A substantial rise in the incidence of bacterial antibiotic resistance has been reported by the National Nosocomial Infection Surveillance System report.[16] Methicillin-resistant *S aureus* (MRSA) and methicillin-resistant *Staphylococcus epidermidis* (MRSE) are the most common antibiotic-resistant organisms isolated for prosthetic knee infection. In one study, these two pathogens accounted for 14% of the infected TKAs presenting to a referral practice.[17] Another study reported that 34% of periprosthetic infections over a 5-year period were caused by either MRSA or MRSE.[18] This rise in incidence is important because of the higher treatment failure rate and limitations in intravenous and oral medications available for cost-effective use. It is likely that the incidence of these infections will continue to rise, and new prevention strategies must be developed.

Classification

In order to classify TKA infection, the temporal relationship between the index procedure and the onset of symptoms must be established, as well as the route by which the infecting organism gains access to the joint space. A classification of periprosthetic infections and recommendations for the proposed management of these patients has been developed,[19] as described in Table 2.

Diagnosis

The surgeon must have a high index of suspicion for infection in any patient with a painful TKA. A detailed history and physical examination are paramount. Acute postoperative infections may be accompanied by prolonged wound drainage, pain, erythema, swelling, induration, heat, and adenopathy. Systemic symptoms such as fevers, night sweats, and chills may occur but are frequently absent early. Late infections may be accompanied by pain or stiffness, and symptoms may have been present for weeks or months before presentation. A history of postoperative antibiotic use or prolonged incisional drainage may be helpful in the diagnosis of infection.

Currently, there is no universally accepted single diagnostic test or modality that is absolutely accurate or reliable for the determination of infection. The accepted definition of infection in the orthopaedic literature is demonstration of at least two of the following three criteria: growth of the same organism in two or

2: Knee

Table 2

Segawa Classification of TKA Infection

Infection Type	Onset	Description
Type 1	Positive intraoperative cultures	Two or more positive intraoperative cultures
Type 2	Early postoperative	Less than 4 weeks postoperatively
Type 3	Late chronic	More than 4 weeks postoperatively
Type 4	Acute hematogenous	Seeding from a distant site with documented or suspected bacteremia

more cultures on solid media obtained by aspiration of deep tissue specimens at the time of surgery; finding of acute inflammation on final histology; and gross purulence or actively draining sinus at the time of surgery.

Serologic Studies

Several recent studies have evaluated the usefulness of preoperative C-reactive protein (CRP), erythrocyte sedimentation rate (ESR), and joint aspiration (cell count with differential and culture). A 2008 study retrospectively reviewed the preoperative evaluation of 670 revision TKAs with respect to ESR and CRP.[20] The sensitivity, specificity, positive predictive value (PPV), and negative predictive value (NPV) of preoperative ESR greater than 30 mm/h were 0.91, 0.72, 0.68, and 0.93, respectively, whereas those of preoperative CRP greater than 10 mg/L were 0.94, 0.74, 0.70, and 0.95, respectively. These values are presently the generally accepted cutoff values in the orthopaedic literature. The combined cost for the two tests was $79. It was recommended that every patient with painful TKA be evaluated with ESR and CRP testing as a cost-effective screening tool to rule out infection. Another study prospectively evaluated the use of ESR and CRP before 151 revision TKAs. An optimal cutoff point for ESR and CRP was identified to be 22.5 mm/h and 13.5 mg/L, respectively, with higher values considered positive for infection. These thresholds for ESR and CRP provided high sensitivity (0.93 and 0.91, respectively) and good specificity (0.83 and 0.86, respectively), with increasing values if both were positive.[21]

Synovial Fluid Aspiration

Synovial fluid aspiration is the most valuable tool in the diagnosis of infection in TKA. Synovial fluid should be aspirated on the basis of clinical suspicion, or when serologic markers are elevated in the setting of an unexplained painful TKA. To achieve optimal results, antibiotic use should be discontinued at least 3 weeks before aspiration. Standard studies of the synovial fluid include white blood cell (WBC) count, differential, and culture. A significant difference between the mean WBC counts (645 versus 25,951 cells/10^{-3} cm³) and neutrophil differentials (27.3% versus 72.8%) in aspiration fluid in knees without and with infection has been reported.[22] Aspiration fluid with 2,500 or more WBC/10^{-3} cm³ (2,500/mm³) and 60% or more neutrophils was highly suggestive of infection. A 2007 study reported that a synovial WBC count greater than 3,000 WBC/10^{-3}cm³ (3,000/mm³) was the most precise test, with a sensitivity of 100%, specificity of 98%, and accuracy of 99%.[23] In a recent multicenter review, optimum cutoff values for both WBC count and polymorphonuclear cell differential were determined rather than testing arbitrary values.[24] The cutoff values for optimal accuracy in the diagnosis of infection were greater than 1,100 WBC/10^{-3}cm³ (1,000/mm³) and greater than 64% for the polymorphonuclear cell differential. When both tests were below their cutoff values, the NPV was 98.2%, whereas when both tests were above their cutoff values, infection was confirmed in 98.6%. The clinical utility of fluid analysis in diagnosing infection could be improved by combining either of the two aspiration results with the ESR and CRP levels. Based on these studies, a rational approach to preoperative evaluation of a painful TKA would include obtaining ESR and CRP levels, and if either is elevated or clinical suspicion is high, aspiration with synovial fluid analysis should be performed.

Imaging

Plain radiographs should be obtained in all patients with a painful TKA. Infection can cause radiographic changes at either the bone-prosthesis or bone-cement interface. Periosteal reaction, endosteal reaction, osteopenia, and osteolysis may occur. Rapid and progressive loosening seen in the first few years should herald the diagnosis of infection (**Figure 1**). However, most patients with prosthetic infection, especially those with an acute presentation, do not have obvious radiographic findings as previously described, or these findings may be indistinguishable from changes seen in aseptic loosening. Plain radiographs are neither sensitive nor specific in detecting prosthetic infection. Their largest role is to rule out other conditions such as wear, osteolysis, or periprosthetic fractures.[25]

Radionuclide studies have been used in the evalua-

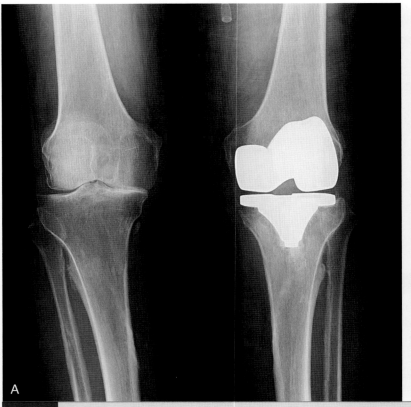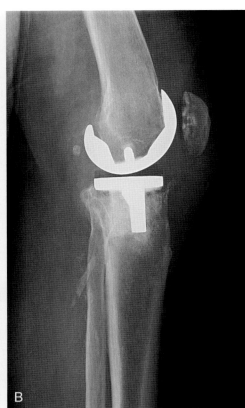

Figure 1 | AP (**A**) and lateral (**B**) radiographs showing an infected TKA.

tion of patients with a painful TKA. In a study of 72 total joint arthroplasties, it was reported that technetium Tc-99m bone scans had a sensitivity of 33%, a specificity of 86%, a PPV of 30%, and a NPV of 88%.[26] Using an indium-111 leukocyte scan, the sensitivity was 77%; specificity, 86%; PPV, 54%; NPV, 95%; and accuracy, 84%.[27] The low PPV (54%) represents a multitude of false-positive results, typically because of aseptic loosening. The combination of bone and leukocyte scans resulted in improved diagnostic value, with a PPV of 100%, eliminating false-positive results. However, the sensitivity dropped to 46%, which represented several false-negative examinations. The authors of this study abandoned nuclear imaging as a preoperative test for prosthetic infection.[28] Nuclear imaging often remains positive longer than 1 year following routine joint arthroplasty, and these tests should only be used as an adjunct to other diagnostic modalities.

The role of fluorodeoxyglucose positron emission tomography (FDG-PET) scans for the diagnosis of prosthetic infection has been studied. FDG reflects glucose utilization and can indicate areas of inflammation. This study uses a single injection, and treatment with antibiotics is not likely to affect the sensitivity in delineating sites of infections because FDG does not rely on leukocyte migration. A recent meta-analysis rated the overall diagnostic performance of FDG-PET as moderate to high.[29] Across 11 studies, sensitivity and specificity ranged from 22.2% to 100% and from 61.5% to 100%, respectively. Pooled estimates from these studies totaling 635 prostheses revealed a sensitivity of 82.1% and specificity of 86.6%. Performance of the FDG-PET was better in the hip than in the knee. The authors caution that the results of the individual studies were heterogeneous with a wide range of values reported,[29] and therefore, its efficacy remains unclear.

Intraoperative Studies

Intraoperative testing with frozen section analysis and Gram stain and culture for the diagnosis of infected TKA is commonly used. The specificity and sensitivity of frozen sections may depend on the area and number of tissue samples that are obtained, as well as the number of WBCs seen per high-power field. In a series of 36 failed prostheses, it was reported that more than five polymorphonuclear leukocytes (PMNLs) per high-power field on analysis of tissue from around each of the 15 implants were associated with infection.[30] There was no acute inflammatory response in association with the 21 prostheses that were not associated with clinical or bacteriologic evidence of infection, including those associated with extensive particles of debris. It has been reported that the criterion of more than five

PMNLs per high-power field had a sensitivity of 100% and a specificity of 96% for the detection of infection.[31] Diagnostic value with the use of 10 PMNLs per high-power field is increased, with a sensitivity of 84% and a specificity of 99%; the PPV was 89% and the NPV of the frozen sections was 98%.[32] Authors of one study cautioned against using a strict quantitative number of PMNLs as a diagnostic tool in their review of frozen section as a guide to infection, stating that the overall histologic picture was more important than an isolated number of PMNLs from one field.[33] For example, a patient with six PMNLs per high-power field in only one microscopic field may not be infected, but a patient with four PMNLs per high-power field in every microscopic field probably is infected.[33]

Intraoperative Gram stains have traditionally been used but their sensitivity has recently been questioned. The ability of intraoperative Gram stains in revision hip and knee arthroplasty was studied. In a series of 413 revision joint arthroplasties, the Gram stain demonstrated only 14.7% sensitivity and 98.9% specificity, with 58 false-negative studies.[34] In a 2009 study of 921 consecutive revision TKAs, intraoperative Gram staining had a sensitivity of 27% and a specificity of 99.9%. The PPV was 98.5% and the NPV was 79%, whereas the test accuracy was 80%.[35] Intraoperative Gram staining does not have adequate sensitivity and NPV to be used on a routine basis.

Prevention Strategies

Preoperative, intraoperative, and postoperative prevention strategies have lowered the rate of TKA infection. Some of these strategies have sound scientific basis, whereas others have theoretic benefit.

Preoperative

Identification and optimization of patient-specific risk factors is the first step in prevention of TKA infection. Evaluation of the surgical site as well as remote sites for infection limits the opportunity for local or blood-borne bacterial contamination. Management of immunosuppressive medications by the surgeon or treating physician if tolerated may decrease infection rates. However, large studies have documented no increase in perioperative infection rates in patients using immunosuppressive medications such as methotrexate and etanercept. A literature review on the perioperative management of medications in patients with rheumatoid arthritis discusses the lack of scientific data regarding the management of disease-modifying antirheumatic drugs and biologic agents. For TKA, holding one to two doses of methotrexate is recommended as a consideration. Biologic agents such as etanercept and anakinra should be held preoperatively in accordance with their half-life and held 10 days postoperatively.[36]

The Centers for Disease Control and Prevention recommends that hair removal immediately before surgery be done if necessary for surgical exposure, and with clippers rather than a razor.[37] A meta-analysis in 2006 found no difference in infection rates in patients with or without preoperative hair removal.[38] Additionally, if hair is removed, depilatory creams and clippers demonstrated a lower infection risk than razors. Timing of hair removal did not impact infection rate in this meta-analysis.[38]

Most clinical studies evaluating the efficacy of skin preparations involve general surgery procedures. The most recent studies documented lower infection rates when using 2% chlorhexadine and 70% isopropyl alcohol versus povidone-iodine.[39] Bacterial counts after skin preparation for foot surgery have also shown less bacterial growth when using 2% chlorhexidine and 70% isopropyl alcohol compared with 0.7% iodine and 74% isopropyl alcohol.[40]

Antibiotic prophylaxis is mandatory in most surgical circumstance. The 2003 National Institutes of Health Consensus Statement on Total Knee Replacement determined there is strong evidence for the routine use of antibiotic prophylaxis.[41] The AAOS issued an information statement in 2004 recommending the routine use of antibiotic prophylaxis with three components: (1) the antibiotic used for prophylaxis should be carefully selected, consistent with current recommendations in the literature, taking into account the issues of resistance and patient allergies; (2) timing and dosage of antibiotic administration should optimize the efficacy of the therapy; and (3) duration of prophylactic antibiotic administration should not exceed the 24-hour postoperative period. Currently, cefazolin or cefuroxime are the preferred antibiotics for patients undergoing orthopaedic procedures. Clindamycin or vancomycin may be used for patients with a confirmed β-lactam allergy. Vancomycin may be used in patients with known colonization with MRSA or in facilities with recent MRSA outbreaks. Prophylactic antibiotics should be administered within 1 hour before skin incision and should be discontinued within 24 hours of the end of surgery.[42] A recent literature review identified 26 studies concerning antibiotic prophylaxis. The data showed an 81% risk reduction and overall 8% reduction in postoperative infection rates.[43]

Intraoperative

Laminar air flow and ultraviolet light in the operating room have been shown to lower the amount of bacterial contamination in the air as well as on surgical wounds. Lower infection rates were demonstrated in a randomized controlled trial evaluating laminar flow;[44] however, the trial was not well controlled and involved a large number of sites, surgeons, treatment regimens, and types of ventilation. It also did not control for the use of antibiotic prophylaxis, which was not routine at the time. More recent literature has called into question the usefulness and cost-effectiveness of laminar air flow systems. Ultraviolet light eliminates bacteria on the surfaces of objects in contact with it. One study demonstrated 90% reduction in airborne bacteria at the wound and 60% reduction in airbone bacteria in the operating room.[45]

The routine use of antibiotic-loaded bone cement (ALBC) in primary TKA is controversial. Support for the use of ALBC is based mainly on registry data. In the Finnish Arthroplasty Registry, 43,149 primary and revision knee arthroplasties were followed for a median of 3 years. Three hundred eighty-seven reoperations were performed because of infection. Both partial and complete revision TKA increased the risk of infection compared with primary knee replacement. Male patients, patients with seropositive rheumatoid arthritis or with a previous fracture around the knee, and patients with constrained and hinged prostheses had increased rates of infection after primary arthroplasty. Wound-related complications increased the risk of deep infection. The combination of parenteral antibiotic prophylaxis and prosthetic fixation with antibiotic-impregnated cement protected against septic failure, especially after revision TKA.

In a smaller community-based registry study, outcomes in patients who underwent primary TKA from May 2003 to March 2007 were reviewed.[46] Infection rates were compared in patients undergoing TKA with ALBC and regular cement. A total of 22,889 primary TKAs were performed, with 2,030 (8.9%) using ALBC. Two thousand four hundred forty-nine patients had diabetes (10.7%), and ALBC was used in 295 (12%). The rate of deep infection was 1.4% for ALBC TKA (28 cases) and 0.7% (154 cases) with regular cement ($P = 0.002$). Among patients with diabetes, the infection rate was 1.7% (5 patients) with ALBC and 0.9% (19 patients) with regular cement ($P = 0.199$). In patients considered at higher risk for infection, ALBC did not appear to reduce TKA infection rates.[46]

A randomized controlled trial investigated the use of cefuroxime-impregnated cement in 340 primary TKAs. There was a significantly lower rate of infection at intermediate-term follow-up.[47] Another study showed a decreased infection rate in a randomized controlled trial of vancomycin-impregnated cement in 180 revision TKAs.[48] In a review of available data, it was suggested that low-dose ALBC be considered a reasonable method of prophylaxis for certain high-risk patients undergoing primary or revision total joint arthroplasty.[49]

Postoperative

Persistent postoperative wound drainage has been shown to be a predictor of infection after total joint arthroplasty.[50] The factors associated with prolonged wound infection were examined and it was reported that obesity, drain output, and use of low-molecular-weight heparin were associated with prolonged wound drainage and infection. The use of either aspirin combined with mechanical prophylaxis or warfarin was associated with less wound drainage.[9]

Treatment

Once the diagnosis of TKA infection is established, treatment decisions are based on several factors, including the classification of the infection, the pathogen and its antibiotic sensitivities, host factors, the status of the soft-tissue envelope, and the status of the prosthesis (Figure 2).

Antibiotic Suppression

Antibiotic treatment alone will not eliminate deep infection, and empiric antibiotic treatment of patients with a potentially infected arthroplasty is strongly discouraged. In certain selected clinical settings, removal of the prosthesis may not be technically feasible or associated with unacceptable morbidity to the patient. Long-term oral suppressive antibiotic therapy may be a reasonable alternative to surgery in this setting, although the optimal duration of antibiotics and the outcome of prosthetic joint infections treated in this manner are not well established. The goal of suppressive therapy is to achieve a functioning prosthesis without pain or drainage, not eradication of infection. Thirty-two patients underwent chronic antibiotic suppression with a mean therapy time of 52.6 months.[51] Criteria for long-term suppressive oral therapy included patients who refused surgery; patients with chronic prosthetic infections who were not surgical candidates for staged reimplantation, resection arthroplasty, or arthrodesis because of a poor general condition and a stable functioning prosthesis; microbiologically documented infection with a sensitive organism; ability to tolerate oral antibiotics once or twice daily; and good compliance and close follow-up as an outpatient. Long-term suppressive antibiotic therapy in this setting had favorable results in 86% of patients (31 of 36) in terms of maintenance of functioning prostheses, with a mean follow-up of more than 60 months.[51]

A second role for antibiotic therapy alone is that of the type 1 infection: unexpected positive intraoperative culture at the time of revision TKA. Type 1 infections are relatively rare, reportedly constituting only 6% of 81 infections in one study[18] and 3% of 509 periprosthetic infections at the Mayo Clinic over a 4-year period.[52] A 2007 study reported on the treatment of 41 type 1 infections; 29 of these had one positive culture and were assumed to be falsely positive.[53] Of these, 24 were treated with antibiotics during the hospital stay only, whereas five patients had a 4- to 6-week course of antibiotics. The remaining 12 patients had some intraoperative sign of infection, including two positive cultures, and were treated with antibiotics for 6 weeks; one required revision surgery. It was recommended that treatment of a single positive intraoperative culture is not necessary in the absence of any other evidence of infection.

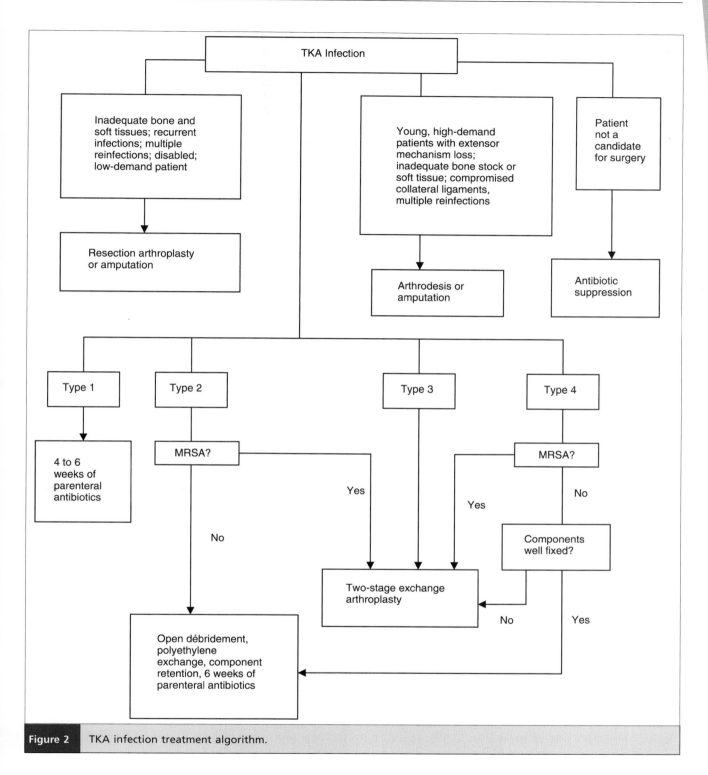

Figure 2 TKA infection treatment algorithm.

Open Débridement, Polyethylene Exchange, and Antibiotic Therapy

Historically, type 2 infections and type 4 infections without implant loosening have been treated by open débridement, polyethylene exchange, and organism-directed antibiotic therapy. The advantages of débridement and retention of components include limited sur-gery with preservation of the prosthesis and bone stock along with a faster recovery. However, the failure rate of the procedure is unacceptably high, averaging 71%. Staphylococcal species (both methicillin-sensitive and -resistant) seem particularly ill suited to débridement and retention of components. In a review of 31 patients with acute *S aureus* TKA infection treated with open débridement, polyethylene exchange, and parenteral antibiotics, only 8% of S aureus infections were eradicated at 4 years, compared with 56% of S epidermidis infections.[54] In a 2009 study, 19 MRSA-infected TKAs were treated with open débridement, polyethylene exchange, parenteral antibiotics, and retention of components.[55] The success rate at 2-year follow-up was only 14%. The authors cautioned against retention of components in the setting of MRSA infection.

Midterm outcomes of open débridement and antibiotic therapy in 10 infected TKAs have been reported.[56] Eight of 10 were functioning well at average 6.8-year follow-up; two knees had recurrence of infection at 3 and 4 years. In a 2007 study of 40 consecutive infected TKAs treated with surgical débridement and parenteral antibiotics at minimum 3-year follow-up, success varied by type of infection.[57] Infection was eradicated in 70% of Segawa type II infections, 50% of type IV, and 0% of type III. Débridement and component retention were recommended for type II and IV infections, and exchange arthroplasty for type III infections. A recent study examined the results of two-stage reimplantation after a failed irrigation and débridement against historic controls for two-stage reimplantation.[58] At 44-month follow-up, 28 of 92 knees (30%) in the irrigation and débridement group failed, and required a second two-stage reimplantation. The two-stage reimplantation failure rate according to the literature was only 9%. It was concluded that irrigation and débridement for periprosthetic knee infection should be avoided. The rate of success for débridement and antibiotic suppression for more sensitive organisms (such as streptococcus) is not reported, but assumed to be better.

One- and Two-Stage Exchange Arthroplasty

Loose components in the setting of acute or chronic total joint infections are best managed with component revision and parenteral antibiotics. A two-stage revision is advantageous because of its good midterm and long-term results, along with the reproducibility of the procedure. One-stage reimplantation describes the removal of an infected TKA with irrigation and débridement and reimplantation of a new TKA during the same surgery. Although much data exist for one-stage exchange for infected THA, there are few data on one-stage exchange for TKA. A literature review detailed 37 infected TKAs treated with one-stage exchange arthroplasty.[59] Infection was controlled in 33 of 37 infected TKAs (89.2%) that were treated with one-stage revision. Factors associated with successful one-stage exchange arthroplasty included infections by gram-positive organisms, absence of sinus formation, aggressive débridement of all infected tissues, use of ALBC for fixation of the new prosthesis, and long-term use of antibiotic therapy. Two of the four failures were in patients with severe rheumatoid arthritis who required corticosteroids.[59] One study reported on 22 infected TKAs treated with one-stage revision.[60] At an average of 10.2 years (range, 1.4 to 19.6 years), 90.9% were free of infection. The wide range of follow-up, however, lessens the applicability of this study.

Two-Stage Revision Arthroplasty

The technique and timing of two-stage revision for the infected TKA is described.[61] In the first stage, the diagnosis of infection is established with removal of the infected implant, infected or devitalized material, and all cement and foreign material. Irrigation and débridement is performed, and an antibiotic-loaded spacer with intramedullary antibiotic-impregnated cement dowels is placed. Intravenous antibiotic therapy for 6 weeks begins after irrigation and débridement. Once the patient has completed a 6-week outpatient course of intravenous antibiotics, the ESR and CRP level are assessed and wound healing is reevaluated. The ESR and CRP level do not need to normalize before reimplantation. However, the values need to trend down sequentially after an antibiotic holiday of at least 3 weeks before aspiration. If cultures from the aspirate are negative, the wound has healed, and the tissues have softened, reimplantation may ensue provided the CRP level and ESR have responded favorably.

During the second stage, intraoperative cultures and frozen sections are sent routinely at the time of reimplantation. Antibiotic-impregnated bone cement is recommended for fixation. Antibiotic therapy is not prolonged after the second stage unless there is a concern about chronic infection that requires chronic antibiotic suppression. If during the second stage there is clinical evidence of ongoing infection and/or the frozen sections are positive for acute inflammation, débridement is repeated with new culture specimens for microbiology, and either the antibiotic spacer is exchanged or a resection is performed.

The survivorship of 96 knees treated with two-stage revision was reportedly 93.5% at 5 years and 85% at 10 years, with reinfection as the end point.[62] In another report on patient function, at 2-year follow-up, patients undergoing revision TKA for infection had 36-item Short Form physical, mental health, and pain scores identical to those of patients with aseptic revisions. The two groups were similar on the Western Ontario and McMaster Universities Osteoarthritis Index functional scale. Infected patients showed improvement in mental health that approached three times that of the noninfected group.[63] If reinfection recurs, it is possible to perform a second two-stage revision. A 2009 study reported on 18 patients with a failed two-stage revision undergoing a second two-stage revision.[64] Infection was eradicated in 14 of 18 patients.

ALBC Spacers

ALBC spacers are useful to stabilize or tension the soft tissues, potentially facilitate the second-stage procedure, and reduce bone loss between stages. ALBC spacers are either static and nonarticulating or articulating in design. The maintenance of appropriate soft-tissue

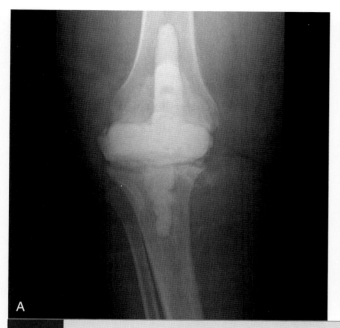
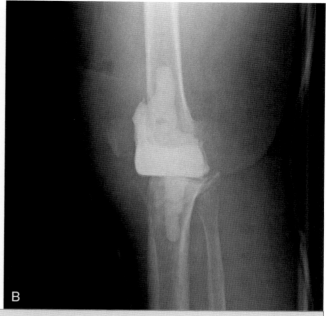

Figure 3   AP (**A**) and lateral (**B**) radiographs showing a static spacer.

tension and joint range of motion may reduce the need for more extensile exposures at the second-stage reimplantation if articulating spacers are used.[65] A recent review of static and mobile antibiotic-impregnated cement spacers used in two-stage exchange arthroplasty demonstrated similar success rates with either type of implant.[66] The authors concluded that more research needs to be conducted to determine the optimum antiobotic spacer in the setting of two-stage exchange arthroplasty.

The original tibiofemoral spacer was preformed in the shape of a disk, L-shaped block, or a disk with a supracondylar separate spacer, inserted loosely into the joint space after the cement had polymerized (**Figure 3**). Limitations of this method include inability to match the shape of the distal femur with the proximal tibia, spacer subluxation with secondary extensor mechanism erosion, wound breakdown, and progressive bone loss.[67] Static spacers are useful in patients with severe soft-tissue complications (such as poor wound healing, open sinus excised, skin necrosis) or bone loss where stability and healing are priority. Advantages of static spacers are immobilization, reduced debris generation, and a concomitant reduction in inflammation. The disadvantage of a static/nonmobile spacer is that it does not allow motion of the joint, which may lead to more scarring of the soft tissues surrounding the knee and may require more extensile exposures at the time of reimplantation. The advantages of mobile cement spacers include the option of allowing an element of physiologic joint motion (**Figure 4**). Mobile articulating spacers may reduce bone loss and preserve function in association with second-stage reimplantation surgery in comparison with static spacers.[63] High doses of antibi-

otics (6 to 8 g), delivered by hand-mixed cement, has been shown to be clinically safe. The use of this high dose is important for the sustained elution of antibiotics at levels that are therapeutic for the pathogenic organisms being treated during the first stage of a two-stage exchange arthroplasty. However, high doses of antibiotics lessen the mechanical characteristics of the cement. Low-dose antibiotic cement (commercially available) is indicated for prophylaxis. It is appropriate for the second stage of two-stage arthroplasty, where optimum mechanical characteristics of the cement are desired.[49] Mobile spacers may be either fabricated in the operating room by the surgeon or prefabricated. Mobile spacers formed in the operating room are inexpensive and provide the option for adjustable antibiotic dosing. Disadvantages of mobile spacers formed in the operating room include additional time to construct the implant in the operating room, a limited number of sizes, and additional cost. The disadvantages of preformed mobile spacers include cost, limitation in implant sizes, antibiotic type, and antibiotic dose. Most preformed spacers often allow delivery of only a single antibiotic agent at a very low dose.

Resection Arthroplasty

Removal of all components with aggressive débridement of all infected tissues without reimplantation of new components or cement spacers defines resection arthroplasty. The indications for resection arthroplasty are inadequate bone and soft tissues, recurrent infections particularly with drug-resistant organisms, and failure of multiple previous attempts at exchange arthroplasty in the setting of a disabled, low-demand patient. The primary disadvantages of this technique are

2: Knee

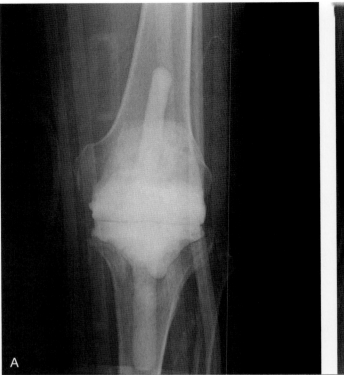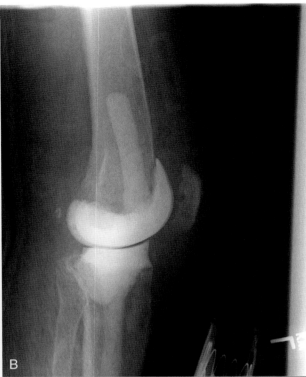

Figure 4   AP (**A**) and lateral (**B**) radiographs showing an articulating spacer.

the frequent occurrence of knee instability with pain during ambulation or transfer, limb-length discrepancy, poor function, and high patient dissatisfaction. The success of eradication of infection has been reported from 50% to 89%.[68,69]

Arthrodesis

Arthrodesis has become less common in North America with the success of two-stage arthroplasty. Knee arthrodesis is indicated in young, high-demand patients and in those with extensor mechanism loss, inadequate bone stock or soft tissue for reimplantation, compromised collateral ligaments, and multiple reinfections particularly with drug-resistant organisms. Disadvantages of arthrodesis include persistent pain, functional limitation, and limb-length inequality. Current methods for arthrodesis include intramedullary nails, double plating, and external fixation. Eighty-five consecutive patients who underwent knee arthrodesis were followed until union, nonunion, amputation, or death occurred. External fixation facilitated successful fusion in 41 of 61 patients and was associated with a 4.9% rate of deep infection. Fusion was successful in 23 of 24 patients with intramedullary nailing and was associated with an 8.3% rate of deep infection. Thirty-four patients (40%) had complications. Knee arthrodesis remains a reasonable salvage alternative for the difficult infected TKA, but the complication rates are high. Intramedullary nailing appears to have a higher rate of successful union but a higher risk of recurrent infection compared with external fixation knee arthrodesis.[70]

Amputation

Above-knee amputation is indicated for recalcitrant TKA infections when all other options have been exhausted. In a review of the Mayo Clinic total joint registry, 67 of 18,443 primary TKAs (0.36%) were eventually followed by above-knee amputation. Thus, the prevalence of above-knee amputations directly related to complications of total knee replacement was 0.14% (25 of 18,443), with uncontrollable infection in 19 knees (76%). After amputation, only nine knees were fitted with a prosthesis. At the time of the last follow-up, only five patients wore the prosthesis for walking. The functional outcome after amputation above a total knee replacement is very poor, and few are able to obtain functional independence.[71]

Summary

Infection in TKA is an infrequent event, but the consequences can be severe. The cost to the patient and health care system is burdensome, and outcomes of revision TKA following infection are not as good as after primary TKA. Although no test is perfect in diagnosing periprosthetic infection, the combination of ESR, CRP level, and joint fluid analysis appears to provide the most accuracy. Despite extended treatment regimens, appropriately treated TKA infection does not preclude an acceptable long-term outcome for the patients.

Annotated References

1. Jämsen E, Huhtala H, Puolakka T, Moilanen T: Risk factors for infection after knee arthroplasty: A register-based analysis of 43,149 cases. *J Bone Joint Surg Am* 2009;91(1):38-47.

   The authors analyzed the Finnish Arthroplasty Register for reoperations related to deep infection and performed an analysis for risk factors. The overall infection rate was 0.90%.

2. Phillips JE, Crane TP, Noy M, Elliott TS, Grimer RJ: The incidence of deep prosthetic infections in a specialist orthopaedic hospital: A 15-year prospective survey. *J Bone Joint Surg Br* 2006;88(7):943-948.

   The authors prospectively followed 4,788 knee arthroplasties, with a 0.86% infection rate. The most common infecting organism was coagulase-negative staphylococcus, followed by *S aureus*. Twenty-nine percent of infections developed during the first 3 months, 35% between 3 months and 1 year, and 36% after 1 year.

3. Suarez J, Griffin W, Springer B, Fehring T, Mason JB, Odum S: Why do revision knee arthroplasties fail? *J Arthroplasty* 2008;23(6, suppl 1)99-103.

   Five hundred sixty-six index revision knee arthroplasties were studied. Of index revisions, 12% failed at an average of 40.1 months. Predominant revision failure modes included infection (46%), aseptic loosening (19%), and instability (13%). Revision knee arthroplasty was more likely to fail in younger patients and in those who underwent polyethylene exchanges. Level of evidence: IV.

4. Chiu FY, Lin CF, Chen CM, Lo WH, Chaung TY: Cefuroxime-impregnated cement at primary total knee arthroplasty in diabetes mellitus: A prospective, randomised study. *J Bone Joint Surg Br* 2001;83(5):691-695.

5. Yang K, Yeo SJ, Lee BP, Lo NN: Total knee arthroplasty in diabetic patients: A study of 109 consecutive cases. *J Arthroplasty* 2001;16(1):102-106.

6. Chesney D, Sales J, Elton R, Brenkel IJ: Infection after knee arthroplasty: A prospective study of 1509 cases. *J Arthroplasty* 2008;23(3):355-359.

   This group prospectively followed 1,509 TKAs for 5 years. The overall deep infection rate was 1%. Coagulase-negative staphylococcus and *S aureus* were the most common isolated organisms. No significant differences were found among age, sex, obesity, rheumatoid arthritis, diabetes, transfusion, or type of TKA.

7. Namba RS, Paxton L, Fithian DC, Stone ML: Obesity and perioperative morbidity in total hip and total knee arthroplasty patients. *J Arthroplasty* 2005;20(7, suppl 3):46-50.

   The authors retrospectively reviewed a prospective registry for outcomes of 1,813 consecutive TKA patients; 52% had a BMI > 30. These patients were significantly younger and had higher rates of diabetes, hypertension, and postoperative infection, particularly with BMI > 35.

8. Winiarsky R, Barth P, Lotke P: Total knee arthroplasty in morbidly obese patients. *J Bone Joint Surg Am* 1998;80(12):1770-1774.

9. Patel VP, Walsh M, Sehgal B, Preston C, DeWal H, Di Cesare PE: Factors associated with prolonged wound drainage after primary total hip and knee arthroplasty. *J Bone Joint Surg Am* 2007;89(1):33-38.

   This is a retrospective observational study of 1,211 primary THAs and 1,226 primary TKAs. Morbid obesity was strongly associated with prolonged wound drainage in the THA group (*P* = 0.001) but not in the TKA group (*P* = 0.590).

10. Amin AK, Patton JT, Cook RE, Brenkel IJ: Does obesity influence the clinical outcome at five years following total knee replacement for osteoarthritis? *J Bone Joint Surg Br* 2006;88(3):335-340.

    A total of 370 consecutive primary TKAs performed for osteoarthritis were followed up prospectively at 6, 18, 36, and 60 months. There was no statistically significant difference between patients with a BMI greater or less than 30 for superficial and deep wound infection, deep venous thrombosis, perioperative mortality, or the number of revisions at 5 years. Level of evidence: IV.

11. Silva M, Luck JV Jr: Long-term results of primary total knee replacement in patients with hemophilia. *J Bone Joint Surg Am* 2005;87(1):85-91.

    The results of 90 primary TKAs performed between 1975 and 2001 in 68 patients with hemophilia were retrospectively reviewed. The overall prevalence of infection was 16%. Level of evidence: IV.

12. Peersman G, Laskin R, Davis J, Peterson M: Infection in total knee replacement: A retrospective review of 6489 total knee replacements. *Clin Orthop Relat Res* 2001;392:15-23.

13. American Academy of Orthopaedic Surgeons: Information Statement: Antibiotic Prophylaxis for Bacteremia in Patients with Joint Replacements. Feb 2009. Accessed September 2009. http://www.aaos.org/about/papers/advistmt/1033.asp.

    This information statement discusses patients at increased risk for hematogenous infection of total joint arthroplasties and what antibiotic prophylaxis is appropriate.

14. Gaston G, Ogden J: Candida glabrata periprosthetic infection: A case report and literature review. *J Arthroplasty* 2004;19(7):927-930.

    A review of the literature on fungal periprosthetic infection is presented. Diagnosis, treatment options, and outcomes of cases are reviewed. Level of evidence: IV.

2: Knee

15. Lee CL, Wei YS, Ho YJ, Lee CH: Postoperative mycobacterium tuberculosis infection after total knee arthroplasty. *Knee* 2009;16(1):87-89.

    The authors describe a case of tuberculosis infection and review the known literature on periprosthetic joint infection with tuberculosis.

16. National Nosocomial Infections Surveillance (NNIS) System: I National Nosocomial Infections Surveillance (NNIS) System Report, data summary from January 1992 through June 2004, issued October 2004. *Am J Infection Control* 2004;32:470-485.

17. Mittal Y, Fehring TK, Hanssen A, Marculescu C, Odum SM, Osmon D: Two-stage reimplantation for periprosthetic knee infection involving resistant organisms. *J Bone Joint Surg Am* 2007;89(6):1227-1231.

    This is a multicenter study reviewing MRSA/MRSE infections. Over a 16-year period, 37 of 263 TKA infections were caused by a resistant organism. All patients were treated with two-stage exchange. Nine (24%) failed with reinfection. The authors recommend two-stage revision for antibiotic-resistant organisms.

18. Parvizi J, Azzam K, Ghanem E, Austin MS, Rothman RH: Periprosthetic infection due to resistant staphylococci: Serious problems on the horizon. *Clin Orthop Relat Res* 2009;467(7):1732-1739.

    The authors examined 127 periprosthetic infections with MRSA/MRSE strains. Two-stage exchange arthroplasty controlled infection in 60% of TKAs, whereas débridement alone controlled only 37% of cases.

19. Segawa H, Tsukayama DT, Kyle RF, Becker DA, Gustilo RB: Infection after total knee arthroplasty: A retrospective study of the treatment of eighty-one infections. *J Bone Joint Surg Am* 1999;81(10):1434-1445.

20. Austin MS, Ghanem E, Joshi A, Lindsay A, Parvizi J: A simple, cost-effective screening protocol to rule out periprosthetic infection. *J Arthroplasty* 2008;23(1):65-68.

    The authors outline a preoperative screening protocol used before revision TKA evaluating sensitivity, specificity, PPV, and NPV. They recommend the combined use to rule out periprosthetic infection.

21. Greidanus NV, Masri BA, Garbuz DS, et al: Use of erythrocyte sedimentation rate and C-reactive protein level to diagnose infection before revision total knee arthroplasty: A prospective evaluation. *J Bone Joint Surg Am* 2007;89(7):1409-1416.

    The authors prospectively examined the statistical characteristics of the preoperative ESR and CRP level in the setting of revision TKA.

22. Mason JB, Fehring TK, Odum SM, Griffin WL, Nussman DS: The value of white blood cell counts before revision total knee arthroplasty. *J Arthroplasty* 2003;18(8):1038-1043.

23. Della Valle CJ, Sporer SM, Jacobs JJ, Berger RA, Rosenberg AG, Paprosky WG: Preoperative testing for sepsis before revision total knee arthroplasty. *J Arthroplasty* 2007;22(6, suppl 2)90-93.

    This study presents results of preoperative testing on 105 revision TKAs, demonstrated excellent sensitivity, specificity, and accuracy of WBC greater than 3,000/mL, and define statistics for ESR and CRP level.

24. Ghanem E, Parvizi J, Burnett RS, et al: Cell count and differential of aspirated fluid in the diagnosis of infection at the site of total knee arthroplasty. *J Bone Joint Surg Am* 2008;90(8):1637-1643.

    Synovial fluid from 429 knees was analyzed finding > 1,100 $WBC/10^{-3}cm^3$ and > 64% for the polymorphonuclear differential to have sensitivity, specificity, PPV, and NPV of 90.7, 88.1, 87.2, 91.5 and 95.0, 94.7, 91.6, and 96.9, respectively. Diagnostic accuracy increased when either or both positive/negative tests were combined with the positive/negative ESR or CRP level.

25. Bauer TW, Parvizi J, Kobayashi N, Krebs V: Diagnosis of periprosthetic infection. *J Bone Joint Surg Am* 2006;88(4):869-882.

    A literature review of diagnostic modalities for periprosthetic infection, including preoperative screening and testing, intraoperative testing, and newer techniques such as polymerase chain reaction examination is presented. Level of evidence: II.

26. Levitsky KA, Hozack WJ, Balderston RA, et al: Evaluation of the painful prosthetic joint: Relative value of bone scan, sedimentation rate, and joint aspiration. *J Arthroplasty* 1991;6(3):237-244.

27. Scher DM, Pak K, Lonner JH, Finkel JE, Zuckerman JD, Di Cesare PE: The predictive value of indium-111 leukocyte scans in the diagnosis of infected total hip, knee, or resection arthroplasties. *J Arthroplasty* 2000;15(3):295-300.

28. Joseph TN, Mujtaba M, Chen AL, et al: Efficacy of combined technetium-99m sulfur colloid/indium-111 leukocyte scans to detect infected total hip and knee arthroplasties. *J Arthroplasty* 2001;16(6):753-758.

29. Kwee TC, Kwee RM, Alavi A: FDG-PET for diagnosing prosthetic joint infection: Systematic review and metaanalysis. *Eur J Nucl Med Mol Imaging* 2008;35(11):2122-2132.

    A meta-analysis with final review of 11 studies and 635 combined hip and knee prostheses is presented. A wide range of reported sensitivity and specificity was found, with varying proportions of hip and knee infections. Pooled estimates revealed a sensitivity of 82.1% and a specificity of 86.6%.

30. Mirra JM, Amstutz HC, Matos M, Gold R: The pathology of the joint tissues and its clinical relevance in prosthesis failure. *Clin Orthop Relat Res* 1976;117:221-240.

31. Feldman DS, Lonner JH, Desai P, Zuckerman JD: The role of intraoperative frozen sections in revision total joint arthroplasty. *J Bone Joint Surg Am* 1995;77(12):1807-1813.

32. Lonner JH, Desai P, Dicesare PE, Steiner G, Zuckerman JD: The reliability of analysis of intraoperative frozen sections for identifying active infection during revision hip or knee arthroplasty. *J Bone Joint Surg Am* 1996;78(10):1553-1558.

33. Fehring TK, McAlister JA Jr: Frozen histologic section as a guide to sepsis in revision joint arthroplasty. *Clin Orthop Relat Res* 1994;304:229-237.

34. Della Valle CJ, Scher DM, Kim YH, et al: The role of intraoperative Gram stain in revision total joint arthroplasty. *J Arthroplasty* 1999;14:500-504.

35. Morgan PM, Sharkey P, Ghanem E, et al: The value of intraoperative Gram stain in revision total knee arthroplasty. *J Bone Joint Surg Am* 2009;91(9):2124-2129.

   The intraoperative Gram stain was found to have poor sensitivity and a poor NPV, and its results did not alter the treatment of any patient undergoing revision TKA for suspected infection. These data suggest a much more limited role for this test.

36. Howe CR, Gardner GC, Kadel NJ: Perioperative medication management for the patient with rheumatoid arthritis. *J Am Acad Orthop Surg* 2006;14:544-551.

   The authors note improvements in the treatment of rheumatoid arthritis with disease-modifying antirheumatic drugs; however, surgery is sometimes needed to reduce pain and improve function. Perioperative management of drug regimens is necessary to optimize surgical outcome.

37. Mangram AJ, Horan TC, Pearson ML, Silver LC, Jarvis WR, Centers for Disease Control and Prevention (CDC) Hospital Infection Control Practices Advisory Committee: Guideline for prevention of surgical site infection, 1999. *Am J Infect Control* 1999;27(2):97-134.

38. Tanner J, Woodings D, Moncaster K: Preoperative hair removal to reduce surgical site infection. *Cochrane Database Syst Rev* 2006;2:CD004202.

   A meta-analysis and literature review of preoperative hair removal, examining 11 randomized controlled trials, is presented. The authors found no differences in surgical site infections among patients who have had hair removed prior to surgery or on the day of surgery. Both clipping and depilatory creams result in fewer surgical site infections than shaving using a razor. Level of evidence: II.

39. Darouiche RO, Wall MJ Jr, Itani KM, et al: Chlorhexidine-alcohol versus Povidone-iodine for surgical-site antisepsis. *N Engl J Med* 2010;362(1):18-26.

   A total of 849 subjects undergoing clean-contaminated surgery were randomized to preoperative skin preparation with either chlorhexidine-alcohol scrub or povidone-iodine scrub and paint. The overall rate of surgical site infection was significantly lower in the chlorhexidine-alcohol group than in the povidone-iodine group (9.5% versus 16.1%; *P* = 0.004).

40. Ostrander RV, Botte MJ, Brage ME: Efficacy of surgical preparation solutions in foot and ankle surgery. *J Bone Joint Surg Am* 2005;87(5):980-985.

   A prospective randomized study was done to evaluate 125 consecutive patients undergoing surgery of the foot and ankle. Of the three solutions tested, 2% chlorhexidine gluconate and 70% isopropyl alcohol was most effective for eliminating bacteria from the forefoot prior to surgery, when comparing cultures obtained from the surgical site. Level of evidence: I.

41. US Department of Health and Human Services National Institutes of Health: NIH Consensus Statement on Total Knee Replacement. December 2003. Accessed December 22, 2009. http://consensus.nih.gov/2003/2003TotalKneeReplacement117html.htm.

   A consensus statement on TKA research and developments from the National Institutes of Health is presented.

42. American Academy of Orthopaedic Surgeons: Information Statement: Recommendations for the use of intravenous antibiotics in primary total joint replacement. June 2004. Accessed December 22, 2009. http://www.aaos.org/about/papers/advistmt/1027.asp.

   This Website is an information statement from the AAOS recommending type, dosage, timing, and duration of intravenous antibiotics for total joint arthroplasty.

43. AlBuhairan B, Hind D, Hutchinson A: Antibiotic prophylaxis for wound infections in total joint arthroplasty: A systematic review. *J Bone Joint Surg Br* 2008;90(7):915-919.

   The literature for antibiotic prophylaxis is reviewed, resulting in a meta-analysis of seven studies (3,065 participants) demonstrating antibiotic prophylaxis reduced the absolute risk of wound infection by 8% and the relative risk by 81% compared with no prophylaxis (*P* < 0.00001).

44. Lidwell OM, Lowbury EJ, Whyte W, Blowers R, Stanley SJ, Lowe D: Effect of ultraclean air in operating rooms on deep sepsis in the joint after total hip or knee replacement: A randomised study. *Br Med J (Clin Res Ed)* 1982;285(6334):10-14.

45. Ritter MA: Operating room environment. *Clin Orthop Relat Res* 1999;369:103-109.

46. Namba RS, Chen Y, Paxton EW, Slipchenko T, Fithian DC: Outcomes of routine use of antibiotic-loaded cement in primary total knee arthroplasty. *J Arthroplasty* 2009;24(6, suppl)44-47.

   Infection rates were compared in patients undergoing TKA with ALBC and regular cement. A total of

2: Knee

22,889 primary TKAs were performed, with 2,030 cases (8.9%) using ALBC. The rate of deep infection was 1.4% for ALBC TKA (28 cases) and 0.7% (154 cases) with regular cement (*P* = 0.002).

47. Chiu FY, Chen CM, Lin CF, Lo WH: Cefuroxime-impregnated cement in primary total knee arthroplasty: A prospective, randomized study of three hundred and forty knees. *J Bone Joint Surg Am* 2002; 84(5):759-762.

48. Chiu FY, Lin CF: Antibiotic-impregnated cement in revision total knee arthroplasty: A prospective cohort study of one hundred and eighty-three knees. *J Bone Joint Surg Am* 2009;91(3):628-633.

   At an average of 89 months postoperatively, no deep infection had developed in 93 knees with vancomycin cement, whereas a deep infection had developed in 6 of the 90 knees (7%) with regular cement. This difference was significant (*P* = 0.0130).

49. Jiranek WA, Hanssen AD, Greenwald AS: Antibiotic-loaded bone cement for infection prophylaxis in total joint replacement. *J Bone Joint Surg Am* 2006;88(11): 2487-2500.

   The use of ALBC for prophylaxis against infection is not indicated for patients not at high risk for infection in routine cemented primary TKA. The mechanical properties are superior in commercially mixed ALBC over hand-mixed ALBC. Low doses of antibiotic in commercially mixed ALBC is used in second-stage revision TKA, whereas high-dose, hand-mixed ALBC is used for active infection.

50. Saleh K, Olson M, Resig S, et al: Predictors of wound infection in hip and knee joint replacement: Results from a 20 year surveillance program. *J Orthop Res* 2002;20(3):506-515.

51. Rao N, Crossett LS, Sinha RK, Le Frock JL: Long-term suppression of infection in total joint arthroplasty. *Clin Orthop Relat Res* 2003;414:55-60.

52. Marculescu CE, Berbari EF, Hanssen AD, Steckelberg JM, Osmon DR: Prosthetic joint infection diagnosed postoperatively by intraoperative culture. *Clin Orthop Relat Res* 2005;439:38-42.

   The authors present a retrospective analysis of 16 cases of type 1 infections treated with various regimens of intravenous and oral antibiotics. The 5-year survival rate (free of treatment failure) for the 16 cases was 89%. Level of evidence: IV.

53. Barrack RL, Aggarwal A, Burnett RS, et al: The fate of the unexpected positive intraoperative cultures after revision total knee arthroplasty. *J Arthroplasty* 2007; 22(6, suppl 2):94-99.

   The authors performed a retrospective examination of 41 positive intraoperative cultures in revision TKA; of these, 29 (71%) had a single positive intraoperative culture and were determined to be a probable false-positive, of which 24 were not treated and none of which manifested any sign of infection at follow-up.

The authors concluded that single positive intraoperative culture after revision TKA does not mandate further treatment in the absence of any other signs of infection.

54. Deirmengian C, Greenbaum J, Lotke PA, Booth RE Jr, Lonner JH: Limited success with open debridement and retention of components in the treatment of acute Staphylococcus aureus infections after total knee arthroplasty. *J Arthroplasty* 2003;18(7, suppl 1):22-26.

55. Bradbury T, Fehring TK, Taunton M, et al: The fate of acute methicillin-resistant *Staphylococcus aureus* periprosthetic knee infections treated by open debridement and retention of components. *J Arthroplasty* 2009;24(6, suppl):101-104.

   This multicenter retrospective study identified 19 patients with acute periprosthetic MRSA knee infections managed by open débridement and retention of components and at least 4 weeks of postoperative intravenous vancomycin therapy. At minimum follow-up of 2 years, the treatment failed to eradicate the infection in 16 patients (84% failure rate).

56. Morrey BF, Westholm F, Schoifet S, Rand JA, Bryan RS: Long-term results of various treatment options for infected total knee arthroplasty. *Clin Orthop Relat Res* 1989;248(248):120-128.

57. Chiu FY, Chen CM: Surgical débridement and parenteral antibiotics in infected revision total knee arthroplasty. *Clin Orthop Relat Res* 2007;461:130-135.

   The authors report the long-term outcomes with one type of treatment strategy for all types of TKA infection, finding it to be most successful in type II and without success in type III.

58. Sherrell JC, Fehring TK, Odum S, et al: The Chitranjan Ranawat Award: Fate of two-stage reimplantation after failed irrigation and débridement for periprosthetic knee infection. *Clin Orthop Relat Res* 2011;469: 18-25.

   The authors determinded the rerevision rate as a result of infection that occurred after two-stage reimplantation to address failed irrigation and débridement of an infected TKA. Level of evidence: III, therapeutic study.

59. Silva M, Tharani R, Schmalzried TP: Results of direct exchange or debridement of the infected total knee arthroplasty. *Clin Orthop Relat Res* 2002;404:125-131.

60. Buechel FF: The infected total knee arthroplasty: Just when you thought it was over. *J Arthroplasty* 2004; 19(4, suppl 1):51-55.

   In 22 infected TKAs treated with a one-stage revision and followed for an average of 10.2 years (range, 1.4 to 19.6 years), 90.9% were free of recurrent infection. Knee scores averaged 79.5, with 85.7% good or excellent results.

61. Burnett RS, Kelly MA, Hanssen AD, Barrack RL, Barrack R: Technique and timing of two-stage exchange for infection in TKA. *Clin Orthop Relat Res* 2007;

464:164-178.

The authors perform a literature review and describe a method of two-stage exchange with the associated methods, complications, and success rate.

62. Haleem AA, Berry DJ, Hanssen AD: Mid-term to long-term followup of two-stage reimplantation for infected total knee arthroplasty. *Clin Orthop Relat Res* 2004; 428:35-39.

A retrospective analysis of 96 knees undergoing a two-stage reimplantation for treatment of an infected TKA demonstrated at final follow-up that 15 knees (16%) required reoperation. Nine knees (9%) had component removal for reinfection, and six knees (6%) were revised for aseptic loosening.

63. Fehring TK, Odum S, Calton TF, Mason JB: Articulating versus static spacers in revision total knee arthroplasty for sepsis: The Ranawat Award. *Clin Orthop Relat Res* 2000;380:9-16.

64. Azzam K, McHale K, Austin M, Purtill JJ, Parvizi J: Outcome of a second two-stage reimplantation for periprosthetic knee infection. *Clin Orthop Relat Res* 2009;467(7):1706-1714.

The authors describe a series of patients undergoing a second two-stage revision TKA for infection, demonstrating acceptable Knee Society scores and eradication of infection in 14 of 18 patients.

65. Durbhakula SM, Czajka J, Fuchs MD, Uhl RL: Antibiotic-loaded articulating cement spacer in the 2-stage exchange of infected total knee arthroplasty. *J Arthroplasty* 2004;19(6):768-774.

An antibiotic-loaded articulating cement spacer was used in the two-stage exchange of 24 infected TKAs. Twenty-two patients (92%) underwent a successful two-stage exchange. The antibiotic-loaded articulating cement spacer preserved knee function between stages, resulting in effective treatment of infection, facilitation of reimplantation, and improved patient satisfaction.

66. Jacobs C, Christensen C, Berend ME: Static and mobile antibiotic-impregnated cement spacers for the management of prosthetic joint infection. *J Am Acad Orthop Surg* 2009;17:356-367.

The authors discuss the advantages of mobile spacers in comparison with static cement spacers.

67. Calton TF, Fehring TK, Griffin WL: Bone loss associated with the use of spacer blocks in infected total knee arthroplasty. *Clin Orthop Relat Res* 1997;345: 148-154.

68. Falahee MH, Matthews LS, Kaufer H: Resection arthroplasty as a salvage procedure for a knee with infection after a total arthroplasty. *J Bone Joint Surg Am* 1987;69(7):1013-1021.

69. Wasielewski RC, Barden RM, Rosenberg AG: Results of different surgical procedures on total knee arthroplasty infections. *J Arthroplasty* 1996;11(8):931-938.

70. Mabry TM, Jacofsky DJ, Haidukewych GJ, Hanssen AD: Comparison of intramedullary nailing and external fixation knee arthrodesis for the infected knee replacement. *Clin Orthop Relat Res* 2007;464:11-15.

Intramedullary nailing and external fixation were compared for knee arthrodesis. Intramedullary nailing demonstrated a better fusion rate but higher complication rate compared with external fixation.

71. Sierra RJ, Trousdale RT, Pagnano MW: Above-the-knee amputation after a total knee replacement: Prevalence, etiology, and functional outcome. *J Bone Joint Surg Am* 2003;85(6):1000-1004.

2: Knee

Section 3

Hip

SECTION EDITORS:
ANDREW H. GLASSMAN, MD, MS
MICHAEL TANZER, MD, FRCSC

Implications of Female Sex/Osteoporosis on Femoral Implant Selection and Restoration of Biomechanics of the Hip

Venessa A. Stas, HonBSc, MD, FRCSC   Jesse E. Templeton, MD   Wayne G. Paprosky, MD

Introduction

Although total hip arthroplasty (THA) has proved to be one of the most successful procedures in orthopaedics, many authors have recognized sex-related disparities related to procurement of treatment and clinical outcomes.[1] The prevalence of degenerative joint disease of the hip is higher among women; however, women who are appropriate surgical candidates are less likely than men to undergo THA.[2] There is evidence in the literature to suggest that women tend to delay surgical intervention until a more advanced stage in their disease course; this behavior may be related to increased willingness to accept disability, apprehension regarding the risks of surgery, and the desire to avoid disruption of normal family and social roles.[3] These findings have been corroborated by studies examining preoperative functional capacity, which have confirmed increased pain with activities, decreased walking distances, and greater use of ambulatory aids among women.[1,4] These sex-based differences persisted after adjustment for age, medical comorbidities, sociodemographic variables, and other clinical characteristics.[3,4]

Compared with males, females patients have demonstrated significantly lower physical performance measure scores in the immediate postoperative period, as well as poorer functional status (for example, decreased walking distance and stair climbing capacity) in the intermediate and long-term periods.[5,6]

Overall revision rates after THA have not been shown to differ between men and women.[7] Nevertheless, sex has been shown to influence the profiles of specific intraoperative and postoperative complications. In one reported series, 74% of intraoperative femoral fractures occurred in females (female:male ratio of 2.9:1).[8] This increased incidence of intraoperative femoral fractures may be a reflection of thinner cortices and decreased intraosseous dimensions in female femora.[8-12] Rates of postoperative dislocation and revision for instability are also significantly higher among women.[7,13] Early postoperative dislocations are twice as common in females and have been attributed to mechanical factors such as cup malposition and inadequate femoral offset.[13] Late dislocations are four times more common in females and may be related to poor soft-tissue integrity.[13] Clinically significant limb-length discrepancies and lateral trochanteric pain after THA have been reported more commonly among women.[14,15]

Although sex-based disparities in outcomes for THA have been recognized, the reasons for these differences have not been fully elucidated. There is compelling evidence to implicate sexual dimorphism in native acetabular and femoral anatomy, as well as sex-specific changes in proximal femoral geometry related to osteoporosis and aging. These insights have been derived from the literature of orthopaedics, forensics, and anthropology.

Sexual Dimorphism in Native Acetabular and Femoral Anatomy

Acetabular anatomy is closely associated with femoral head size and sphericity, as well as morphology of the femoral neck (**Table 1**). Mean acetabular diameter is

Dr. Paprosky or an immediate family member has received royalties from Wright Medical Technology and Zimmer; is a member of a speakers' bureau or has made paid presentations on behalf of Zimmer; is a paid consultant for or is an employee of Zimmer; has received research or institutional support from Rush University; and serves as a board member, owner, officer, or committee member of the Bone and Joint Decade, USA and the Hip Society. Neither of the following authors nor any immediate family member has received anything of value from or owns stock in a commercial company or institution related directly or indirectly to the subject of this chapter: Dr. Stas and Dr. Templeton.

3: Hip

Table 1

Comparison of Acetabular Anatomy Between Adult Females and Males

Parameter	Study	Population	Females*	Males*	P Value†	Comments
Diameter (mm)	Papaloucas et al[16] (2008)	Greek, deceased	49.1 ± 2.7	55.7 ± 2.7	< 0.00001	↓ in females
	Köhnlein et al[17] (2009)	Swiss, deceased	47.5 ± 2.7	54.0 ± 2.8	< 0.00001	
Depth (mm)	Papaloucas et al[16] (2008)	Greek, deceased	20.4 ± 1.9	24.2 ± 2.2	< 0.00001	↓ in females
Depth of articular surface	Köhnlein et al[17] (2009)	Swiss, deceased	-	-	< 0.033	↓ in females at cranial acetabulum and adjacent to acetabular notch
Width of acetabular notch	Köhnlein et al[17] (2009)	Swiss, deceased	-	-	0.00007	↑ in females
Offset	Purkait[18] (2003)	Indian, deceased	-	-	-	More lateral and anterior in females
Anteversion (°)	Köhnlein et al[17] (2009)	Swiss, deceased	21.7 ± 6.6	17.0 ± 4.7	0.013	↑ in females (via direct rim measurements)
Inclination (°)	Köhnlein et al[17] (2009)	Swiss, deceased	49.8 ± 4.1	48.1 ± 4.1	NS	No difference

*All values presented as mean ± standard deviation.
†Statistical significance defined as $P \leq 0.05$.
NS = not significant.

significantly decreased among women (48 to 49 ± 3 mm) compared with men (54 to 56 ± 3 mm).[16,17] The female acetabulum is relatively shallow, and the depth of the articular surface is decreased in the vicinity of the cranial acetabulum and adjacent to the wide acetabular notch.[16,17] The female acetabulum demonstrates greater lateral and anterior offset, increased anteversion on direct rim measurements (22° ± 7° versus 17° ± 5° among males, $P < 0.013$), and similar abduction (50° ± 4°) compared with the male acetabulum.[17,18]

Femoral Anatomy

Mean femoral head diameter is decreased by 5 to 7 mm in females, which corresponds with sex-related differences in acetabular diameter[9,16-19] (Table 2). Femoral head height, defined as the vertical distance between the femoral head center and the midportion of the lesser trochanter, is approximately 5 mm lower in females than in males.[9] Females also exhibit significantly lower femoral offset, with an average deficit of 7 mm.[9]

Femoral neck lengths are, on average, 3 to 5 mm shorter in women than in men.[12,20] The female femoral neck is also characterized by a narrow outer diameter and thin cortices.[10,12] Similar femoral neck-shaft angles have been reported from cadaver series analyzing women and men of similar age.[9]

The cortices of the intertrochanteric region are thinner in women than in men, and this thinness is more pronounced at the calcar femorale.[10,12] The outer diam-

eter in this region is narrower in females than in males.[12]

The trend toward a relative decrease in outer diameter and cortical thickness is also observed along the female diaphysis.[9,10] The anterior bow of the femoral diaphysis is less pronounced in females (8.2° ± 0.4° versus 10.5° ± 0.6° in males, $P < 0.01$).[9] The isthmus, defined as the narrowest portion of the intramedullary canal, has a more proximal location in women.[9] Whereas the anterior-posterior diameter of the isthmus is similar in males and females, the medial-lateral diameter of the isthmus is slightly decreased and the canal less tapered in females.[9,10]

Classification of Proximal Femoral Morphology

Variation in proximal femoral morphology (Table 3) has been described qualitatively by the Dorr classification and quantitatively by the canal flare index (CFI).[9,21] Three femoral types have been identified based on AP and lateral plain radiographs of the hip; demographic and histomorphometric factors have been characterized for each type.[21] The CFI is defined as the ratio of the intracortical diameter (measured 20 mm proximal to the geometric center of the lesser trochanter) divided by the canal width of the isthmus.[9]

Type A femora (Figure 1) are distinguished by funnel-shaped or "champagne flute" proximal femoral geometry, as well as a narrow canal diameter at the

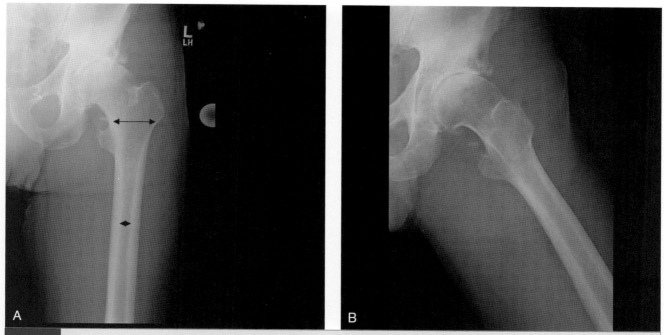

Figure 1   **A** and **B**, Radiographic views of a Dorr type A femur in a 50-year-old man. Thick, dense cortices with a well-defined endosteal surface are seen. Arrows in **A** indicate that the diaphyseal canal is funnel-shaped proximally and narrow at the isthmus (CFI = 4.8).

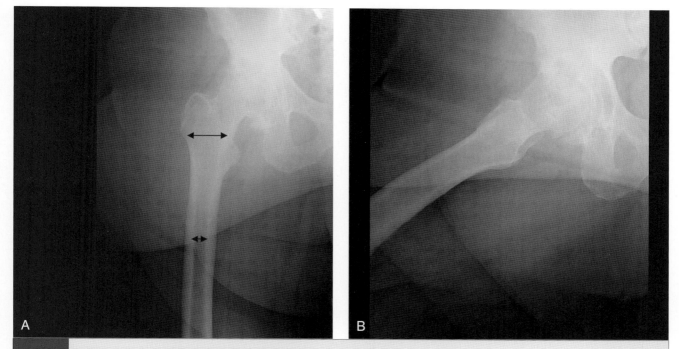

Figure 2   **A** and **B**, Radiographic views of a Dorr type B femur in a 55-year-old man. Arrows in **A** indicate increased diaphyseal intramedullary width at the isthmus (CFI = 3.5) and relatively thin posterior cortices.

isthmus (corresponding with a CFI greater than 4.7).[9,21] Diaphyseal cortices are thick and the endosteal surface well defined.[21] These patients predominantly tend to be male and relatively young, and have a higher body weight.[21]

Type B femora (**Figure 2**) demonstrate intermediate canal diameter (corresponding with a CFI between 3.0 and 4.7), relatively thin medial and posterior cortices, and a scalloped or striated endosteal surface.[9,21] Male predominance is noted but less pronounced with type B

3: Hip

Table 2

Comparison of Femoral Anatomy Between Adult Females and Males

Parameter	Study	Population
Femoral Head		
Diameter (mm)	Noble et al[9] (1995)	North American, deceased, > 60
	Mall et al[19] (2000)	German, deceased
	Purkait[18] (2003)	Indian, deceased
	Papaloucas et al[16] (2008)	Greek, deceased
Head height (mm)	Noble et al[9] (1995)	North American, deceased, > 60
Medial femoral head offset (mm)	Noble et al[9] (1995)	North American, deceased, > 60
Femoral Neck		
Outer diameter (mm)	Peacock et al[10] (1998)	Caucasian, ≥ 60
	Yates et al[12] (2007)	≥ 72
Length (mm)	Nelson et al[20] (2000)	African American and Caucasian, postmenopausal (≥ 50)
	Yates et al[12] (2007)	≥ 72
Cortical thickness (mm)	Yates et al[12] (2007)	≥ 72
Femoral neck-shaft angle (°)	Noble et al[9] (1995)	North American, deceased, > 60
	Noble et al[9] (1995)	North American, deceased, 40-60
	Nelson et al[20] (2000)	African American and Caucasian, postmenopausal (≥ 50)
Intertrochanteric Region		
Outer diameter (mm)	Yates et al[12] (2007)	≥ 72
Cortical thickness (mm)	Yates et al[12] (2007)	≥ 72
Calcar femorale thickness (mm)	Peacock et al[10] (1998)	Caucasian, ≥ 60
Femoral Diaphysis		
Outer diameter (mm)	Noble et al[9] (1995)	North American, deceased, > 60
	Peacock et al[10] (1998)	Caucasian, ≥ 60
Canal width, proximal to lesser trochanter (mm)	Noble et al[9] (1995)	North American, deceased, > 60
Canal width, at isthmus (mm)	Noble et al[9] (1995)	North American, deceased, > 60
	Peacock et al[10] (1998)	Caucasian, ≥ 60
Anterior bow angle (°)	Noble et al[9] (1995)	North American, deceased, > 60
Isthmus position (mm)	Noble et al[9] (1995)	North American, deceased, > 60
Cortical thickness (mm)	Peacock et al[10] (1998)	Caucasian, ≥ 60

NS = not significant; ML = mediolateral; AP = anteroposterior.
*All values presented as mean ± standard deviation, unless otherwise specified.
† Statistical significance defined as $P \leq 0.05$.
‡ Values presented as mean +/– standard error.

(male to female ratio 2:1) compared with type A femora (male to female ratio 9:1).[21]

In contrast, type C or "stovepipe" femora (Figure 3) are predominantly seen in older (postmenopausal) women with lower body weight.[21] Hallmarks include cortical thinning, expansion of the intramedullary canal, a CFI less than 3.0, and an irregular endosteal surface.[9]

Implications of Aging on Femoral Anatomy

Bones have both periosteal and endosteal (endocortical, trabecular, and intracortical) surfaces. Periosteal bone formation defines the cross-sectional area of the bone, whereas endocortical bone formation or resorption determine cortical thickness.[22] During the aging process in both sexes, periosteal bone formation is slowed. When coupled with endosteal resorption, there is net bone

Table 2

Comparison of Femoral Anatomy Between Adult Females and Males (continued)

Females*	Males*	P Value†	Comments
42.8 ± 0.8	49.8 ± 0.4	< 0.001	↓ in females
44 ± 3	49 ± 3	< 0.005	
38 ± 2	44 ± 3	< 0.0001	
41.6 ± 1.9	48.5 ± 2.3	< 0.0001	
47.7 ± 1.2	53.0 ± 1.1	< 0.05	↓ in females
42.8 ± 0.8	49.8 ± 0.4	< 0.05	↓ in females
32.6 ± 3.3	37.7 ± 2.8	< 0.001	↓ in females
30.0 ± 0.1‡	32.7 ± 0.2‡	< 0.001	↓ in females
43.7 ± 5.4	-	-	No difference between African American and Caucasian women
46.8 ± 0.4‡	52.3 ± 0.5‡	< 0.001	↓ in females
1.3 ± 0.01‡	1.4 ± 0.02‡	< 0.001	↓ in females
124.4 ± 1.0	123.4 ± 1.2	NS	No difference
128.3 ± 1.4	125.5 ± 1.1	NS	No difference
131.4 ± 4.5	-	-	No difference between African American and Caucasian women
53.7 ± 0.02‡	56.7 ± 0.03‡	< 0.0001	↓ in females
2.5 ± 0.03‡	3.1 ± 0.06‡	< 0.0001	↓ in females
5.5 ± 1.3	7.1 ± 1.9	< 0.001	↓ in females
26.6 ± 0.6	29.4 ± 0.5	< 0.01	↓ in females
32.8 ± 2.7	37.9 ± 3.0	< 0.001	
42.7 ± 0.9	48.2 ± 0.9	< 0.001	↓ in females
12.3 ± 0.4 (ML)	13.0 ± 0.4 (ML)	< 0.01	ML diameter ↓ in females
16.3 ± 0.5 (AP)	16.3 ± 0.5 (AP)	NS	No difference in AP diameter
14.7 ± 2.5 (ML)	15.7 ± 2.5 (ML)	< 0.001	
8.2 ± 0.4		< 0.01	↓ in females
114.9 ± 2.9	127.8 ± 4.0	< 0.001	More proximal in females
9.06 ± 1.34	11.1 ± 1.4	< 0.001	↓ in females

loss and widening of both periosteal and endocortical diameters.[12] The net amount of bone loss in men is less than in women because periosteal apposition is greater in men.[23]

Two major components of bone strength are bone mass and bone structure, both of which can be measured by noninvasive methods. Bone mass at the hip is measured by dual-energy x-ray absorptiometry (DEXA) to give values of bone mineral density (BMD) and bone mineral content (BMC). Measurements are taken from multiple sites in the proximal femur (femoral neck, greater trochanter, the Ward triangle, femoral shaft, total upper femur).[10] BMD and BMC can be used to estimate fracture predication and disease/treatment effects. Bone structure, represented by the architectural arrangement of cortical and cancellous bone and by the size and shape of the proximal femur, is assessed by radiographs and/or from images obtained by DEXA. Structural variables that can be measured include cortical thickness, femoral and medullary width, width of the

Table 3

Classification of Proximal Femoral Morphology

Parameter	Type A	Type B	Type C
Proximal femoral geometry	Funnel shaped ("champagne flute")	N/A	"Stovepipe"
Canal width at the isthmus	Narrow	Intermediate	Wide
Canal flare index	> 4.7	3.0 - 4.7	< 3.0
Diaphyseal cortical thickness	Thick medial, lateral, and posterior cortices (1.70 ± 0.30 mm)	Thin medial and posterior cortices (0.95 ± 0.10 mm)	Very thin medial and posterior cortices (0.50 ± 0.08 mm)
Endosteal surface	Sharp, well-defined	Scalloped or striated posteriorly	Irregular and/or poorly defined
Common patient characteristics	Younger Higher body weight	N/A	Older (postmenopausal) Lower body weight
Sex distribution	Males > females (9:1)	Males > females (2:1)	Females > males (7:3)

N/A = not applicable.
(Adapted from Dorr LD, Faugere M, Mackel AM, Gruen TA, Bognar B, Malluche HH: Structural and cellular assessment of bone quality of proximal femur. *Bone* 1993;14:231-242.)
(Adapted from Noble PC, Box GG, Kamaric E, Fink MJ, Alexander JW, Tulos HS: The effect of aging on the shape of the proximal femur. *Clin Orthop Relat Res* 1995;316:31-44.)

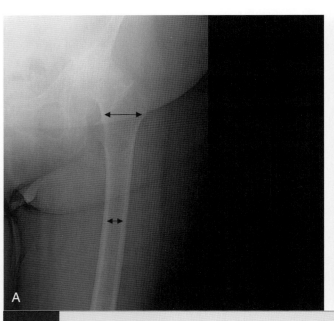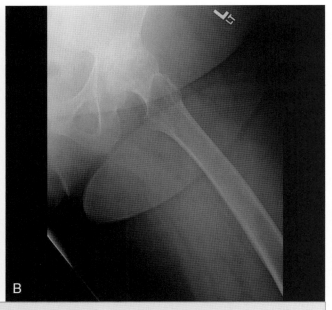

Figure 3 **A** and **B**, Radiographic views of a Dorr type C femur in a 76-year-old woman. The characteristic "stovepipe" appearance is seen. Arrows in **A** indicate manifestation of decreased cortical thickness and increased diaphyseal intramedullary diameter (CFI = 2.9).

femoral head and neck, hip and femoral axis length, Singh grade, and center of mass of the femoral neck.[10]

Bone mass is negatively related to age and positively related to height and weight in both women and men. Women have diminished BMD and BMC compared with men. Age-related loss of bone mass occurs at all sites in both sexes.[10]

Although similarities exist, there are significant sex differences in hip structural geometry, and the differ-

ences increase with advancing age.[10,12] At the femoral neck and intertrochanteric regions of the femur, cross-sectional area, outer diameter, cortical thickness, and section modulus are all statistically significantly lower in females than in males even after adjustment for age, height, and weight.[12] At the level of the femoral shaft, males have wider periosteal diameters than females because of greater periosteal rather than endocortical apposition in the peripubertal period.[24]

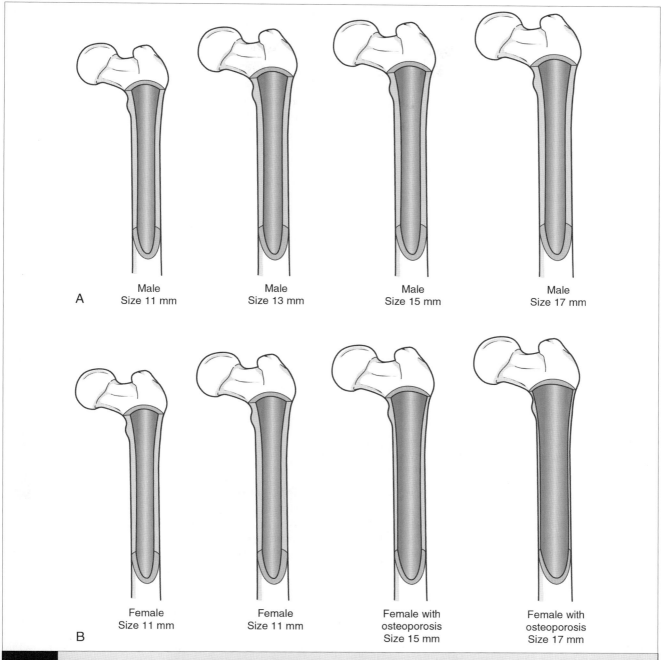

Figure 4 In men (**A**) and in women without osteoporosis (**B**), intraosseous and extraosseous dimensions of the femur increase proportionally. In females with osteoporosis, there is intraosseous enlargement of the femoral canal, without corresponding extraosseous enlargement, resulting in wider canals with thinner cortices.

Unlike men, who show significant aging differences only at the femoral neck, women reveal a consistent and progressively worsening pattern of hip structural geometry at the femoral neck, intertrochanteric region, and femoral shaft with increasing age.[12] Statistically significant changes in men older than 85 years compared with men in their early 70s show increased outer diameter and reduced cortical thickness at the femoral neck. Statistically significant changes in women of the same age groups show reduced outer diameter and cortical thickness at the femoral neck with aging.[12] According to one study,[12] women showed changes in the intertrochanteric region with aging as evidenced by a reduced cross-sectional area and cortical thickness, whereas males did not. In contrast, another study showed no age-related differences in the intertrochanteric region in both women and men.[9]

Bone structure measurements that involve the femo-

3: Hip

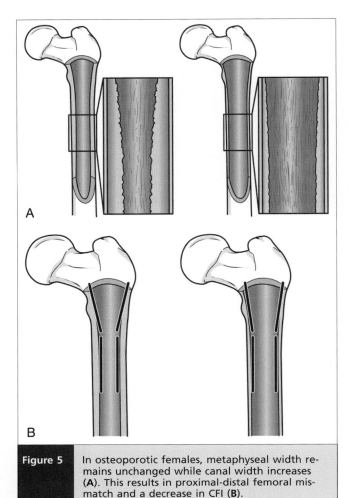

Figure 5 In osteoporotic females, metaphyseal width remains unchanged while canal width increases (**A**). This results in proximal-distal femoral mismatch and a decrease in CFI (**B**).

Osteoporosis

Osteoporosis is defined as a decrease in bone mass and alteration of microarchitecture leading to increased bone fragility.[25] Osteoporosis is diagnosed when BMD is reduced by 2.5 standard deviations below the mean value for young normal individuals (T score <−2.5).[26] Although both women and men lose bone minerals during aging, the effect is more profound in women, and is accelerated because of the rapid decline in estrogen during menopause.[27] Approximately 25% of postmenopausal white women with advanced osteoarthritis scheduled to undergo THA meet the World Health Organization's criterion for osteoporosis.[28]

In most men and in women without osteoporosis, the intraosseous dimensions of the femur increase proportionally with the extraosseous dimensions. Osteoporosis causes intraosseous femoral canal enlargement without the corresponding proportional extraosseous enlargement, resulting in wider canals with thinner cortices[29] (**Figure 4**).

Furthermore, in men, metaphyseal width increases proportionally as canal width increases. In osteoporotic women, metaphyseal width remains relatively unchanged as canal width increases, resulting in a proximal-distal femoral mismatch and a decrease in CFI[29] (**Figure 5**).

Osteoporosis has a significant impact on preoperative planning for THA. Osteoporosis and Dorr type C bone are relative contraindications for the use of proximally coated uncemented prostheses.[30] Fully porous-coated uncemented implants, cemented stems, and impaction grafting are often chosen in osteoporotic individuals.

The risk of intraoperative complications, such as periprosthetic femur fracture, is increased in females and with older age and is confounded by osteoporosis.[31,32] Some have suggested the use of temporary cerclage wires before preparation of the osteoporotic femoral canal for an uncemented prosthesis.[33] Osteoporosis also increases the likelihood of postoperative stress shielding, thigh pain, and femoral fracture.[34-36]

Because of the significant variability among female hips, a classification system was devised specifically for female hips, dividing them into six categories based on stature, neck-shaft angle, degree of osteoporosis, canal diameter, metaphyseal width, and head height/offset[29] (**Table 4**). This classification system helps to emphasize the differences among female hips and serves as an alert for potential pitfalls that can be encountered when using traditional implants. It serves as a guide for implant selection to improve outcomes for females undergoing THA.

ral shaft cortex width and medullary width show a substantial difference between aging men and women. In men, there is no change in shaft cortical thickness or medullary width with age; however, in women, shaft cortical thickness is strongly age related and decreases because of the expanding medullary width.[9,10]

Diaphyseal expansion in females with aging is the main factor influencing the change in cross-sectional shape of the femur. The CFI was found to be the largest in the young female group (age 40 to 60 years) corresponding to a champagne-fluted canal shape (CFI = 4.49), whereas significantly smaller values were observed in older female femora (CFI = 3.86) corresponding to a stovepipe canal shape. Males did not show this trend of proximal flare reduction with aging.[9]

Aging affects the femoral neck-shaft angle in women and men. Both women and men experience slight varus inclination of 3° with age (40 to 60 years old versus 60 to 90 years old) without any difference between sexes.[9]

With aging, the height of the femoral head above the lesser trochanter decreases in females but does not change in males.[9]

Table 4

Female Hip Types

	Type 1	Type 2	Type 3	Type 4	Type 5	Type 6
Stature	Tall	Tall	Short	Short	Short	Short
Neck Angle (°)	135	> 135	135	135	125	125
Osteoporosis	+/–	+/–	–	+	––	+
Canal Diameter (mm)	11-16	11-16	11-14	13-20	11-13	13-20
Metaphysis	Progressive	Progressive	Progressive	Reduced	Progressive	Reduced
Head Height/Offset	Progressive	Nonprogressive	Progressive	Reduced	Progressive	Reduced

(Adapted from Hartman CW, Gilbert BJ, Paprosky WG: Gender issues in total hip arthroplasty: Length, offset, and osteoporosis. *Semin Arthroplasty* 2009;20(1):62-65.)

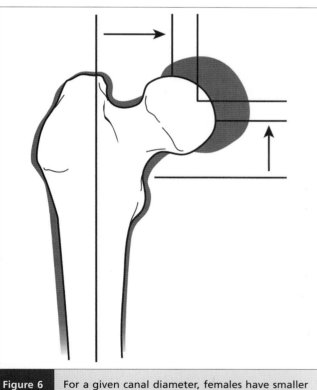

Figure 6 For a given canal diameter, females have smaller metaphyses, lower head heights, and less femoral offset.

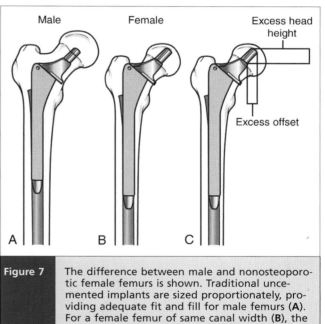

Figure 7 The difference between male and nonosteoporotic female femurs is shown. Traditional uncemented implants are sized proportionately, providing adequate fit and fill for male femurs (**A**). For a female femur of same canal width (**B**), the offset may be too large and the head height too high (**C**).

3: Hip

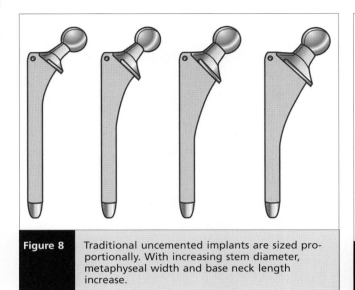

Figure 8 Traditional uncemented implants are sized proportionally. With increasing stem diameter, metaphyseal width and base neck length increase.

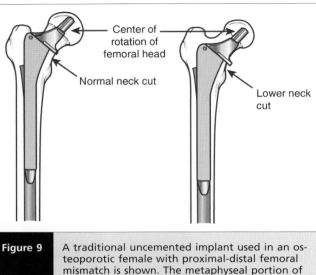

Figure 9 A traditional uncemented implant used in an osteoporotic female with proximal-distal femoral mismatch is shown. The metaphyseal portion of the implant impinges against the medial femoral cortex, remaining proud (**A**). To accommodate the larger implant metaphysis, a lower neck cut can be made, allowing the implant to seat more distally (**B**).

Restoration of Hip Biomechanics and Implant Selection

With canal diameter as the independent variable, females have smaller metaphyses, lower head heights, and less femoral offset[29] (**Figure 6**). The female hip averages 3° more anteversion than the male hip.[37]

Traditional uncemented implants are sized proportionally, providing adequate fit and fill for male femurs. Using a traditional uncemented implant in a female of similar canal width, the head height and offset may be too high, resulting in leg lengthening and nonanatomic offset (**Figure 7**). In one study,[14] 4 of 21 revisions for limb-length discrepancy were in females with proud femoral components or nonanatomic offset. Leg lengthening is the most common reason for litigation against the orthopaedic community.[38] It seems that increasing femoral offset would lead to trochanteric bursitis, but no study to date has found a statistically significant correlation.[15]

In men, extraosseous and intraosseous dimensions increase proportionally (**Figure 4**). Therefore, as the diaphyseal dimensions increase, metaphyseal width and neck length increase accordingly.[29] Traditional uncemented implants are sized proportionally, meaning that metaphyseal width and base neck length increase with stem diameter (**Figure 8**).

Both aging and osteoporosis have a significant impact on the geometry of the female femur. Whereas there is essentially no change in the size of the metaphysis proximal to the lesser trochanter with aging, at the level of the femoral isthmus, osteoporotic female bones expand to such an extent that they are of similar size compared with male femora.[9] The reduction of proximal flare corresponds to a change from a Dorr type A or B to type C femur. This proximal-distal femoral mismatch has a significant implication for choice of femoral prosthesis design.

Cementless fixation relies on direct apposition of the prosthesis to the endosteal surface. Biologic incorporation is maximized when the proximal and distal contour of the prosthetic component match the corresponding dimensions of the medullary cavity.[9] Traditional uncemented implants are made to fit a Dorr type A or B femur. If this implant is used in an older, osteoporotic female with proximal-distal femoral mismatch and a wide diaphysis (Dorr type C), the use of a larger traditional stem with its coexistent larger metaphyseal portion would appear oversized proximally, impinge against the medial femoral cortex at the level of the femoral neck osteotomy site (increasing the risk of proximal femur fracture), remain proud, and result in an inappropriate increase in leg length and offset.[9,29] To accommodate the differences in the older female femur, the surgeon may make intraoperative adjustments, such as a lower neck cut, in an attempt to reduce the amount of limb-length discrepancy and increased offset (**Figure 9**).

An ideal femoral prosthesis for an older female with osteoporosis would not only have less offset and head height, but would have less metaphyseal flare to accommodate the stovepipe type of femur. If this implant were used in a younger female without osteoporosis, the use of a smaller stem to fit the diaphysis would result in inadequate metaphyseal fill unless the femur was excessively reamed to expand the medullary canal, effectively converting the young femur type to an old one.[9]

An ideal female femoral stem is one with a smaller metaphysis, shorter head height, smaller offset, and more anteversion. Enlarging stem size would not result in a proportional increase in base neck length or metaphyseal size. Custom-made prostheses are an option, but these are expensive and production is time-consuming. Modular components are a viable alternative and allow for independent fit of the metaphyseal and diaphyseal areas, resulting in a semi–custom-made device. Modularity does come at a cost: implants are more expensive and component interface stress and micromotion can lead to fretting, wear debris, and, ultimately, loss of junctional mechanical integrity.[39] Implant variety is currently the gold standard option. Implants with reduced neck length, low head center, low offset options, and anteverted stems are available.

Summary

Although there are small sex-related differences in acetabular morphology, the main sexual dimorphism is seen in the geometry of the proximal femur. Women have smaller metaphyses, shorter head heights, smaller offset, and increased anteversion. One must be cognizant of these differences when performing THA with traditional implants so as not to increase leg length and offset.

Unlike aging in males where there are no changes in metaphyseal or femoral shaft geometry, aging and osteoporosis in females result in relative preservation of metaphyseal width but significant endosteal enlargement at the isthmus, resulting in proximal-distal femoral mismatch. Traditional implants assume proportional increases in base neck length and metaphyseal width with increasing canal size. When used in women with osteoporosis and large canals, traditional implants cause metaphyseal impingement, leading to proud placement of the component and resultant leg lengthening and nonanatomic increased offset. Sex-specific femoral stems with smaller metaphyses and shorter base neck lengths would be ideal for women, especially those with osteoporosis. There is a significant difference between the hips of men and women that should not be ignored in implant selection in THAs.

Annotated References

1. Holtzman J, Saleh K, Kane R: Gender differences in functional status and pain in a Medicare population undergoing elective total hip arthroplasty. *Med Care* 2002;40(6):461-470.

2. Hawker GA, Wright JG, Coyte PC, et al: Differences between men and women in the rate of use of hip and knee arthroplasty. *N Engl J Med* 2000;342(14):1016-1022.

3. Karlson EW, Daltroy LH, Liang MH, Eaton HE, Katz JN: Gender differences in patient preferences may underlie differential utilization of elective surgery. *Am J Med* 1997;102(6):524-530.

4. Katz JN, Wright EA, Guadagnoli E, Liang MH, Karlson EW, Cleary PD: Differences between men and women undergoing major orthopedic surgery for degenerative arthritis. *Arthritis Rheum* 1994;37(5):687-694.

5. Röder C, Parvizi J, Eggli S, Berry DJ, Müller ME, Busato A: Demographic factors affecting long-term outcome of total hip arthroplasty. *Clin Orthop Relat Res* 2003;417:62-73.

6. Kennedy DM, Hanna SE, Stratford PW, Wessel J, Gollish JD: Preoperative function and gender predict pattern of functional recovery after hip and knee arthroplasty. *J Arthroplasty* 2006;21(4):559-566.

   Multiple variables were evaluated as predictors of recovery after total hip and knee arthroplasty in 152 patients. Sex ($P < 0.003$) and preoperative score ($P < 0.001$) were found to be significant predictors of postoperative physical performance measure scores.

7. Kostamo T, Bourne RB, Whittaker JP, McCalden RW, MacDonald SJ: No difference in gender-specific hip replacement outcomes. *Clin Orthop Relat Res* 2009;467(1):135-140.

   The authors compared implant survivorship, clinical outcomes, revision rates, and sizing/offset differences between men and women in 4,114 primary THAs at minimum 2-year follow-up. Survivorship and revision rates were not found to be significantly different between men and women. Level of evidence: II.

8. Schwartz JT Jr, Mayer JG, Engh CA: Femoral fracture during non-cemented total hip arthroplasty. *J Bone Joint Surg Am* 1989;71(8):1135-1142.

9. Noble PC, Box GG, Kamaric E, Fink MJ, Alexander JW, Tullos HS: The effect of aging on the shape of the proximal femur. *Clin Orthop Relat Res* 1995;316(316):31-44.

10. Peacock M, Liu G, Carey M, et al: Bone mass and structure at the hip in men and women over the age of 60 years. *Osteoporos Int* 1998;8(3):231-239.

11. Moroni A, Faldini C, Piras F, Giannini S: Risk factors for intraoperative femoral fractures during total hip replacement. *Ann Chir Gynaecol* 2000;89(2):113-118.

12. Yates LB, Karasik D, Beck TJ, Cupples LA, Kiel DP: Hip structural geometry in old and old-old age: Similarities and differences between men and women. *Bone* 2007;41(4):722-732.

    The authors evaluated hip structural geometry to determine sex-based differences in men and women older than 72 years.

13. Morrey BF: Difficult complications after hip joint replacement: Dislocation. *Clin Orthop Relat Res* 1997;344:179-187.

14. Parvizi J, Sharkey PF, Bissett GA, Rothman RH, Hozack WJ: Surgical treatment of limb-length discrepancy

3: Hip

following total hip arthroplasty. *J Bone Joint Surg Am* 2003;85(12):2310-2317.

15. Iorio R, Healy WL, Warren PD, Appleby D: Lateral trochanteric pain following primary total hip arthroplasty. *J Arthroplasty* 2006;21(2):233-236.

    The incidence of lateral trochanteric pain (LTP) after THA was reported at 4.4% (6.2% among women). Female sex ($P < 0.04$) and direct lateral approach ($P < 0.01$) were associated with LTP. Limb-length discrepancy and femoral offset were not associated with LTP.

16. Papaloucas C, Fiska A, Demetriou T: Sexual dimorphism of the hip joint in Greeks. *Forensic Sci Int* 2008; 179(1):83.e1-83.e3.

    Two hundred pelvic and femoral bones (100 male, 100 female) with mean age of 63 to 65 years were measured in this anatomic study. Comparison of male and female geometry demonstrated significant differences in acetabular diameter, acetabular depth, and femoral head diameter ($P < 0.00001$ for all).

17. Köhnlein W, Ganz R, Impellizzeri FM, Leunig M: Acetabular morphology: Implications for joint-preserving surgery. *Clin Orthop Relat Res* 2009;467(3):682-691.

    Measurements were performed on 66 acetabula (16 female, 42 male) of similar age. Reported findings included decreased acetabular diameter ($P < 0.00001$), increased acetabular anteversion ($P < 0.013$), and shallower acetabula in females.

18. Purkait R: Sex determination from femoral head measurements: A new approach. *Leg Med (Tokyo)* 2003; 5(Suppl 1):S347-S350.

19. Mall G, Graw M, Gehring KD, Hubig M: Determination of sex from femora. *Forensic Sci Int* 2000;113(1-3):315-321.

20. Nelson DA, Barondess DA, Hendrix SL, Beck TJ: Cross-sectional geometry, bone strength, and bone mass in the proximal femur in black and white postmenopausal women. *J Bone Miner Res* 2000;15(10): 1992-1997.

21. Dorr LD, Faugere MC, Mackel AM, Gruen TA, Bognar B, Malluche HH: Structural and cellular assessment of bone quality of proximal femur. *Bone* 1993; 14(3):231-242.

22. Seeman E: Pathogenesis of bone fragility in women and men. *Lancet* 2002;359(9320):1841-1850.

23. Duan Y, Turner CH, Kim BT, Seeman E: Sexual dimorphism in vertebral fragility is more the result of gender differences in age-related bone gain than bone loss. *J Bone Miner Res* 2001;16(12):2267-2275.

24. Seeman E: Clinical review 137: Sexual dimorphism in skeletal size, density, and strength. *J Clin Endocrinol Metab* 2001;86(10):4576-4584.

25. Peck WA, Burkhardt P, Christiansen C: Consensus development conference: Diagnosis, prophylaxis, and treatment of osteoporosis. *Am J Med* 1993;94(6):646-650.

26. Kanis JA, Melton LJ III, Christiansen C, Johnston CC, Khaltaev N: The diagnosis of osteoporosis. *J Bone Miner Res* 1994;9(8):1137-1141.

27. Ahlborg HG, Johnell O, Nilsson BE, Jeppsson S, Rannevik G, Karlsson MK: Bone loss in relation to menopause: A prospective study during 16 years. *Bone* 2001;28(3):327-331.

28. Glowacki J, Hurwitz S, Thornhill TS, Kelly M, LeBoff MS: Osteoporosis and vitamin-D deficiency among postmenopausal women with osteoarthritis undergoing total hip arthroplasty. *J Bone Joint Surg Am* 2003; 85(12):2371-2377.

29. Hartman CW, Gilvert BJ, Paprosky WG: Gender issues in total hip arthroplasty: Length, offset, and osteoporosis. *Semin Arthroplasty* 2009;20(1):62-65.

    The authors explore anatomic differences between males and females and the effect of these differences on reconstructing leg length and offset in THA. A classification system describing six female femoral subtypes is presented.

30. LaPorte DM, Mont MA, Hungerford DS: Proximally porous-coated ingrowth prostheses: Limits of use. *Orthopedics* 1999;22(12):1154-1162.

31. Franklin J, Malchau H: Risk factors for periprosthetic femoral fracture. *Injury* 2007;38(6):655-660.

    A review of the etiologies for late periprosthetic femoral fractures is presented. The implications of age, sex, index diagnosis, and compromised bone quality (osteoporosis) are specifically addressed.

32. Davidson D, Pike J, Garbuz D, Duncan CP, Masri BA: Intraoperative periprosthetic fractures during total hip arthroplasty: Evaluation and management. *J Bone Joint Surg Am* 2008;90(9):2000-2012.

    The authors review risk factors for intraoperative periprosthetic femoral fractures. It is noted that certain risk factors, including female sex and increased age, may be confounded by the presence of osteoporosis.

33. Martell JM, Pierson RH III, Jacobs JJ, Rosenberg AG, Maley M, Galante JO: Primary total hip reconstruction with a titanium fiber-coated prosthesis inserted without cement. *J Bone Joint Surg Am* 1993;75(4): 554-571.

34. Moreland JR, Bernstein ML: Femoral revision hip arthroplasty with uncemented, porous-coated stems. *Clin Orthop Relat Res* 1995;319(319):141-150.

35. Engh CA, Bobyn JD, Glassman AH: Porous-coated hip replacement: The factors governing bone ingrowth, stress shielding, and clinical results. *J Bone Joint Surg Br* 1987;69(1):45-55.

36. Wu CC, Au MK, Wu SS, Lin LC: Risk factors for post-operative femoral fracture in cementless hip arthroplasty. *J Formos Med Assoc* 1999;98(3):190-194.

37. Jain AK, Maheshwari AV, Nath S, Singh MP, Nagar M: Anteversion of the femoral neck in Indian dry femora. *J Orthop Sci* 2003;8(3):334-340.

38. Hofmann AA, Skrzynski MC: Leg-length inequality and nerve palsy in total hip arthroplasty: A lawyer awaits! *Orthopedics* 2000;23(9):943-944.

39. Patel A, Bliss J, Calfee RP, Froehlich J, Limbird R: Modular femoral stem-sleeve junction failure after primary total hip arthroplasty. *J Arthroplasty* 2009;24(7): 1143.e1-1143.e5.

Three cases of stem-sleeve junction failure in primary THA are presented. The authors conclude that stresses at modular component interfaces may result in a sequence of micromotion, production of wear debris, and catastrophic failure.

3: Hip

Chapter 18

Total Hip Arthroplasty in Unusual Medical and Surgically Challenging Conditions

Steven J. MacDonald, MD, FRCSC   Javad Parvizi, MD   Elie Ghanem, MD   Dana C. Mears, MD, PhD

Total Hip Arthroplasty for Developmental Dysplasia
Steven J. MacDonald, MD, FRCSC

Developmental dysplasia of the hip (DDH) is one of the most complex scenarios faced by reconstructive surgeons when performing a primary total hip arthroplasty (THA). It has been long understood, and recently confirmed with large databases, that DDH is the most common hip pathology that leads to secondary coxarthrosis.[1,2]

The term DDH represents a broad spectrum of a disease process. Case presentation can range from a minimally dysplastic acetabulum with mild femoral head uncoverage to a complete hip dislocation with the femoral head articulating with the ilium. Many classification systems have been developed[3,4] primarily based on the position of the femoral head relative to the true acetabulum. These classification systems have been demonstrated to be reliable and reproducible.[5]

Dr. MacDonald or an immediate family member has received royalties from DePuy; serves as a paid consultant for or is an employee of DePuy; has received research or institutional support from DePuy, Smith & Nephew, and Stryker; and serves as a board member, owner, officer, or committee member for The Knee Society. Dr. Parvizi or an immediate family member serves as a paid consultant for or is an employee of Biomet, Covidien, National Institutes of Health (NIAMS & NICHD), Salient Surgical, Smith & Nephew, Stryker, TissueGene, and Zimmer; has received research and institutional support from 3M, Musculoskeletal Transplant Foundation, National Institutes of Health (NIAMS & NICHD), Stryker, and Zimmer; and serves as a board member, owner, officer, or committee member for the American Association of Hip and Knee Surgeons, American Board of Orthopaedic Surgery, British Orthopaedic Association, CD Diagnostics, The Hip Society, Orthopaedic Research and Education Foundation, the Orthopaedic Research Society, SmartTech, and United Healthcare. Neither of the following authors nor a member of their immediate families has received anything of value from or owns stock in a commercial company or institution related directly or indirectly to the subject of this chapter: Dr. Ghanem and Dr. Mears.

There may be anatomic abnormalities of multiple structures. Acetabular deficiency, in various degrees, is the most obvious finding. The acetabulum itself is often poorly developed and has a much smaller diameter than normally seen, with a thin anterior and relatively thicker posterior column. Changes commonly found on the femoral side include increased femoral anteversion, a valgus femoral neck, metaphyseal-diaphyseal mismatch, and posterior positioning of the greater trochanter. The soft-tissue structures are also often involved, with the hip capsule and multiple muscles being tight and shortened, creating a more difficult exposure. Neurovascular structures (profunda femoris artery, femoral nerve, sciatic nerve) are at an increased risk of injury during a THA for DDH, and excessive leg lengthening (> 4 cm) must be avoided.

Preoperative Planning

Preoperative planning begins with a complete and detailed physical examination with documentation of any soft-tissue contractures and assessment of true and apparent limb-length discrepancies. Standard radiographs should include an AP view of both the pelvis and the hip, as well as a lateral view of the hip. Judet views or a CT scan may help in evaluating acetabular bone stock.

On the acetabular side, the templating and planning should have the acetabular component ideally placed in the location of the true acetabulum. Acetabular component coverage will determine the requirement for any bone grafting. If greater than 30% of the component is uncovered, normally autogenous femoral head will be used to augment this deficiency. Commonly the acetabular component will be a smaller diameter (< 50 mm) and preoperative planning for the various bearing options (for example, metal on highly cross-linked polyethylene of adequate thickness, ceramic on ceramic, ceramic on polyethylene) available for that proposed cup must occur (**Figure 1**).

On the femoral side, planning must include addressing issues of increased femoral anteversion, a narrower

3: Hip

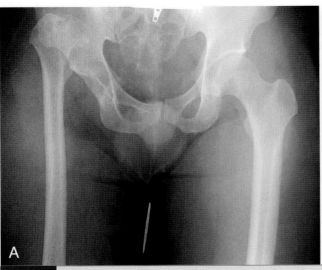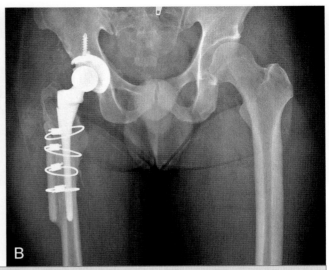

Figure 1 **A**, Preoperative radiograph of a 50-year-old man with DDH. **B**, Radiograph 1 year postoperatively demonstrating a healed subtrochanteric osteotomy (augmented with a strut graft), with a modular femoral component and a small (44-mm) acetabular component (26-mm head on highly cross-linked polyethylene).

diaphysis relative to the metaphysis, posterior location of the greater trochanter, and the potential need for a femoral shortening osteotomy. Component selection options include cemented, cementless nonmodular, and cementless modular stems. Cementless modular stems are particularly useful in the DDH application by providing a decoupling of the metaphyseal and diaphyseal portions of the components and allowing for anteversion orientation independent of the femoral anatomy. If a femoral shortening osteotomy is performed, cementless components prevent cement extravasation into the osteotomy site.

Surgical Considerations

THA in a patient with DDH presents several challenges related to THA, including exposure, the potential need for an extensile approach, bone stock deficiency, component selection and positioning, leg lengthening, offset restoration, and hip stability. Regardless of the approach used, the surgeon must understand the interplay of decisions and how they affect each other. The decision to place the acetabular component in the true acetabulum in a patient with high-riding DDH will create challenges on limb lengthening and increase the potential need for a femoral shortening osteotomy. The decision to slightly medialize the acetabular component to improve component coverage will create less offset in the reconstruction and increase the potential need for an offset femoral component.

Standard approaches to the hip can be used for mild to moderate dysplasia (Crowe I, II, and III); however, for severe dysplasia an approach that is extensile should be performed. The transtrochanteric approach,[6]

a trochanteric slide, or a subtrochanteric osteotomy[7,8] have all been described. The subtrochanteric osteotomy offers the advantages of shortening and derotation simultaneously. A trochanteric osteotomy is avoided, thereby preserving the abductor sleeve in continuity, and the femoral metaphysis is intact, facilitating cementless femoral component fixation. The use of both modular and nonmodular cementless femoral components has been described in combination with a subtrochanteric osteotomy.

The acetabular component should ideally be located in the true acetabulum, which will commonly have the best host bone stock. Positioning of the component in a more superior location, a so-called high hip center, has also been advocated, although this may be associated with an increased incidence of acetabular and femoral component loosening.[9] Once the true acetabulum is located, careful exposure and identification of both anterior and posterior columns and the inferior border of the acetabulum must be performed. Although the bone stock in this location is commonly of maximal volume, it may also be relatively osteopenic because of lack of direct loading in a patient with high-riding DDH. Reaming must proceed slowly, and dedicated smaller-sized reamers are commonly required. The final acetabular component size is often less than 50 mm. The medial wall will be thinned by the reaming procedure, and often intentionally slightly perforated, to maximize coverage of the acetabular component. Acetabular reamings can be placed medially before cup insertion for bone grafting of the medial deficiency (**Figure 1**). A portion of the acetabular component can be left uncovered superolaterally; however, with larger deficiencies a structural graft using the patient's own resected femoral head is recommended.

Good long-term results using both cemented and cementless acetabular components have been reported.[10-12] Component loosening has been more commonly seen with cemented reconstructions and issues with polyethylene wear and osteolysis with cementless series. Although the long-term fate of autogenous femoral head grafts in patients with DDH undergoing THA has been variable, a recent series has demonstrated excellent survivorship.[13]

Historically, cemented narrow straight stems (so-called CDH stems) or custom stems were commonly used. These were often coupled with the technique of a higher hip center and progressive removal of proximal femoral bone, thereby creating a more cylindrical shape to the femur until a reduction of the construct could be achieved. Alternate reconstructive techniques currently are used, and stem selection is often based on surgeon preference, quality of host bone, degree of femoral deformities present, and the need for a femoral osteotomy. Modular cementless stems offer several advantages as discussed previously, but also introduce the theoretic concerns of fretting wear, corrosion, and fracture. Published reports using different modular design systems in DDH cases have been promising.[14,15]

THA, when performed for DDH, is usually associated with a rise in complications such as postoperative dislocation, nerve injury, and implant-related failures such as aseptic loosening, polyethylene wear, and osteolysis. These complications are increased relative to the severity of the dysplasia. Procedurally related complications, such as trochanteric nonunion, osteotomy site nonunion or delayed union, abductor weakness, femoral perforation, or fracture, also occur.

Recent publications[16,17] have challenged the premise that patients undergoing THA for DDH have poorer implant survivorship than those with osteoarthritis. Two registry-based database reviews found no differences in revision risk when adjustments for age and implants were performed. This is encouraging and may demonstrate the benefits of newer techniques, implants, and materials in these challenging cases.

Classification Systems
Javad Parvizi, MD
Elie Ghanem, MD

The severity of hip dysplasia varies widely, ranging from cases of shallow acetabuli to completely dislocated hips. Several classifications have been proposed for DDH in adults that are helpful during preoperative planning and useful academically for comparing the results of different studies. An objective method to measure the degree of subluxation that organized dysplastic hips into four groups according to increasing severity of dysplasia has been described in the literature.[3] The amount of proximal femoral head migration is calculated on an AP radiograph of the pelvis by measuring the vertical distance between the inter-teardrop line and

the femoral head–medial neck junction (Figure 2). The amount of subluxation is the ratio between this distance and the vertical diameter of the undeformed femoral head. In the presence of a deformed contralateral head (not unusual in patients with dysplasia), the predicted femoral head vertical diameter for all practical purposes is 20% of the height of the pelvis as measured from the highest point of iliac crest to the inferior margin of the ischial tuberosity. The investigators compared the vertical distance between the inter-teardrop line and the femoral head–neck junction to the predicted vertical diameter of the femoral head to obtain the degree of dislocation (Table 1).

A simple and effective classification has been described for three distinct types of adult hip dysplasia: dysplasia, low dislocation, and high dislocation[4] (Table 1). With dysplasia, the femoral head, despite some degree of subluxation, is still contained within the original acetabulum. With low dislocation, the femoral head articulates with a false acetabulum that partially covers the true acetabulum. Radiographically, there appear to be two overlapping acetabuli with the inferior part of the false acetabulum being an osteophyte that begins at the level of the superior rim of the true acetabulum. With high dislocation, the femoral head has migrated superiorly and posteriorly. The true acetabulum is inferior and anterior to the depression in the iliac wing with which the femoral head articulates and may have the appearance of a false acetabulum.

Acetabular Reconstruction

Acetabular reconstruction in patients with hip dysplasia is important because it determines the surgical approach used, the type of bone graft needed, and the type of acetabular reconstruction that should be performed. The exposure can be performed through a standard anterolateral or posterolateral approach or with extensile approaches in difficult reconstructions according to the preference of the surgeon, but with a few caveats kept in mind. The gluteus medius split should be performed during an anterolateral approach within the determined safe zone to avoid nerve damage.[18] This safe zone is defined as the distance between the inferior branch of the superior gluteal nerve and the tip of the greater trochanter, which was determined to be 3 cm in all but two severely dysplastic hips (Crowe type III) at the anterior third of the gluteus medius. The authors found that the distance between the superior gluteal nerve and the greater trochanter is influenced by the severity of hip dysplasia, and therefore recommended splitting the posterior portion of the gluteus medius or using a nerve stimulator in high-grade dysplasias.[18]

The key step in acetabular reconstruction in patients with a dysplastic acetabulum is obtaining satisfactory acetabular coverage. The Crowe classification is useful in determining the appropriate type of acetabular reconstruction in patients with hip dysplasia. At each

3: Hip

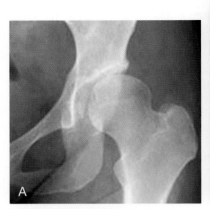
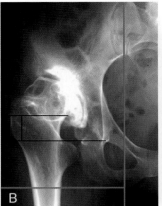
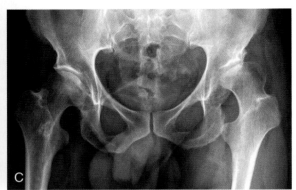
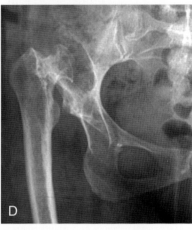

Figure 2 AP radiographs of dysplastic hips graded according to the Crowe classification depending on the severity of superior displacement. **A**, Type I. **B**, Type II. **C**, Type III. **D**, Type IV. The amount of proximal femoral head migration is calculated on an AP pelvis by measuring the vertical distance between the interteardrop line and the femoral head–neck junction (black lines). The predicted vertical femoral head diameter is 20% of the height of the pelvis (red lines).

Table 1

The Degree of Severity of DDH According to the Crowe and Hartofilakidis Classifications

Hartofilakidis Classification	Crowe Type	Percentage of Vertical Diameter of Femoral Head	Percentage of Pelvic Vertical Height
Dysplasia	Type I	< 50%	< 0.1
Low dislocation	Type II	50% -75%	0.1-0.15
	Type III	75% - 100%	0.15-0.2
High dislocation	Type IV	> 100%	> 0.2

level of subluxation, the typical acetabular deformities vary and the reconstruction needs to be planned based on that deformity.

Crowe I

In this cohort of patients, dysplasia of the hip is mild and the bone quality is preserved. Reconstruction in most patients can be done with standard acetabular components placed at the site of the true acetabulum[19] (**Figure 3**). Medial wall thickness can be assessed with a drill and a measuring depth gauge, and medialization can be performed safely to improve coverage of the cup if the need arises.

Crowe II or III

Acetabular deformities present in Crowe types II and III are slightly more challenging to reconstruct because of the marked anterolateral rim deficiency. In these patients, if a standard acetabular component is placed at the site of the true acetabulum, a portion of the component may be left uncovered and therefore unsupported, which can lead to early loosening. Several alternatives exist to achieve primary stability and improve acetabular coverage, including a small cup placed in an anatomic location or high hip center position,[20] bulk femoral head autograft with cement or cementless cup fixation,[21] a medial wall displacement osteotomy,[22]

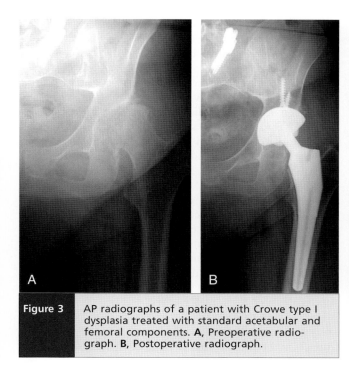

Figure 3   AP radiographs of a patient with Crowe type I dysplasia treated with standard acetabular and femoral components. **A**, Preoperative radiograph. **B**, Postoperative radiograph.

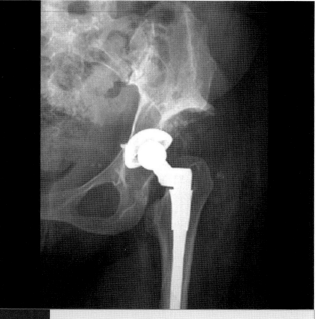

Figure 4   AP radiograph of a patient with low dislocation treated with a small acetabular component (44 mm) and femoral head (22 mm) with a high hip center.

overreaming the medial wall of the acetabulum to obtain better cup coverage,[4,23] or acetabular reinforcement rings.[24]

Small Acetabular Component
Downsizing the acetabular component poses a simple solution that is less technically demanding in the presence of poor acetabular bone stock. Acetabular components with an outside shell diameter of 42 to 46 mm provide excellent long-term results (**Figure 4**). Long-term follow-up on 60 hips with congenital dysplasia treated with small cemented acetabular cups has been reported.[10] The 10- and 25-year survival rates were 97% and 58%, respectively. Recent data support the use of uncemented, small acetabular components fixed with transacetabular screws in Crowe I dysplasia with improved survivorship compared with their cemented counterparts.[14]

Cotyloplasty
Cotyloplasty or socket medialization is another effective method of reducing bone insufficiency. It entails intentionally overreaming or deliberately fracturing the medial wall of the acetabulum to place the acetabular component in the available iliac bone. This technique improves lateral coverage for the component and decreases joint reactive forces by medializing the hip's center of rotation.[4] Although cotyloplasty has shown promising results in the short term, its application has not been without consequences. Intentional violation of the medial acetabular wall may increase intraoperative and postoperative morbidity and compromise the success of later revision surgery; it is also associated with the risk of early acetabular migration into the pelvis.[23]

Medial Wall Displacement Osteotomy
A technique of displacing the circumferential acetabular medial wall via an osteotomy in patients with hip dysplasia who required THA has been described.[22] This technique was developed to medialize the acetabular component toward the optimal center of rotation and to maximize bony coverage. The method preserves medial wall trabecular bone stock and maintains the uniformity of the entire bone floor with the use of standard cementless components.

High Hip Center
Placing the acetabular component superior to its true anatomic location allows the component to be covered more completely by native bone, which facilitates biologic fixation and avoids the need for bone grafting. This alteration in the center of hip rotation is associated with some disadvantages. It has been reported that a high hip center leads to a high rate of dislocation after surgery, limb-length discrepancy, and a limp.[20]

A high hip center dramatically changes the hip biomechanics, which may influence the survival of the THA. Authors of a 2009 study reported that for every millimeter of lateral displacement of the acetabular cup relative to the ideal center of rotation, an increase of 0.7% in hip load should be expected, and for every millimeter of proximal displacement an increase of 0.1% in hip load should be expected.[25] A three-dimensional biomechanics model was used in another study and it was reported that superolateral displacement of the hip center decreased the abductor moment arm by 28%, and this effect could not be overcome by increasing the

3: Hip

neck length of the femoral component.[26] It was suggested that superior and superomedial positioning of the hip center without lateral placement does not have major adverse effects on abduction moment when the neck length is appropriately increased.

However, there is no consensus regarding the long-term survivorship of acetabular components placed at a high hip center, with clinical studies showing contradictory results. One study demonstrated that superior (> 15 mm from its anatomic location) and lateral placement of the acetabular cup is associated with substantially higher rates of loosening and revision of both the acetabular and femoral components.[9] On the other hand, authors of a 2009 study reported no acetabular failures at 15 years of follow-up of porous-coated acetabular components placed more than 20 mm above the teardrop for dysplastic hips (Crowe types I to III).[27]

Acetabular Augmentation With Cement
Cement was previously used to fill the superolateral acetabular defects, but this technique was soon abandoned because long-term follow-up revealed high rates of acetabular component loosening, especially among patients in whom a large quantity of cement is used.[28] Conversely, a 2005 study reported that placing the cup in the anatomic position and using cement rather than bone graft to fill the superolateral bone defect can lead to a durable THA in patients with severe hip dysplasia at a minimum 20-year follow-up. These authors attributed their good outcome to the placement of the hip center at its anatomic position and to the lateralization of the greater trochanter.[11]

Acetabular Augmentation With Bulk Graft
The most common problem encountered with DDH is insufficient acetabular bone coverage, that is, coverage of less than 60% of the cup, which has been shown to compromise the durability of cup fixation.[29] Acetabular augmentation with bulk bone graft seems to be an appealing alternative for reconstruction of the acetabulum in dysplastic hips. The patient's femoral head acts as a source for bulk autograft during index arthroplasty and provides osteoconductive support with the potential for enhanced bone stock if revision surgery is required.[21] Furthermore, bulk grafting has the capacity to restore the anatomic hip center with placement of the acetabular component in a reconstructed "true" acetabulum, which precludes the negative impact of a high hip center on hip biomechanics.[26]

Despite the numerous cited advantages, it is important to examine the long-term outcomes of bulk allografting and autografting. Although early results generally are favorable, with grafts rarely failing during the first 5 years, longer-term results have been discouraging. As the extent of the coverage of the acetabular component by the graft increases, the late failure rates of the component also increase.[30] The authors of this study found that 60% of the cups implanted with autograft or allograft were loose after a mean of 16.5 years.[30] Reconstruction of the acetabulum with an uncemented cup and structural bone graft shows more promising long-term results compared with cemented reconstruction.[31]

Although metallic screws are more commonly used to fix the bulk bone graft to the wing of ilium, concerns have been raised regarding their role in graft absorption and third-body wear with screw pullout. Hence, other biodegradable and biocompatible materials such as poly-L-lactic acid (PLLA) have been introduced in place of metallic and ceramic screws in the fixation of acetabular bone grafts. Stronger bioabsorbable screws made of composites of hydroxyapatite and PLLA have been used to fix the structural bone graft augmentation of the acetabulum in a series of 104 cases of DDH reconstructed using cemented THA.[32] There were no adverse effects including foreign-body inflammatory reaction to the implants, and bony union of the graft was achieved in all cases, with an acetabular component survivorship of 90% at 15 years.

Impaction Bone Grafting
Impaction bone grafting with a cemented cup is another option used to reconstruct the acetabulum at the level of the transverse ligament when massive bone loss is present.[33] In contrast to reconstructions with structural grafts, resorption of the bone graft was not observed at 10- to 15-year follow-up of 28 consecutive dysplastic hips, possibly because the bulk allografts may not fully incorporate, whereas revascularization of the small-fragment grafts used in impaction grafting is easier from the host bone bed.

Acetabular Cage and Ring
Given the high failure rate of bulk bone graft, some authors have recommended using an acetabular reinforcement ring or cage to reconstruct the dysplastic acetabulum.[24]

Cemented Versus Cementless Cups
There is increasing evidence favoring the use of uncemented acetabular components in patient with dysplasia. Long-term follow-up of cemented acetabular cups show high rates of second-decade loosening and the need for acetabular component revision.[28] According to a 2006 study, acetabular revision in cemented cups is associated with younger age and accelerated polyethylene wear.[12] Given that most patients with hip dysplasia undergo THA at a young age, it would seem prudent that press-fit techniques would be more appropriate. Long-term results of uncemented hemispheric acetabular sockets were found to have better outcomes compared with those of their cemented counterparts.[34]

Insufficient bone stock and osseous coverage frequently necessitate inserting acetabular screw fixation to improve the stability of the acetabular cup. Some authors have recommended that fixation should be achieved using at least two secure screws.[35] The safe zone for transacetabular screw fixation in patients with osteoarthritis has been defined as the posterior superior and posterior inferior quadrants.[36] Because the true acetabulum of a hip with a high dislocation is located more anterior and inferior than a nondysplastic hip, screw placement in these safe zones by the quadrant system places the obturator and femoral vessels at risk.[37] The posterior superior safe zone had shifted, and it was recommended that surgeons use multihole cups rather than cluster hole cups to increase their options for screw placement.[37]

Crowe IV

In high-dislocation hips, the best bone to support an acetabular component is at the anatomic hip center because the femoral head lies superiorly and does not erode the anterolateral portion of the true acetabulum. Therefore, in most instances, the acetabulum can be reconstructed using a small acetabular cup at the level of the true acetabulum. The acetabular fovea, teardrop, and transverse ligament can be used as internal landmarks during the reaming process. Most of the socket coverage should be obtained from the posterior column, and careful attention is required to avoid overreaming the anterior and medial walls. The surgeon should also remember that the bone quality in this area is quite soft; to account for this, the last reamers should be used in reverse mode to preserve bone stock by expanding the acetabulum and compacting rather than removing bone.[19]

However, anatomic socket placement can result in a hip that is difficult to reduce, and reduction can be associated with considerable limb lengthening and an increased risk of neurologic traction injury.[3] The traditional method has been to use an osteotomy of the greater trochanter with associated proximal femoral shortening. The osteotomized greater trochanter needs to be advanced and attached to the diaphyseal part of the femur, but this procedure has a high likelihood of nonunion.[38] Additionally, an osteotomy at this level changes the anatomy of the proximal femur that becomes a small straight tube without a metaphyseal flare. An alternative technique is to perform a shortening subtrochanteric osteotomy; this provides the advantages of preserving the proximal femoral anatomy, avoiding the problems associated with reattachment of the greater trochanter, and facilitating a cementless femoral reconstruction in young patients.[39]

Indications and Techniques of Subtrochanteric Osteotomy

If the center of hip rotation is brought down to its normal level or to a nearly normal level, the femur may have to be shortened to avoid nerve injury. Femoral subtrochanteric shortening derotational osteotomy decreases the soft-tissue tension around the hip and the chance of neurovascular injury during lengthening, especially injury to the sciatic nerve with lengthening of more than 4 cm.[7] The exact site of the shortening osteotomy varies according to the patient's anatomy, but

it is generally 8 to 10 cm distal to the tip of the greater trochanter and always distal to the lesser trochanter. Autologous cancellous bone graft can be used at the osteotomy site, whereas cortical autograft struts cut from the resected femoral bone fragment provide additional stabilization.[8] If the osteotomy site is unstable, plate and screw fixation can be applied.

Femoral Reconstruction

The diameter of the femoral canal in dysplastic patients is quite small and will only accept narrow (8- or 9-mm) components. Excessive anteversion may also cause some problems in determining the proper orientation of the femoral component. The canal rotation should be evaluated based on the position of the lesser trochanter.[19] Also, the anteversion of the implanted acetabular component will influence how much anteversion can be accepted on the femoral side without compromising hip stability. It is not difficult to correct femoral component position in cemented implants; however, for cementless implants, it is usually more problematic to obtain the desired femoral component anteversion. When there is more than 40° of anteversion, a corrective rotational osteotomy or a modular implant in which the version of the femoral neck can be varied may be necessary[7] (Figure 5).

In severe cases of dysplasia, the femur loses its metaphyseal flare and the femoral component should be placed in the diaphysis, rather than across the metaphysis and into the diaphysis. The contour of ordinary cemented and uncemented femoral components with metaphyseal and diaphyseal portions do not fit in femurs with this degree of deformity, and attempts to use these components may lead to fracture of the femur. The femoral component needs to be straight without metaphyseal flare, short, and small.[8] Previous subtrochanteric osteotomies make varus or valgus diaphyseal deformities that sometimes need additional osteotomies to restore normal alignment before insertion of femoral components.

Cemented Versus Uncemented Femoral Component

Cemented stems allow the surgeon to deal with moderate degrees of deformity, particularly problems related to the excessive anteversion of the femur.[10] However, serious concerns regarding their long-term longevity have been raised. The probability of survival of a cemented Charnley low-friction femoral component 25 years postoperatively with aseptic loosening as the end point was 60% for patients undergoing THA for hip dysplasia.[40] Hence, uncemented femoral components are appealing because many patients with dysplastic hips undergo THA at a young age. However, nonmodular, proximally coated, uncemented femoral components should be considered only for patients with mild deformity.[19] Extensively coated implants that bypass

3: Hip

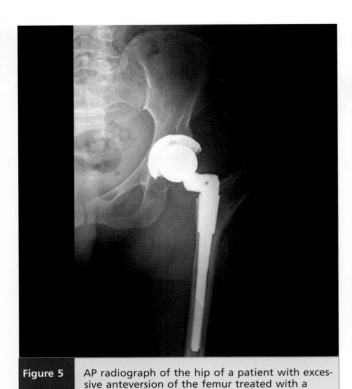

Figure 5 AP radiograph of the hip of a patient with excessive anteversion of the femur treated with a modular stem (S-ROM).

the metaphyseal region and gain distal purchase can be used in the presence of metaphyseal deformities, provided that their metaphyseal cross section is reduced.[8] Modular designs including the S-ROM system (DePuy, Warsaw, IN) allow the surgeon to mix and match metaphyseal and diaphyseal sizes and to achieve optimal implant orientation and anteversion. Authors of a 2009 study used the modular cementless S-ROM system in 28 hips with Crowe III or IV DDH; these hips were revision free at 10-year follow-up with improvement in Medical Outcomes Study 36-Item Short Form and Western Ontario and McMaster Universities Osteoarthritis Index (WOMAC) scores.[41]

Although cemented stems can be used in conjunction with subtrochanteric osteotomies, uncemented femoral stems with extensive porous coating or distal fixation systems are preferable. Twenty-eight consecutive primary THAs for Crowe type IV hip dysplasia were studied.[8] All patients underwent subtrochanteric osteotomy and placement of acetabular component at the level of the true acetabulum and received uncemented femoral and acetabular components. The authors concluded that this technique was associated with high rates of successful implant fixation and healing of the osteotomy site and good functional outcomes. Authors of a 2009 study reported on 20 DDH Crowe type IV hips followed up at 8 years treated with subtrochanteric shortening derotational osteotomy and a cementless porous-coated cylindrical femoral component.[42] No nerve palsies were observed, and bony union to the femoral component was observed in all cases 4 to 6

months after surgery, except one that required revision surgery.

Complications and Outcome

THA performed for a dysplastic hip has been associated with higher complication rates, including increased risk of revision during the first 6-month postoperative period compared with patients undergoing THA for primary osteoarthritis.[16] The rate of hip dislocation in patients with dysplastic hips has varied from 2% to 10%, with some authors attributing this high incidence to the posterolateral approach.[43]

The postoperative functional result of patients with DDH is also believed to be inferior compared with that of patients treated with routine primary THA for osteoarthritis, possibly because of long-standing abductor muscle deconditioning and gait abnormalities.[8] However, it represents a substantial improvement compared with the functional results that were achieved with earlier methods of treatment of this complex problem. On the contrary, no significant difference was found with respect to Harris hip scores or limp between conventional osteoarthritis and those with a Crowe I dysplastic acetabulum.[20] Although the number of complications increased significantly with the severity of DDH, there was no significant difference in Harris hip score or limp as the Crowe types progressed from II to IV.

Reconstruction of the acetabulum still represents a major challenge, and the incidence of complications and poor results appears to correlate with the severity of hip deformity, lack of lateral osseous support, and inclination and position of the acetabular cup.[3,9] It has been reported that the more severe the dysplasia, the higher the rates of failure and complications.[20] It has been noted that the clinical results of femoral stems were equivalent in the group of patients with dysplasia, low dislocation, and high dislocation types, but the results of acetabular components were significantly worse in the hips with a high dislocation type mainly caused by polyethylene wear and osteolysis and subsequent cup loosening at 10-year follow-up.[29] The rate of osteolysis has a significant relation to the polyethylene wear rate and has varied from 13% up to 25% at 7- to 10-year follow-up.[29]

THA After an Acetabular Fracture
Dana C. Mears, MD, PhD

Despite the initial method of treatment, a patient with an acetabular fracture may develop features of a poor clinical outcome, including the onset of incapacitating hip pain secondary to posttraumatic arthrosis or osteonecrosis of the hip.[44-47] Subsequently, the principal therapeutic option is THA.[48,49] Although in selected cases an arthrodesis of the hip may be feasible, this type of fusion can be challenging in the presence of displaced, osteopenic, or avascular bone.[50] In the United States, even when such a procedure is a viable option, many patients are reluctant to consider it. For many years, a THA after an acetabular fracture has been recognized as a potentially difficult procedure.[45-47] In the presence of an acetabular fracture, which possesses little displacement and limited extra-articular hardware, generally an uncomplicated THA can be performed using diverse surgical approaches similar to a procedure performed for degenerative arthritis. Whether initial nonsurgical or surgical treatment was used to manage an acute and highly displaced acetabular fracture, complications such as a nonunion or the presence of a bone defect, interposed hardware, or heterotopic bone may affect the arthroplasty.[49] One long-standing question is whether such a secondary arthroplasty is technically easier to perform and potentially more durable if an acute open reduction of a displaced acetabular fracture is undertaken. Studies have shown that an open reduction and internal fixation (ORIF) provided not only the optimal potential for a favorable clinical outcome, but also the best potential for late arthroplastic reconstruction if posttraumatic arthrosis or osteonecrosis is present.[44] It has been suggested that an unreduced acetabular fracture that occurred after nonsurgical treatment was susceptible to nonunion, a large acetabular defect, or a pelvic malunion. Any of these late complications could jeopardize the outcome of a secondary THA. More recent studies[48,49] have evaluated various reconstructive techniques for THA after an acetabular fracture that initially was managed either nonsurgically or surgically. A second objective of these studies was the determination of whether an initial nonsurgical or surgical course of treatment for an acute acetabular fracture provided a superior environment for a secondary THA. The criteria for success included the technical ease and reproducibility of the arthroplasty, along with the degree of clinical success (including the longevity of function). Such an evaluation was intended to address the contention that initial surgical treatment of an acetabular fracture provided the optimal environment for a successful late reconstruction. The presence of an acute acetabular fracture might lead to complications that virtually ensured a poor outcome whether nonsurgical treatment or an open reduction was performed. In this situation, the potential therapeutic options might include a method of acute THA.

Clinical and Radiographic Assessment of Acetabular Fracture

An acetabular fracture may occur after a major traumatic event such as a motor vehicle crash, a fall from a height, or an industrial accident.[44,45,47] Most acetabular fractures in the elderly currently occur after minor trauma, such as a fall from a standing position, in which moderately or markedly osteopenic bone is a major contributor to the injury.[51] In the presence of osteopenic bone, marked impaction of the femoral head or the acetabulum may occur and thereby a poor prog-

nosis is expected regardless of whether an open reduction is performed.[52] Occasionally, a history of symptomatic degenerative or inflammatory arthritis of the hip or osteonecrosis is documented as another indicator of a compromised prognosis after nonsurgical management or ORIF of an acute acetabular fracture. After a major traumatic event, a patient is susceptible to conditions such as sciatic nerve palsy. Even if a minor degree of posttraumatic neurologic deficit is documented at the time of an open reduction or a late THA, the patient may experience exacerbation of the nerve deficit, which may become a permanent source of dysesthesia, motor weakness, or sensory impairment.[53,54] These complications are most likely to arise in the patient who undergoes a posterior approach to the hip and acetabulum in which the sciatic nerve is manipulated even to a minor degree. This concern influences the preoperative planning for a THA, including the optimal surgical approach.

For the preoperative planning of a THA after an acetabular fracture, other relevant features of the history include an evaluation for drug and alcohol abuse, and assessment of the nature of vocational activities or hobbies that may provide a high likelihood for falls, major accidents, heavy lifting, or other abuse of the hip. For an elderly patient, the presence of posturing of the hip, marked weakness of the hip abductor muscles, or a comorbidity that culminates in recurring falls merits consideration as a contraindication to an acute arthroplasty.

In addition to a general evaluation of the patient, the clinical examination includes an examination of the relevant hip and the pelvis for features of deformity and for traumatic or surgical scars.[48,55] A potential hip deformity or limb-length discrepancy is documented along with the range of motion of the hip. The examination attempts to identify any clinical features of a sciatic or femoral nerve palsy, even of a subtle degree. If an open reduction was previously performed, the hip is evaluated for features of possible occult infection and heterotopic bone.

A radiographic evaluation of the hip and pelvis includes the standard AP, iliac, and obturator oblique views, along with a CT scan[49,55] (Figures 6 through 8). The images are assessed carefully for the presence of impaction that is optimally seen in sagittal and coronal reconstructions. On the standard CT transaxial images, even a large area of impaction involving 30% of the femoral head or of the acetabular dome may be difficult to appreciate. In an osteoporotic patient who sustains a fracture after a simple fall, a large area of impaction or of abrasive damage to the joint may be encountered at the time of the open reduction despite minimal preoperative radiographic evidence (Figure 8). Three-dimensional CT (Figure 9) with supplementary disarticulated images of the acetabulum and the femoral head provides the optimal means to accurately characterize a complex deformity of the hemipelvis and potentially the entire pelvic ring where it is involved in the deformity.

3: Hip

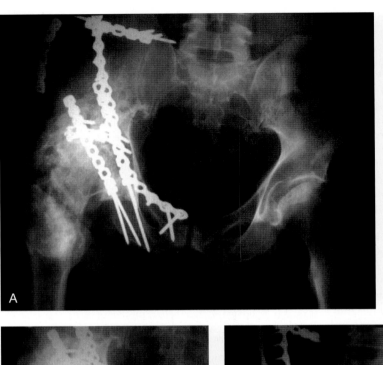
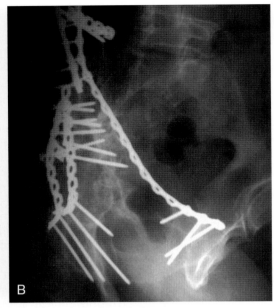
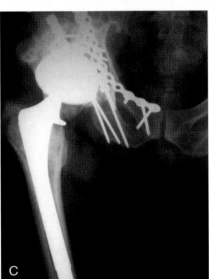
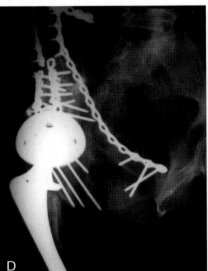
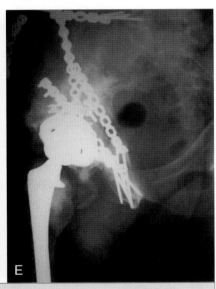

Figure 6 Radiographs of the pelvis of a 52-year-old man show a complex acetabular fracture seen 2 years after a primary ORIF of a both-column posterior wall fracture. For the subsequent posttraumatic arthritis, THA was performed with the use of the minimally invasive two-incision technique. **A** and **B**, Preoperative AP and obturator oblique views. **B** shows the substantial space available for the cup. AP (**C**), obturator (**D**), and iliac oblique (**E**) views, 2 years after surgery. The ample space for the cup between the column plates is documented.

If a prior open reduction of an acetabular fracture was performed, the location of hardware (possibly trochanteric screws) is noted in the AP and the oblique radiographs (**Figures 6** and **10**). An obturator oblique view highlights the position of an anterior column screw, which may interfere with the reaming of the acetabulum and insertion of the cup. The iliac oblique view is indicative of the position of hardware attached to the posterior column and wall. The images are assessed for features of a residual acetabular or pelvic ring deformity, including the magnitude and vector of the displacement. Subsequently, a postoperative evalua-

tion of comparable post-THA images and a comparison with the preoperative images enables the surgeon to assess the adequacy of the preoperative plan (**Figures 6** and **10**).

Timing of THA After Acetabular Fracture

This section evaluates the indications for a THA after an acetabular fracture, the timing of the procedure, and the technical considerations, along with the appropriate clinical protocol and potential complications. Three distinct time periods after an acute acetabular fracture when THA should be considered have been identified:

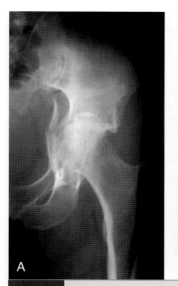
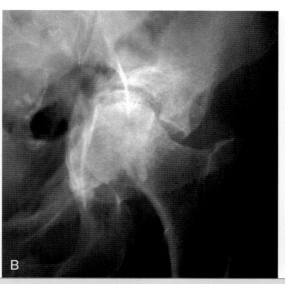
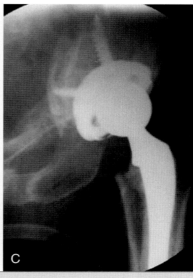

Figure 7 Radiographs of the hip of a 68-year-old woman confirm the presence of an anterior wall, column, and quadrilateral fracture 3 months after initial nonsurgical treatment with a THA along with impaction grafting to the central acetabular defect. **A,** Initial AP view. **B,** Radiographic view 2 months after injury when severe hip pain secondary to severe posttraumatic degenerative arthritis was present; a central acetabular nonunion/malunion is seen. **C,** Radiographic view 3 years after THA showing central acetabular impaction grafting and hybrid THA.

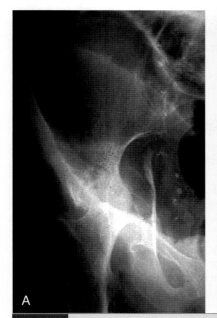
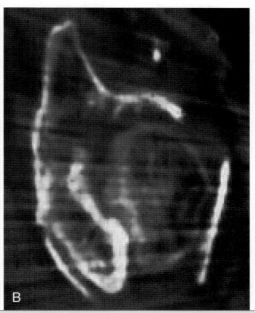
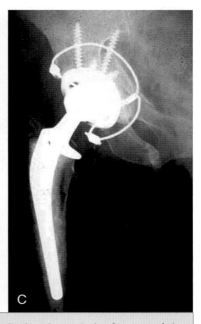

Figure 8 Radiographs and CT scan of the hip of a 92-year-old woman who had a simple, displaced acetabular fracture of the anterior wall, column, and quadrilateral surface that occurred after a fall. Three days later, a primary hybrid THA was performed with cerclage cable fixation of the acetabulum, using an anterolateral approach. **A,** Preoperative AP view. **B,** Preoperative CT view with central acetabular impaction. **C,** Two-year postoperative AP view.

3 months or longer, 3 weeks to 3 months, and within 3 weeks of the injury.[49,56]

THA 3 Months or Longer After the Time of the Injury
Typically, at 3 months after the time of injury, the fracture has united with or without a residual deformity.

The principal indications for the procedure are posttraumatic arthritis and osteonecrosis. Associated considerations include the presence of an acetabular nonunion and/or a potential acetabular deformity, which may be complicated by a deformity of the ipsilateral or contralateral pelvic ring. If an ORIF of the acetabulum

3: Hip

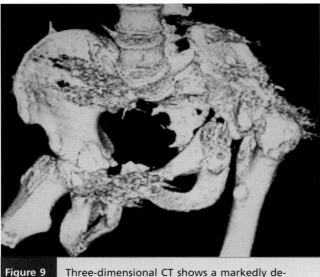

Figure 9 Three-dimensional CT shows a markedly deformed pelvis in a 32-year-old man 2 years after a motor vehicular crash in which he was an unrestrained driver. Two months after the injury, ORIF of the right posterior ilium, right rami, left sacrum, and left acetabulum culminated in multiple major displaced nonunions. The complex painful deformities that persist 2 years after the surgical reconstructions are confirmed. Posttraumatic arthritis of the left hip was considered an indication for a THA.

is performed acutely, then a secondary THA may have to address one or more problematic factors, including the presence of interposed hardware, heterotopic bone, dense scar tissue, frank or occult infection, a sciatic nerve palsy, or entrapment of the sciatic nerve in scar tissue (**Figure 6**). Special preoperative diagnostic tests may be indicated in an attempt to identify and characterize these problematic factors.

THA 3 to 12 Weeks After the Acute Injury

In some instances, after an apparently uneventful acute presentation and course of management of a displaced acetabular fracture, some complicating clinical or radiographic features become apparent. Following initial nonsurgical treatment, the fracture may undergo displacement later, which provokes a secondary mechanical erosion of the femoral head. Susceptible fracture patterns include a transverse or T-type fracture, a posterior fracture-dislocation, or an anterior wall/anterior column fracture with displacement of the quadrilateral surface (**Figure 7**). Following acute ORIF, failure to achieve an accurate reduction or a loss of fixation with a secondary displacement may culminate in the precipitous onset of erosive damage to the femoral head. Once incapacitating pain is accompanied by radiographic confirmation of extensive erosion of the femoral head and an incongruent hip joint, the likelihood for a successful clinical outcome is remote. THA can be considered the most realistic treatment to achieve relief of pain and a functional clinical outcome.

THA Less Than 3 Weeks After Injury

The most controversial situation is an acute presentation of an acetabular fracture, which is associated with an intrinsically abysmal outcome.[56] Provocative factors include marked impaction or erosion of the femoral head and/or acetabulum, an associated displaced subcapital femoral neck fracture, and occasionally extensive comminution (**Figure 8**). The age and potential presence of medical comorbidities is an additional factor.

THA in a Young and Fit Adult Patient

In a young, active adult patient with a potentially long life expectancy who has a displaced acetabular fracture, primary ORIF should be carefully considered in an attempt to defer THA. In some young adults, however, the extensive damage and deformity of the hip precludes the realization of a painless and functional hip joint after closed treatment or ORIF. In such a situation, THA may be inevitable. Whether a primary THA or an initial nonsurgical course or ORIF should be undertaken in the presence of a highly comminuted acetabular fracture with marked displacement and bony impaction is controversial[44,47,56] (**Figure 11**). In such a situation, an acute open reduction is associated with a poor prognosis, whereas it may be difficult to achieve a stable cup in the disrupted acetabulum during acute THA. Likewise, the third therapeutic option of a primary nonsurgical course may be hampered by the concern for a late displaced and ununited acetabulum. For a young adult with a highly complex acetabular fracture, the optimal therapeutic option remains controversial and unclear. The principal complicating factors are impaction and marked comminution of the articular surface as opposed to displacement.

Inevitably, the acute ORIF is followed by some degree of scar tissue formation, muscle injury, the potential for heterotopic bone formation, and conceivably infection (**Figure 10**). A more extensive initial surgical exposure makes these complications more likely to occur, and they may hamper the completion of a subsequent THA to further jeopardize the late clinical outcome.

THA in an Elderly Patient

In the elderly patient with various medical comorbidities, including osteopenia, an acetabular fracture typically occurs after a simple fall and has limited displacement but extensive impaction and comminution (**Figure 8**). One example is an elderly, osteopenic patient with a posterior wall fracture, typified by extensive impaction of the femoral head and the acetabulum so that a rapid destruction of the hip joint follows nonsurgical treatment or an ORIF[51] (**Figure 12**). The insurmountable complication that prevents an effective ORIF is the impaction rather than the modest displacement. If the area of impaction mostly involves the femoral head and the posterior wall, a primary THA using a cementless multiscrew cup and a cemented or cementless stem is technically realistic. The modest acetabular deformity does not increase the technical difficulty of the arthroplasty.

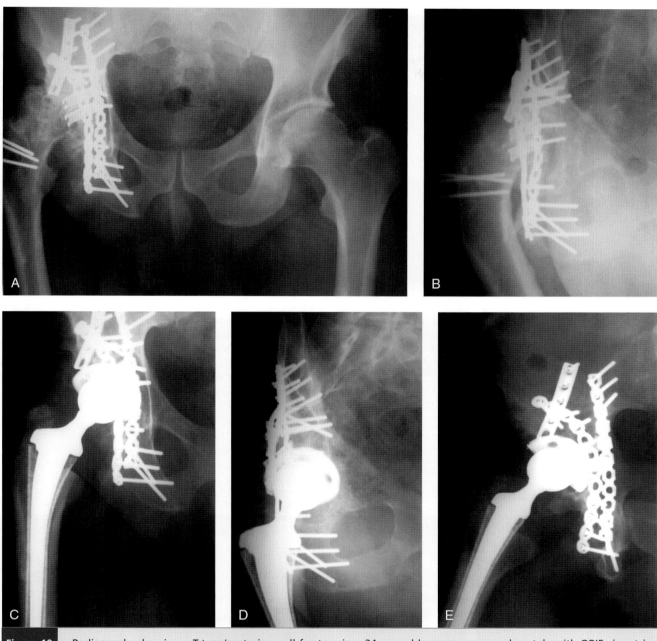

Figure 10   Radiographs showing a T-type/posterior wall fracture in a 34-year-old woman managed acutely with ORIF via a triradiate incision. One year later, incapacitating pain secondary to posttraumatic arthritis culminated in a THA performed through a minimally invasive two-incision approach. During the latter procedure, one screw was cut with a power burr to remove a segment, which occupied the site needed for the cup. **A,** The AP pelvis is shown. **B,** Preoperative obturator oblique view. **C,** AP view 2 years after THA. **D,** Corresponding obturator oblique view. **E,** Corresponding iliac oblique view.

Exceptions occur in an elderly patient who has a more violent injury, whereby a marked deformity poses a considerable technical challenge (**Figure 8**). Several authors have recommended that an acute ORIF should be performed, even when the prognosis for the procedure was predictably poor.[44,57] An initial nonsurgical approach with a late THA, after a bony union has occurred, has

recently been favored.[48,49,51] A major societal change is the increase in the population of patients older than 75 years. Clinical documentation for this age group was minimal in earlier studies. The typical medical comorbidities, including dementia and profound osteopenia, favor the role of primary nonsurgical treatment and a late THA if incapacitating hip pain occurs.

Preoperative Planning and the Formation of a Surgical Strategy

The degree of appropriate preoperative planning correlates with the nature of complications related to the injury and the type of initial management. A procedure for THA for posttraumatic degenerative arthritis or osteonecrosis in which the initial fracture was minimally displaced and was treated nonsurgically may be identical to that of a standard THA. In this situation, the prior experience of the surgeon will dictate the type of surgical exposure, bony preparation, and the types of cementless or hybrid implants used. The presence of one or more complications may call for modification of the surgical procedure.[55]

Prior Posterior Surgical Approach and/or Sciatic Nerve Palsy

To minimize the risk of iatrogenic sciatic nerve palsy or recurrence of neurologic deficit, THA is optimally performed using an anterolateral or anterior approach to avoid manipulation of the sciatic nerve or a dissection of the nerve from adjacent scar tissue.[48,55] If a posterior or posterolateral approach is required, possibly to remove an errant intra-articular screw, the use of intraoperative neurologic monitoring with continuous electromyelographic monitoring, nerve conduction velocities, and somatosensory-evoked potentials is recommended.[58,59] In this way, the surgeon can be alerted to subtle neurologic changes that accompany a limited manipulation of the hip or of a provocative adjustment of a posterior column retractor so that a postoperative deterioration of sciatic nerve function is avoided.

The Presence of Periacetabular Hardware

The hardware may have been placed using a standard posterior (Kocher-Langenbeck) approach, an ilioinguinal approach, or an extended lateral (extended iliofem-

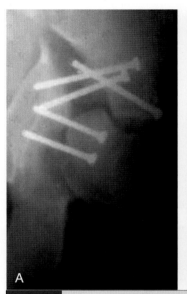
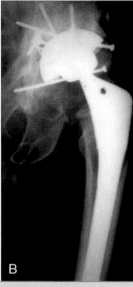

Figure 11 Radiographs of the hip of a 25-year-old man who sustained a transverse acetabular fracture managed acutely with an ORIF. Two months later, a painful malaligned nonunion was documented. At that time, a THA was performed along with a revised reduction and internal fixation of the fracture. **A,** AP view 2 months after the ORIF. **B,** AP view 4 years after the THA.

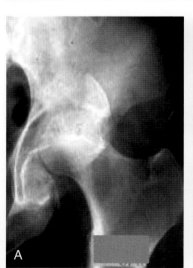
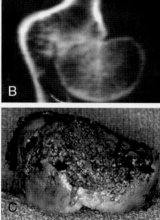
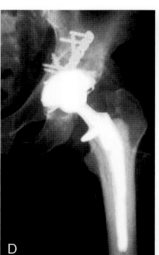
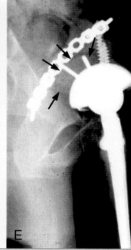

Figure 12 Radiographs and CT images are indicative of a displaced posterior wall fracture with marked impaction of the femoral head in a 62-year-old man. Two weeks after initial nonsurgical management, an open reduction of the posterior wall was accompanied by a THA and the application of a structural femoral head bone graft to the defective posterior wall. The graft was harvested from the excised femoral head. **A,** Preoperative AP view showing the displaced wall fragments and femoral head. **B,** CT with femoral head impaction. **C,** CT with impaction of the femoral head and acetabulum. **D,** Postoperative AP view 6 months later. **E,** Corresponding iliac oblique view to highlight structural graft (arrows).

oral or a triradiate) exposure.[60-63] The initial exposure dictates the sites and orientations of fixation screws and considerations for screw removal. The preoperative obturator and iliac oblique radiographs permit a general assessment of the regions of the screws and the likelihood for a screw to occupy a site needed for the acetabular cup (**Figures 6 and 10**). An errant screw may be managed in one of several ways. If the screw head is readily exposed, especially by the incision used for the arthroplasty, the screw may be removed. Occasionally, a screw may be removed by a limited percutaneous approach along with the use of intraoperative fluoroscopy. If the screw was inserted using an ilioinguinal approach, or potentially by an alternative exposure, direct visualization of the screw head may be impractical unless a large dissection is performed. As an alternative strategy, the segment of the screw that traverses the region of the acetabulum to be occupied by the cup can be removed within the acetabular recess under direct exposure using a diamond burr or wheel.

A fixation plate previously inserted to buttress the posterior wall may impinge upon the femoral head. This situation may result from errant placement of the plate or in the aftermath of an erosive or avascular loss of the articular portion of the wall. The plate can be removed by direct exposure of the posterior column, or the exposed undersurface of the plate can be covered using an impaction grafting technique within the acetabulum.[64] After débridement of membrane and scar tissue within the acetabulum, morcellized cancellous allograft is placed in the acetabular recess to cover the exposed hardware. Reverse reaming is performed to pack the graft material before cup insertion (**Figure 7**).

Displacement of an Acetabular Wall

In the presence or absence of internal fixation, a portion of the acetabular wall may be displaced by several millimeters. After cup insertion, the acetabular deformity compromises the anticipated bony support of the implant. As part of the THA, the wall fragment can be reduced through an open exposure (**Figure 11**). A plate can be applied to the posterior column to immobilize the wall fragment. If the surgical reconstruction is performed more than 1 month after the time of injury, the reduction is hampered by the presence of proliferative scar tissue. Unlike an acute open reduction of a displaced wall fragment, the late reduction is likely to denude the bone, eliminate its blood supply, and make osteonecrosis more likely to occur. As an alternative strategy, an impaction grafting of the acetabular recess may be preferred. In this scenario, the fracture lines at sites of displacement are débrided. Morcellized cancellous allograft is placed into the acetabulum for impaction and thereby restoration of a hemispherical recess suitable for a cup.

Displacement of an Acetabular Column or a Transverse Fracture

An anterior or posterior column may be displaced by various degrees as a linear, rotational, or combined deformity. The magnitude of the deformity may vary from small (< 1 cm) to medium (1 to 2 cm) to large (> 2 cm).[49,55,65] A large cup or impaction bone grafting can be used to treat a small deformity. For a medium to large deformity, a partial or complete correction of the deformed column or transverse fracture merits consideration (**Figure 9**). As the magnitude of the deformity increases, the surgical procedure becomes progressively more involved. Typically, the wall segment is scarified, possibly with callus formation. To mobilize the fragment, a sufficient release of the scar and callus is needed so that a correction of the deformity is feasible. Generally, the fragment does not fit precisely into the site of the defect so that stabilization of the bone with the use of screws, plates, or screws anchored to the cup is impaired.

Multicolumn Deformity

Following a both-column fracture and other associated injury patterns, a complex displacement of multiple acetabular segments may occur in which the segments can be directly united, indirectly united with callus, or ununited.[49,55,65] If a limited displacement of the segments (< 1 cm) is documented, the application of a jumbo cup or of impaction bone grafting may suffice. In the presence of a large displacement (> 2 cm) as part of the THA, correction of the deformity is necessary. Although the acetabular reconstruction could be undertaken as a preliminary procedure before the THA, the completion of both stages under a single anesthetic agent is preferred to make full use of the extensive surgical exposure. When the stages are separated, then scar tissue and potentially heterotopic bone formation following the first procedure hampers the second exposure and increases the risk of an iatrogenic neurovascular injury.

Heterotopic Bone Formation

Following an acetabular fracture and subsequent ORIF, heterotopic bone (heterotopic ossification [HO]) may form spontaneously.[44,66,67] Well-recognized predisposing factors include a concomitant closed head injury and an obese middle-aged male patient.[68] The extent of HO formation varies widely, from a limited area or areas of capsule or hip muscle (Brooker grade 1 or 2) to a circumferential mass of bone that completely surrounds the hip joint (Brooker grade 3 or 4).[67] The potential functional implications include stiffness of the hip and pain. The heterotopic bone may arise in an otherwise functional hip joint or one with varying degrees of posttraumatic arthritis. In terms of management, this distinction is crucial. If the hip joint with symptomatic HO is substantially arthritic, then an effective attempt to remove the HO necessitates a THA. When a THA is planned, the surgical strategy involves a plan to expose and remove the HO. From the preoperative radiographs and CT, the extent and location of the HO is identified[64] (**Figure 13**). A suitable surgical approach is identified. If the HO is circumferentially disposed

3: Hip

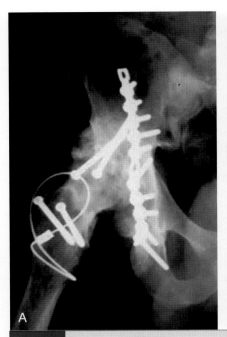
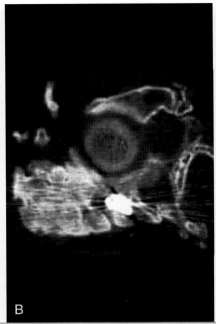
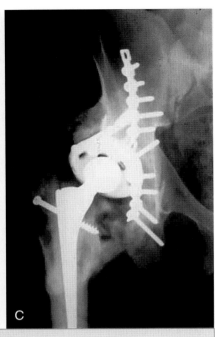

Figure 13 Radiographs and CT showing a transverse/posterior wall fracture in a morbidly obese 46-year-old man who sustained a concomitant closed head injury and was managed with an acute ORIF. Four years later, symptomatic posttraumatic degenerative arthritis with stiffness and pain in the hip culminated in a THA along with limited excision of the HO and partial hardware removal. One day later, irradiation therapy with 7cGy was applied to the hip. One year later the patient had much improved pain relief but no improvement in mobility of the hip. **A**, AP view 4 years after ORIF and immediately preceding the THA. **B**, CT taken immediately before the THA to highlight extensive HO. **C**, AP view taken 3 years after the THA when recurrent Brooker grade 3 HO markedly limited the motion of the hip.

around the hip as Brooker grade 3 or 4, a triradiate incision with preservation of the greater trochanteric attachment of the hip abductors merits serious consideration.[63] Intraoperative fluoroscopy is valuable to permit a radiographic distinction of HO from the intact acetabular and proximal femoral bone. Otherwise, inadvertently, intact pelvic bone may be removed. When the HO infiltrates the adjacent hip muscles and tendons, the principal muscle mass and adjacent tendons are preserved, notably with respect to the insertions of ossified gluteus medius and minimus tendons on the greater trochanter. Usually the ossified hip capsule is a discrete layer so that the more peripheral muscles can be distinguished. In a patient with Brooker grade 3 or 4 HO, despite an extensive resection the restoration of effective motion of the hip may be limited by the combination of scarring and stiffness of the adjacent muscles. Also, postoperative recurrence of HO around the hip may further compromise hip mobility (**Figure 13**).

Following the surgical resection of HO, various strategies have been used in an attempt to stifle recurrent HO formation. The principal examples include bisphosphonates, indomethacin, and low-dose irradiation therapy (such as 7 to 10 cGy in 1 to 10 single-dose fractions).[69-71] The reported results are difficult to rigorously document in view of the paucity of experimental studies using a control group. Irradiation therapy has been an effective modality. Nevertheless, in a patient with a prior closed head injury, virtually complete recurrence of the HO is not unusual.

Occult Infection of the Hip

Especially in the presence of Brooker grade 3 or 4 HO, an occult infection of the hip may be a source of pain, which is attributed to posttraumatic degenerative arthritis. The typical clinical presentation follows an ORIF of a comminuted fracture, especially after an extensile approach, such as an extended iliofemoral or a triradiate incision, or two approaches. In the aftermath of an associated fracture, a large surgical exposure, and potentially the formation of extensive scar tissue including HO, the presence of a deep wound infection may be difficult to document. Although clinical features of an abscess formation, along with fever and chills, may simplify the diagnosis, particularly in the presence of Brooker grade 3 or 4 HO, an occult infection within the hip joint may be more difficult to confirm. Although routine blood tests including a white blood cell count, erythrocyte sedimentation rate, and C-reactive protein level may indicate infection, confirmatory imaging is difficult or impossible.[72] With the acetabular hardware, the results of CT, MRI, and radionuclide imaging are likely to be inconclusive.[72] Aspiration of the hip may be impossible to perform because of the HO. At the time of the THA, a preoperative suspicion of an occult infection should encourage

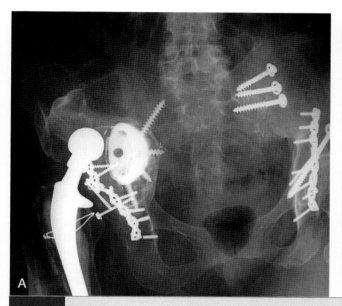
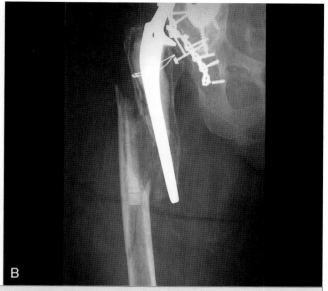

Figure 14   Radiographs confirm extensive pelvic deformity after the last ORIF and proximal femoral views confirm persistent pelvic deformity in a woman who had an ORIF 9 years earlier and 3 years after the THA. At this stage, incapacitating hip pain was complicated by a simple fall when the patient sustained a periprosthetic proximal femoral fracture. **A,** A large acetabular defect and malrotated cup along with a dislocated THA are seen. **B,** AP radiographic view of the hip confirms periprosthetic femoral fracture.

an appropriate explanation to the patient of the therapeutic plan if an infection is confirmed during the surgical approach for the THA. If sepsis of the hip, is confirmed, a two-stage arthroplasty is preferred.[73] The initial procedure becomes a débridement of the hip, including an excision of the femoral head and the insertion of a cement spacer. A course of culture-specific intravenous antibiotic therapy follows. Prior to the THA and after completion of the antibiotic regimen, a closed trephine biopsy of the hip is done to procure culture specimens. If the cultures are negative, the THA is performed. If the THA is a primary procedure and the culture specimens taken then are positive, a course of culture-specific antibiotics is administered.

Osteonecrosis of the Acetabulum

Approximately 25 years ago, extensile exposures of the acetabulum were first introduced, characterized by extensive dissection on both the inner and outer pelvic surfaces along with a correspondingly extensive devascularization of bone. During the following decade when a secondary THA was performed for many of these patients, a devastating complication ensued in a few patients that was characterized by migration of a cementless cup through the acetabulum to protrude into the true pelvis[74] (**Figure 14**). Surgical attempts at correction led to a high failure rate, with additional bone loss and recurrent loosening of the cup. When repeat revisions followed, ultimately many of these situations culminated in a discontinuity or dissociation of the acetabulum and often a nonreconstructable pseudarthrosis of the hip joint.[75] At the time of initial cup failure, biopsies of the acetabulum confirmed the pres-

ence of extensive areas of avascular bone, even in arthroplastic procedures performed years after the initial ORIF of the acetabulum. If a reconstructive procedure is planned, a strategy for an extensive replacement of structural acetabulum and adjacent ilium may be necessary (**Figures 15** and **16**). The procedure is comparable to an exchange arthroplasty for a failed primary THA in which a dissociation is documented. Although extensile approaches are used less frequently now, problematic acetabular fixation and premature cup failure remain potential problems after a major acetabular exposure. The surgeon is advised to relay this concern to a patient before the THA is performed.

Standard Surgical Technique

The procedure may be performed under general, spinal, or epidural anesthesia. Following a fracture initially treated nonsurgically or with limited ORIF and uncomplicated by a persistent deformity, extensive HO, or remotely situated and protruding acetabular hardware, a conventional posterolateral or anterolateral surgical approach can be used as dictated by the surgeon's preference.[76] Whichever approach is used, the procedure is performed with the patient in a full lateral decubitus position. The ipsilateral limb is carefully positioned with extension of the hip and flexion of the knee beyond a right angle to minimize tension on the sciatic nerve and lumbosacral plexus. If a posterolateral approach is used, one of two strategies can be used. The exposure can be developed deep to the split in the gluteus maximus through the piriformis tendon adjacent to the greater trochanter, with progression through the underlying hip capsule. This strategy maximizes the

3: Hip

distance from the hip joint to the sciatic nerve where the nerve overlies the posterior column. If the posterior column is exposed for removal of a plate or to address a nonunion, then the overlying sciatic nerve is vulnerable to injury. Especially if a prior open reduction was performed, the nerve is embedded in scar tissue, which

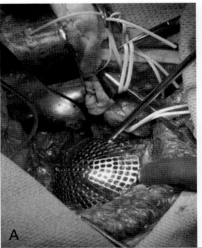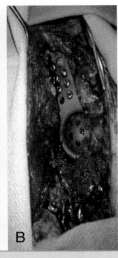

Figure 15 Intraoperative photographs show the acetabular reconstruction. **A,** A large titanium mesh is viewed through an ilioinguinal incision, which replenishes the inner pelvic table. **B,** An acetabular cage is viewed through an anterolateral hip incision. Approximately 500 mL of morcellized cancellous autograft obliterated the defect between the inner and outer pelvic tables.

is continuous with the scar tissue overlying the posterior column. The entrapped nerve is vulnerable to an iatrogenic laceration or a traction injury when it is retracted away from the underlying bone. Therefore, the nerve is formally exposed starting distally at the site of insertion of the gluteus maximus to the proximal femoral shaft. With a sharp release of the maximus insertion from the femur, the sciatic nerve can be directly seen. The nerve is progressively exposed in a proximal direction until the greater sciatic notch is reached. Vessel loops are used to facilitate gentle manipulation of the nerve. The scarified short external rotators are preserved as a biologic covering of the posterior column for when the sciatic nerve is repositioned over the bone. During an exposure of the posterior column, a sciatic nerve retractor can be placed in the lesser sciatic notch.[48] Although the retractor optimizes visualization, it is vulnerable to apply excessive tension on the sciatic nerve, unless intermittent gentle retraction is undertaken.

In an effort to see the superior acetabular wall or the adjacent column, a Hohmann-type retractor typically is placed under the glutei to retract the muscle mass. This technique may cause a traction injury of the superior gluteal nerve. Because the position of the nerve and its branches within the musculature is variable, a fully safe site for the retractor or vector of displacement of the muscle mass does not exist.[71,72] A gentle displacement of the gluteal muscles is necessary.

In the presence of a large malalignment of the acetabulum, such as a prior displaced transverse or T-type fracture, as a part of the arthroplastic procedure, an open reduction of the deformed segment may be neces-

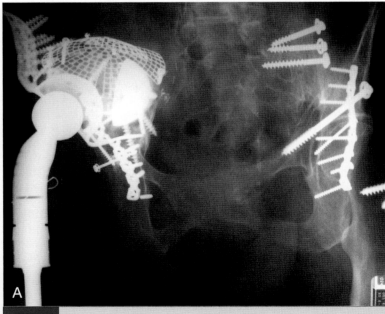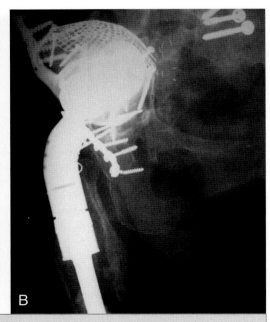

Figure 16 AP (**A**) and obturator oblique (**B**) views taken 3 years after injury confirm the THA with a segmental proximal femoral replacement stem, when the patient had minimal hip pain and ambulated with a cane.

sary (**Figure 11**). To adequately see and correct the deformity, the use of an extensile approach such as a triradiate or extended iliofemoral incision can be made.[62,63] An attempt is made to preserve the gluteal insertions on the greater trochanter and the greater trochanter itself. The excised femoral head and neck is saved for autograft, which typically is needed to obliterate a residual acetabular gap. The subsequent procedural steps are tailored to the particular fracture pattern.

Minimally Invasive Two-Incision Approach

As an alternative to the conventional approach, two small incisions are advantageous after an acetabular fracture because of the limitation of the surgical field.[77-79] The patient is placed supine on a radiolucent table. Image intensification permits excellent radiographic visualization of the acetabulum and adjacent hardware. The anterior exposure provides a direct view into the acetabular recess to highlight the fracture deformity. The sciatic nerve is well separated from the surgical field to minimize the risk of a direct neurologic injury. When a two-incision approach is used, the hip is briefly hyperextended during the femoral preparation. For a posterolateral or an anterolateral approach, the hip has to be flexed and adducted briefly during femoral preparation to create a position that might provoke an iatrogenic injury to the sciatic nerve. This provocative position is a potential aggravating factor for a so-called "second crush" or traction injury to a nerve that may have been subjected to contusion during the initial traumatic event or a subsequent open reduction, especially after a posterior fracture-dislocation.[53] The use of a radiolucent Jupiter Operating Table (Trumpf Inc, Charleston, SC) or a similar model that permits independent hyperextension of either hip and lower extremity is recommended.[77,79] A suitable short-acting spinal or general anesthetic regimen is used.[80,81] A 12- or 15-inch image intensifier is used to identify the critical landmarks of the hip. Using an AP view of the hip joint, the site for a 6- to 7-cm incision overlying the intertrochanteric ridge of the proximal femur is identified. The incision is extended sharply to the deep fascia. The classic interval between the tensor fascia lata and the sartorius is used to expose the hip joint and remove the femoral head. A direct view into the acetabulum facilitates the removal of a segment of an obstructive intra-articular screw or the application of morcellized bone graft to obliterate an acetabular defect. In the presence of a neighboring plate with screws, the acetabular reaming under fluoroscopy permits precise positioning of the cup without impingement of the reamer on the hardware (**Figures 6 and 10**). If the residual bone covering the adjacent screws is deficient, morcellized autograft from the femoral head is packed via reverse reaming. A standard cementless cup is inserted along with two anchoring screws and a standard polyethylene liner. Then, the proximal femur is prepared for the insertion of a conventional cementless stem.

Strategies to Address Acetabular Defects Encountered in Late THA After an Acetabular Fracture

The presence of an acetabular defect is a frequent feature of a late THA after an acetabular fracture. The defect may be highly variable in size and location. Overall the strategies for obliteration of the defect are based on the long-standing prior experience of revision THA for large lytic defects. A small and contained defect can be filled with autograft that is harvested from the femoral head.[82] Either morcellized graft or a structural graft harvested from the excised femoral head can be used. For a moderate defect, impaction grafting with or without the use of mesh reinforcement merits consideration. (**Figure 7**). This technique was used for an exchange arthroplasty and in conjunction with cancellous allograft.[64] For a large, contained central defect, initially morcellized bone graft harvested from the excised femoral head is placed in the base of the defect. Then a circular preformed titanium mesh of the appropriate size is placed over the bone graft so that its circular edge rests on supportive bone. As an alternative supportive device, a Trabecular Metal–covered titanium disk (Zimmer, Warsaw, IN) may be used. If the defect is very large, the mesh can be anchored with small screws around its periphery. Additional cancellous graft is placed on the exposed surface of the mesh. An acetabular reamer of the appropriate size is used in reverse mode to impact the graft. This step may be repeated until a complete bony bed can be seen. Then a cup of the corresponding size is impacted into the acetabulum and supplementary screw fixation is undertaken. For a defective posterior wall, a crescentic mesh of appropriate size can be anchored over the defect with multiple screws. Impaction autografting is undertaken followed by the insertion of the cementless cup with multiple holes for screws.

In the presence of a posttraumatic acetabular nonunion, as a counterpart to an acetabular dissociation, an alternative technique involves the use of a ring or cage.[83,84] The fracture gap is débrided to viable bone and obliterated with bone graft. Then the cage is placed into the acetabular recess for anchorage with multiple screws (**Figures 15 and 16**). In the clinical example provided here, the large size of the defect necessitated the application of a supplementary titanium mesh on the inner pelvic table. The mesh was anchored with screws to the adjacent bone. The large intervening space was obliterated with 500 mL of morcellized cancellous bone allograft. To minimize the risk of premature loosening of the cage, newer designs (Biomet, Warsaw, IN) possess an ingrowth surface to oppose the acetabulum. Typically, an acetabular component is cemented into the cage. Although a cage is conceptually a solution for a traumatic dissociation, premature loosening and fracture of the cage are well-documented problems.[77]

As a recent alternative to the use of a cage, Trabecular Metal augment blocks (Zimmer) have recently become available in various sizes and shapes (**Figure 17**). This variability and the potential to apply these blocks to multiple sites around the cup greatly simplifies the

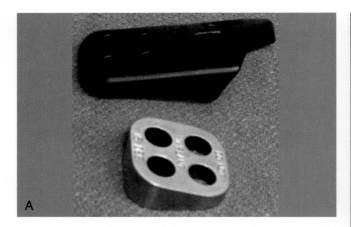
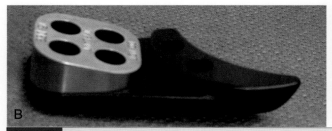
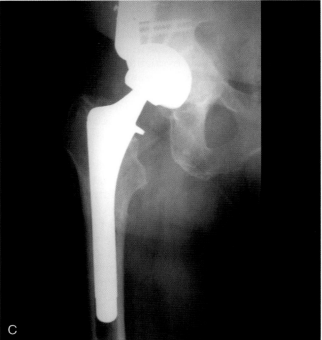

Figure 17 Augment blocks are used to reconstruct an large peripheral acetabular defect. **A,** A posterior wall augment block with a 15° shim. **B,** The shim is positioned beneath the augment block to facilitate the optimal contact of the augment upon the irregular pelvic table. The augment is cemented to both the shim and the cup. **C,** AP radiograph of a THA including an augment block and shim.

reconstruction. A wedge-shaped "shim" is available in three sizes and is positioned on the undersurface of the buttress plate. The shim facilitates the fitting of the buttress plate onto the irregular pelvic surface. The augment block is anchored to both the shim and a Trabecular Metal cup with the use of bone cement.[80] Structural or morcellized bone graft may be placed under a portion of the augment to restore the acetabular bone stock. The augment block is attached to the pelvis with multiple screws. The acetabular recess is prepared with reaming and potentially with impaction grafting. A trial fitting of the cup is undertaken to ensure its appropriate size and position. The cement is mixed and placed on the adjacent surface of the augment block. The cup is inserted into the acetabular recess and anchored with multiple screws. A shortcoming of the current technique is the essential sequence of a preliminary attachment of the augment block before the insertion of the cup to ensure that a compressive load is applied to the cement during its solidification. If the sequence is reversed, during the tightening of the screws in the augment block, the block tends to be displaced by a small distance from the cup, thereby placing the solidifying cement under tension. In this situation, the cement usually cracks during the impaction of the polyethylene liner into the cup or the location of the hip.

Large Acetabular Defects
The most capacious acetabulum is encountered in the presence of pelvic malunion or nonunion accompanying a displaced acetabular fracture. Where the acetabular defect exceeds 3 cm of medial displacement, generally an effective reconstructive solution requires a realignment of the pelvic ring deformity[65] (**Figure 9**). Surgeons performing such a technical exercise must be knowledgeable about surgical exposures, realignment strategies, and pelvic ring fixation. Either the entire procedure may be undertaken under a single anesthetic agent or as sequential procedures, including the THA.

Retained Hardware
Femoral hardware is usually limited to greater trochanteric screws that were used to stabilize a trochanteric osteotomy as part of an extensile acetabular exposure. The screws are removed to facilitate the femoral preparation. The acetabular hardware may consist of screws and one or more plates, typically applied to the posterior column. In many instances, the lengthy posterior plate(s) extends distally to the ischial tuberosity or further down the ischium. To insert the plate, the sciatic nerve has to be elevated and gently displaced. As part of removal of the plate, the nerve has to be carefully elevated from its scarified attachment to the bursa, overlying the plate. Particularly if nerve contusion occurred at the time of the acute injury or as part of the retraction during the ORIF, the nerve is especially susceptible to further injury to provoke a foot drop and hypoesthesia and/or dysesthesia of the foot. From this perspective, the plate should be retained un-

less the associated screws are confirmed to be situated within the region that will be occupied by the cup. As an alternative to plate removal, two practical alternatives merit consideration. Where one or two screws through the plate occupy the acetabular dome in the space needed for the cup, the offending screws can be removed from the posterior wall by resorting to a limited deep dissection without a retraction of the sciatic nerve. Alternatively, the two-incision technique can be used (**Figures 6** and **10**). The posterior fixation is unlikely to violate the space needed for the cup. Furthermore, the sciatic nerve does not have to be exposed.

Occasionally, a posterior plate is covered with a thick layer of HO, which would complicate hardware removal. In the presence of erosion of the periarticular acetabular bone, upon exposure of the hip for the THA, the denuded plate may be seen. To provide a bony surface for the acetabular cup and as an alternative to a complex plate removal, impaction bone grafting merits consideration as a simpler technical option.

Deep Infection
Particularly in the presence of extensive HO formation that occurred after an acute ORIF of an acetabular fracture, an occult infection in the hip may be difficult or impossible to detect before the secondary THA. The conventional radiographic features of osteomyelitis are obscured by the surrounding HO. An element of suspicion may be helpful. If an infection is documented, a débridement of the hip with the insertion of a cement spacer is preferred, along with the administration of culture-specific antibiotic therapy. THA may be considered later.[73]

Femoral Components
Apart from the two-incision technique, which requires the use of a cementless stem, the other surgical approaches are consistent with the use of either a conventional cementless or cemented component. If the patient has been incapacitated for a prolonged period before the arthroplasty, a substantial degree of osteopenia is likely to be encountered. This situation may favor the use of a longer cementless stem with a more extensive area of "scratch fit."

THA for an Acetabular Fracture 3 to 12 Weeks After the Injury
Within 3 to 12 weeks after injury, usually the fracture has at least partly or completely united. The indications for a THA within this time period are complicating features such as impaction or abrasive damage to the femoral head or acetabular impaction, factors that do not materially alter the technical difficulty of the procedure[49,55] (**Figures 7, 11,** and **12**). If the lack of a union of the fracture is a material factor whereby an anticipated union would simplify the THA, then a deferral of the procedure is advisable. Typical features would include a contained acetabular defect suitable for impaction grafting. If a partial union of a transverse fracture

is encountered, the residual fracture gap is obliterated with bone graft. A multiholed cup can be used as a hemispherical fixation plate, with screws anchored to the superior and inferior bone fragments.

Acute THA for an Acetabular Fracture
An acute THA creates the complicating factor of an unstable acetabulum for the insertion of the cup.[49,55,56] Although this factor may be of minor concern for a posterior wall fracture, it becomes a formidable challenge if the acetabulum is highly comminuted. For an injury pattern that is more comminuted than an isolated posterior wall, the surgical team should be experienced in acetabular fracture fixation as well as with THA. In the presence of a comminuted both-column fracture, a deferral of the arthroplasty until after union of the fracture has occurred is a prudent course. Specific reconstructive techniques for particular fracture patterns follow.

Posterior Wall Fracture
Visualization of this injury can be achieved from a posterolateral or anterolateral incision or the anterior portion of a two-incision approach incision. If a posterior approach is used, the capsular attachment to the principal wall fragment is carefully preserved so that the fragment serves as a vascularized bone flap for a bulk autograft of femoral head. Following the removal of the femoral head and acetabular reaming, a small acetabular defect is filled with morcellized bone graft from the femoral head and impacted with reverse reaming. If a large acetabular defect in the posterior wall is encountered, the femoral head is carefully shaped to fit accurately into the defect. The graft can be anchored with free screws, a posterior column plate (**Figure 9**), or screws that extend through the acetabular component.

Transverse or T-Type Fracture
From the perspective of an exchange arthroplasty, a transverse fracture is an example of a dissociation that is simplified by the preservation of the acetabular roof. With the use of a standard multiscrew cup or a cage or ring, effective anchorage of an acetabular component can be readily achieved.[49,55,56] The technical challenge pertains to the reduction and immobilization of the inferior half of the acetabulum (**Figure 11**). Following a standard exposure to remove the femoral head and to view the acetabulum, the fracture is reduced by use of large pelvic bone-holding forceps with one jaw placed on the inner acetabular surface, either by a passage through the greater sciatic notch or around the anterior pelvic brim.

To eliminate an associated rotational component of the deformity, a Steinmann pin or a Schanz screw can be inserted into the tubercle of the ischial tuberosity and manipulated to realign the fracture. For definitive fixation, lag screws and/or plate fixation can be used. A 3.5-mm reconstruction plate applied to the posterior column also can be used as a reduction device to correct the deformity.

3: Hip

Another method of fixation involves one or two cables or heavy wires that serve both to reduce and to stabilize the fracture[85] (**Figure 8**). A free-ended 2-mm cable or a large wire is passed along the inner pelvic surface by the use of a Statinski clamp and passed along the quadrilateral surface to the greater sciatic notch. The cable rests directly on the inner pelvic table and away from the roof of the greater sciatic notch, in proximity to the sciatic nerve and the superior gluteal neurovascular bundle. Depending on the fracture pattern, a second cable can be passed through the lesser sciatic notch or the obturator foramen. The two ends of each cable are connected above the acetabular roof. The acetabulum is then reamed and prepared for insertion of the cup. Multiple screws may be inserted through the cup to augment the fracture stabilization.

Anterior Column Fracture

This fracture variant occurs most often in elderly patients and possesses a large fragment of quadrilateral surface as well as separate pieces of anterior column and wall.[44] In the initial posttraumatic radiographs, the presence of a so-called gull sign is indicative of extensive impaction of the anterior acetabulum and thereby an abysmal prognosis irrespective of whether closed or conventional open management is used (**Figure 7**). An impaction grafting technique can be used to stabilize the fracture. Alternatively, in the presence of a large and inevitably exceedingly thin quadrilateral fragment, the cabling technique (**Figure 8**) can be used to stabilize the fracture.[85] After the exposure and removal of the femoral head, the quadrilateral fragment is reduced under fluoroscopy with eccentric pelvic forceps. Image intensification can be used to confirm the reduction. Then the cabling technique is undertaken. Morcellized femoral head autograft is applied to the central acetabulum. After reverse reaming, a cementless cup is inserted into the acetabulum and anchored with multiple screws.

Both-Column Fracture

This injury pattern usually possesses a high and a low anterior column fragment as well as a posterior column fragment that includes the quadrilateral surface. In contrast with the previously described procedures, the high anterior column fragment requires an initial stabilization. After the exposure and removal of the femoral head, the high anterior fragment is reduced under image intensification with tenaculum forceps. For fixation, two large cannulated screws are inserted into the anterior-inferior iliac spine and advanced along the greater sciatic buttress. The two principal inferior fracture fragments are then reduced and immobilized as described for a T-type fracture.

Postoperative Management

Prophylactic antibiotic therapy continues for 1 day after the surgical procedure.[86,87] Routine prophylaxis with deep venous thrombosis is initially done using various mechanical means, including pneumatic compression devices or compression stockings. Therapeutic anticoagulation is done for 1 month with a low-molecular-weight heparin, warfarin, or aspirin.[88,89] Postoperative pain management is facilitated with a continuous nerve block.[81] On the day after surgery, physical and occupational therapy are initiated with gait and transfer training along with active motion exercises for the hip and strengthening activities. In the presence of an apparently stable acetabulum and cup, weight bearing to tolerance is encouraged. If an ORIF of the acetabulum was performed, then partial weight bearing is advised for 1 month after the surgery. A strengthening program for the hip muscles, including the use of aerobic techniques and weight machines, is suggested for 1 year after the reconstruction.

Results of THA After an Acetabular Fracture

Previous authors have reported highly diverse clinical and radiographic outcomes after late THA to treat an acetabular fracture.[48,49,90] The diversity of the results is not surprising in view of the heterogeneity of the fracture patterns and the many methods of primary fracture management. In most studies, the primary complication was the premature loosening of cups. In one study, a matched cohort of patients with acetabular fracture was compared with a similarly matched group of 49 patients with primary degenerative arthritis.[48] The study also evaluated the fracture group by initial nonsurgical or surgical treatment. With respect to the functional outcome as documented by WOMAC, Musculoskeletal Function Assessment, and Medical Outcomes Study 36-Item Short Form ratings, the results were statistically worse in the fracture group. The complication rate was significantly higher in the ORIF patients than in the nonsurgical group with respect to iatrogenic sciatic nerve palsy, postoperative wound infection, and dislocation. One average, the time to revision was much shorter in the fracture group than in the elective THA group of patients with degenerative arthritis, secondary to acetabular loosening. Within the fracture group, the ORIF patients progressed to cup revision for loosening in a shorter time than the nonsurgical group. In that regard the results of the nonsurgical group were similar to the elective THA group of patients with degenerative arthritis. After ORIF of an acetabular fracture, the presence of scarring, devascularization, and HO serve as precursors of postoperative infection, sciatic nerve injury, and premature cup loosening. As a general observation, the ORIF group pertains to generally more forceful injuries with a greater degree of initial fracture displacement, comminution, and devascularization. From these considerations, the late results for THA after acetabular fractures are not surprising.

The results for 57 patients who underwent an acute THA within 21 days after an acetabular fracture were reported.[56] The patients were followed for a mean duration of 8.1 years (range, 2 to 12 years). At the latest clinical evaluation, 49 patients (86%) had no or slight and intermittent pain and 18 undertook some degree of laboring activities. Forty-five patients (79%) had an excellent or good Harris hip score. When the Harris hip scores were categorized by the patient age in decades, a strong correlation was evident, with the highest scores achieved in the youngest patients and a progressive deterioration of the scores with advancing age, notably in those patients 70 to 89 years old. All of the fractures united within 12 weeks. Late surgical procedures included single instances of HO removal, late cup revision for malalignment, and trochanteric wire removal.

Complications After THA for an Acetabular Fracture

Overall, the complications after a THA performed following an acetabular fracture are similar to those that may follow a conventional THA.[86] The most typical ones, including postoperative wound infection, deep venous thrombosis and pulmonary embolus, dislocation, secondary loosening of the implants, and as well as general medical complications, are reviewed elsewhere. A few complications most relevant to this focal topic are reviewed here.

Sciatic Nerve Palsy

A sciatic nerve palsy after a THA performed for an acetabular fracture is less likely to fully recover and is associated with a prolonged or indefinite period of dysesthetic pain. Contributing factors include the potential for an immediate posttraumatic nerve injury, and iatrogenic components associated with an acute ORIF and the secondary THA. Even if the posttraumatic neurologic deficit fully recovers, the nerve is more vulnerable to another injury at the time of the THA, even when a less forceful manipulation occurs. After the secondary insult, the nerve is less likely to fully recover. The conventional types of management for late nerve deficit include the use of an ankle-foot orthosis along with pain management for dysesthetic pain. Surgical exploration of the nerve is rarely beneficial.

Recurrent HO Formation

Immediately after surgical excision of HO, 700-cGy irradiation therapy may diminish the likelihood of recurrent HO formation.[71] Although prophylactic use of indomethacin has been suggested, the results have been disappointing.[70] In a high-risk patient such as an obese male with a head injury and grade 3 or 4 HO following the initial ORIF, and despite the use of postoperative radiation therapy after a THA with HO removal, a high likelihood for recurrent HO formation even of a grade 3 or 4 magnitude can be anticipated.

Failed, Loose, or Displaced Acetabular Component

Following the THA, the cup sometimes loosens and displaces within a period of months. Several factors may be implicated, including an inadequate size and frictional fit or bony coverage of the cup, or insufficient supplementary screw fixation or avascularity of the adjacent acetabular bone. Multiple radiographic views including a comparison with the initial images taken after the THA may facilitate an identification of the relevant factors. If inadequate acetabular bone stock is documented, at the time of the revision arthroplasty, the use of an augment block for the cup may permit a secure anchorage to be achieved. Alternative strategies may include the use of an acetabular roof ring or a cage. If the inadequate acetabular bone stock is secondary to an acetabular deformity from an acetabular malunion or residual pelvic ring deformity, a reconstructive procedure may require an open reduction of the involved acetabular and pelvic segments. The expertise of a pelvic surgeon may be needed to plan and perform the complex reconstructive procedure.

Complex Situations

When a THA after an acetabular fracture fails, in certain circumstances the likelihood for a successful revision arthroplasty becomes a remote possibility. Although these situations are uncommon, the typical scenario follows multiple prior hip procedures, with culmination in a loose cup, marked HO formation, bone loss, scarification, and/or the absence of effective hip muscles. A point is reached whereby a resectional arthroplasty with or without the insertion of a cement spacer may afford the best likelihood for optimal functional recovery. That procedure minimizes the risk of additional postoperative complications. When such a clinical and radiographic situation is documented, a review by a highly experienced hip specialist may aid in the recognition of this situation.

Summary

Performing a THA in a patient with hip dysplasia presents a unique scenario. Dependent on the degree of dysplasia and deformity, case complexity can range from relatively straightforward to extremely challenging. A thorough knowledge of the anatomic variabilities allows the surgeon to address these challenges while minimizing intraoperative and postoperative complications. There have been many advances in techniques and implant design that have translated into more reproducible results with better outcomes and improved midterm to long-term implant survivorship.

Overall, THA after an acetabular fracture is a viable therapeutic option to manage posttraumatic degenerative arthritis or osteonecrosis. Typically, the procedure is more complex than that undertaken for degenerative arthritis. If the acetabular fracture patient has other injuries, such as a sciatic nerve palsy, the clinical outcome may be substantially impaired by that complicating factor. Where a late THA is performed after a primary ORIF was undertaken for the acetabular fracture, the clinical outcome and anticipated longevity of the ar-

3: Hip

throplasty is compromised. This concern culminated in the development of acute THA for highly selective acetabular fractures. The acute arthroplastic procedure is complicated by the presence of an unstable acetabulum, potentially as a traumatic counterpart to a dissociation. Although the technical challenges may be substantial and necessitate considerable surgical experience in both arthroplasty and pelvis trauma surgery, nevertheless, the acute THA has been documented as a valuable therapeutic method for selective displaced fractures.

The wide range of anatomic abnormalities involving the acetabulum and femur that characterize hip dysplasia in its different severities dictate the need for different reconstructive techniques, including osteotomies and bone grafting when THA is pursued. The young age and active lifestyle of this patient population, coupled with the increased complexity of surgery and potential complications, explain the elevated historic failure rate of acetabular and femoral implants in patients with dysplasia and emphasize the need for a case-by-case appraisal and appropriate selection of implants and reconstructive/surgical techniques.

Annotated References

1. Harris WH: Etiology of osteoarthritis of the hip. *Clin Orthop Relat Res* 1986;213(213):20-33.

2. Jacobsen S, Sonne-Holm S, Søballe K, Gebuhr P, Lund B: Hip dysplasia and osteoarthrosis: A survey of 4151 subjects from the Osteoarthrosis Substudy of the Copenhagen City Heart Study. *Acta Orthop* 2005;76(2):149-158.

   The authors evaluated more than 4,000 patients' pelvic radiographs. They also evaluated the center edge angle, Sharp angle, femoral head extrusion index, and acetabular depth ratio in each radiograph and concluded that hip dysplasia is an etiologic factor in the development of hip osteoarthritis.

3. Crowe JF, Mani VJ, Ranawat CS: Total hip replacement in congenital dislocation and dysplasia of the hip. *J Bone Joint Surg Am* 1979;61(1):15-23.

4. Hartofilakidis G, Stamos K, Karachalios T, Ioannidis TT, Zacharakis N: Congenital hip disease in adults: Classification of acetabular deficiencies and operative treatment with acetabuloplasty combined with total hip arthroplasty. *J Bone Joint Surg Am* 1996;78(5):683-692.

5. Yiannakopoulos CK, Chougle A, Eskelinen A, Hodgkinson JP, Hartofilakidis G: Inter- and intra-observer variability of the Crowe and Hartofilakidis classification systems for congenital hip disease in adults. *J Bone Joint Surg Br* 2008;90(5):579-583.

   This study evaluated the reliability of the two most commonly used classification systems for DDH. Three experienced hip surgeons from three different countries evaluated the radiographs. Excellent intraob-

server and interobserver reliability was seen with both classification systems.

6. Dunn HK, Hess WE: Total hip reconstruction in chronically dislocated hips. *J Bone Joint Surg Am* 1976;58(6):838-845.

7. Masonis JL, Patel JV, Miu A, et al: Subtrochanteric shortening and derotational osteotomy in primary total hip arthroplasty for patients with severe hip dysplasia: 5-year follow-up. *J Arthroplasty* 2003;18(3, suppl 1):68-73.

8. Krych AJ, Howard JL, Trousdale RT, Cabanela ME, Berry DJ: Total hip arthroplasty with shortening subtrochanteric osteotomy in Crowe type-IV developmental dysplasia: Surgical technique. *J Bone Joint Surg Am* 2010;92(suppl 1, pt 2):176-187.

   The authors describe the technique of a subtrochanteric osteotomy in 28 Crowe IV dysplastic hips, followed for a mean of 4.8 years, when used with cementless acetabular and femoral components. Overall high rates of success were achieved; however, the authors also emphasize the higher complication rates found (two nonunions, one acetabular and one femoral component loosening, and one polyethylene liner disengagement) compared with primary THA in patients with degenerative arthritis. Level of evidence: IV.

9. Pagnano W, Hanssen AD, Lewallen DG, Shaughnessy WJ: The effect of superior placement of the acetabular component on the rate of loosening after total hip arthroplasty. *J Bone Joint Surg Am* 1996;78(7):1004-1014.

10. Hampton BJ, Harris WH: Primary cementless acetabular components in hips with severe developmental dysplasia or total dislocation: A concise follow-up, at an average of sixteen years, of a previous report. *J Bone Joint Surg Am* 2006;88(7):1549-1552.

    The authors report on a series of 20 patients with an average 16-year follow-up. Only one shell was revised for aseptic loosening, leading to a reported 92% survivorship. Level of evidence: IV.

11. Klapach AS, Callaghan JJ, Miller KA, et al: Total hip arthroplasty with cement and without acetabular bone graft for severe hip dysplasia: A concise follow-up, at a minimum of twenty years, of a previous report. *J Bone Joint Surg Am* 2005;87(2):280-285.

    The authors report on a series of 66 Charnley total hip replacements followed for a minimum of 20 years. All acetabular components were placed at the anatomic hip center. The reported survivorship of the acetabular component was 86% with revision because of aseptic loosening as the end point.

12. Chougle A, Hemmady MV, Hodgkinson JP: Long-term survival of the acetabular component after total hip arthroplasty with cement in patients with developmental dysplasia of the hip. *J Bone Joint Surg Am* 2006;88(1):71-79.

    The authors report on a series of 292 cemented total

hip replacements with an average follow-up of 15.7 years. Acetabular component survivorship was reported as 90.6% at 10 years and 63% at 20 years.

13. Kim M, Kadowaki T: High long-term survival of bulk femoral head autograft for acetabular reconstruction in cementless THA for developmental hip dysplasia. *Clin Orthop Relat Res* 2010;468(6):1611-1620.

The authors report on a series of 83 cementless total hip reconstructions with an average follow-up of 11 years. No femoral head autograft collapse was seen and a 10-year survival rate of 97% was reported with aseptic loosening as the end point.

14. Cameron HU, Botsford DJ, Park YS: Influence of the Crowe rating on the outcome of total hip arthroplasty in congenital hip dysplasia. *J Arthroplasty* 1996;11(5):582-587.

15. Sakai T, Ohzono K, Nishii T, Miki H, Takao M, Sugano N: A modular femoral neck and head system works well in cementless total hip replacement for patients with developmental dysplasia of the hip. *J Bone Joint Surg Br* 2010;92(6):770-776.

The authors evaluated two groups of 74 DDH total hip reconstructions comparing a modular neck system with a nonmodular system, at a mean follow-up of 14.5 years. They report a higher mean total Harris hip score, greater abduction, decreased osteolysis, and better restoration of leg lengths in the modular group.

16. Thillemann TM, Pedersen AB, Johnsen SP, Søballe K, Danish Hip Arthroplasty Registry: Implant survival after primary total hip arthroplasty due to childhood hip disorders: Results from the Danish Hip Arthroplasty Registry. *Acta Orthop* 2008;79(6):769-776.

A total of 56,087 THA procedures (96% osteoarthritis, 1.6% acetabular dysplasia, 1.0% congenital hip dislocation, 0.5% epiphysiolysis, 0.4% Legg-Calvé-Perthes disease) were compared with respect to the underlying diagnosis at the time of surgery for implant survivorship. Patients with acetabular dysplasia had an increased early risk of revision due to dislocation. Late risk of revision was not dependent on hip disorder diagnosis.

17. Engesaeter LB, Furnes O, Havelin LI: Developmental dysplasia of the hip—good results of later total hip arthroplasty: 7135 primary total hip arthroplasties after developmental dysplasia of the hip compared with 59774 total hip arthroplasties in idiopathic coxarthrosis followed for 0 to 15 years in the Norwegian Arthroplasty Register. *J Arthroplasty* 2008;23(2):235-240.

The results of THA for DDH were the same as for idiopathic osteoarthritis after adjustments for younger age and implant types. This article emphasizes the need to evaluate carefully the data as the risk of revision was 1.5 times higher for DDH cases before adjustments for age and implant types, demonstrating the importance of comparing like groups.

18. Ikeuchi M, Kawakami T, Yamanaka N, Okanoue Y, Tani T: Safe zone for the superior gluteal nerve in the transgluteal approach to the dysplastic hip: Intraoperative evaluation using a nerve stimulator. *Acta Orthop* 2006;77(4):603-606.

The superior gluteal nerve can be damaged during the transgluteal approach to the hip in THA. This article emphasizes a 3-cm safe zone in most dysplastic hips, whereas in severely dysplastic hips the superior gluteal nerve occasionally coursed within 3 cm of the tip of the greater trochanter. A nerve stimulator can be used to identify the nerve in these severe cases.

19. Sanchez-Sotelo J, Berry DJ, Trousdale RT, Cabanela ME: Surgical treatment of developmental dysplasia of the hip in adults: II. Arthroplasty options. *J Am Acad Orthop Surg* 2002;10(5):334-344.

20. Morsi E, Garbuz D, Gross AE: Total hip arthroplasty with shelf grafts using uncemented cups: A long-term follow-up study. *J Arthroplasty* 1996;11(1):81-85.

21. Zhang H, Huang Y, Zhou YX, Zhou YX, Lv M, Jiang ZH: Acetabular medial wall displacement osteotomy in total hip arthroplasty: A technique to optimize the acetabular reconstruction in acetabular dysplasia. *J Arthroplasty* 2005;20(5):562-567.

A total of 30 hips with acetabular dysplasia were operated on using circumferential acetabular medial wall displacement osteotomy to reconstruct the acetabulum during THA and obtain an optimal hip center of rotation. The authors state that their short-term follow-up suggests that this technique is reliable and reproducible and generally avoids the use of bone graft and graft site morbidity.

22. Dorr LD, Tawakkol S, Moorthy M, Long W, Wan Z: Medial protrusio technique for placement of a porous-coated, hemispherical acetabular component without cement in a total hip arthroplasty in patients who have acetabular dysplasia. *J Bone Joint Surg Am* 1999;81(1):83-92.

23. Siebenrock KA, Tannast M, Kim S, Morgenstern W, Ganz R: Acetabular reconstruction using a roof reinforcement ring with hook for total hip arthroplasty in developmental dysplasia of the hip-osteoarthritis minimum 10-year follow-up results. *J Arthroplasty* 2005;20(4):492-498.

The authors evaluate the acetabular reinforcement ring with hook in the treatment of acetabular deformity.

24. Sochart DH, Porter ML: The long-term results of Charnley low-friction arthroplasty in young patients who have congenital dislocation, degenerative osteoarthrosis, or rheumatoid arthritis. *J Bone Joint Surg Am* 1997;79(11):1599-1617.

25. Bicanic G, Delimar D, Delimar M, Pecina M: Influence of the acetabular cup position on hip load during arthroplasty in hip dysplasia. *Int Orthop* 2009;33(2):397-402.

The authors evaluate hip load change in respect to various acetabular cup positions in female patients who underwent total hip replacement surgery because of hip dysplasia. The calculation suggests that for every

3: Hip

millimeter of lateral displacement of the acetabular cup an increase of 0.7% in hip load should be expected, and for every millimeter of proximal displacement an increase of 0.1% in hip load should be expected (or decreased if displacement is medial or distal). Also, for every millimeter of neck length increase, 1% decrease is expected and for every millimeter of lateral offset, 0.8% decrease is expected.

26. Delp SL, Wixson RL, Komattu AV, Kocmond JH: How superior placement of the joint center in hip arthroplasty affects the abductor muscles. *Clin Orthop Relat Res* 1996;328:137-146.

27. Kaneuji A, Sugimori T, Ichiseki T, Yamada K, Fukui K, Matsumoto T: Minimum ten-year results of a porous acetabular component for Crowe I to III hip dysplasia using an elevated hip center. *J Arthroplasty* 2009;24(2):187-194.

    The investigators conducted a retrospective study of the placement of porous-coated acetabular components using screws at more than 20 mm above the teardrop without structural bone graft for dysplastic hips to determine long-term outcome. No acetabular components showed loosening. One metal shell was revised for wear and osteolysis.

28. MacKenzie JR, Kelley SS, Johnston RC: Total hip replacement for coxarthrosis secondary to congenital dysplasia and dislocation of the hip: Long-term results. *J Bone Joint Surg Am* 1996;78(1):55-61.

29. Kim YH, Kim JS: Total hip arthroplasty in adult patients who had developmental dysplasia of the hip. *J Arthroplasty* 2005;20(8):1029-1036.

    This study evaluated the hypothesis that the clinical results are equivalent in the group of patients with dysplasia, low dislocation, and high dislocation types using a contemporary technique for hip arthroplasty. In the high dislocation group, seven hips (17%) had a revision of one or both components. In the low dislocation group, three hips (9%) had a revision of one or both components. In the dysplastic group, two hips (5%) had a revision of one or both components.

30. Shinar AA, Harris WH: Bulk structural autogenous grafts and allografts for reconstruction of the acetabulum in total hip arthroplasty: Sixteen-year-average follow-up. *J Bone Joint Surg Am* 1997;79(2):159-168.

31. Spangehl MJ, Berry DJ, Trousdale RT, Cabanela ME: Uncemented acetabular components with bulk femoral head autograft for acetabular reconstruction in developmental dysplasia of the hip: Results at five to twelve years. *J Bone Joint Surg Am* 2001;83(10):1484-1489.

32. Goto K, Akiyama H, Kawanabe K, So K, Morimoto T, Nakamura T: Long-term results of cemented total hip arthroplasty for dysplasia, with structural autograft fixed with poly-L-lactic acid screws. *J Arthroplasty* 2009;24(8):1146-1151.

    This study reviewed a series of cemented THA for dysplasia, with structural autograft fixed with poly-L-lactic acid screws. The results of this study indicated that poly-L-lactic acid screws are safe and useful for

the fixation of acetabular bone graft similar to cemented THA with a careful rehabilitation program.

33. Somford MP, Bolder SB, Gardeniers JW, Slooff TJ, Schreurs BW: Favorable survival of acetabular reconstruction with bone impaction grafting in dysplastic hips. *Clin Orthop Relat Res* 2008;466(2):359-365.

    The bone impaction grafting technique in combination with a cemented total hip can restore the bone stock in dysplastic patients. The investigators report on 28 hips performed using this technique. The cumulative survival of the cup with revision for any reason as the end point was 96% at 10 years and 84% at 15 years.

34. Harris WH: Results of uncemented cups: A critical appraisal at 15 years. *Clin Orthop Relat Res* 2003;417:121-125.

35. Hendrich C, Mehling I, Sauer U, Kirschner S, Martell JM: Cementless acetabular reconstruction and structural bone-grafting in dysplastic hips. *J Bone Joint Surg Am* 2006;88(2):387-394.

    Forty-seven patients who had DDH underwent 56 THAs and received a structural graft in combination with a cementless Harris-Galante type I cup. The 11-year survival rate for the spherical press-fit cups in combination with bulk bone grafting is satisfactory given the complexity of these reconstructions. Level of evidence: IV.

36. Wasielewski RC, Cooperstein LA, Kruger MP, Rubash HE: Acetabular anatomy and the transacetabular fixation of screws in total hip arthroplasty. *J Bone Joint Surg Am* 1990;72(4):501-508.

37. Liu Q, Zhou YX, Xu HJ, Tang J, Guo SJ, Tang QH: Safe zone for transacetabular screw fixation in prosthetic acetabular reconstruction of high developmental dysplasia of the hip. *J Bone Joint Surg Am* 2009;91(12):2880-2885.

    The quadrant system, although helpful in determining screw placement in hips with a normal center of rotation, can be misleading and of limited value in guiding screw insertion to augment acetabular shells for hips with a high dislocation. Screws guided by the quadrant system frequently injured the obturator blood vessels in the hips with a high dislocation. In these patients, the safe zone shifted as a result of moving the prosthetic cup.

38. Eskelinen A, Helenius I, Remes V, Ylinen P, Tallroth K, Paavilainen T: Cementless total hip arthroplasty in patients with high congenital hip dislocation. *J Bone Joint Surg Am* 2006;88(1):80-91.

    The study included 68 THAs performed between 1989 and 1994 in 56 consecutive patients with high congenital hip dislocation. The cup was placed at the level of the true acetabulum, and a shortening osteotomy of the proximal part of the femur and distal advancement of the greater trochanter were performed in 90% of the hips. With revision because of aseptic loosening as the end point, the 10-year survival rate for press-fit, porous-coated acetabular components was 94.9% and the rate of survival for the femoral components, with

3: Hip

revision because of aseptic loosening as the end point, was 98.4%.

39. Archibeck MJ, Rosenberg AG, Berger RA, Silverton CD: Trochanteric osteotomy and fixation during total hip arthroplasty. *J Am Acad Orthop Surg* 2003;11(3): 163-173.

40. Georgiades G, Babis GC, Hartofilakidis G: Charnley low-friction arthroplasty in young patients with osteo-arthritis: Outcomes at a minimum of twenty-two years. *J Bone Joint Surg Am* 2009;91(12):2846-2851.

    The authors concluded that long-term results of Charnley low-friction arthroplasty can be used as a benchmark to compare outcomes of various designs in young patients with congenital hip disease undergoing THA.

41. Biant LC, Bruce WJ, Assini JB, Walker PM, Walsh WR: Primary total hip arthroplasty in severe develop-mental dysplasia of the hip: Ten-year results using a ce-mentless modular stem. *J Arthroplasty* 2009;24(1):27-32.

    The authors report the average 10-year clinical and ra-diographic results of 28 hips with Crowe III or IV DDH that had hip arthroplasty using the cementless modular S-ROM stem. None of the S-ROM stems had been revised or were loose at an average 10-year follow-up.

42. Nagoya S, Kaya M, Sasaki M, Tateda K, Kosukegawa I, Yamashita T: Cementless total hip replacement with subtrochanteric femoral shortening for severe develop-mental dysplasia of the hip. *J Bone Joint Surg Br* 2009; 91(9):1142-1147.

    The authors describe their experience using cementless THA combined with a subtrochanteric femoral short-ening osteotomy in 20 hips with Crowe type IV dislo-cation with a mean follow-up of 8.1 years. THA com-bined with subtrochanteric shortening femoral osteotomy in this situation is beneficial in avoiding nerve injury and still permits valuable improvement in inequality of leg length.

43. Ito H, Matsuno T, Minami A, Aoki Y: Intermediate-term results after hybrid total hip arthroplasty for the treatment of dysplastic hips. *J Bone Joint Surg Am* 2003;85(9):1725-1732.

44. Letournel E, Judet R: *Fractures of the Acetabulum*, ed 2. New York, NY, Springer-Verlag, 1993, pp 137-155.

45. Matta JM: Fractures of the acetabulum: Accuracy of reduction and clinical results in patients managed op-eratively within three weeks after the injury. *J Bone Joint Surg Am* 1996;78(11):1632-1645.

46. Mears DC, Velyvis JH, Chang CP: Displaced acetabu-lar fractures managed operatively: Indicators of out-come. *Clin Orthop Relat Res* 2003;407(407):173-186.

47. Moed BR, McMichael JC: Outcomes of posterior wall fractures of the acetabulum: Surgical technique. *J Bone*

Joint Surg Am 2008;90(suppl 2, pt 1):87-107.

    The authors outline their surgical technique for surgi-cal management of posterior wall fractures. The sa-lient observation is significant of poor late clinical re-sults for what is often errantly perceived as the simplest type of acetabular fracture.

48. Tile M, Jimenez ML, Borkhoff C: Delayed total hip ar-throplasty following acetabular fracture, in Tile M, Helfet DL, Kellam JF, eds: *Fractures of the Pelvis and Acetabulum*, ed 3. Philadelphia, PA, Lippincott Wil-liams & Wilkins, 2003, pp 786-794.

49. Mears DC, Velyvis JH: Primary total hip arthroplasty after acetabular fracture. *J Bone Joint Surg Am* 2000; 82:1328-1353.

50. Callaghan JJ, McBeath AA: Arthrodesis, in Callaghan JJ, Rosenberg JJ, Rubash HE, eds: *The Adult Hip*. Philadelphia, PA, Lippincott Williams & Wilkins, 1998, pp 749-759.

51. Mears DC: Surgical treatment of acetabular fractures in elderly patients with osteoporotic bone. *J Am Acad Orthop Surg* 1999;7(2):128-141.

52. Mears DC, Mears SC: Internal fixation of osteoporotic acetabular and pelvic fractures, in An Y, ed: *Internal Fixation of Osteoporotic Bone*. New York, NY, Thieme Medical Publishers, 2002, pp 137-155.

53. Osterman AL: The double crush syndrome. *Orthop Clin North Am* 1988;19(1):147-155.

54. Russell GV Jr, Nork SE, Chip Routt ML Jr: Perioper-ative complications associated with operative treat-ment of acetabular fractures. *J Trauma* 2001;51(6): 1098-1103.

55. Mears DC, Velyvis JH: Primary total hip replacement for an acetabular fracture, in Tile M, Helfet DL, Kel-lam JF, eds: *Fractures of the Pelvis and Acetabulum*, ed 3. Philadelphia, PA, Lippincott Williams & Wilkins, 2003, pp 770-785.

56. Mears DC, Velyvis JH: Acute total hip arthroplasty for selected displaced acetabular fractures: Two to twelve-year results. *J Bone Joint Surg Am* 2002;84(1):1-9.

57. Helfet DL, Borrelli J Jr, DiPasquale T, Sanders R: Sta-bilization of acetabular fractures in elderly patients. *J Bone Joint Surg Am* 1992;74(5):753-765.

58. Vrahas M, Gordon RG, Mears DC, Krieger D, Scla-bassi RJ: Intraoperative somatosensory evoked poten-tial monitoring of pelvic and acetabular fractures. *J Orthop Trauma* 1992;6(1):50-58.

59. Helfet DL, Anand N, Malkani AL, et al: Intraoperative monitoring of motor pathways during operative fixa-tion of acute acetabular fractures. *J Orthop Trauma* 1997;11(1):2-6.

60. Moed BR: Acetabular fractures: The Kocher-

3: Hip

Langenbeck approach, in Wiss DA, ed: *Fractures: Master Techniques in Orthopaedic Surgery*. Philadelphia, PA, Lippincott Williams & Wilkins, 1998, pp 631-655.

61. Matta JM, Reilly MC: Acetabular fractures: The ilioinguinal approach, in Wiss DA, ed: *Fractures: Master Techniques in Orthopaedic Surgery*. Philadelphia, PA, Lippincott Williams & Wilkins, 1998, pp 657-673.

62. Helfet DL, Bartlett CS, Malkani AL: Acetabular fractures: The extended iliofemoral approach, in Wiss DA, ed: *Fractures: Master Techniques in Orthopaedic Surgery*. Philadelphia, PA, Lippincott Williams & Wilkins, 1998, pp 675-695.

63. Mears DC, MacLeod MD: Surgical approaches: Triradiate and modified triradiate, in Wiss D, ed: *Master Techniques in Orthopaedic Surgery: Fractures*. New York, NY, Lippincott Raven Press, 1997, pp 701-728.

64. Sloof TJ, Scheurs BW, Buma P, Gardeniers JW: Impaction morselized allografting and cement. *Instr Course Lect* 1999;48:79-89.

65. Mears DC, Velyvis JH: Surgical reconstruction of late pelvic post-traumatic nonunions and malalignments. *J Bone Joint Surg Br* 2003;85(1):21-30.

66. Moed BR, Smith ST: Three-view radiographic assessment of heterotopic ossification after acetabular fracture surgery. *J Orthop Trauma* 1996;10(2):93-98.

67. Brooker AF, Bowerman JW, Robinson RA, Riley LH Jr: Ectopic ossification following total hip replacement: Incidence and a method of classification. *J Bone Joint Surg Am* 1973;55(8):1629-1632.

68. Cipriano CA, Pill SG, Keenan MA: Heterotopic ossification following traumatic brain injury and spinal cord injury. *J Am Acad Orthop Surg* 2009;17(11):689-697.

    The extraordinary predilection for marked HO formation in the hip joint in a patient with a concomitant head and hip trauma is documented. The precipitating factor after the head injury that provokes HO formation remains unclear.

69. Banovac K: The effect of etidronate on late development of heterotopic ossification after spinal cord injury. *J Spinal Cord Med* 2000;23(1):40-44.

70. Matta JM, Siebenrock KA: Does indomethacin reduce heterotopic bone formation after operations for acetabular fractures? A prospective randomized study. *J Bone Joint Surg Br* 1997;79(6):959-963.

71. Burd TA, Lowry KJ, Anglen JO: Indomethacin compared with localized irradiation for the prevention of heterotopic ossification following surgical treatment of acetabular fractures. *J Bone Joint Surg Am* 2001; 83(12):1783-1788.

72. Fitzgerald RH, Davis LP, Rajan DK: Radionucleide imaging, in Callaghan JJ, Rosenberg JJ, Rubash HE, eds: *The Adult Hip*. Philadelphia, PA, Lippincott Williams & Wilkins, 1998, pp 373-391.

73. Masri BA, Duncan CP: Sepsis: Two-stage exchange, in Callaghan JJ, Rosenberg JJ, Rubash HE, eds: *The Adult Hip*. Philadelphia, PA, Lippincott Williams & Wilkins, 1998, pp 1317-1330.

74. Mears DC: Avascular necrosis of the acetabulum. *Oper Tech Orthop* 1997;7:241-249.

75. Berry DJ, Lewallen DG, Hanssen AD, Cabanela ME: Pelvic discontinuity in revision total hip arthroplasty. *J Bone Joint Surg Am* 1999;81(12):1692-1702.

76. McGann WA: Surgical approaches, in Callaghan JJ, Rosenberg JJ, Rubash HE, eds: *The Adult Hip*. Philadelphia, PA, Lippincott Williams & Wilkins, 1998, pp 663-718.

77. Mears DC, Mears SC, Chelly JE: Two-incision hip replacement in the morbidly obese patient. *Semin Arthroplasty* 2007;18:272-279.

    The two-incision technique is described in detail. The description also highlights the specific modifications that are used for a large and morbidly obese patient.

78. Weeden SH, Schmidt R: Early results of minimally invasive two-incision total hip arthroplasty: A review at 24-month follow-up. *Semin Arthroplasty* 2007;18: 246-250.

    The authors present favorable results for short-term follow-up evaluation after the use of the two-incision technique. This analysis is more favorable for the clinical outcomes in contrast to several earlier publications by authors who possessed modest surgical experience, which was related to higher incidences of intraoperative complications.

79. Mears DC, Mears SC, Chelly JE, Dai F, Vulakovich KL: THA with a minimally invasive technique, multimodal anesthesia, and home rehabilitation: Factors associated with early discharge? *Clin Orthop Relat Res* 2009;467(6):1412-1417.

    Detailed short-term results for 676 patients are provided along with the multimodal pain management regimen and accelerated therapeutic program. The results document that approximately 40% of the patients were discharged to home after a 23-hour admission.

80. Ben-David B, Frankel R, Arzumonov T, Marchevsky Y, Volpin G: Minidose bupivacaine-fentanyl spinal anesthesia for surgical repair of hip fracture in the aged. *Anesthesiology* 2000;92(1):6-10.

81. Chelly JE, Ben-David B, Mears DC: Anesthesia and acute pain management for minimally invasive hip surgery. *Tech Reg Anesth Pain Manage* 2004;8:70-75.

82. Issack PS, Figgie MP, Helfet DL: Treatment of acetab-

ular nonunion and posttraumatic arthritis with bone grafting and total hip arthroplasty. *Am J Orthop (Belle Mead NJ)* 2009;38(3):138-141.

The surgical techniques and clinical results for patients who progressed to various patterns of acetabular nonunion complicated by posttraumatic arthritis are reported. The complexity of the surgical procedures is highlighted.

83. Peters CL, Curtain M, Samuelson KM: Acetabular revision with the Burch-Schnieder antiprotrusio cage and cancellous allograft bone. *J Arthroplasty* 1995;10(3): 307-312.

84. Paprosky WG, O'Rourke M, Sporer SM: The treatment of acetabular bone defects with an associated pelvic discontinuity. *Clin Orthop Relat Res* 2005;441: 216-220.

The authors discuss the treatment of pelvic discontinuity in patients with severe acetabular bone loss. Level of evidence: III.

85. Mears DC, Shirahama M: Stabilization of an acetabular fracture with cables for acute total hip arthroplasty. *J Arthroplasty* 1998;13(1):104-107.

86. Berry DJ: Primary total hip arthroplasty, in Chapman MW, ed: *Chapman's Orthopaedic Surgery*. Philadelphia, PA, Lippincott Williams & Wilkins, 2001, pp 2769-2794.

87. Bhattacharyya T, Hooper DC: Antibiotic dosing before primary hip and knee replacement as a pay-for-performance measure. *J Bone Joint Surg Am* 2007; 89(2):287-291.

The authors provide a quantitative guideline to antibiotic selection and dosage as prophylactic agents for THA. The analysis serves as a guideline for cost-effective use of prophylactic antibiotics for arthroplastic surgery.

88. Colwell CW Jr, Collis DK, Paulson R, et al: Comparison of enoxaparin and warfarin for the prevention of venous thromboembolic disease after total hip arthroplasty: Evaluation during hospitalization and three months after discharge. *J Bone Joint Surg Am* 1999; 81(7):932-940.

89. Johanson NA, Lachiewicz PF, Lieberman JR, et al: Prevention of symptomatic pulmonary embolism in patients undergoing total hip or knee arthroplasty. *J Am Acad Orthop Surg* 2009;17(3):183-196.

A clinical practice guideline on the management of adults with pulmonary embolus prophylaxis after total hip and total knee replacements is presented. The guideline is based on a systematic review of numerous published studies. It evaluates the roles of various prophylactic agents with respect to patient risk factors for a postoperative pulmonary embolus.

90. Romness DW, Lewallen DG: Total hip arthroplasty after fracture of the acetabulum: Long-term results. *J Bone Joint Surg Br* 1990;72(5):761-764.

Chapter 19

Minimally Invasive Total Hip Arthroplasty

Gregg R. Klein, MD   Mark A. Hartzband, MD   Soheil Najibi, MD, PhD   Joel M. Matta, MD
Douglas E. Padgett, MD

Introduction
Gregg R. Klein, MD
Mark A. Hartzband, MD

The long-term success of total hip arthroplasty (THA) has been well documented. Historically, multiple surgical approaches to the hip for THA, including the anterior, anterolateral, direct lateral, transtrochanteric, and posterolateral approaches, have been described. Although each approach has its own advantages and disadvantages, all have well-documented success.

During the late 1990s the concept of reducing incision size and soft-tissue dissection in THA was studied. The earliest investigator of minimally invasive procedures implanted several different prostheses through a limited anterior approach, often with small secondary incisions for insertion of acetabular or femoral instrumentation.[1,2] The field of minimally invasive THA has been controversial, with multiple questions raised about the safety, reproducibility, and applicability of the procedure to various patients with different bony anatomy and body habitus.

A true definition of minimally invasive or mini-incision surgery does not exist. Commonly, mini-incision surgery has been defined as an incision length of less than 10 cm.[3] Minimally invasive THA has essentially been grouped into two main categories: mini-incision approaches and minimally invasive procedures. Mini-incision approaches are modifications of traditional approaches with limited incisions and soft-tissue dissection, the most popular of which are the mini-posterior and mini-direct lateral (Hardinge) approaches. Proponents of these approaches like that they

are familiar, easy to learn without the steep learning curve associated with the other minimally invasive surgical approaches, reproducible, and allow precise implantation of various types of hip implants. In addition, these procedures are believed to be extensile if complications or unforeseen problems occur. The ability to considerably shrink incision size and limit deep surgical dissections has been reported. For example, with the mini-posterior approach, the direct head of the gluteus maximus tendon is no longer divided and the piriformis is not divided when the anatomy allows.

With minimally invasive surgical procedures, the common denominator in all the variations is to minimize soft-tissue damage and avoid cutting muscles and tendons during the surgical exposure. These procedures are either new intramuscular muscle-sparing approaches or new renditions of long-standing internervous approaches to the hip, which include the anterolateral, direct anterior, and two-incision approaches.[4-7] The proposed advantage of these procedures is that they are truly internervous and can be performed without cutting muscle. When these procedures are performed by experienced surgeons, patients have rapid recovery, less blood loss, less pain, shorter hospital stays, and faster return to function, ultimately leading to improved patient satisfaction. In addition, maximum stability has been cited as an advantage of these approaches because they are all based on an anterior exposure of the acetabulum.

Critics of these procedures have reported issues such as wound-healing complications, component malposition, muscle damage, femoral fractures, and a steep

Dr. Klein or an immediate family member is a member of a speakers' bureau or has made paid presentations on behalf of Zimmer; is a paid consultant for or is an employee of Biomet and Zimmer; and has received research or institutional support from Zimmer. Dr. Hartzband or an immediate family member has received royalties from Zimmer, is a member of a speakers' bureau or has made paid presentations on behalf of Zimmer; is a paid consultant for or is an employee of Zimmer; and has received research or institutional support from Zimmer. Dr. Matta or an immediate family member has received royalties from OSI; is a member of a speakers' bureau or has made paid presentations on behalf of DePuy; and is a paid consultant for or is an employee of DePuy and Stryker. Dr. Matta or an immediate family member is a paid consultant for or is an employee of Mako and Stryker; owns stock or stock options in Mako; and serves as a board member, owner, officer, or committee member of the American Association of Hip and Knee Surgeons. Neither Dr. Najibi nor any immediate family member has received anything of value from or owns stock in a commercial company or institutional related directly or indirectly to the subject of this chapter.

3: Hip

learning curve. Another drawback cited is the requirement for a second generation of specialized instrumentation to avoid damage to the greater trochanter during broach and component insertion. Some techniques require additional surgical assistants and/or specialized and expensive operating tables, which may have limited appeal or availability to many surgeons.

Multimodal Pathways/Protocols

A by-product of the initial development of minimally invasive and mini-incision surgery, and perhaps the factor most responsible for significant reductions in length of hospital stay, has been the development of new and aggressive perioperative patient management protocols including modified anesthesia, complex polypharmacy pain management pathways, and aggressive rehabilitation techniques.[8,9] These techniques have been developed in conjunction with the surgical techniques. Thus, it may be difficult to distinguish between the contributions of the less invasive surgical approach and those of the modified clinical pathways.[8,9]

All of these pathways use polypharmacy to interrupt pain pathways at multiple levels, and to minimize or avoid parenteral narcotics. A combination of cyclooxygenase-1 (COX-1) and cyclooxygenase-2 (COX-2) inhibitors and oral narcotics usually is given preoperatively to minimize postoperative pain. Additionally, antiemetics and gastrointestinal motility enhancers are frequently administered. Some cocktails include the intraoperative use of an intravenous bolus of steroids.

Additional variables are the accelerated in-hospital rehabilitation pathways and rapid mobilization. Patients are typically out of bed and ambulating on the day of surgery. Preoperative patient education outlining the expected postoperative protocol often makes obtaining these goals easier. In addition, the hospital staff is reeducated in terms of expectations regarding milestones and timing of discharge.

Authors of a 2007 study reported that patient preconditioning, family education, preemptive analgesia, and accelerated preoperative and postoperative rehabilitation all play major roles in better outcomes after minimally invasive surgery.[10] Authors of a 2008 study compared 44 patients with a traditional care pathway with 38 patients with a new rehabilitation protocol and with 40 patients who had a minimally invasive technique with a modified protocol. They found that the new rehabilitation protocol alone reduced the length of hospital stay and improved the speed of rehabilitation. The minimally invasive surgical technique further improved the short-term outcomes.[11] Similarly, patients with a standard incision and a minimal incision posterior approach were compared in another study and the groups subdivided based on either a routine or intensive therapy program; it was concluded that the length of hospital stay was substantially shorter in the inten-

sive therapy group. Incision length did not have an effect on length of hospital stay in this study.[12] In a study of 50 THAs with either standard perioperative management or advanced therapy and anesthesia protocols, it was concluded that there was a dramatic reduction in the time that it took to achieve discharge goals in the advanced protocol group.[13] The authors of a systematic review reported that multimodal pain control with revised anesthesia protocols and accelerated rehabilitation improves recovery after minimally invasive THA compared with traditional methods. Preoperative physical therapy also may improve postoperative functional recovery.[14]

Safety (Component Position and Complications)

The development of new techniques and approaches has raised concern regarding the safety of less invasive THA. An ideally performed arthroplasty should be reproducible and have appropriate component interfaces, positioning, and alignment along with a low complication rate. There is controversy in the literature as to whether less invasive procedures result in optimal component positioning. Some authors have experienced greater degrees of component malpositioning with certain approaches.

Most published articles on mini-incision and minimally invasive THA are focused on the mini-posterior approach.[15] Authors of a 2004 study presented an early report of 50 mini-incision THAs with a posterior approach and compared them with 85 standard THAs.[16] There were no specific selection criteria, and three different surgeons with little or no experience in mini-incision THA performed the procedures. The authors found a higher risk of wound complications, acetabular component malposition, and poor fit of the femoral components in the mini-incision group and therefore did not recommend the mini-incision technique. Cemented and uncemented THAs performed through either a standard or mini-incision approach were compared; the authors found no difference in component positioning on the acetabular side, but there was varus positioning of approximately 2° of the cemented stems in the mini-incision group.[17] Numerous authors have reported more favorable results with the mini-posterior approach.[17-21] In a study of 1,000 consecutive single-incision mini-posterior approach THAs with a minimum of 2 years of follow-up, a low rate of complications and component malposition was found, leading to the conclusion that satisfactory results can be consistently achieved.[21] In another study, 219 hips were randomized to either a short or standard incision group. Patients were blinded to which group they were in. The authors found that there was no difference in component placement or cement-mantle quality between the groups.[22] The clinical and radiographic results of 90 THAs performed with a mini-posterior approach at 10 to 13 years were reviewed in a 2006 study; these results were comparable to those of conventional techniques.[18]

The anterior minimally invasive surgical exposures have been less frequently evaluated. A prospective randomized cadaver study evaluated the results of cementing a femoral component through either a standard anterolateral transgluteal approach or a direct anterior approach. The authors found no difference between the cement mantles in the two approaches and concluded that a direct anterior minimally invasive approach did not adversely affect the results of cementation of the femoral component.[23] Exposure and implant positioning in primary THA using the anterolateral and posterior minimally invasive approaches were prospectively compared. There were no significant differences in regard to component positioning or limb-length discrepancy. However, the femoral exposure was more difficult in the anterolateral approach, resulting in more trochanteric fractures and femoral perforations.[24]

The authors of a 2006 study evaluated 102 primary THAs performed through either a standard or limited direct lateral approach and found comparable component position in both groups, but more intraoperative femoral fractures in the limited-incision group.[25] Patients undergoing direct lateral THA were randomized into four groups (standard incision and standard rehabilitation protocols, small incision and standard protocols, standard incision and accelerated protocols, and small incision and accelerated protocols). The authors did not find a difference in complications or other surgical parameters regardless of the size of the incision.[10] Forty patients treated with a transgluteal THA with either a small or standard incision were reviewed; the authors found that there were significant variations in implant positions and more complications such as dislocation, fracture, or limb-length discrepancy in the small-incision group.[26]

The two-incision minimally invasive THA has generated great debate in the literature. Critics of the two-incision technique cite a steep learning curve and high complication rates.[27,28] One study reported a 2% incidence of femoral fracture.[7] The surgeon developers of the two-incision technique reported their results in 375 hips and showed a minor complication rate of 2.1% and a major complication rate of 1.3%.[29] Authors of a 2005 study reported the results of 80 patients with a mean age of 70.5 years who were treated with the two-incision technique and found a much greater complication rate including fractures.[28] These two studies differed in the femoral stem design used, and the 2005 study included a much higher proportion of older, osteoporotic obese women. This older female cohort experienced most of the fractures. Authors of a 2006 study also reported a relatively high complication rate with the two-incision technique but found that the complications decreased as the surgeon gained experience with the procedure.[30] This study also found a statistically higher rate of component malposition in the two-incision group. The number of cup outliers (< 30° or > 50°) was 28% in the two-incsion group and 10%

in the single-incision group. Furthermore, the number of stem grades with a poor fit and fill was 10% in the two-incision group and 1% in the single-incision group.[27,30]

A recent study reported the results of 400 initial two-incision THAs and found that the complication rate decreased with each 100 hips. There were two fractures in the first 100 hips, a third fracture in the next 100 hips, and no fractures in the next 200.[31] In a retrospective comparison of 43 matched pairs of patients having either a mini-posterior THA or a two-incision THA, the two-incision THA was associated with better function and decreased length of stay. There were no differences in complications between the two techniques.[32] Component position for 67 minimally invasive two-incision THAs and 28 THAs with a standard direct lateral approach was compared and no significant differences were found; there was acceptable placement with both techniques, and there were no differences in intraoperative or postoperative complications.[33]

Muscle Damage

A proposed advantage of less invasive THA is the minimization of muscle damage. Conflicting evidence exists in the literature. Some studies report greater muscle damage with minimally invasive surgical procedures,[34] others report no difference,[35] and yet others have shown less muscle damage.[36] All of these studies used different methods to assess muscle damage. Twenty cadaver hips were randomly assigned to two groups: a two-incision approach and a mini-posterior approach. After insertion of the arthroplasty components the authors quantitatively assessed the muscle damage in each group. The authors found that damage to the gluteus medius and minimus was greater with the two-incision technique.[34] Limitations of this study include the differing behaviors of cadaver versus living soft tissues and bone, and quantitative measurements do not necessarily translate into functional injury to muscle.[37] A more scientific approach was taken in a 2009 study, whereby serum markers for skeletal muscle damage were measured in 30 consecutive patients undergoing THA. They were divided into three groups: mini-incision Watson-Jones, mini-posterior, and two-incision groups. The authors found similar trends in serum enzyme markers consistent with skeletal muscle damage in all three groups.[35] The authors of a 2008 study randomly performed MRIs on 32 patients who had primary THA with either the two-incision, standard posterolateral, or standard direct lateral techniques.[36] The hip musculature was compared with that of the contralateral unreplaced hip using MRI with metal subtraction at least 18 months after the surgical procedure. The authors found that the posterior and direct lateral approaches had an increased incidence of muscle damage compared with the two-incision hips.[37]

Functional Recovery

The initial goals of minimally invasive and limited-incision surgery were faster recovery and rehabilitation and less pain than traditional techniques. There are multiple studies that either support or refute these claims.

Mini-incision and standard incision THA were compared in a prospective, randomized, blinded study; the authors found that there was no difference in component placement, cement mantle quality, or functional outcomes at 6 weeks.[22] The only variables associated with early hospital discharge were patient age and preoperative hemoglobin levels.[22] Gait analysis was used to compare four different types of THA approaches: mini-posterior, anterolateral, anterior Judet, and traditional posterior long incisions.[38] There was no difference between the groups in velocity, cadence, stride length, single-limb support time, or double-limb support time at 6 weeks or 3 months. However, this study had a small number of patients in each group. A systematic review of 16 level I and II studies found that multimodal pain control with revised protocols and accelerated rehabilitation speeds recovery after minimally invasive THA compared with the standard approaches, but small incisions or minimally invasive approaches do not themselves demonstrate improved outcomes.[14]

Other studies have found that these newer surgical exposures result in improved short-term functional recovery compared with the standard exposures. A prospective, randomized study comparing standard posterior approach THA and small-incision posterior approach THA (< 8 cm) found that fewer patients limped in the minimally invasive group at 6 weeks postoperatively.[39] At 1 to 2 years there were no differences between the groups. Another study compared THA with an anterolateral standard and anterolateral mini-incision technique and found that patients with the mini incision had better hip muscle strength, walking speed, and functional score.[40] At 1 year, there was no difference between the groups. In a prospective, randomized, blinded study, the authors compared traditional long-incision THA with mini-incision posterior approach THA and found that the small-incision group showed better early pain control, earlier discharge home, and less use of assistive devices.[41] At 6 weeks and 3 months there were no differences between the groups.

Whether minimally invasive or mini-incision THA results in the quickest and most functional recovery is a topic of debate. In a retrospective matched pair analysis the mini-posterior approach was compared with the two-incision THA; length of hospital stay was shorter and function was regained earlier in the two-incision group.[3] The author did note that the posterior mini-incision procedure was easier to perform. The same two procedures were compared in a randomized clinical trial; patients recovered more slowly after the two-incision procedure.[42] Two additional studies compared the two-incision THA, the mini-posterior, and mini-anterolateral techniques.[43,44] In terms of early discharge and recovery, there was no difference in hospital discharge, functional recovery milestones, or outcome measures.[43] In a different randomized prospective study, gait analysis on these three groups found that there were no differences between the two-incision and mini-posterior approaches, but the anterolateral approach showed a gait pattern consistent with abductor muscle injury in the early postoperative period.[44]

Minimally invasive THA has resulted in shortened hospital stays and rapid recovery. Results of a multimodal approach, including a minimally invasive surgical technique, preoperative teaching, regional anesthesia, preemptive oral analgesia and antiemetic therapy, rapid rehabilitation protocols, and same-day discharge from the hospital has recently been reported.[9] The authors assessed the feasibility and safety of this approach in 150 consecutive patients. All were discharged home the same day. There was one readmission for fracture and nine emergency department evaluations in the 3-month postoperative period.[9] Outpatient THA has also been shown to be financially advantageous. The cost of surgery in patients with outpatient and inpatient THA was compared; the average hospital bill was less for the outpatient surgery.[45]

Patient Expectations/Cosmesis

Three goals of less invasive THA have been described: pain relief, improvement in function, and patient satisfaction.[46] A proposed benefit of minimally invasive or mini-incision surgery is improved cosmesis and thus the perception of a more successful operation. Patients seem to equate a small incision with less body violation that may lead to less pain, easier recovery, and greater satisfaction.[47] A psychological survey was administered to 165 patients who were treated with THA.[48] One hundred nine patients had a small incision and 56 had long incisions. Preoperatively, the patients expected that small-incision surgery would positively influence their primary goals and satisfaction. At 6 weeks after surgery, patients in both groups had similar feelings that small incisions would positively affect outcomes. At 6 to 12 months postoperatively, all patients had achieved their goals and the length of incision was less important. However, 40% of patients with long incisions were not satisfied because they wished they had received a small incision. These patients felt this way because they were self-conscious and believed that they had difficulty reincorporating the replaced hip into their whole-body image.[48]

Authors of a 2004 study reported on 135 unilateral THAs (50 mini-incision and 85 with a standard incision) and found a higher wound complication rate in the mini-incision group.[16] This series was very early in the authors' experience with mini-incision THA. Another study reported on 34 THAs with either standard or mini-incision THA and had the scars evaluated by two blinded plastic surgeons using a standardized rating system.[49] The plastic surgeons found that more mini-incision patients had scars rated as poor than did patients with a standard incision. All patients believed that their hip scar was acceptable. The authors speculated that the small-incision scars might be inferior because of skin and soft-tissue damage from high retractor pressures during exposure.

Mini-incision posterior approach THA was performed in a group of 115 consecutive patients without predetermining the incision length; there was a correlation between incision size and patient weight, height, and sex.[50] The authors concluded that larger patients can expect a longer incision, and for a given body weight women will have longer incisions than men.[50]

Technique

The surgical paradigm changes significantly with both the mini-incision and minimally invasive hip approaches. The first assistant is integral in moving the extremity to allow the surgeon to have improved visualization. All of the concepts of less invasive THA involve the mobile window concept, which is based upon the principle that excellent visualization of the deep structures may be obtained by manipulating either the soft-tissue window or the tissues below the window (the femur) into multiple positions during the arthroplasty. For example, the entire acetabulum may not be visualized in one viewing, but with manipulation of the femur and/or the mobile window during the exposure the entire acetabulum can be well visualized. One approach (the anterolateral approach) describes five distinct positions required for the limb as the THA evolves.[51] Poor visualization is rarely dealt with by pulling harder or adding retractors, but rather by removing retractors, pulling less forcibly, and/or changing the position of the limb.

Instrumentation

As less invasive procedures evolved, it became apparent that new specific instruments are required to maximize exposure, minimize soft-tissue injury, and ensure proper component position. Retractors with rounded edges and contoured surfaces with light attachments to illuminate the deep recesses of the wound have afforded comparable or better visualization than that afforded by conventional open procedures. Modified reamers, offset reamer handles, offset cup inserters, and offset broach handles minimize soft-tissue injury and maximize the ability to correctly orient the components on a consistent basis.

Learning Curve

Similar to adopting any new surgical technique, there is a learning curve before the surgeon is comfortable with and can accurately and safely perform the desired procedure. The reported learning curve for the two-incision technique has ranged from modest to steep.[27] One study has reported that the learning curve for "trained" surgeons for the two-incision technique may last beyond the tenth case.[52] The learning curve for the anterior-supine minimally invasive THA reportedly is approximately 40 cases and 6 months in a high-volume joint surgeon's practice.[53]

Anterior Approach for THA
Soheil Najibi, MD
Joel M. Matta, MD

The first THA through a single anterior incision was performed by Robert Judet in 1947 using the Hueter anterior approach with the patient supine on the Judet table. This approach involved the removal of the anterior tensor fascia lata from the anterolateral iliac crest, sectioning the reflected head of the rectus and release of the piriformis.

Since the initial description, the approach has been modified to allow exposure of the acetabulum and proximal femur through a single anterior incision without release of any muscles or tendons from the pelvis or the femur.

There are several advantages to the anterior approach of the hip. Anatomically, the hip joint is closer to the skin anteriorly than posteriorly. The anterior approach uses the internervous interval between the sartorius muscle medially (innervated by the femoral nerve) and the tensor facia lata muscle laterally (innervated by the superior gluteal nerve), also known as a short or modified Smith-Peterson approach. The anterior approach preserves the attachment of all the muscles around the hip including the short external rotators, which function as dynamic stabilizers of the hip joint much like the rotator cuff functions as a dynamic stabilizer of the shoulder joint. Moreover, the anterior approach preserves the attachment of the gluteus medius and minimus on the greater trochanter and avoids the abductor dysfunction and postoperative limp associated with lateral and posterior approaches.[54]

In addition to the anatomic advantages of a shallow dissection and muscle preservation, the anterior approach to THA has several advantages over the traditional posterior (Kocher) and lateral (Hardinge) approaches, including a shorter hospital stay postoperatively and a faster return to function, no postoperative hip precautions, overall lower complication rates (including postoperative dislocation, nerve injury, and deep infection), the accurate placement of the acetabular and femoral components, intraoperative comparison and matching of the leg lengths, and the ability to perform bilateral THAs safely in one setting. Moreover,

3: Hip

hip resurfacing can also be performed through the anterior approach.

The overall rate of major complications appears to be lower in anterior THA compared with that in posterior and lateral approaches. In a series of 2,100 primary anterior THAs, the rate of deep infection is 0.05% and the rate of motor neurapraxia is 0.1% (one case of femoral and one case of sciatic nerve neurapraxia, both of which resolved 3 months after the surgery).[5,55] More importantly, the overall rate of dislocation after primary THA through the anterior approach is a fraction of that reported in posterior and lateral approaches.[5] In the 2005 study, the rate of dislocation is 0.15% (three cases).[5] All dislocations occurred in the first 500 primary anterior THAs. In the last 1,600 primary THAs, no dislocation was reported. Ankle fractures have been reported as a complication of anterior THA when traction is used. During the initial 500 cases, there were three cases of ipsilateral nondisplaced ankle fractures that occurred over a 2-month period. Fractures occurred at the initiation of hip dislocation, with external rotation of the leg. Since then, modifications of the technique have included capsular release from the medial femoral neck and use of a corkscrew in the femoral head to aid in dislocation. Since the implementation of this modification, there have been no other cases of ankle fractures in the last 1,600 primary THAs performed using the anterior approach.

One of the most serious complications associated with THA is dislocation, reported in 0.4% to 11% of patients.[56,57] Recent Medicare data show a 4% rate of dislocation overall after THA through the posterior and lateral approaches. The risk of dislocation is minimized with the anterior approach. Preservation of the short external rotators of the hip contributes to a very low dislocation rate associated with the anterior approach compared with other approaches.[5,55] The potential for postoperative limb-length discrepancy is a concern with both the posterior and lateral approaches when performed in the lateral decubitus position. A major advantage of the anterior approach is preservation of all the muscle attachments to the femur and the pelvis, and hence preservation of the dynamic stability of the hip. An equally important advantage is the ability to adjust the acetabular component inclination and version, and to accurately match the leg lengths intraoperatively with the use of an orthopaedic table and fluoroscopy.

THA using the anterior approach can be performed successfully with or without a specially designed radiolucent orthopaedic table.[50,58-61] However, the use of a standard table limits the applicability of the anterior approach and should be avoided in large or obese patients and those in whom femoral exposure and preparation is anticipated to be difficult. The use of a specially designed orthopaedic table is advocated by several authors.[5,62] This type of table enables use of the anterior approach for almost all patients regardless of height, weight, or body mass index. Femoral exposure

is easily achieved, even in obese patients. The main indication for a posterior approach usually is the presence of posterior column and/or wall fracture or defect requiring reconstruction or bone grafting. Specially designed orthopaedic traction tables allow the intraoperative use of fluoroscopy for precise acetabular component positioning as well as leg-length determination. These tables facilitate delivery and preparation of the proximal femur, as well as trial reductions. Use of the specialized table facilitates bilateral simultaneous THAs.

Disadvantages of the specialized table include the possibility of intraoperative ankle fractures and postoperative knee pain. In one series, three nondisplaced ankle fractures occurred intraoperatively.[5] The presumed mechanism is the external rotation force used for hip dislocation during the procedure. This risk is minimized by taking additional measures to reduce the torque on the ankle and the tibia during the dislocation step of the procedure, including insertion of a corkscrew into the femoral head before the dislocation to apply external rotation and force lateral displacement of the femoral head. Also, a scrubbed assistant can aid the dislocation by grasping the femoral condyles and applying additional rotation, therefore decreasing the torque on the distal aspect of the extremity. These steps are particularly important in elderly patients with osteoporotic bone.

The major contraindication to performing THA using an anterior approach is the presence of posterior acetabular bone defect requiring bone grafting and reconstruction.

Technique

Preoperative Planning
Preoperative templating is performed to assess several parameters, including acetabular shell size, level of the femoral neck cut, femoral stem size, and head-neck length and the hip offset.

Positioning
The patient is placed supine on the orthopaedic table. Both legs are attached to a mobile spar capable of traction, rotation, and angulation in all directions (Figure 1, A). The contralateral hip is placed in neutral rotation, extension, and abduction-adduction to serve as a radiographic control for the surgically treated side. The hip undergoing surgery is placed in slight internal rotation to enhance the natural bulge of the tensor fascia lata muscle.

Incision and Approach
The short Smith-Peterson approach is used. The incision starts 3 cm posterior and 1 cm distal to the anterior superior iliac spin. A straight incision is carried distal and slightly posterior for a total of 8 to 10 cm (Figure 1, B). The tensor fascia lata is identified. It is opened sharply in line with the incision at the junction of the anterior third and posterior two thirds of the ten-

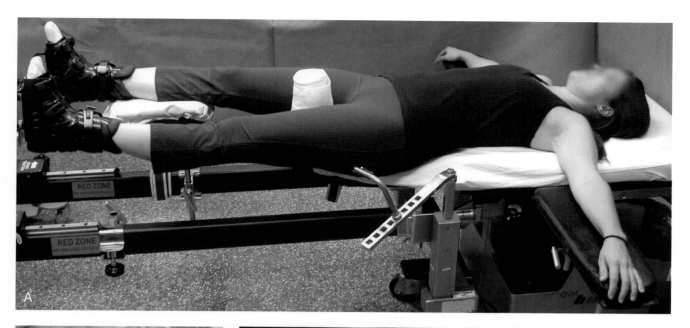

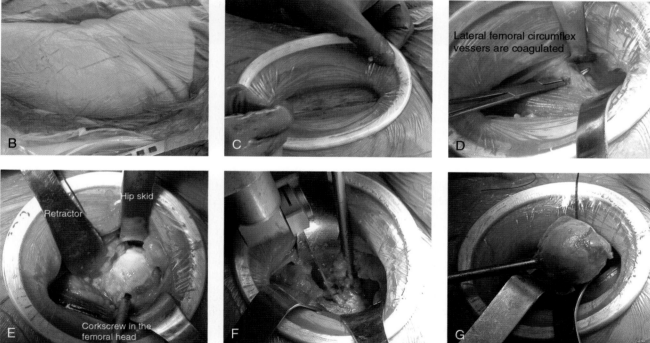

Figure 1 The short Smith-Peterson approach is shown. **A,** The patient is positioned supine on the orthopaedic table. The trochanteric hook and the attachment for the motorized lift are visible. These tools are placed after sterile prepping and draping of the patient. **B,** The attachment of the femoral lift is inserted through the drapes and sealed with plastic drape. The incision site is marked with a ruler, 3 cm lateral and 1 cm distal to the anterior-superior iliac spine. **C,** After skin incision, a protractor is inserted in the wound to protect the skin edges and subcutaneous tissues during the operation. The fascia of the tensor is identified and divided in line with its fibers. **D,** After placement of blunt cobra retractors medial and lateral to the femoral neck, the lateral femoral circumflex vessels are identified, clamped, and coagulated with Bovie cautery. The deep fascia is then divided distally to expose the vastus lateralis origin and intertrochanteric ridge. **E,** After the capsulotomy, the cobra retractors are replaced inside the capsule, the superior lateral labrum is excised, and a hip skid and corkscrew are used to dislocate the femoral head. **F,** After the femoral head dislocation and release of medial capsule from the inferior aspect of the femoral neck and exposure of the lesser trochanter, the hip is reduced and the femoral neck is cut with an oscillating saw. The osteotomy is completed with a straight osteotome. Care should be taken to avoid damage to the greater trochanter during this step. **G,** The femoral head is then removed with the use of the corkscrew. The acetabulum can now be seen.

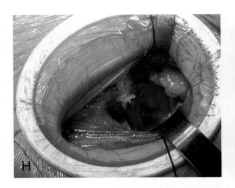
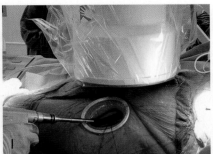
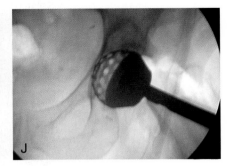

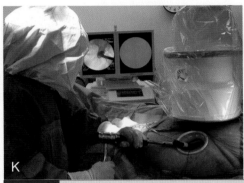
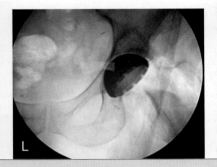
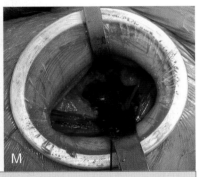

Figure 1 *(Continued)* The short Smith-Peterson approach is shown. **H,** The placement of a cobra retractor posteriorly and a curved Hohmann retractor anteriorly aids in visualization of the acetabulum. Remnants of the labrum are excised and removed. The reaming of the acetabulum. Remnants of the labrum are excised and removed. The reaming of the acetabulum is initiated under direct vision and completed under fluoroscopic guidance. **I** and **J,** The acetabulum is reamed under fluoroscopic visualization. **K,** The acetabular cup is inserted and the inclination and version are adjusted under fluoroscopic visualization. **L,** The cup inclination and version are verified with fluoroscopy. **M,** The anterior and posterior retractors are reinserted and the liner is placed under direct vision.

sor muscle belly (**Figure 1, C**). Care is taken to avoid injury to the tensor muscle. Once the tensor fascia lata is opened, blunt dissection in the medial aspect of the tensor within the tensor sheet is performed. This dissection develops the interval between the tensor fascia lata and sartorius superficially. Dissection along the medial border of the tensor fascia lata in the proximal and posterior direction allows for exposure of the lateral hip capsule. A blunt cobra retractor is placed outside the superolateral hip capsule. Next, a Hibbs retractor is used to retract the sartorius and the direct head of the rectus femoris medially, hence exposing the reflected head of the rectus femoris (which follows the anterior acetabular rim laterally). The rectus femoris is retracted medially by placement of a Hohmann retractor on the anterior hip capsule. A Cobb elevator is placed just distal to the reflected head of the rectus and directed distal and medial to elevate the iliopsoas and the rectus femoris muscle from the anterior capsule. A second blunt cobra retractor is now placed medial to the hip capsule. Using the Hibbs retractor, the distal aspect of the tensor muscle is retracted laterally to expose the lateral femoral circumflex vessels (**Figure 1, D**). These vessels are clamped, coagulated using cautery, and divided. The deep aponeurosis overlying the anterior capsule is identified and sharply divided distally to allow for enhanced exposure of the anterior capsule and the origin

of the vastus lateralis muscle. An L-shaped capsulotomy is performed. The proximal aspect of the lateral capsule is detached from the sulcus between the anterolateral neck and the greater trochanter. The distal anterior capsule is released from the proximal femur and the anterior inter-trochanteric line. The anterior and lateral capsular flaps are tagged with suture for repair at the end of the procedure.

The lateral and medial cobra retractors are now placed inside the capsule to aid in exposure of the femoral neck. A hip skid is initially inserted between the femoral head and the roof of the acetabulum and then placed medially. The ligamentum teres is cut using the hip skid or a curved osteotome. External rotation of the leg exposes the femoral head. A corkscrew is then drilled into the femoral head. The traction on the leg is released on the orthopaedic table. With anterior traction on the corkscrew and simultaneous external rotation of the femoral head using the hip skid as a lever, the hip is dislocated (**Figure 1, E**). Once the femoral head is dislocated, the leg is externally rotated to expose the inferior femoral neck. To avoid excessive torque on the ankle, manual external rotation of the foot is done by the surgeon. In elderly and osteoporotic patients, the torque on the ankle is reduced by manual rotation of the distal femur. The leg is then extended

3: Hip

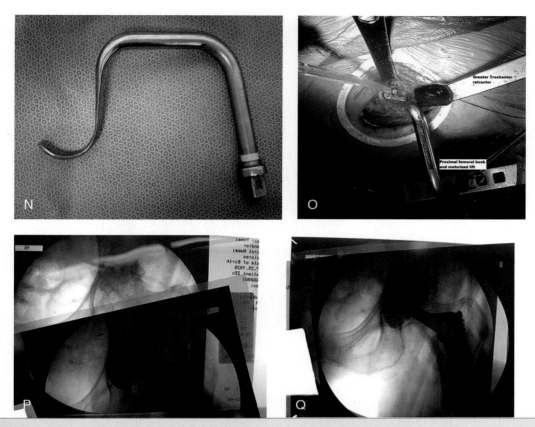

Figure 1 *(Continued)* The short Smith-Peterson approach is shown. **N,** The trochanteric hook, which is used to lift the proximal femur, is shown. **O,** The trochanteric hook is inserted with the leg in neutral rotation; the leg is then externally rotated. The hip is extended and abducted. The trochanteric hook is attached to the motorized lift, and a greater trochanter retractor is placed at the tip of the greater trochanter to protect the soft tissues during the broaching process. Once the appropriate size broach is inserted, the motorized lift is brought down, the trochanteric hook and retractors are removed, and a trial reduction is performed by traction and internal rotation of the hip. **P** and **Q,** Fluoroscopic images of both hips are taken and printed. The image of the contralateral hip is flipped and the image of the surgically treated hip with the trial femoral components is superimposed. Then bony landmarks are matched to the pelvis, including the teardrop, ilioischial, and iliopectineal lines. The position of the surgically treated greater and lesser trochanters are then compared between the surgically treated and contralateral hips. The length and offset are compared on the radiographs. The hip is dislocated, and adjustments are made to the femur. The hip is reduced again and the measurement is repeated. This step is repeated until the offset and length are matched to the contralateral hip.

and abducted to expose the inferior femoral neck. The capsular attachment is released from the inferior neck. The lesser trochanter can be palpated. The hip is then reduced and the femoral neck is cut with an oscillating saw (Figure 1, F), and the osteotomy is completed with a 0.5-inch straight osteotome. The femoral head is then removed using the corkscrew (Figure 1, G). The acetabulum can now be seen with placement of the cobra retractor posteriorly and a curved Hohmann retractor anteriorly (Figure 1, H).

The acetabulum is reamed to the appropriate size. A fluoroscopic check is made on the final depth and diameter of the reaming (Figure 1, I and J). The appropriate acetabular cup is inserted under fluoroscopic guidance (Figure 1, K). The adjustments to the inclination and version of the cup can be made with fluoroscopic guidance. The acetabular component version and inclination are checked with fluoroscopy (Figure 1, L). The

acetabular liner is then inserted under direct vision (Figure 1, M).

After insertion of the cup, the femoral preparation is undertaken. The trochanteric hook (Figure 1, N) is inserted around the proximal femur. The leg is externally rotated, extended, and abducted to expose the proximal femur. The trochanteric hook is engaged to the motorized lift. Using the motorized lift and the trochanteric hook, proximal femoral visualization and preparation are improved. A greater trochanter retractor is placed at the proximal tip of the greater trochanter during the broaching to protect the soft tissues (Figure 1, O). The femur is then broached to appropriate size and the trial reduction is performed. Fluoroscopic anterior-posterior image of the contralateral and the surgically treated hip are printed and superimposed to compare the length and offset of both hips. Appropriate adjustments to the length and offset are then

3: Hip

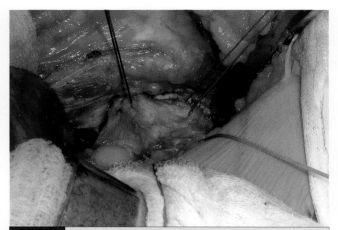

Figure 2 The upper corners of the trapezoidal capsulotomy are seen tagged with nonabsorbable sutures and pulled toward the posterior borders of the trochanter. The capsule as well as the short rotators will be reattached through drill holes in the trochanter to enhance posterior stability.

made in the femur to match the length and offset of the surgically treated hip with that of the contralateral hip (**Figure 1, P and Q**). Once the length and offset of the hips are matched, the femoral components are inserted and final reduction is performed. The closure of the capsule, fascia of the tensor, and skin is then performed.

Posterior Approach for THA
Douglas E. Padgett, MD

The posterior approach to the hip has been a popular method to gain access to the hip joint for decades. Classically described by Moore with modifications attributable to Langenbeck and then with Kocher, this approach provides ready access to the hip joint for the treatment of posterior acetabular wall/column fractures, excision of loose bodies, and insertion of endoprostheses, including total hip and surface replacement arthroplasty. Regardless of subtle differences in technique, posterior approaches involve internervous plane dissection that superficially is centered about the greater trochanter. The proximal aspect of the approach begins at the posterior-superior iliac spine and is directed to the greater trochanter and then extended distally either anterior or parallel to the shaft of the femur. After skin incision, the fascia overlying the gluteus maximus is incised in line with the raphe of the gluteal fibers. After separation of the gluteal fibers and removal of the trochanteric bursa, the external rotators of the hip are encountered: the piriformis, the superior/inferior gemelli, and the obturator internus. Distal to these is the quadratus femoris with its accompanying branches of the medial femoral circumflex artery, which provides the major source of blood supply to the proximal femur. Beneath these structures

lies the posterior capsule. Traditionally the incision for hip arthroplasty is 12 to 14 cm in length. It should be recognized that the proximal extent of the incision is the key for femoral exposure and preparation, whereas the distal limb of the incision will influence visualization and ability to access the acetabulum.

Numerous advantages of the posterior approach for THA have been cited; surgeon familiarity is the most common. Ease of dislocation, bone resection, and subsequent bony preparation when performing hip arthroplasty account for its widespread popularity. In addition, the approach is extensile should either proximal or distal exposure be required. In addition, it has been proposed that the posterior approach minimizes trauma to the hip abductor muscles (gluteus medius/minimus) and limits the risk of superior gluteal nerve injury compared with other approaches.[63] However, cadaver studies evaluating posterolateral, minimally invasive two-incision as well as Smith-Peterson approaches have all documented some degree of insult with each procedure.[37] Recent laboratory analysis of gait suggests that although THA rarely reestablishes a normal gait pattern, the posterolateral approach results in a more normal pattern compared with the anterolateral approach.[64] This supports the commonly held notion that gait and limp are improved with the posterolateral approach compared with other commonly used approaches.

The ideal approach for hip resurfacing is controversial. Clearly hip resurfacing is a technically demanding procedure and execution is paramount to success. The ability to mobilize the proximal femur for both femoral and acetabular preparation requires the ability to convert any approach into an extensile one. A criticism of the posterolateral approach for resurfacing is potential compromise of the blood supply to the femoral head.[65] Investigators have documented a significant reduction in femoral head perfusion with the posterolateral versus the transgluteal approach.[66] The authors postulate that long-term viability of the femoral head and possible late osteonecrosis could be a consideration.

When comparing surgical approaches for THA, the most controversial issue is the risk of postoperative instability. Recent studies suggest that hip dislocation is the most common reason for revision THA in the United States.[67] Surgical approach is one of the commonly cited surgical factors that influence the risk of dislocation. In a Mayo Clinic study of dislocation after THA in the 1970s-1980s, surgical approach appeared to be the predominant predictor of the risk of instability with an almost 6% dislocation rate using the posterior approach independent of head size.[68] However, it appears that this paradigm is changing. Recent larger cohort studies show that trends in cumulative instability are influenced by not only approach but also head size. It appears that a larger femoral head diameter decreases risk of instability, with the effect most pronounced when associated with the use of the posterolateral approach.[69] In addition to head size, soft-tissue reconstruction appears to be an independent factor associated with a lower risk of instability when using the posterior approach.[70] The enhanced repair uses an anatomic reattachment of the posterior capsular, short external rotators, and quadratus femoris through drill holes in the posterior trochanter[71] (Figure 2). Ultrasound as well as MRI confirm that these posterior structures can incorporate as an intact soft-tissue restraint.[72,73] In initial reports of consecutive patients undergoing primary THA at two institutions, surgeons were able to reduce dislocation rates of 4% to 6% before enhanced soft-tissue repair techniques to 0% to 0.8% following adoption of this technique.[71] Even in groups at higher risk for injury such as the elderly, authors report a substantial reduction in the incidence of dislocation using this enhanced soft-tissue reconstruction in combination with a larger diameter head (11% dislocation without repair, 0% dislocation with repair, and either 32-mm head or 28-mm head with elevated liner).[74] It appears that a combination of surgical strategies including posterior soft-tissue repair in conjunction with a larger diameter head have greatly reduced the incidence of hip dislocation using the posterior approach, making the rates of instability comparable to those of other surgical approaches.

Much has been written about the so-called minimally invasive surgical approaches to THA. The claims of less pain, expedited recovery, and an increased incidence of complications such as periprosthetic fracture and component malposition are supported by some studies and refuted by others.[29] Results of the minimally invasive posterior approach from several institutions have been somewhat consistent. By using smaller incisions and limiting the posterior dissection to the piriformis, conjoined tendon, and capsule, authors have demonstrated lower pain scores, earlier discharge, and less reliance on assistive devices for the minimally invasive surgical group compared with incisions of traditional length and posterior approaches.[39,41] However, by 6 weeks, there were equivalent functional results for both groups. It is now apparent that the use of minimally invasive techniques is of short-term benefit to patients. Although reduction in pain and improvement in mobilization are worthy goals, the precision and accuracy of the reconstruction should never be compromised by limited surgical site visualization.

Annotated References

1. Keggi KJ, Huo MH, Zatorski LE: Anterior approach to total hip replacement: Surgical technique and clinical results of our first one thousand cases using noncemented prostheses. *Yale J Biol Med* 1993;66(3):243-256.

2. Kennon RE, Keggi JM, Wetmore RS, Zatorski LE, Huo MH, Keggi KJ: Total hip arthroplasty through a minimally invasive anterior surgical approach. *J Bone Joint Surg Am* 2003;85(suppl 4):39-48.

3. Levine BR, Klein GR, Di Cesare PE: Surgical approaches in total hip arthroplasty: A review of the mini-incision and MIS literature. *Bull NYU Hosp Jt Dis* 2007;65(1):5-18.

   The authors review the classic, minimally invasive, and less invasive approaches to THA. The available literature to date is summarized.

4. Bertin KC, Röttinger H: Anterolateral mini-incision hip replacement surgery: A modified Watson-Jones approach. *Clin Orthop Relat Res* 2004;429:248-255.

5. Matta JM, Shahrdar C, Ferguson T: Single-incision anterior approach for total hip arthroplasty on an orthopaedic table. *Clin Orthop Relat Res* 2005;441:115-124.

   The surgical technique and results of a single-incision anterior approach using an orthopaedic table are presented. Level of evidence: IV.

6. Berger RA: The technique of minimally invasive total hip arthroplasty using the two-incision approach. *Instr Course Lect* 2004;53:149-155.

7. Berger RA, Duwelius PJ: The two-incision minimally invasive total hip arthroplasty: Technique and results. *Orthop Clin North Am* 2004;35(2):163-172.

8. Berger RA: A comprehensive approach to outpatient total hip arthroplasty. *Am J Orthop (Belle Mead NJ)* 2007;36(9, suppl):4-5.

9. Berger RA, Sanders SA, Thill ES, Sporer SM, Della Valle C: Newer anesthesia and rehabilitation protocols enable outpatient hip replacement in selected patients. *Clin Orthop Relat Res* 2009;467(6):1424-1430.

   The feasibility and safety of outpatient THA in 150 consecutive patients is presented. A comprehensive perioperative anesthesia and rehabilitation protocol including preoperative teaching, regional anesthesia, and preemptive oral analgesia and antiemetic therapy was implemented around a minimally invasive surgical technique. Level of evidence: IV.

10. Pour AE, Parvizi J, Sharkey PF, Hozack WJ, Rothman RH: Minimally invasive hip arthroplasty: What role does patient preconditioning play? *J Bone Joint Surg Am* 2007;89(9):1920-1927.

    One hundred THAs were randomized into four groups based on the size of the incision, preoperative counseling, the type of preoperative and postoperative rehabilitation, and the analgesia protocol. The functional improvement at the time of discharge to home, patient satisfaction, and walking ability at discharge were better in patients who had received an accelerated preoperative and postoperative rehabilitation regimen regardless of the size of the incision.

11. Lilikakis AK, Gillespie B, Villar RN: The benefit of modified rehabilitation and minimally invasive techniques in total hip replacement. *Ann R Coll Surg Engl* 2008;90(5):406-411.

    New rehabilitation protocol alone can reduce the length of hospital stay and facilitate rehabilitation.

3: Hip

Combining rehabilitation protocols with modified anesthesia and minimally invasive surgical techniques can further improve short-term outcome after total hip replacement.

12. Peck CN, Foster A, McLauchlan GJ: Reducing incision length or intensifying rehabilitation: What makes the difference to length of stay in total hip replacement in a UK setting? *Int Orthop* 2006;30(5):395-398.

A standard posterior approach was compared with minimal-incision approach. In both groups, physiotherapy involved either a routine or intensive regimen. In the UK setting, intensive physiotherapy can significantly decrease in-patient stay, but reducing the incision length does not.

13. Nuelle DG, Mann K: Minimal incision protocols for anesthesia, pain management, and physical therapy with standard incisions in hip and knee arthroplasties: The effect on early outcomes. *J Arthroplasty* 2007;22(1):20-25.

Fifty patients underwent total joint arthroplasty with standard incisions. The first 25 patients had standard perioperative management, whereas the second 25 had advanced protocols. The advanced group showed a reduction in the time it took to achieve the goals for discharge.

14. Sharma V, Morgan PM, Cheng EY: Factors influencing early rehabilitation after THA: A systematic review. *Clin Orthop Relat Res* 2009;467(6):1400-1411.

A systematic review of 16 level I and II studies is presented. Multimodal pain control with revised anesthesia protocols and accelerated rehabilitation speeds recovery after minimally invasive THA compared with standard-approach THA, but a smaller incision length or minimally invasive approach does not demonstrably improve the short-term outcome. Level of evidence: II.

15. Wall SJ, Mears SC: Analysis of published evidence on minimally invasive total hip arthroplasty. *J Arthroplasty* 2008;23(7, suppl):55-58.

The literature was reviewed to analyze various types of minimally invasive THA. The mini-posterior approach was the only approach with good-quality randomized controlled study evidence. The overall length of follow-up and quality of reports for minimally invasive THA is low.

16. Woolson ST, Mow CS, Syquia JF, Lannin JV, Schurman DJ: Comparison of primary total hip replacements performed with a standard incision or a mini-incision. *J Bone Joint Surg Am* 2004;86(7):1353-1358.

17. Teet JS, Skinner HB, Khoury L: The effect of the "mini" incision in total hip arthroplasty on component position. *J Arthroplasty* 2006;21(4):503-507.

Cemented and uncemented THA performed through either a standard or mini-incision were compared. The mini incision did not compromise THA results on the acetabular side, but varus positioning of the cemented femoral component nearing 2° was concerning.

18. Flören M, Lester DK: Durability of implant fixation after less-invasive total hip arthroplasty. *J Arthroplasty* 2006;21(6):783-790.

The results of 90 THAs performed with a mini-posterior approach at 10 to 13 years was reviewed and found to be comparable to those of conventional techniques.

19. Khan RJ, Fick D, Khoo P, Yao F, Nivbrant B, Wood D: Less invasive total hip arthroplasty: Description of a new technique. *J Arthroplasty* 2006;21(7):1038-1046.

A less invavisive approach was found to result in less blood loss and a shorter length of hospital stay compared with a standard posterior approach.

20. Procyk S: Initial results with a mini-posterior approach for total hip arthroplasty. *Int Orthop* 2007;31(suppl 1): S17-S20.

Preliminary results with a mini-posterior approach in 60 patients showed rapid functional recovery, minimal postoperative pain, a reduced length of stay, few complications, and optimal component positioning.

21. Swanson TV: Early results of 1000 consecutive, posterior, single-incision minimally invasive surgery total hip arthroplasties. *J Arthroplasty* 2005;20(7, suppl 3):26-32.

One thousand mini-posterior THAs were followed prospectively for a minimum of 2 years. Complications and component malpositioning were within accepted standards.

22. Ogonda L, Wilson R, Archbold P, et al: A minimal-incision technique in total hip arthroplasty does not improve early postoperative outcomes: A prospective, randomized, controlled trial. *J Bone Joint Surg Am* 2005;87(4):701-710.

Two hundred nineteen THAs were prospectively randomized to either a short incision or standard incision. There were no significant differences between the two groups in regard to postoperative or functional outcomes.

23. Mayr E, Krismer M, Ertl M, Kessler O, Thaler M, Nogler M: Uncompromised quality of the cement mantle in Exeter femoral components implanted through a minimally-invasive direct anterior approach: A prospective, randomised cadaver study. *J Bone Joint Surg Br* 2006;88(9):1252-1256.

Cemented femoral components implanted through either a standard anterolateral transgluteal approach or in angulated fashion through a direct anterior approach were reviewed. The direct anterior insertion did not adversely affect the quality of the cement mantle.

24. Laffosse JM, Accadbled F, Molinier F, Chiron P, Hocine B, Puget J: Anterolateral mini-invasive versus posterior mini-invasive approach for primary total hip replacement: Comparison of exposure and implant positioning. *Arch Orthop Trauma Surg* 2008;128(4):363-369.

There were no significant differences between an anterolateral minimally invasive approach compared with a posterior minimally invasive approach in regard to limb-length discrepancy and component position. However, there were more femoral fractures in the anterior approach.

25. Asayama I, Kinsey TL, Mahoney OM: Two-year experience using a limited-incision direct lateral approach in total hip arthroplasty. *J Arthroplasty* 2006;21(8):1083-1091.

    One hundred two patients were blinded to either a limited or standard direct lateral approach. At 2 years, there was no evidence or a clinical benefit for the limited incision.

26. Han KY, Garino JP, Rhyu KH: Gains and losses of small incision lateral total hip arthroplasty: What the patients want and its index case result. *Arch Orthop Trauma Surg* 2009;129(5):635-640.

    Forty transgluteal THAs with either a small or standard incision were compared. There were significant variations in implant positions and more complications such as dislocation, fracture, or limb-length discrepancy in the small incision group.

27. Bal BS, Haltom D, Aleto T, Barrett M: Early complications of primary total hip replacement performed with a two-incision minimally invasive technique. *J Bone Joint Surg Am* 2005;87(11):2432-2438.

    The early results of 89 two-incision THAs are presented. The early complication rate was higher than single-incision approaches, but the complication rate decreased significantly as more experience was gained.

28. Pagnano MW, Leone J, Lewallen DG, Hanssen AD: Two-incision THA had modest outcomes and some substantial complications. *Clin Orthop Relat Res* 2005;441:86-90.

    Forty-five women and 35 men with a mean age of 70.5 years treated with a two-incision technique had longer surgical times and substantially more complications than did the patients treated with a standard posterior approach. Level of evidence: III.

29. Berry DJ, Berger RA, Callaghan JJ, et al: Minimally invasive total hip arthroplasty: Development, early results, and a critical analysis. Presented at the Annual Meeting of the American Orthopaedic Association, Charleston, South Carolina, USA, June 14, 2003. *J Bone Joint Surg Am* 2003;85(11):2235-2246.

30. Bal BS, Haltom D, Aleto T, Barrett M: Early complications of primary total hip replacement performed with a two-incision minimally invasive technique: Surgical technique. *J Bone Joint Surg Am* 2006;88(suppl 1, pt 2): 221-233.

    The surgical technique for two-incision THA is presented. The authors report a relatively high early complication rate that decreased as experience was gained.

31. Hartzband MA, Klein GR: Two-incision total hip arthroplasty: The Hackensack experience. *Semin Arthroplasty* 2007;18(4):251-256.

    The surgical technique and a single surgeon's initial experience with 400 consecutive two-incision THAs are presented. There was a significant decrease in surgical time, fluoroscopic usage, and complication rates as experience was gained. Modifications to the original technique are presented.

32. Duwelius PJ, Burkhart RL, Hayhurst JO, Moller H, Butler JB: Comparison of the 2-incision and mini-incision posterior total hip arthroplasty technique: A retrospective match-pair controlled study. *J Arthroplasty* 2007;22(1):48-56.

    A matched-pair analysis of the mini-posterior and two-incision THA approaches was performed. Function was regained earlier with the two-incision procedure. Posterior mini-incision patients had a shorter operating time and less blood loss. Complications were similar.

33. Williams SL, Bachison C, Michelson JD, Manner PA: Component position in 2-incision minimally invasive total hip arthroplasty compared to standard total hip arthroplasty. *J Arthroplasty* 2008;23(2):197-202.

    Radiographic assessment of component position of THA in two-incision minimally invasive surgery and a standard direct lateral approach reveals no significant differences.

34. Mardones R, Pagnano MW, Nemanich JP, Trousdale RT: The Frank Stinchfield Award: Muscle damage after total hip arthroplasty done with the two-incision and mini-posterior techniques. *Clin Orthop Relat Res* 2005;441:63-67.

    A cadaver study compared the two-incision and mini-posterior approach with regard to muscle damage. Every two-incision total hip replacement caused measurable damage to the abductors, the external rotators, or both. Every mini-posterior hip replacement caused damage to the external rotators and abductors.

35. Cohen RG, Katz JA, Skrepnik NV: The relationship between skeletal muscle serum markers and primary THA: A pilot study. *Clin Orthop Relat Res* 2009; 467(7):1747-1752.

    There was no difference in serum markers for skeletal muscle damage in three different minimally invasive approaches: Watson-Jones, mini-posterior, and a minimally invasive two-incision technique.

36. Bal BS, Lowe JA: Muscle damage in minimally invasive total hip arthroplasty: MRI evidence that it is not significant. *Instr Course Lect* 2008;57:223-229.

    MRI with a metal subtraction protocol compared the musculature of a surgically treated hip with that of the normal contralateral hip. The standard posterolateral and direct lateral approaches showed more postoperative alterations in the hip muscles compared with the two-incision approach.

37. Parratte S, Pagnano MW: Muscle damage during minimally invasive total hip arthroplasty: Cadaver-based evidence that it is significant. *Instr Course Lect* 2008; 57:231-234.

3: Hip

This article reviews a series of cadaver studies that indicate that it is not possible to routinely perform minimally invasive THA without causing some measureable degree of muscle damage.

38. Ward SR, Jones RE, Long WT, Thomas DJ, Dorr LD: Functional recovery of muscles after minimally invasive total hip arthroplasty. *Instr Course Lect* 2008;57: 249-254.

    A gait analysis compared multiple surgical approaches and found that patients undergoing THA recover muscle function to preoperative levels within 6 weeks. No advantage was shown with the use of different small-incision approaches.

39. Chimento GF, Pavone V, Sharrock N, Kahn B, Cahill J, Sculco TP: Minimally invasive total hip arthroplasty: A prospective randomized study. *J Arthroplasty* 2005; 20(2):139-144.

    Patients were randomized to either small or standard incisions. The small-incision group had less blood loss and limped less. There was no difference at 1- and 2-year follow-up.

40. Lin DH, Jan MH, Liu TK, Lin YF, Hou SM: Effects of anterolateral minimally invasive surgery in total hip arthroplasty on hip muscle strength, walking speed, and functional score. *J Arthroplasty* 2007;22(8):1187-1192.

    Fifty-three patients who underwent a mini-incision THA were matched with 53 patients who underwent conventional anterolateral THA. In the first year the mini-incision THA had significantly better hip muscle strength, walking speed, and functional score. At 1 year there were no differences.

41. Dorr LD, Maheshwari AV, Long WT, Wan Z, Sirianni LE: Early pain relief and function after posterior minimally invasive and conventional total hip arthroplasty: A prospective, randomized, blinded study. *J Bone Joint Surg Am* 2007;89(6):1153-1160.

    Sixty patients were randomized to have either a posterior mini-incision or a traditional incision. At the end of the surgery the mini-incision group had extension of the skin incision. The mini-incision group had better early pain control, earlier discharge to home, and less use of assistive devices. Level of evidence: I.

42. Pagnano MW, Trousdale RT, Meneghini RM, Hanssen AD: Slower recovery after two-incision than mini-posterior-incision total hip arthroplasty: A randomized clinical trial. *J Bone Joint Surg Am* 2008;90(5):1000-1006.

    Seventy-two hips were randomized to either the two-incision or mini-posterior THA. The clinical outcome as measured on the basis of the 12-Item Short Form scores was similar at both 2 months and 1 year postoperatively. The rate of complications was the same in both groups.

43. Meneghini RM, Smits SA: Early discharge and recovery with three minimally invasive total hip arthroplasty approaches: A preliminary study. *Clin Orthop Relat Res* 2009;467(6):1431-1437.

    Twenty-four consecutive patients were randomized to a two-incision, mini-posterior, or mini-anterolateral approach and enrolled in an aggressive postoperative rehabilitation program. There was no difference in hospital discharge, functional milestone recovery, or validated outcome measures during the first year after surgery. Level of evidence: IV.

44. Meneghini RM, Smits SA, Swinford RR, Bahamonde RE: A randomized, prospective study of 3 minimally invasive surgical approaches in total hip arthroplasty: Comprehensive gait analysis. *J Arthroplasty* 2008; 23(6, Suppl 1)68-73.

    Twenty-four consecutive hips were randomized to a two-incision, mini-posterior, or mini-anterolateral approach. Gait analysis showed the anterolateral approach consistent with abductor muscle injury in the early recovery period. There were no differences between the two-incision and posterior approaches.

45. Bertin KC: Minimally invasive outpatient total hip arthroplasty: A financial analysis. *Clin Orthop Relat Res* 2005;435:154-163.

    The cost of outpatient THA was compared with the cost of a matched group of patients having inpatient THAs. Outpatient THA was financially advantageous. Level of evidence: IV.

46. Dorr LD, Chao L: The emotional state of the patient after total hip and knee arthroplasty. *Clin Orthop Relat Res* 2007;463:7-12.

    The emotional state and expectations of the patient play a factor in recovery after THA.

47. Malik A, Dorr LD: The science of minimally invasive total hip arthroplasty. *Clin Orthop Relat Res* 2007; 463:74-84.

    The science of minimally invasive hip surgery is reviewed including the effects of anesthesia, pain management, and rapid recovery protocols.

48. Dorr LD, Thomas D, Long WT, Polatin PB, Sirianni LE: Psychologic reasons for patients preferring minimally invasive total hip arthroplasty. *Clin Orthop Relat Res* 2007;458:94-100.

    A 14-question patient-perception questionnaire was administered to patients preoperatively and 6 weeks postoperatively and a follow-up survey at 6 months to 1 year postoperatively. A small incision influences a patient's satisfaction postoperatively.

49. Mow CS, Woolson ST, Ngarmukos SG, Park EH, Lorenz HP: Comparison of scars from total hip replacements done with a standard or a mini-incision. *Clin Orthop Relat Res* 2005;441:80-85.

    Using a standardized rating system, two plastic surgeons independently graded the scars after THA. More scars following the mini incision were rated poor than standard scars. More mini-incision patients had wound-healing problems. All the patients believed that their hip scar was acceptable in appearance. Level of evidence: II.

50. McGrory BJ, Finch ME, Furlong PJ, Ruterbories J: Incision length correlates with patient weight, height, and gender when using a minimal-incision technique in total hip arthroplasty. *J Surg Orthop Adv* 2008;17(2): 77-81.

Incision size using a mini-posterior approach was correlated with patient weight, height, and sex. Larger patients can expect a longer incision, and for a given weight, women will have longer incisions than men.

51. Rahman W, Richards CJ, Duncan CP: Surgical nuances to minimize muscle damage during the anterolateral intermuscular approach in minimally invasive hip replacement. *Instr Course Lect* 2008;57:243-247.

Details to minimize muscle damage during minimally invasive anterolateral THA are described.

52. Archibeck MJ, White RE Jr: Learning curve for the two-incision total hip replacement. *Clin Orthop Relat Res* 2004;429:232-238.

53. Seng BE, Berend KR, Ajluni AF, Lombardi AV Jr: Anterior-supine minimally invasive total hip arthroplasty: Defining the learning curve. *Orthop Clin North Am* 2009;40(3):343-350.

A learning curve of 40 cases and 6 months in a high-volume joint surgeon's practice is demonstrated for performing the anterior-supine approach.

54. Robbins GM, Masri BA, Garbuz DS, Greidanus N, Duncan CP: Treatment of hip instability. *Orthop Clin North Am* 2001;32(4):593-610, viii.

55. Restrepo C, Mortazavi SM, Brothers J, Parvizi J, Rothman RH: Hip dislocation: Are hip precautions necessary in anterior approaches? *Clin Orthop Relat Res* 2011;469(2):417-422.

Study results indicated a low incidence of hip dislocation after primary THA when early postoperative restrictions were absent. Level of evidence: II.

56. Coventry MB: Late dislocations in patients with Charnley total hip arthroplasty. *J Bone Joint Surg Am* 1985;67(6):832-841.

57. DeWal H, Su E, DiCesare PE: Instability following total hip arthroplasty. *Am J Orthop (Belle Mead NJ)* 2003;32(8):377-382.

58. Mast NH, Muñoz M, Matta JM: Simultaneous bilateral supine anterior approach total hip arthroplasty: Evaluation of early complications and short-term rehabilitation. *Orthop Clin North Am* 2009;40(3):351-356.

Study results indicated that simultaneous bilateral anterior approach total hip arthroplasty had acceptable complication rates that compare favorably with previously published series.

59. Benoit B, Gofton W, Beaulé PE: Hueter anterior approach for hip resurfacing: Assessment of the learning curve. *Orthop Clin North Am* 2009;40(3):357-363.

The authors evaluated safety and learning curve of Hueter hip resurfacing using an anterior approach and concluded that it is a reasonable alternative to other surgical approaches. Additional long-term studies are needed.

60. Bender B, Nogler M, Hozack WJ: Direct anterior approach for total hip arthroplasty. *Orthop Clin North Am* 2009;40(3):321-328.

The authors state that the direct anterior approach for THA is advantageous because it causes minimal soft-tissue trauma, which results in accelerated postoperative mobilization and rehabilitation.

61. Light TR, Keggi KJ: Anterior approach to hip arthroplasty. *Clin Orthop Relat Res* 1980;152(152):255-260.

62. Rachbauer F, Kain MS, Leunig M: The history of the anterior approach to the hip. *Orthop Clin North Am* 2009;40(3):311-320.

The authors discuss the advantages of the anterior approach for THA.

63. Kenny P, O'Brien CP, Synnott K, Walsh MG. Damage to the superior gluteal nerve after two different approaches to the hip. *J Bone Joint Surg Br* 1999;81(6): 979-981.

64. Madsen MS, Ritter MA, Morris HH, Meding JB, Berend ME, Faris PM, Vardaxis VG: The effect of total hip arthroplasty surgical approach on gait. *J Orthop Res* 2004;22(1):44-50.

65. Steffen RT, Fern D, Norton M, Murray DW, Gill HS. Femoral oxygenation during hip resurfacing through the trochanteric flip approach. *Clin Orthop Relat Res* 2009;467(4):934-939.

The authors determined that oxygen preservation with the trochanteric flip approach was similar to that seen with the anterolateral approach, but with less variation.

66. Khan A, Yates P, Lovering A, Bannister GC, Spencer RF: The effect of surgical approach on blood flow to the femoral head during resurfacing *J Bone Joint Surg Br* 2007;89(1):21-25.

The authors used cefuroxime as a marker of femoral head perfusion during 20 hip resurfacing arthroplasties using either the posterolateral or transgluteal approach. Bone samples demonstrated significantly reduced levels of cefuroxime in the posterolateral group, suggesting a reduction in femoral head perfusion. These findings may have implications regarding long-term femoral head viability when performing hip resurfacing via the posterolateral approach.

67. Bozic KJ, Kurtz SM, Lau E, Ong K, Vail TP, Berry DJ: The epidemiology of revision total hip arthroplasty in the United States. *J Bone Joint Surg Am* 2009;91(1): 128-133.

The authors determined that hip instability and mechanical loosening are the most common reasons for revision THA.

3: Hip

68. Woo RY, Morrey BF: Dislocations after total hip arthroplasty. *J Bone Joint Surg Am* 1982;64(9):1295-1306.

69. Berry DJ, von Knoch M, Schleck CD, Harmsen WS: Effect of femoral head diameter and operative approach on risk of dislocation after primary total hip arthroplasty. *J Bone Joint Surg Am* 2005;87(11):2456-2463.

    An analysis of more than 20,000 primary THAs was performed to evaluate the effect of surgical approach and femoral head diameter on the risk of dislocation. By approach, the 10-year dislocation risk was: 3.1% for anterolateral, 3.4% for transtrochanteric, and 6.9% for posterolateral approaches. Across all approaches, larger head size (32 mm) led to a reduced risk of dislocation, with the greatest effect on reduction in dislocation occurring in the posterolateral approach group.

70. Weeden SH, Paprosky WG, Bowling JW: The early dislocation rate in primary total hip arthroplasty following the posterior approach with posterior soft-tissue repair. *J Arthroplasty* 2003;18(6):709-713.

71. Pellicci PM, Bostrom MP, Poss R: Posterior approach to total hip replacement using enhanced posterior soft tissue repair. *Clin Orthop Relat Res* 1998;335(355):224-228.

72. Su EP, Mahoney CR, Adler RS, Padgett DE, Pellicci PM: Integrity of repaired posterior structures after THA. *Clin Orthop Relat Res* 2006;47:43-47.

    The authors found that ultrasonography can be used to effectively assess the integrity of posterior repair after THA; posterior structures were intact in most patients studied.

73. Pellicci PM, Potter HG, Foo LF, Boettner F: MRI shows biologic restoration of posterior soft tissue repairs after THA. *Clin Orthop Relat Res* 2009;467(4):940-945.

    Study results indicated that repaired posterior soft tissues provide a biologic scaffold that allows a posterior pseudocapsule to form.

74. Sierra RJ, Raposo JM, Trousdale RT, Cabanela ME: Dislocation of primary THA done through a posterolateral approach in the elderly. *Clin Orthop Relat Res* 2005;441:262-267

    The authors used a posterolateral approach to assess the rate of dislocation of THA and suggest the use of a 32-mm head in combination with posterior capsule repair to reduce the incidence of dislocation. Level of evidence: III-1.

Chapter 20

Hip Impingement

Michael Leunig, MD   John C. Clohisy, MD   J.W. Thomas Byrd, MD

Diagnosis and Classification
Michael Leunig, MD

Introduction

Osteoarthritis (OA) of the hip is one of the major causes of pain and disability in developed countries.[1] Resulting therapeutic interventions and socioeconomic costs pose a considerable burden on health and social services.[2] The etiology of OA is multifactorial. Recently it was proposed that most, if not all, so-called idiopathic OA is secondary, due to subtle developmental abnormalities.[3-5] Based on experimental and clinical studies, including in situ evaluation of adolescents and young adults undergoing surgical dislocations of the hip, femoroacetabular impingement (FAI) was proposed to cause early OA in the nondysplastic hip.

More than a century ago, hip damage caused by a femoroacetabular conflict was first anecdotally reported in orthopaedic textbooks and publications as sequelae of childhood disease, mainly slipped capital femoral epiphysis (SCFE). The current concept of FAI dates back to the early 1990s with the recognition of FAI in retroverted, malunited femoral neck fractures. But it was not until the development of an open surgical technique to safely dislocate the hip and allow direct observation of the joint that the concept of FAI was introduced as a mechanical cause of OA. In comparison with previous studies relating secondary OA to grossly visible deformities, (acetabular dysplasia, femoral pistol grip, or head tilt),[6-8] the originality and distinction of the FAI concept previously proposed is that subtle, often unrecognized developmental alterations and spatial malorientation of the hip in the absence of overt childhood disease might instigate OA.[5]

Dr. Leunig or an immediate family member serves as a paid consultant for or is an employee of Smith & Nephew; serves as an unpaid consultant for Pivot; and owns stock or stock options in Pivot. Dr. Clohisy or an immediate family member has received research or institutional support from Wright Medical Technology and is a board member, owner, officer, or committee member of the Mid-America Orthopaedic Association. Dr. Byrd or an immediate family member serves as a paid consultant for or is an employee of Smith & Nephew; has received research or institutional support from Smith & Nephew; and is a board member, owner, officer, or committee member of Baptist Plaza Surgicare.

Diagnosis
Clinical Presentation

FAI typically presents in young, active adults, two thirds of whom report an insidious onset of symptoms. Initially the pain is intermittent, but may be exacerbated by high-demand activities that require forceful or excessive hip flexion and internal rotation. Flexion/adduction and extension/external rotation are further degrees of motion that can cause pain. In most patients, the chief symptom is anterior groin pain made worse by prolonged periods of standing, sitting, walking, and many other activities. In a small cohort of 56 patients, it was demonstrated that, in addition to the groin (in 88% of patients), the pain also can be referred to the lateral hip (67% of patients), the anterior thigh (35% of patients), and, less frequently, the buttock, knee, low back, and lateral and posterior thigh.[9] Pain is a major complaint in young and active patients and its severity is described as moderate, severe, or disabling in 81% of the hips. Aching and sharp pain were both present in 73% of the hips. A mechanical component to the pain (65%) and exacerbation with sitting (65%) are also common. The most effective means of alleviating the pain was rest (67%) and frequent changing of position.

Male patients with FAI often experience a lifelong decrease in hip range of motion (ROM), most commonly decreased flexion/internal rotation. In comparison, female patients with FAI often report a rather normal or even increased ROM during adolescence that decreases as symptoms occur later in life. Because of subtle findings on routine radiographs, these patients may experience a delay of up to 3 years in establishing the diagnosis of FAI. As a consequence, they often undergo extensive orthopaedic workup and some even undergo surgical intervention for FAI at another anatomic site. When obtaining a further history, it is critical to inquire about childhood hip diseases such as hip dysplasia, Legg-Calvé-Perthes disease, and SCFE, which are known causes of labral tears as well as hip arthritis. In most patients, however, no such diagnosis will be found.

As symptoms progress, most patients experience moderate to marked pain and substantial limitations of activity. The relatively active patient population underscores the concept that high-demand activity may be a risk factor for development of symptomatic FAI in the mechanically jeopardized hip. Activity limitations seem

3: Hip

© 2011 American Academy of Orthopaedic Surgeons

Orthopaedic Knowledge Update: Hip and Knee Reconstruction 4

279

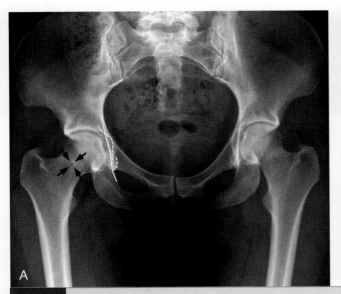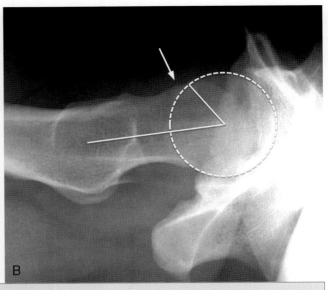

Figure 1 AP pelvic and cross-table radiographs of a 26-year-old woman with global pincer FAI. **A,** The AP pelvic radiograph shows a normal acetabular version but inclusion of almost the entire femoral head within the acetabular socket. The acetabular fossa (dotted line) is medial to the Kohler (ilioischial) line (solid line), suggesting coxa profunda. A secondary impingement cyst (arrows) is visible in the central femoral neck. **(B)** The cross-table lateral view reveals an almost spherical femoral head with an α angle of 52° and an indentation groove (arrow).

to have a substantial negative impact on these patients because 74% reported their physical activity level to be less than average.[9] Patients presenting with symptoms indicating FAI should undergo a basic physical examination to ensure that other pain sources in addition to the hip are not overlooked. In contrast to joints such as the elbow or shoulder, there is no recognized structured evaluation protocol for the hip. In an attempt to provide some guidelines, a 2010 study recently reported the 10 most common clinical tests used by experienced surgeons when assessing patients for unexplained hip pain.[10] As with other joints, basic tests such as inspection, neurovascular assessment, palpation, ROM assessment, and strength assessment need to be performed on the hip. An experienced examiner will be guided by the findings of the presenting patient, whereas the inexperienced examiner must not be too quick to omit tests from an examination. Key information can be obtained by assessing flexion/internal rotation, flexion, and abduction of the hip as well as flexion, adduction, and internal rotation (impingement test), supposing that these limitations caused some discomfort. For flexion/internal rotation, a quantitative device has recently been proposed.[11]

Radiographic Evaluation

For decades, only an AP pelvic or hip radiograph was used for grading disease severity (hip dysplasia, Legg-Calvé-Perthes disease) or determining the presence of OA. Subtle alterations, particularly of the femur, often escaped detection because they would become obvious only on a lateral view.[12] In other cases, these subtle alterations may have been missed altogether with conventional radiographic assessment.[13] Nevertheless, conventional radiographs (in two planes) are the mainstay in radiographic assessment.

Diagnostic imaging of the hip should begin with a standardized AP pelvic radiograph, with care to ensure that the rotation and pelvic inclination are appropriate.[14] Slight alterations in either of these parameters can lead to an inaccurate assessment and interpretation of acetabular coverage. Even in the routine setting at specialized centers, only 15% of radiographs meet these standards.[15] Once the adequacy of the radiograph is ensured, an evaluation should be conducted to rule out underlying hip disease or OA. A femoral head or medial acetabular wall that is close to or medial to the ilioischial line (Kohler line) is characteristic for protrusio acetabuli and coxa profunda, respectively (**Figure 1**). The anterior and posterior acetabular walls should then be outlined. These lines should maintain a separation throughout their entire course. Overlap of the anterior and posterior walls at the superolateral margin of the acetabulum is called the figure-of-8 or crossover sign[16] and has been validated to represent local overcoverage or retroversion of the acetabulum[17] (**Figure 2**). In addition, the ischial spine sign has recently been introduced and validated for detecting cranial acetabular retroversion.[15,18]

The next step is to assess for femoral alterations, which are less obvious or can even be missed on AP pelvic views[12,13] (**Figure 3, A**). Given its anterosuperior location, insufficient head-neck offset is underappreciated on a standard AP radiograph and/or may be obstructed by the greater trochanter on a frog lateral view. The aspherical head-neck junction is best visualized on either a 45° Dunn view or a cross-table lateral view with the leg in 15° of internal rotation (**Figure 3, B**). The internally rotated cross-table lateral view is often more practical for routine use, because positioning for the Dunn view requires a leg holder or assistant. Either image can be used to measure the head-neck offset and the α angle, which are both abnormal in cam FAI. When comparing cross-table view derived α angles with those initially described in the literature[19] based on MRI (abnormal, 74° versus normal, 42°), similar values (71° versus 50°) were found on cross-table radiographs for abnormal and normal hips.[12]

Magnetic Resonance Arthrography

For many years, conventional MRI of the pelvis has been performed in three planes to identify hip pathologies such as osteonecrosis, loose bodies, and labral pathologies. Recently, there has been a need for more detailed information to help diagnose early stages of OA, which are not well visualized on standard radiographs or conventional MRI. Magnetic resonance arthrography (MRA) of the hip has been used with increasing frequency to identify hip pathomorphologies such as FAI (**Figure 4**) and hip dysplasia. MRA, the combination of MRI with intra-articular injection of gadolinium-based contrast agents, is a minimally invasive method to provide additional information on the status of the cartilage and labrum. The extent of cartilage and labral damage has profound implications for both the surgeon and patient in developing and understanding the treatment plan.

Based on findings by hip arthroscopy, MRA has revealed both a high sensitivity and accuracy to detect labral tears (**Figure 4**) ranging from 92% to 100% and

93% to 96%, respectively.[20,21] Pitfalls may be caused by a sublabral sulcus or cleft.[22] Although MRA is currently the best available imaging tool for hip evaluation with respect to the acetabular labrum in terms of cartilage evaluation, study results are still moderate.[23] In particular, the detection of cartilage delamination remains difficult.[24] The relatively thin cartilage, the sphe-

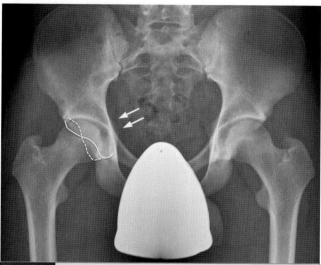

Figure 2   AP pelvic radiograph of a 17-year-old patient who plays professional hockey and who has local pincer FAI caused by acetabular retroversion. The anterior acetabular rim (solid line) is in the cranial aspect of the acetabulum lateral to the posterior acetabular rim (dotted line). The point at which both rims meet is called the crossover sign.

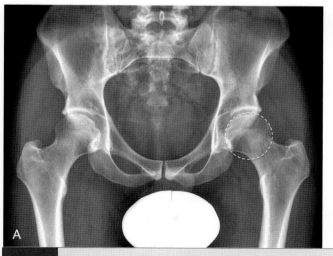
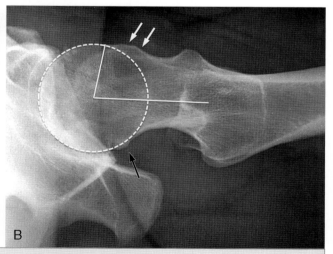

Figure 3   AP pelvic and cross-table radiographs of a 38-year-old patient with cam FAI caused by an anterolateral asphericity of the femoral head. **A,** Although the AP pelvis only shows a mild acetabular retroversion, with an almost spherical femoral head (dotted white line), the anterior and posterior deformities of the proximal femur are visible on the cross-table radiograph. **B,** Anteriorly (white arrows) and posteriorly (black arrow), the femoral head shows non-spherical extension causing cam FAI (dotted line indicates a sphere). The α angle is 78°, which is very high.

3: Hip

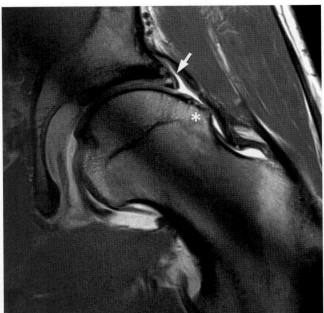

Figure 4   Proton density-weighted sequence of a radial MRA. This technique allows not only the identification of the bony femoral head deformity (asterisk) but also secondary changes at the acetabular labrum (arrow). The acetabular roof also reveals a significant hypersclerosis indicated by the low-intensity signal.

rical joint shape, and narrowness of tissue structures pose logistical difficulties and demand high magnetic resonance technology standards.

Recent developments in high-resolution isotropic imaging, cartilage-specific magnetic resonance sequences, local gradient and radiofrequency coils, and high-field magnetic resonance systems potentially improve diagnostic capabilities, thereby reducing the need for a contrast agent. In addition to morphologic MRI, biochemical magnetic resonance (delayed gadolinium-enhanced MRI of cartilage and T2 mapping) approaches that characterize cartilage microstructure and biochemical content will contribute to a better understanding of cartilage degeneration. In patients for whom MRI is contraindicated (because of claustrophobia, electronic implanted devices, cardiac pacing wires, or orbital metal bodies), CT or even CT arthrography is an acceptable alternative with equally high sensitivity, specificity, and accuracy. Gonadal radiation exposure is a concern in these mainly young patients.

Classification

FAI is a pathomechanical process by which the human hip can fail. The hip joint is an approximation of a socket joint; however, the human hip is not completely congruent. Even very subtle structural abnormalities of the femur and acetabulum combined with terminal and/or rigorous hip motion can lead to repetitive

stresses at the acetabular rim that damage the adjacent soft-tissue structures such as the labrum and/or cartilage. The site of hip damage in FAI is similar to the acetabular rim damage recently described for hip dysplasia; however, the failure mechanisms are almost the opposite. In hip dysplasia, the unstable femoral head migrates and subluxates in regions of the least coverage of the femoral head. In FAI, the femoral head remains well centered, but the free arc of hip motion is limited by either an acetabulum that is functionally excessive (deep or maloriented, causing pincer FAI), a misshaped proximal femur (insufficient head-neck offset, nonspherical head causing cam FAI), and/or a combination of the two.[4] A summary of findings/characteristics in cam and pincer FAI is presented in Table 1.

The damage patterns of pincer and cam FAI differ substantially when one of these two types exists as an isolated deformity, with pincer FAI (Figure 5, A) being more localized at the labrum and cam FAI (Figure 5, B) taking place at the cartilage with outside-in abrasion and/or delamination.[25] Extremes of hip motion and, to a lesser degree, variations in the tissue quality of the labral/chondral junction might contribute to an enhanced vulnerability at the anterosuperior rim; however, the main damage in FAI is caused by bony abnormalities.[25] Central parts of the joint and the femoral head are only involved in the development of more advanced OA or in pincer FAI. Although childhood diseases such as Legg-Calvé-Perthes disease, SCFE, hip dysplasia, and bladder extrophy are associated with an increased incidence in pincer- and cam-type FAI, the etiology of most FAI-causing abnormalities has not been identified. Acetabular protrusion leading to global pincer FAI might be caused by metabolic or inflammatory disease, although for some patients no such explanation can be postulated. For acetabular retroversion (focal pincer FAI), representing a posterior opening of the acetabulum rather than a deficiency of the posterior acetabular wall, the etiology is even less understood. For most cam FAI, the etiology of the proximal femoral malformation or malorientation remains a topic of debate. Although sequelae of childhood disease, in particular SCFE, were initially considered and still are etiologic factors, most patients with cam FAI do not have orientational growth plate abnormalities, which suggests a different developmental etiology.[26] Physeal stresses (such as from trauma or rigorous sports) during development (extrinsic factors) and genetics (intrinsic factors) represent potential sources for the development of proximal femoral abnormalities. Finally, there are a substantial number of posttraumatic (acetabular dysplasia, femoral retrotorsion) and iatrogenic deformities (femoral varus osteotomy, retroversion after pelvic osteotomy such as a Salter) of the hip joint leading to FAI. Without appreciating the etiology of malformations leading to FAI, preventive measures are unlikely to become effective.

Table 1

Summary of Findings/Characteristics in Cam and/or Pincer FAI

Location of Deformity	Femoral Alterations	Acetabular Alterations
Frequent signs and symptoms	Key: Groin pain Male > female (3:1) Younger than 30 – 35 yrs Activity level above average Poor stretching in adolescence Stop-and-go sport (high impact) Insidious onset but activity related Traumatic event rare	Key: Groin pain Female > male (14:1) Older than 30 – 35 yrs Activity level above average Decreasing range of hip motion Insidious onset but activity related Traumatic event rare
Clinical findings	Key: Reduced internal rotation Functional impairment Gait mostly unaltered ROM, flexion/IR and abduction reduced Positive impingement test	Key: Reduced rotation Functional impairment Gait mostly unaltered ROM, flexion/IR, extension/ER and abduction reduced Positive impingement test
Radiographic findings	Key: Asphericity in lateral hip radiograph Femoral head asphericity Pistol grip deformity Horizontal growth plate sign Epiphyseal retrotilt/translation Coxa magna/plana Low center column diaphyseal angle < 125° Alpha angle > 55° Femoral head-neck offset < 8 mm Offset ratio < 0.18 Os acetabuli Impingement cysts (herniation pits)	Key: Deep socket in anteroposterior pelvis Coxa profunda Protrusio acetabuli Focal acetabular retroversion (figure-of-8 configuration) Lateral center edge angle > 39° Reduced extrusion index Acetabular index < 0° Posterior wall sign Linear indentation sign Ossification of acetabular rim Appositional bone sign Posterior inferior joint space loss
MRA	Key: Triad of abnormal head-neck anterosuperior labral, and cartilage morphology	Key: Labral cysts and/or rim ossification Contre coup lesion
Damage mechanism	Key: Inclusion with outside-in damage	Key: Impaction with rim damage
Location	Key: Anterosuperior with deep extension	Key: Circumferential, located at the rim
Associated deformities	Slipped capital femoral epiphysis Legg-Calvé-Perthes disease Coxa vara Postslip deformity Femoral retroversion Growth abnormality of femoral epiphysis	Bladder extrophy Proximal femoral focal deficiency Posttraumatic dysplasia Chronic residual dysplasia of acetabulum Legg-Calvé-Perthes disease Slipped capital femoral epiphysis Idiopathic and iatrogenic retroversion
Progression	Rapid	Slow
Classification	Cam-FAI	Pincer-FAI

ROM = range of motion; IR = internal rotation; ER = external rotation.

Open Surgery
John C. Clohisy, MD

Introduction

Joint preservation surgery for hip impingement disorders has evolved markedly over the past several years. This has resulted from improved understanding of hip OA pathophysiology and appreciation of the etiologic role of FAI.[27] Additionally, introduction and refinement of alternative surgical techniques has improved the ability to correct prearthritic structural abnormalities and to treat associated intra-articular disease (articular cartilage and labrum).[28] Currently, there are several surgical techniques to manage hip impingement, yet the basic goals and concepts of surgical treatment are universal and independent of surgical approach and/or technique. Surgical treatment is directed at relieving symptoms, enhancing function and activity, improving

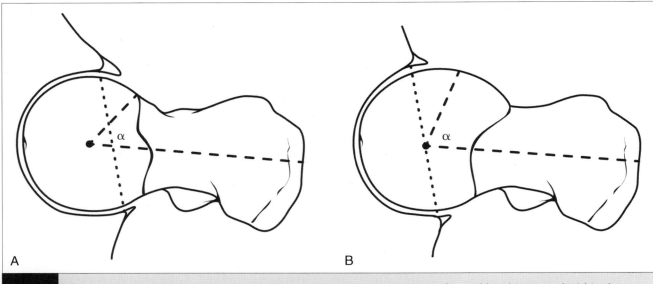

Figure 5 Schematic drawings of (**A**) pincer FAI and (**B**) cam FAI. **A**, In pincer FAI, the femoral head is trapped within the acetabular socket, indicated by the fact that the rotational center of the femoral head (black dot) lies medial to a line connecting the anterior and posterior acetabular rim (dotted line). The α angle in pure pincer FAI is not significantly increased (> 55°); however, there is frequently an indentation line at the head-neck junction. **B**, In cam FAI, the femoral head is not round, but rather oval, with an α angle mostly greater than 55°, whereas the acetabular coverage is not increased, indicated by the fact that the rotational center of the femoral head (black dot) lies lateral to the rim-connecting line.

quality of life, and preserving the hip joint over time. These goals are best achieved by the adherence to basic concepts of treating FAI. First, accurate diagnosis and detailed analysis of hip pathomechanics and associated intra-articular disease are essential for developing an effective surgical treatment plan. Second, surgical treatment should focus on selecting and performing a procedure that provides comprehensive correction of structural disease and concurrent management of intra-articular abnormalities. Third, care is taken to avoid undercorrection, which can result in persistent impingement, or overcorrection, with the potential for iatrogenic structural instability.

Given the broad spectrum of FAI pathomorphologies[29] and diverse patient characteristics, comprehensive treatment of FAI encompasses a spectrum of surgical strategies. Contemporary surgical options include periacetabular osteotomy (PAO), proximal femoral osteotomy, surgical hip dislocation, anterior approaches, hip arthroscopy combined with an anterior approach and all-arthroscopic techniques. Each of these surgical approaches has distinct indications, advantages, and disadvantages. This full armamentarium of surgical approaches enables the surgeon to apply the most appropriate surgical technique to each patient.

Periacetabular Osteotomy
Indications
PAO is a relatively uncommon procedure for the treatment of FAI and is indicated in a very specific subgroup of patients.[30] For treating FAI, PAO is considered in young patients (younger than 30 years) with major ac-

etabular retroversion,[31] posterior acetabular wall deficiency, and healthy anterosuperior acetabular articular cartilage. Precise radiographic imaging and MRI are essential in selecting such patients for PAO. Major acetabular retroversion results in anterosuperior overcoverage of the femoral head (pincer impingement), yet the associated posterolateral acetabular insufficiency puts the hip at risk for worsened instability with acetabular rim trimming. Therefore, acetabular anteversion and flexion correction is performed to relieve anterolateral impingement and improve posterior acetabular coverage of the femoral head.[32] The acetabular correction is frequently combined with an osteochondroplasty of the femoral head-neck junction to ensure decompression of the impingement lesion.

Surgical Technique
A PAO is performed with the patient in the supine position. Surgical exposure can be performed with various modifications of anterior approaches to the hip.[30,33,34] A modified Smith-Peterson approach with abductor sparring is favorable. The rectus tendon origin is released and an anterior arthrotomy is performed to assess the hip after surgical correction. The PAO cuts are made, the acetabular fragment mobilized, and reduction performed. Acetabular correction is achieved by anteversion and flexion of the fragment. Care is taken to avoid overcorrection of the acetabulum, thereby creating posteroinferior impingement of the femoral head-neck junction and acetabular rim. The reoriented acetabulum is provisionally fixed and the reduction analyzed with intraoperative radiographs. Definitive fixation is

performed with 4.5-mm screws. After acetabular reorientation the hip is examined dynamically for residual anterior impingement. In most patients a concurrent osteochondroplasty of the anterolateral femoral head-neck junction is performed. Final hip motion is assessed to confirm relief of impingement and improved flexion and internal rotation in flexion.

Clinical Outcomes

Data regarding the clinical outcomes of the PAO in treating hip impingement disease are limited. One study reported the early outcomes (average, 2.5 years) of 29 hips treated with this technique.[32] Twenty-six hips (90%) had a good or excellent clinical result, and three hips required additional surgery. Additional investigation is needed to better define the appropriate indications and clinical outcomes of this surgical approach for the treatment of this specific subgroup of patients with FAI.

Surgical Hip Dislocation

Indication

Surgical dislocation of the hip is a versatile approach that can be used to treat FAI, articular cartilage defects, unstable SCFEs, tumors, and acute fractures. This surgical technique is based on enhanced understanding of the vascular blood supply to the femoral head[35] (**Figure 6**). Wide exposure of both the acetabulum and proximal femur is achieved via dislocation with preservation of the terminal branches of the medial femoral circumflex artery. This enables precise intra-articular and periarticular hip procedures without limitations from surgical exposure. With respect to FAI, surgical dislocation of the hip is appropriate for most patients and disease patterns. Patients with symptomatic FAI without moderate to advanced secondary OA are candidates for surgery. All impingement pathomorphologies with the exception of major acetabular retroversion can be treated with this procedure. The technique allows circumferential exposure of the acetabulum and labrum as well as access to the femoral head, femoral neck, intertrochanteric region, and greater trochanter. Acetabular rim resection, labral resection/refixation, articular cartilage management, femoral head-neck osteochondroplasty, relative neck lengthening, trochanteric advancement, and proximal femoral osteotomy can all be performed via this approach. Perhaps the most important role of this technique is to correct extensive and/or circumferential FAI disease patterns that are less amenable to arthroscopic management (**Figure 7**). Posterior and posteroinferior acetabular rim lesions and femoral-sided deformities that extend posterior to the retinacular vessels may be better addressed with this technique. Similarly, deformities requiring concurrent relative neck lengthening, trochanteric advancement, and/or proximal femoral osteotomy are effectively treated using this technique.

Surgical Technique

The patient is in the lateral decubitus position with the

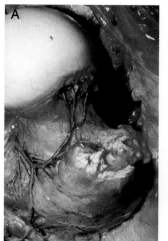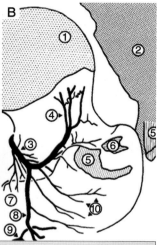

Figure 6 **A**, Photograph showing the perforation of the terminal branches into bone (right hip, posterosuperior view). The terminal subsynovial branches are located on the posterosuperior aspect of the neck of the femur and penetrate bone 2 to 4 mm lateral to the bone-cartilage junction. **B**, Diagram showing (1) the head of the femur; (2) the gluteus medius; (3) the deep branch of the medial femoral circumflex artery; (4) the terminal subsynovial branches of the medial femoral circumflex artery; (5) the insertion and tendon of gluteus medius; (6) the insertion of tendon of piriformis; (7) the lesser trochanter with nutrient vessels; (8) the trochanteric branch; (9) the branch of the first perforating artery; and (10) the trochanteric branches. (Reproduced with permission from Gautier E, Ganz K, Krügel N, Gill T, Ganz R: Anatomy of the medial femoral circumflex artery and its surgical implications. *J Bone Joint Surg Br* 2000;82:679-683.)

extremity draped free for manipulation and ROM testing. A straight lateral, Kocher-Langenbeck, or Gibson-type incision can be used. A trochanteric "flip" osteotomy is performed and the trochanter is retracted anteriorly. A z-shaped capsulotomy allows access to the joint and the hip is assessed for impingement in flexion and combined flexion/internal rotation. Anterior dislocation is then performed and the femoral head is displaced posteroinferiorly, enabling wide exposure of the acetabulum (**Figure 8**). The remainder of the procedure is patient-specific and depends on the intra-articular disease and pathomorphologies of the acetabulum and proximal femur. Most commonly, a disruption of the anterosuperior labrochondral junction is present. The acetabular labrum may require mobilization or detachment for access to perform a rim osteoplasty. The excessive acetabular rim is removed, the labrum refixed with suture anchors, and articular cartilage lesions treated (chondroplasty or microfracture).[36,37] Attention is then turned to the femoral side where lack of offset (or concavity) at the femoral head-neck junction is corrected. The most profound deformity is usually located anterolateral, yet there is significant variability in the

3: Hip

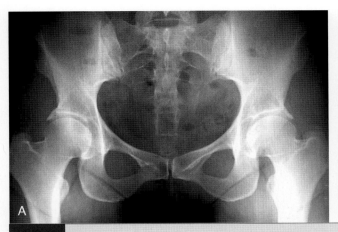
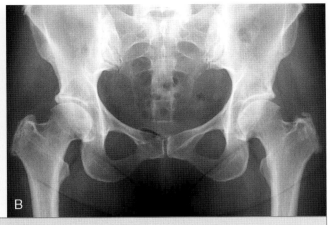

Figure 7 AP radiographs of a 42-year-old woman with a bilateral pincer impingement. This patient presented with progressive bilateral hip pain associated with hip flexion activities. **A**, Preoperative AP radiograph shows appositional bone growth circumferentially around the acetabular rim. The patient had a positive bilateral impingement test and restricted hip flexion and internal rotation in flexion. **B**, Postoperative radiograph. Treatment with bilateral surgical dislocation including acetabular rim osteoplasty and osteochondroplasty of the femoral head-neck junction was associated with an excellent clinical result in both hips at 3 years (right hip) and 4 years (left hip).

location and extent of femoral deformities. In patients with major femoral neck and/or intertrochanteric abnormalities, additional procedures (relative neck lengthening, proximal femoral osteotomy, or trochanteric advancement) can be performed (**Figure 9**). After the reconstruction, intraoperative radiographic evaluation and dynamic ROM examination is performed to confirm adequate surgical correction. Improved hip flexion and flexion/internal rotation should be observed. Trochanteric fixation is achieved with 3.5- or 4.5-mm fixation screws.

Clinical Outcomes

Early to midterm clinical results are published by various surgeons from different institutions.[37-40] Pain relief, improved function, and improved quality of life have been documented for most patients. Good to excellent outcomes are observed in 65% to 90% of patients. Poor clinical results and failures have been associated with older age, more advanced secondary OA, and more severe pain symptoms preoperatively.[39] Clinical failures and the need for conversion to a total hip arthroplasty (THA) occur in approximately 10% to 20% of patients. Major complications are rare but can include trochanteric nonunion and thromboembolic disease. Femoral neck fracture, osteonecrosis, and nerve palsy are extremely uncommon and not observed in most studies. Longer term follow-up studies are needed to discern the impact of these procedures on survivorship of the natural hip joint.

Anterior Approach

Indications

Anterior approaches to the hip have been introduced as less invasive techniques for managing specific patterns of hip impingement disease.[41-43] Nevertheless, intraarticular conditions (labral detachment and articular

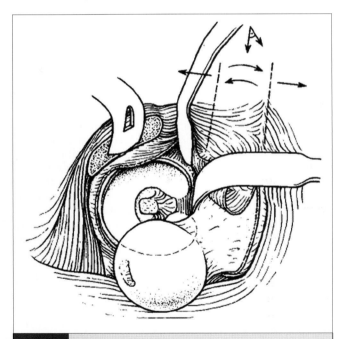

Figure 8 Diagram showing that, for inspection of the acetabulum, one retractor is impacted above the acetabulum. A second retractor hooks on the anterior rim and a third retractor levers the calcar of the neck against the incisura acetabuli. For inspection of the femoral head, no retractors are needed; the knee is lowered and with rotation of the leg (arrows); different surfaces of the head can be visualized. (Reproduced with permission from Ganz R, Gill T, Gautier E, Ganz K, Krügel N, Berlemann U: Surgical dislocation of the adult hip: A technique with full access to the femoral head and acetabulum without the risk of avascular necrosis. *J Bone Joint Surg Br* 2001;83:1119-1124.)

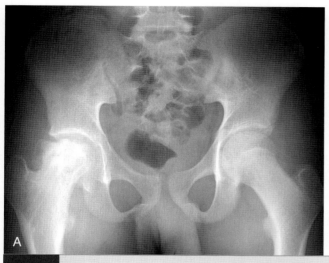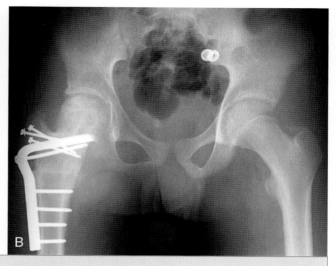

Figure 9 **A,** Anterior radiograph of a 14-year-old boy with a posttraumatic osteonecrosis of the femoral head, femoral head extrusion and severe abduction and flexion impingement. **B,** Posterior view after the patient was treated with a surgical dislocation, recontouring of the femoral head-neck junction, flexion proximal femoral osteotomy, and trochanteric advancement. The patient had an excellent clinical result 1 year after surgery with marked relief of pain and improved gait and function.

cartilage lesions) can be difficult to access through the anterior approach; therefore, many surgeons advocate combined arthroscopy. The arthroscope is used to treat disease of the acetabular rim (labrum, articular cartilage, and pincer deformity), whereas the open exposure provides direct access and visualization of the anterolateral femoral head-neck junction. The best candidates for anterior approaches include patients with symptomatic FAI with anterior and/or anterolateral impingement deformities. These structural abnormalities are the most common and can be readily accessed through a mini-anterior approach. Although combined arthroscopy is preferable for treating the associated acetabular rim disease, some surgeons accomplish this with the open technique alone.

Surgical Technique

The patient is positioned supine; if joint distraction is desired during the procedure, fracture table traction can be used. The incision is placed at the inferior aspect of the anterior superior iliac spine and extended distally 6 to 10 cm. Lateral translation of the incision 1 to 2 cm may lessen the risk of lateral femoral cutaneous nerve sensory deficit. The intramuscular plane between the tensor fascia lata and sartorius is developed to expose the origin of the rectus femoris. The reflected head is released and the arthrotomy performed. The acetabular rim and labrum are best exposed by elevation of the capsular origin and joint distraction. Alternatively, the acetabular rim disease can be managed by arthroscopy before the open procedure. Osteochondroplasty of the anterior femoral head-neck junction is performed with the extremity flexed, abducted, and externally rotated. The anterolateral and lateral regions are accessed with

progressive extension and internal rotation. The retinacular vessels are visualized at the posterolateral head-neck junction and protected as the osteochondroplasty is extended posterolaterally. Radiographic assessment and dynamic ROM examination is performed to confirm adequate decompression of the mechanical impingement and improved hip flexion and flexion/ internal rotation.

Clinical Outcomes

Recent studies have documented the early results associated with the anterior approach for treating FAI.[39,41-43] Most studies combine the approach with arthroscopy to treat intra-articular disease elements. Results with this strategy are similar to those with surgical dislocation; major complications are rare.

Arthroscopic Treatment
J.W. Thomas Byrd, MD

Introduction

The arthroscopic approach to FAI is more than just the technique of arthroscopic correction. This approach is based on the following four premises. (1) FAI is a cause of hip joint pathology causing pain and secondary OA. (2) Abnormal joint morphology may be present as an asymptomatic condition. Thus, impingement morphology may exist in the absence of impingement pathology. (3) Pathologic pincer impingement is most clearly associated with breakdown of the acetabular labrum and then secondarily, over time, the development of chondromalacia. (4) Pathologic cam impingement is most clearly associated with failure of the acetabular articular surface secondary to the shear effect, and the labrum is relatively preserved until later in the disease course.

Based on these premises, the arthroscopic findings of joint pathology are part of the treatment algorithm in proceeding with correction of the bony impingement lesions.[44] There are three arthroscopic parameters of pincer impingement. First is the presence of anterior labral pathology necessary for pathologic pincer impingement. Second, positioning of the anterior portal may be difficult despite adequate distraction resulting from the bony prominence of the anterolateral acetabulum. Third is the presence of bone overhanging the labrum where normally there should just be a capsular reflection when pincer impingement is not present. Over time, acetabular chondromalacia will begin to occur with advancing labral deterioration. The principal feature of cam impingement is articular failure of the anterolateral acetabulum caused by the shear effect of the cam lesion. This ranges from closed grade I chondral blistering to full-thickness grade IV articular delamination. Secondary labral failure will begin to occur, but there is a disproportionate amount of articular loss.

Advantages of Arthroscopic Correction of Impingement

Arthroscopic correction of impingement is substantially less invasive than open procedures. Reported complications with the arthroscopic approach are significantly fewer than with the open technique.[44-48] It can be performed as an outpatient procedure and is associated with easier recovery. Time is needed for healing of the osteoplasty and repaired soft tissues within the joint with any technique, but full release for activities is usually anticipated by 12 to 16 weeks, which is quicker than that normally accomplished with open procedures.

Correction of impingement is contraindicated in the presence of advanced disease, because it is unlikely to alter the natural course. Imaging studies usually underestimate the severity of articular damage.[49] At arthroscopy, extensive articular loss is sometimes identified that was undetected by preoperative studies and would have contraindicated an open approach.

Patient Selection

Most patients with symptomatic FAI can be treated with arthroscopic intervention. Arthroscopy may be contraindicated in the presence of some severe deformities and is specifically contraindicated in those that require a PAO or proximal femoral osteotomy. Some severe cases of acetabular protrusio or profunda may be difficult to correct accurately and may benefit more from an open approach.

Preoperative Planning

The planning is based on a patient with clinical findings of hip disease and radiographic findings of impingement. Evaluating the rotational motion of the hip is important in assessing distractibility of the joint. A limited arc of motion is indicative of a tight joint that may introduce challenges for effective access during the procedure.[50] Radiographs represent a poor two-dimensional image of the three-dimensional anatomy of impingement. CT with three-dimensional reconstructions can be especially helpful in arthroscopic management by precisely defining the abnormal bony architecture. CT is not necessary for open procedures because of the complete exposure of the joint. However, with arthroscopy, CT provides a road map to define precisely the size, shape, and location of abnormal bone to be removed.

Technique

Anesthesia

These procedures are most commonly performed under general anesthesia. Muscle relaxation is important for achieving adequate joint space separation without having to use excessive traction force. Maintaining the systolic blood pressure below 100 mm Hg also helps control hemostasis and maintain optimal visualization during the procedure. Epidural anesthesia is an appropriate alternative, but an adequate motor block is important for distraction.

Distraction Systems

Most standard fracture tables can accommodate arthroscopic hip procedures. The perineal post should be heavily padded to lessen the risk of perineal injury with traction.

Custom distractor systems specifically designed for hip arthroscopy are also available. The important features of any of these methods are that they must be able to achieve adequate traction force across the joint while providing fluoroscopic imaging and access to the hip for portal placements.[51] Additionally, with the traction released, they must allow for the hip to be placed through ROM for access to the peripheral compartment and for assessing the amount of bony resection.[52]

Patient Position

Hip arthroscopy is most commonly performed with the patient positioned supine.[51] Some surgeons prefer the lateral decubitus position, and arthroscopic correction of impingement can be performed effectively with either position.[53]

Pincer Impingement

Arthroscopic management of FAI begins with arthroscopy of the central compartment. Traction is applied and three standard portals provide optimal access for surveying and addressing intra-articular pathology[51] (Figure 10). After determining the damage caused by pincer impingement, diseased labrum is conservatively débrided. Often, this alone exposes the pincer lesion, which is then recontoured with a high-speed burr, switching between the various portals to accurately re-

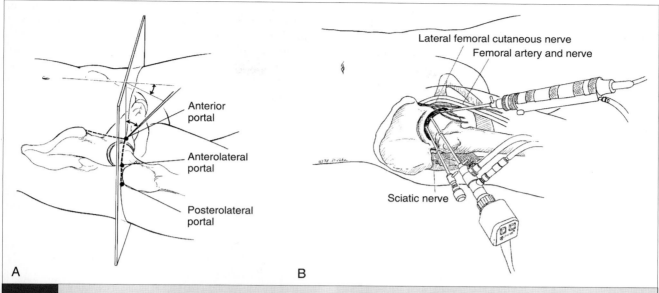

Figure 10 **A,** The site of the anterior portal coincides with the intersection of a sagittal line drawn distally from the anterior superior iliac spine and a transverse line across the superior margin of the greater trochanter. The direction of this portal courses approximately 45° cephalad and 30° toward the midline. The anterolateral and posterolateral portals are positioned directly over the superior aspect of the trochanter at its anterior and posterior borders. **B,** The relationship of the major neurovascular structures to the three standard portals is illustrated. The femoral artery and nerve lie well medial to the anterior portal. The sciatic nerve lies posterior to the posterolateral portal. The lateral femoral cutaneous nerve lies close to the anterior portal. Injury to this structure is avoided by using proper portal placement. The anterolateral portal is established first because it lies most centrally in the safe zone for arthroscopy. (Figure 10A courtesy of Smith & Nephew Endoscopy, Andover, MA. Figure 10B courtesy of J.W. Thomas Byrd, MD, Nashville, TN.)

create the normal curvature of the acetabular rim (**Figure 11**). In some instances, and especially in younger individuals, the quality of the labral tissue may be sufficient for repair. Mobilization of the labrum from the rim of the acetabulum is necessary to preserve the tissue while accurately resecting the pincer lesion. Labral repair is performed with suture anchors (**Figure 12**). These require more distally based portals or percutaneous placement to ensure that the anchors diverge from the articular surface and do not perforate the acetabulum.

Cam Impingement

Management of cam impingement also begins with arthroscopy of the central compartment, assessing for articular failure characteristic of pathologic cam impingement. The articular damage is addressed, commonly ranging from chondroplasty to microfracture, and attention is then turned to the cam lesion via the peripheral compartment. Creation of a capsular window makes it easier to move the instruments from the central to the peripheral compartment as traction is released and the hip is flexed[54] (**Figure 13**). After fully exposing the cam lesion, the abnormal bone is recontoured with a high-speed burr, re-creating the normal concave relationship at the articular junction (**Figure 14**). Care is taken to preserve the lateral retinacular vessels.

Assessing the Adequacy of Bony Resection

There is no perfect system for calculating the amount of bone to be removed or for assessing the amount of bone that has been removed. Relying too much on any one parameter can be hazardous. Overcorrection or undercorrection can be equally problematic and, with poor guidance, both problems can exist in the same patient.

The amount of bone to be removed is assessed by preoperative imaging including plain radiography, and three-dimensional CT can be especially helpful. Intraoperative assessment is mainly guided by good arthroscopic visualization and can be supplemented by intraoperative fluoroscopy and dynamic testing by placing the hip through ROM.[44,55,56] The surgeon should probably not rely solely on any single method for assessing the recontouring.

Results

A 2006 study reported on 183 patients who underwent arthroscopic correction of impingement using the lateral position.[45] The distribution of the types of impingement was not reported, but correction of the pincer and cam lesions in conjunction with labral débridement was described. Preliminary results indicated that the impingement sign was eliminated in 94% and there was a high degree of satisfaction, although no other specific outcome measures were reported. The

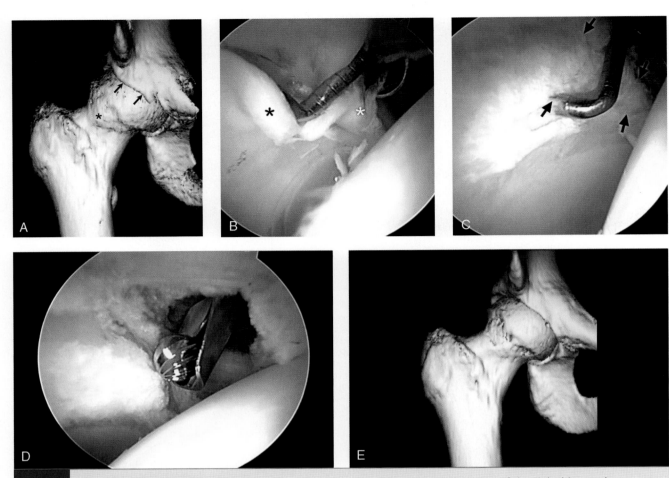

Figure 11 Imaging studies of a 38-year-old woman with progressive pain and loss of motion of the right hip are shown. **A,** Three-dimensional CT scan shows pincer impingement (arrows) as well as a kissing lesion characterized by osteophyte formation on the femoral head (asterisk). **B,** Viewing anteriorly from the anterolateral portal, there is maceration of the anterior labrum (white asterisk) and some associated articular delamination (black asterisk). **C,** Débridement of the degenerate labrum exposes the pincer lesion (arrows). **D,** The pincer lesion is recontoured with a burr. **E,** Postoperative three-dimensional CT scan demonstrates the extent of bony recontouring of the acetabulum and the femoral head. (Courtesy of J.W. Thomas Byrd, MD, Nashville, TN.)

results were generally noted to be poorer in the presence of more extensive articular damage.

A 2008 study reported early outcomes in 96 patients (100 hips) at an average follow-up period of 10 months.[46] There were 26 cam, 21 pincer, and 53 combined lesions. Thirty hips (31%) underwent labral repair or refixation and the rest débridement; 85 hips (86%) had negative or only mildly positive impingement tests postoperatively. The modified Harris hip score was significantly improved an average of 25 points (preoperative, 60; postoperative, 85). Three hips were converted to THA during this early follow-up period. There was one partial transient sciatic nerve neurapraxia and six instances of heterotopic bone formation.

A 2009 study reported on 122 patients with minimum 2-year follow-up.[47] Ten patients refused to participate in the follow-up; of 112 patients, 23 had correction of cam lesions; 3, pincer lesions; and 86, combined lesions. For the 90 patients who remained after excluding those lost to follow-up (12) or converted to THA (10), an average 26-point improvement in the modified Harris hip score was reported (preoperative, 58; postoperative, 84) with no specific reported complications. Higher preoperative hip score, less joint space narrowing, and labral repair were found to be predictors of better outcomes.

Another 2009 study reported on 220 patients (227 hips) with minimum 1-year follow-up.[44] There were 162 cam, 21 pincer, and 44 combined lesions that were corrected. No labral repairs were performed in this early series. The median improvement was 21 points (preoperative, 66; postoperative, 87) with 100% follow-up. One was converted to THA and six underwent repeat arthroscopy. There were three complications including a transient neurapraxia of the pudendal nerve and one of the lateral femoral cutaneous nerve, each of which resolved uneventfully, and one mild heterotopic ossification that did not preclude a successful outcome.

In another 2009 study, 39 patients who underwent

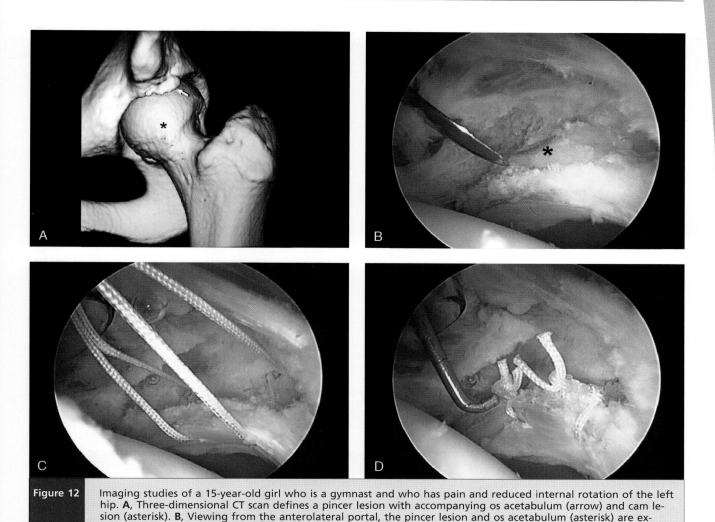

Figure 12 Imaging studies of a 15-year-old girl who is a gymnast and who has pain and reduced internal rotation of the left hip. **A,** Three-dimensional CT scan defines a pincer lesion with accompanying os acetabulum (arrow) and cam lesion (asterisk). **B,** Viewing from the anterolateral portal, the pincer lesion and os acetabulum (asterisk) are exposed with the labrum being sharply released with an arthroscopic knife. **C,** The acetabular fragment has been removed and the rim trimmed with anchors placed to repair the labrum. **D,** The labrum has been refixed. (Courtesy of J.W. Thomas Byrd, MD, Nashville, TN.)

labral repair in conjunction with correction of FAI were identified and compared with a previous matched group of 36 FAI patients in whom the labrum was débrided.[57] The authors reported superior results in the labral repair group at 1-year follow-up, but noted that other variables could have influenced the outcomes. There is certainly a trend toward labral preservation, but these early results of repair versus débridement must be interpreted cautiously because there are significant methodologic biases.

Few but substantial complications have also been reported in conjunction with arthroscopic correction of FAI. Several femoral neck fractures have been encountered, usually associated with poor compliance with postoperative precautions.[48] Also, postoperative dislocation has been reported when rim trimming was performed in a patient in whom dysplasia may have played a role.[58] This emphasizes the importance of accurately interpreting radiographs.

Summary

Contemporary treatment of FAI should include a spectrum of surgical procedures that are applied in a case-specific fashion. Open surgeries have been very effective in providing early to midterm pain relief, enhanced function, and improved quality of life for most patients. Ample exposure, direct visualization, comprehensive deformity correction, low complication rates, and unrestricted capacity to dynamically assess the joint are the main advantages of these techniques. Long-term clinical results are needed to further determine the survivorship of these alternative, joint preservation procedures.

Many patients with FAI can be appropriately managed with arthroscopic surgery. However, the surgeon must be clinically astute in assessing the patient and interpreting the studies to determine the best approach. Meticulous attention to the details of the procedure is necessary. The advantages of this less invasive approach

3: Hip

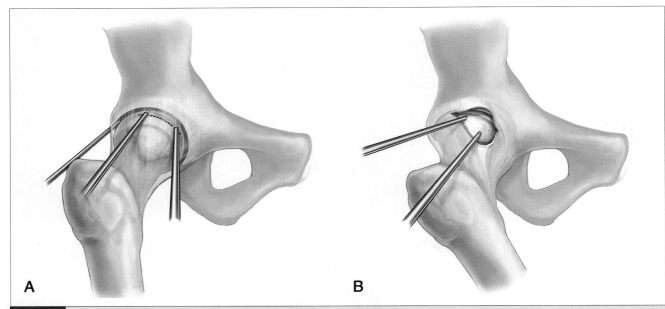

Figure 13   **A**, A capsulotomy is performed by connecting the anterior and anterolateral portals. The capsulotomy is geographically located adjacent to the area of the cam lesion. This capsulotomy is necessary in order for the instruments to pass freely from the central to the peripheral compartment as the traction is released and the hip flexed. **B**, With the hip flexed, the anterolateral portal is now positioned along the neck of the femur. A cephalad (proximal) anterolateral portal has been placed, and the original anterior and posterolateral portals have been removed. These two portals allow access to the entirety of the cam lesion in most cases. Their position also allows an unhindered view with the c-arm. (Courtesy of J.W. Thomas Byrd, MD, Nashville, TN.)

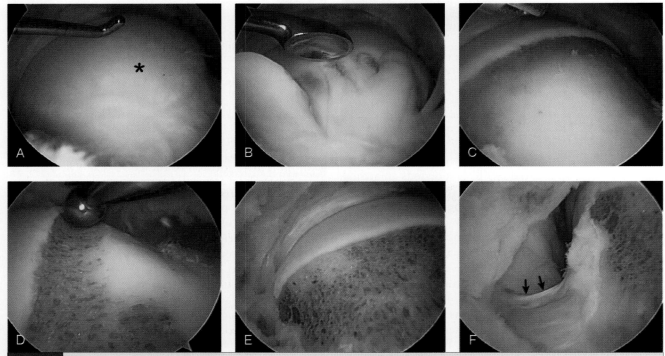

Figure 14   View of a cam impingement from the peripheral compartment. **A.** The cam lesion is identified covered in fibrocartilage (asterisk). **B**, An arthroscopic curet is used to denude the abnormal bone. **C**, The area to be excised has been fully exposed. The soft-tissue preparation aids in precisely defining the margins to be excised. **D**, Bony resection is begun at the articular margin. **E**, The completed recontouring is surveyed. **F**, From a lateral view on the base of the neck, the lateral retinacular vessels are identified (arrows) and preserved during the recontouring. (Courtesy of J.W. Thomas Byrd, MD, Nashville, TN.)

are evident; it is performed as an outpatient procedure with few complications and facilitates postoperative rehabilitation. Also, the imaging studies may underestimate the severity of articular loss, which may only become evident during arthroscopy and which would normally contraindicate open surgical correction of impingement.

Annotated References

1. Reginster JY: The prevalence and burden of arthritis. *Rheumatology (Oxford)* 2002;41(Supp 1):3-6.

2. Elders MJ: The increasing impact of arthritis on public health. *J Rheumatol Suppl* 2000;60:6-8.

3. Ganz R, Leunig M, Leunig-Ganz K, Harris WH: The etiology of osteoarthritis of the hip: An integrated mechanical concept. *Clin Orthop Relat Res* 2008;466(2): 264-272.

   Recent information supports a hypothesis that so-called primary OA is also secondary to subtle developmental abnormalities, and the mechanism in these cases is FAI rather than excessive contact stress.

4. Leunig M, Beaulé PE, Ganz R: The concept of femoroacetabular impingement: Current status and future perspectives. *Clin Orthop Relat Res* 2009;467(3):616-622.

   With an increased recognition and acceptance of FAI, defined standards of assessment and treatment need to be established to provide high accuracy and precision in diagnosis. Early recognition of FAI with subsequent behavioral modification or even surgery may reduce the rate of OA.

5. Ganz R, Parvizi J, Beck M, Leunig M, Nötzli H, Siebenrock KA: Femoroacetabular impingement: A cause for osteoarthritis of the hip. *Clin Orthop Relat Res* 2003;417:112-120.

6. Solomon L, Schnitzler CM: Pathogenetic types of coxarthrosis and implications for treatment. *Arch Orthop Trauma Surg* 1983;101(4):259-261.

7. Harris WH: Etiology of osteoarthritis of the hip. *Clin Orthop Relat Res* 1986;213:20-33.

8. Murray RO: The aetiology of primary osteoarthritis of the hip. *Br J Radiol* 1965;38(455):810-824.

9. Clohisy JC, Knaus ER, Hunt DM, Lesher JM, Harris-Hayes M, Prather H: Clinical presentation of patients with symptomatic anterior hip impingement. *Clin Orthop Relat Res* 2009;467(3):638-644.

   On examination, the anterior impingement test produced pain in 88% of the hips. Hip flexion and internal rotation in flexion were limited to an average 97° and 9°, respectively. The patients were relatively active, yet demonstrated restrictions of function and overall health.

10. Martin HD, Kelly BT, Leunig M, et al: The pattern and technique in the clinical evaluation of the adult hip: The common physical examination tests of hip specialists. *Arthroscopy* 2010;26(2):161-172.

    The authors systematically evaluated the technique and tests used in the physical examination of the adult hip performed by clinicians experienced in the treatment of hip disease. They concluded that patients presenting with groin, abdominal, back, and/or hip pain need to have a basic comprehensive physical examination to ensure that the hip is not overlooked.

11. Reichenbach S, Jüni P, Nüesch E, Frey F, Ganz R, Leunig M: An examination chair to measure internal rotation of the hip in routine settings: A validation study. *Osteoarthritis Cartilage* 2010;18(3):365-371.

    The use of an examination chair revealed a precise assessment of hip internal rotation in a population-based inception cohort study of young asymptomatic males. It was strongly correlated with standard clinical assessment of internal rotation, but was considerably more reliable.

12. Meyer DC, Beck M, Ellis T, Ganz R, Leunig M: Comparison of six radiographic projections to assess femoral head/neck asphericity. *Clin Orthop Relat Res* 2006; 445:181-185.

    Diagnosis of a pathologic femoral head/neck contour depends on the radiologic projection. The Dunn view or a cross-table projection in internal rotation best shows femoral head-neck asphericity, whereas AP or externally rotated cross-table views are likely to miss asphericity.

13. Dudda M, Albers C, Mamisch TC, Werlen S, Beck M: Do normal radiographs exclude asphericity of the femoral head-neck junction? *Clin Orthop Relat Res* 2009; 467(3):651-659.

    Even when conventional radiographs appear normal, an increased α angle can be present anterosuperiorly. Without the use of radial slices in MRA, the asphericity would be underestimated in these patients.

14. Siebenrock KA, Kalbermatten DF, Ganz R: Effect of pelvic tilt on acetabular retroversion: A study of pelves from cadavers. *Clin Orthop Relat Res* 2003;407:241-248.

15. Kalberer F, Sierra RJ, Madan SS, Ganz R, Leunig M: Ischial spine projection into the pelvis: A new sign for acetabular retroversion. *Clin Orthop Relat Res* 2008; 466(3):677-683.

    The high correlation between the ischial spine and the crossover signs showed that in retroversion the affected inferior hemipelvis is rotated posteriorly, which is not caused by a hypoplastic posterior wall or a prominence of the anterior wall only.

16. Reynolds D, Lucas J, Klaue K: Retroversion of the acetabulum: A cause of hip pain. *J Bone Joint Surg Br* 1999;81(2):281-288.

17. Jamali AA, Mladenov K, Meyer DC, et al: Anteroposterior pelvic radiographs to assess acetabular retroversion: High validity of the "cross-over-sign". *J Orthop Res* 2007;25(6):758-765.

    Retroversion is almost exclusively a problem of the cranial acetabulum. The presence of a positive cross-over sign is a highly reliable indicator of cranial acetabular version of less than 4°.

18. Kakaty DK, Fischer AF, Hosalkar HS, Siebenrock KA, Tannast M: The ischial spine sign: Does pelvic tilt and rotation matter? *Clin Orthop Relat Res* 2010;468(3):769-774.

    This study suggests the ischial spine sign is a valid tool for diagnosing acetabular retroversion on plain radiographs taken using a standardized technique regardless of the degree of pelvic tilt and rotation.

19. Nötzli HP, Wyss TF, Stoecklin CH, Schmid MR, Treiber K, Hodler J: The contour of the femoral head-neck junction as a predictor for the risk of anterior impingement. *J Bone Joint Surg Br* 2002;84(4):556-560.

20. Byrd JW, Jones KS: Diagnostic accuracy of clinical assessment, magnetic resonance imaging, magnetic resonance arthrography, and intra-articular injection in hip arthroscopy patients. *Am J Sports Med* 2004;32(7):1668-1674.

21. Chan YS, Lien LC, Hsu HL, et al: Evaluating hip labral tears using magnetic resonance arthrography: A prospective study comparing hip arthroscopy and magnetic resonance arthrography diagnosis. *Arthroscopy* 2005;21(10):1250.

22. Studler U, Kalberer F, Leunig M, et al: MR arthrography of the hip: Differentiation between an anterior sublabral recess as a normal variant and a labral tear. *Radiology* 2008;249(3):947-954.

    Recesses occur as normal variants in the anteroinferior part of the acetabulum. Location in the 8 o'clock position, linear shape of contrast material interposition, partial separation of the labrum, and absence of perilabral abnormalities are characteristics of a recess.

23. Schmid MR, Nötzli HP, Zanetti M, Wyss TF, Hodler J: Cartilage lesions in the hip: Diagnostic effectiveness of MR arthrography. *Radiology* 2003;226(2):382-386.

24. Pfirrmann CW, Duc SR, Zanetti M, Dora C, Hodler J: MR arthrography of acetabular cartilage delamination in femoroacetabular cam impingement. *Radiology* 2008;249(1):236-241.

    Cartilage delamination is common in patients undergoing surgery for FAI. Fluid under the cartilage delamination is a specific but rare finding. Hypointense areas in the acetabular cartilage appear to be helpful diagnostic criteria.

25. Beck M, Kalhor M, Leunig M, Ganz R: Hip morphology influences the pattern of damage to the acetabular cartilage: Femoroacetabular impingement as a cause of

early osteoarthritis of the hip. *J Bone Joint Surg Br* 2005;87(7):1012-1018.

26. Siebenrock KA, Wahab KH, Werlen S, Kalhor M, Leunig M, Ganz R: Abnormal extension of the femoral head epiphysis as a cause of cam impingement. *Clin Orthop Relat Res* 2004;418:54-60.

27. Ganz R, Leunig M, Leunig-Ganz K, Harris WH: The etiology of osteoarthritis of the hip: An integrated mechanical concept. *Clin Orthop Relat Res* 2008;466(2):264-272.

    The authors review the current concepts of structural hip disease as an etiology of secondary OA. Recent information regarding FAI supports the hypothesis that mild impingement abnormalities may be the source of many cases that have been classified as "primary" OA in the past. Pincer- and cam-type disease patterns are reviewed.

28. Clohisy JC, Beaulé PE, O'Malley A, Safran MR, Schoenecker P: AOA symposium: Hip disease in the young adult. Current concepts of etiology and surgical treatment. *J Bone Joint Surg Am* 2008;90(10):2267-2281.

    This article presents an overview of hip disease in the adolescent and young adult patient. Patient evaluation and surgical techniques are summarized to provide general concepts of hip joint preservation surgery.

29. Beck M, Kalhor M, Leunig M, Ganz R: Hip morphology influences the pattern of damage to the acetabular cartilage: Femoroacetabular impingement as a cause of early osteoarthritis of the hip. *J Bone Joint Surg Br* 2005;87(7):1012-1018.

    These authors analyzed 302 hips and defined the underlying structural impingement abnormalities. Their data indicate that combined cam and pincer impingement abnormalities are extremely common, whereas isolated cam or isolated pincer lesions are less common. They demonstrated that cam impingement causes damage to the anterosuperior acetabular cartilage with separation between the labrum and cartilage. Pincer impingement causes localized circumferential cartilage damage along the acetabular rim.

30. Ganz R, Klaue K, Vinh TS, Mast JW: A new periacetabular osteotomy for the treatment of hip dysplasias: Technique and preliminary results. *Clin Orthop Relat Res* 1988;232:26-36.

31. Reynolds D, Lucas J, Klaue K: Retroversion of the acetabulum: A cause of hip pain. *J Bone Joint Surg Br* 1999;81(2):281-288.

32. Siebenrock KA, Schoeniger R, Ganz R: Anterior femoro-acetabular impingement due to acetabular retroversion: Treatment with periacetabular osteotomy. *J Bone Joint Surg Am* 2003;85-A(2):278-286.

33. Clohisy JC, Barrett SE, Gordon JE, Delgado ED, Schoenecker PL: Periacetabular osteotomy in the treatment of severe acetabular dysplasia: Surgical tech-

nique. *J Bone Joint Surg Am* 2006;88(Suppl 1 Pt 1): 65-83.

The authors studied PAO in the treatment of severe acetabular dysplasia in 16 hips and found that early clinical results were very good.

34. Leunig M, Siebenrock KA, Ganz R: Rationale of periacetabular osteotomy and background work. *Inst Course Lect* 2001;50:221-238.

35. Gautier E, Ganz K, Krügel N, Gill T, Ganz R: Anatomy of the medial femoral circumflex artery and its surgical implications. *J Bone Joint Surg Br* 2000;82(5): 679-683.

36. Ganz R, Gill TJ, Gautier E, Ganz K, Krügel N, Berlemann U: Surgical dislocation of the adult hip: A technique with full access to the femoral head and acetabulum without the risk of avascular necrosis. *J Bone Joint Surg Br* 2001;83(8):1119-1124.

37. Espinosa N, Rothenfluh DA, Beck M, Ganz R, Leunig M: Treatment of femoro-acetabular impingement: Preliminary results of labral refixation. *J Bone Joint Surg Am* 2006;88(5):925-935.

This study compares the clinical outcome of 20 patients (25 hips) treated for FAI with labral refixation to that of 32 patients (35 hips) treated with labral resection. All were treated with a surgical dislocation approach. Better outcomes were reported in the group of patients who underwent labral refixation.

38. Beaulé PE, Le Duff MJ, Zaragoza E: Quality of life following femoral head-neck osteochondroplasty for femoroacetabular impingement. *J Bone Joint Surg Am* 2007;89(4):773-779.

This study reports the clinical outcomes of surgical hip dislocation in 34 patients (37 hips) with FAI. At a mean of 3.1 years follow-up, the average Western Ontario and McMaster Universities (WOMAC) score improved 20.1 points, and six patients (16%) had an unsatisfactory outcome with no clinical improvement and/or worsening of the WOMAC score.

39. Clohisy JC, St John LC, Schutz AL: Surgical treatment of femoroacetabular impingement: A systematic review of the literature. *Clin Orthop Relat Res* 2010;468(2): 555-564.

This study is a systematic review of the literature regarding FAI surgery. Eleven studies that met inclusion criteria were reviewed. Clinical results were good to excellent in 65% to 96% of cases. Complications were noted in 0 to 18% of the procedures. Conversion to total hip replacement was reported in 0 to 26% of the cases.

40. Peters CL, Erickson JA: Treatment of femoroacetabular impingement with surgical dislocation and débridement in young adults. *J Bone Joint Surg Am* 2006;88(8):1735-1741.

A series of 96 hips treated with surgical dislocation for FAI was reviewed. At a mean follow-up of 26 months, the average Harris hip score improved 24 points and

six hips (6%) were converted to THA or had a lower postoperative Harris hip score.

41. Clohisy JC, Zebala LP, Nepple JJ, Pashos G: Combined hip arthroscopy and limited open osteochondroplasty for femoroacetabular impingement. *J Bone Joint Surg Am* 2010;92(8):1697-1706.

After a retrospective review of 35 patients, the authors concluded that combined hip arthroscopy and limited open osteochondroplasty of the femoral head-neck junction is effective for treating FAI.

42. Laude F, Sariali E, Nogier A: Femoroacetabular impingement treatment using arthroscopy and anterior approach. *Clin Orthop Relat Res* 2009;467(3):747-752.

The authors reported on a series of 97 patients (100 hips) who underwent osteochondroplasty of the femoral neck for FAI using a mini-open anterior Hueter approach with arthroscopic assistance. At a mean follow-up of 28.6 months, the average nonarthritic hip score improved 29.1 points and 11 hips (11%) were converted to THA.

43. Ribas M, Ledesma R, Cardenas C, Marin-Peña O, Toro J, Caceres E: Clinical results after anterior mini-open approach for femoroacetabular impingement in early degenerative stage. *Hip Int* 2010;20(S7):36-42.

The authors reported the clinical results of 117 consecutive cases treated with an anterior mini-open approach for FAI. Patients were divided into three groups according to preoperative Tönnis OA grades, and at a mean 3.7 years follow-up, satisfactory results were seen in 97.8% of patients with Tönnis grade 0 OA, 93.6% of patients with grade 1 OA, and 50.1% of patients with grade 2 OA. Nine hips (7.7%) were converted to THA.

44. Byrd JW, Jones KS: Arthroscopic management of femoroacetabular impingement. *Instr Course Lect* 2009; 58:231-239.

The role of arthroscopy as part of the treatment algorithm in the management of FAI is described. The arthroscopic technique for correcting impingement is detailed. Preliminary experience in the first 220 patients (227 hips) with minimum 1-year follow-up are reported. Level of evidence: IV.

45. Sampson TG: Arthroscopic treatment of femoroacetabular impingement: A proposed technique with clinical experience. *Instr Course Lect* 2006;55:337-346.

The arthroscopic technique of addressing FAI in the lateral decubitus position is described. Preliminary experience in 183 cases is reported. Level of evidence: IV.

46. Larson CM, Giveans MR: Arthroscopic management of femoroacetabular impingement: Early outcomes measures. *Arthroscopy* 2008;24(5):540-546.

Early outcomes in the arthroscopic management of FAI are reported with an average follow-up of 9.9 months (range, 3 months to 3 years). Level of evidence: IV.

3: Hip

47. Philippon MJ, Briggs KK, Yen YM, Kuppersmith DA: Outcomes following hip arthroscopy for femoroacetabular impingement with associated chondrolabral dysfunction: Minimum two-year follow-up. *J Bone Joint Surg Br* 2009;91(1):16-23.

    Outcomes of hip arthroscopy for FAI with minimum 2-year follow-up are reported in 122 patients. Only 90 patients were available for follow-up, but predictors of better outcomes were higher preoperative scores, less joint space narrowing, and repair of the labrum. Level of evidence: IV.

48. Sampson TG: Arthroscopic treatment of femoroacetabular impingement. *Am J Orthop (Belle Mead NJ)* 2008;37(12):608-612.

    A stepwise approach to arthroscopic treatment of FAI is outlined. Three femoral neck fractures are reported among more than 800 cases. Level of evidence: V.

49. Byrd JW, Jones KS: Diagnostic accuracy of clinical assessment, magnetic resonance imaging, magnetic resonance arthrography, and intra-articular injection in hip arthroscopy patients. *Am J Sports Med* 2004;32(7):1668-1674.

    Clinical assessment, MRI, gadolinium arthrography with MRI, and intra-articular injection of anesthetic are all performed on 40 patients and the results are compared to the arthroscopic findings. Level of evidence: II.

50. Byrd JW: Hip arthroscopy: Patient assessment and indications. *Instr Course Lect* 2003;52:711-719.

51. Byrd JW: Hip arthroscopy by the supine approach. *Instr Course Lect* 2006;55:325-336.

    A detailed description of the technique of hip arthroscopy with the patient in the supine position is reported. Level of evidence: V.

52. Dienst M, Gödde S, Seil R, Hammer D, Kohn D: Hip arthroscopy without traction: In vivo anatomy of the peripheral hip joint cavity. *Arthroscopy* 2001;17(9):924-931.

53. Glick JM: Hip arthroscopy by the lateral approach. *Instr Course Lect* 2006;55:317-323.

    A detailed description of the technique of hip arthroscopy with the patient in the lateral decubitus position is reported. Level of evidence: V.

54. Byrd JW, Jones KS: Arthroscopic femoroplasty in the management of cam-type femoroacetabular impingement. *Clin Orthop Relat Res* 2009;467(3):739-746.

    The details of the arthroscopic management of cam-type FAI are reported, including indications, technique, and outcomes in 200 patients (207 hips) with minimum 1-year, 100% follow-up. Level of evidence: IV.

55. Larson CM, Wulf CA: Intraoperative fluoroscopy for evaluation of bony resection during arthroscopic management of femoroacetabular impingement in the supine position. *Arthroscopy* 2009;25(10):1183-1192.

    This technical note describes a method of using intraoperative fluoroscopy to evaluate bony resection from the acetabular rim and the femoral head-neck junction. Level of evidence: V.

56. Philippon MJ, Stubbs AJ, Schenker ML, Maxwell RB, Ganz R, Leunig M: Arthroscopic management of femoroacetabular impingement: Osteoplasty technique and literature review. *Am J Sports Med* 2007;35(9):1571-1580.

    This technique-oriented article describes the methods of osteoplasty and reviews the current literature. Dynamic assessment of the surgical correction is described by using intraoperative ROM. Level of evidence: IV.

57. Larson CM, Giveans MR: Arthroscopic debridement versus refixation of the acetabular labrum associated with femoroacetabular impingement. *Arthroscopy* 2009;25(4):369-376.

    The results of labral refixation in conjunction with correction of FAI in 39 patients are compared to those of a historic group of 36 patients in whom the labrum was resected in conjunction with correction of FAI. Level of evidence: III.

58. Matsuda DK: Acute iatrogenic dislocation following hip impingement arthroscopic surgery. *Arthroscopy* 2009;25(4):400-404.

    This case report describes iatrogenic dislocation of the hip following arthroscopic acetabular rim trimming. Potential risk factors and methods of avoidance are discussed. Level of evidence: V.

Chapter 21

Alternatives to Total Hip Arthroplasty

Paul E. Beaulé, MD, FRCSC   Thomas Parker Vail, MD
Andrew John Shimmin, MD, MBBS, FAOrthA, FRACS

Patient Selection
Paul E. Beaulé, MD, FRCSC

The ideal patient for hip resurfacing is a young (men younger than 65 years and women younger than 55 years old), active patient with degenerative hip arthritis with no to minimal proximal femoral deformity as well as normal kidney function.[1,2] Hip resurfacing is contraindicated in the elderly patient with osteoporotic bone, patients on long-term steroids, and those who have compromised renal function or proximal femoral tumors.[1] Relative contraindications to hip resurfacing include inflammatory arthritis, severe acetabular dysplasia, poor proximal femoral bone geometry such as a short femoral neck with a high-riding greater trochanter, poor femoral bone stock subsequent to large femoral head cysts, erosive arthritis, known metal sensitivities, and limb-length discrepancy greater than 2 cm.[2,3] The risk to women of childbearing age remains uncertain. Authors of a 2007 study recently confirmed previous reports that both cobalt and chromium ions cross the placenta.[4] In all instances, the maternal metal ions were within the typical range and the effect on the

Dr. Beaulé or an immediate family member has received royalties from Wright Medical Technology; is a member of a speaker's bureau or has made paid presentations on behalf of Wright Medical Technology, Smith & Nephew, and MEDACTA; serves as a paid consultant for or is an employee of Corin USA, Smith & Nephew, Wright Medical Technology, and MEDACTA; owns stock or stock options in Wright Medical Technology; and has received research or institutional support from Corin USA. Dr. Vail or an immediate family member has received royalties from DePuy; serves as a paid consultant for or is an employee of DePuy; owns stock or stock options in Pivot Medical; and serves as a board member, owner, officer, or committee member of the American Board of Orthopaedic Surgeons, the American Association of Hip and Knee Surgeons, and the Knee Society. Dr. Shimmin or an immediate family member is a member of a speaker's bureau or has made paid presentations on behalf of DePuy; serves as a paid consultant for or is an employee of DePuy and Corin UK; and has received research or institutional support from DePuy.

fetus is still unknown. Women of childbearing age should be informed of the theoretic risk and attempt to delay arthroplasty surgery as long as possible, preferably until they no longer want to have children or at least 2 years after a hip resurfacing.[1]

In contrast to total hip replacement, survivorship of hip resurfacing is greatly influenced by the quality and quantity of both femoral and acetabular bone stock. A surface arthroplasty risk index (SARI) based on a group of patients younger than 40 years has been published.[5] The patients were given a numeric value based on the presence of four risk factors: femoral head cysts larger than 1 cm (2 points), weight less than 82 kg (2 points), previous proximal femoral surgery (1 point) and UCLA activity score greater than 6 (1 point). They reported that a SARI greater than 3 represented a 12-fold increase in risk of early failure or adverse radiologic change. This index remained valid regardless of the underlying diagnosis[6] and implant design.[7] Some diagnoses, such as hip dysplasia and osteonecrosis, represent technical surgical difficulties such as proper acetabular component placement with hip dysplasia[8] and femoral fixation with osteonecrosis.[2] Four major series of hip resurfacing in the treatment of hip dysplasia all reported a failure rate of 3% to 10%.[8-11] Most of the failures occurred on the femoral side despite the obvious difficulty in achieving a press fit of an acetabular component with no central screw fixation in a deficient acetabulum. This relatively low failure rate on the acetabular side is largely attributable to the use of the so-called "dysplasia" cups, which have peripheral screws to ensure proper initial stability. Authors of a 2008 study reported no acetabular failures at a mean follow-up of 7.8 years in 103 patients with Crowe II and III dysplasia using a cup with peripheral screws.[11] However, the failure rate was 3% on the femoral side. In a 2007 study, no failures were reported on the acetabular side when a hemispherical press-fit cup in acetabular Crowe I and II deformities was used, but the failure rate on the femoral side was 8%.[8] In both of these series, limb-length discrepancies of less than 2 cm were corrected in most instances.

3: Hip

Table 1

Summary of the Different Surgical Approaches Applicable to Hip Resurfacing

Surgical Approach	Exposure	Femoral Head Blood Flow	Risks/Disadvantages
Posterior	Excellent	Intraoperative compromise	Sciatic nerve palsy
Lateral	Very good	Preserved	Abductor muscle weakness
Transtrochanteric	Excellent	Preserved, if osteotomy extracapsular	Trochanteric nonunion with migration May require removal of screws
Trochanteric flip/slide	Excellent	Preserved	Abductor muscle weakness Trochanteric nonunion without migration May require removal of screws
Anterior	Good	Preserved	Visualization of the socket can be difficult Unfamiliar to many surgeons May require positioning table

With osteonecrosis of the hip, the main concern is the size of the femoral head defect and the remaining area for fixation of the femoral component.[5,12] The importance of these factors on early femoral component failure is also influenced by the size of the femoral component, that is, the impact of a 1-cm[3] lesion with a 42-mm femoral component versus a 52-mm femoral component is different.[5] In addition to the compromised fixation area, these large lesions are usually filled with bone cement. This increases the risk of secondary thermal bone necrosis due to heat generation associated with large volumes of cement, and probably represents a significant contributor to the higher failure rate of hip resurfacing in osteonecrosis.[12-14] On the other hand, two recent studies reported that for the same size femoral component and femoral head deficiency the survivorship was no different between osteonecrosis and other diagnoses.[15,16] These results again would support the initial findings[5,12] where the cumulative score of the SARI takes into account the size of the femoral head lesion as well as patient size.

The ability of hip resurfacing to restore and/or maintain hip biomechanics has been questioned by some authors.[3,17] Two studies documented an average decrease in femoral offset ranging from 4.5 to 8 mm.[3,17] This finding, combined with a limited capacity to correct for limb-length discrepancy greater than 2 cm, has called into question the capacity of hip resurfacing to offer proper restoration of hip biomechanics. In a prospective randomized clinical trial comparing hip resurfacing to total hip replacement, a greater percentage of resurfaced hips were reconstructed within 4 mm in terms of offset (29 of 49 patients [59%] versus 15 of 55 patients [27%]) and leg lengths (42 of 49 patients [86%] versus 33 of 55 patients [60%]) than after total hip replacement.[18] Regarding preexisting hip deformity, one study reported that 57% of patients undergoing hip resurfacing had insufficient femoral head/neck offset consistent with cam-type femoroacetabular impingement,[19] which, if left uncorrected, could lead to persistent impingement causing premature wear of the bearing[20,21] as well as persistent hip pain.[6]

Surgical Approach

The choice of surgical approach for hip resurfacing should be primarily based on the surgeons' experience and comfort level to ensure proper component sizing and orientation.[2] This is critical because varus positioning of the femoral component[22] as well as excessive abduction of the acetabular component[23] both have been associated with early failure of hip resurfacing. Another concern regarding the surgical approach and outcome after hip resurfacing is the risk of femoral neck fracture, which is reported to occur in 1% to 2% of cases with the current generation of implants.[7,24] One of the potential etiologic factors of femoral neck fractures is an osteonecrotic event compromising the structural integrity of the femoral neck and known to occur after hip resurfacing.[13,25,26] In the most recent report of failed resurfacings, the authors found evidence of significant osteonecrosis in 80% of cases, with 60% of the femoral neck fractures associated with osteonecrosis.[25] These findings of osteonecrotic lesions would be consistent with current femoral head blood flow and oxygen tension studies showing significant compromise of the femoral head vascularity with direct damage to the retinacular vessels or their main supply, the ascending branch of the medial circumflex artery.[27-29] In addition, these findings call into question the choice of surgical approach for hip resurfacing, with the posterior approach being the most commonly used[30-32] but also the most detrimental to femoral head blood supply because of the release of the short external rotators, and with it the sacrifice of the ascending branch of the medial circumflex artery. Consequently, some resurfacing surgeons have advocated the use of a vascular–sparing approach[33,34] to minimize the clinical insult to the reamed femoral head and maximize the viability of the interface.[35] The principle of such an approach is an anterior dislocation of the femoral head, preserving the soft-tissue capsule around the posterolateral femoral neck and avoiding contact with the retinacular vessels with the cylindrical femoral head reamers. **Table 1** provides a summary of the different surgical approaches applicable to hip resurfacing. The Ganz surgical dislocation approach[36] has provided surgeons with the ability to treat intra-articular hip disease without placing the femoral head at risk for osteonecrosis. In addition, because of excellent exposure to the acetabulum and femoral head-neck junction, its applicability to hip resurfacing may be reasonable. This approach was used in 116 hip resurfacing procedures in 106 patients where most patients returned to normal and recreational activities.[37] However, significant morbidity was associated with this approach, with an 8.7% nonunion rate and an 18.7% revision surgery rate for removal of painful internal fixation. This complication rate is not dissimilar from that found in a 2006 study using this approach when performing primary total hip replacement.[38] Consequently, this approach is preferable only in patients with a high-riding trochanter, to optimize abductor function by performing a distal transfer, or in the treatment of cam-type femoroacetabular impingement where it is uncertain if the joint can be preserved, thus permitting hip resurfacing if indicated.[37] The other two approaches described for hip resurfacing are the anterior and lateral Hueter approaches.[39] With both approaches, the exposure of the femoral head/neck is very good but acetabular exposure can be more difficult. In terms of patient function, the lateral approach can lead to prolonged limping[40] whereas the anterior Hueter is a truly internervous approach to the hip with the initial experience being quite favorable.[41] It is important to note that a special positioning maybe required for anterior approach hip resurfacing.

Controversy will remain as to which approach is best suited for hip resurfacing until long-term studies comparing the durability of components inserted through different approaches are available. Until then, it is recommended that the surgeon starting hip resurfacing use the approach that he or she is most comfortable with.

Metal-on-Metal Resurfacing
Thomas Parker Vail, MD

Design

Hip resurfacing as a concept dates back to the earliest attempts to treat degenerative and traumatic hip conditions. Its history includes some of the earliest surgical innovators in hip surgery who thought that an anatomic reconstruction of the hip was best achieved by designing a device that was created in the image of the natural hip joint.[42] Early attempts included facial interposition, capping the femoral head with a variety of polymer,[43] ceramic, and metallic materials, temporary femoral head molds,[44,45] and ultimately matching a femoral resurfacing component with a metallic or polyethylene counterface implant fixed by polymethylmethacrylate to the underlying bone. The facial interposition concept did not provide a predictable or durable functional result, and the initial artificial biomaterials did not withstand the harsh axial and torsional loading environment of the hip joint. The result was that the more brittle materials became fragmented, and the polymeric materials failed in smaller pieces because of adhesive wear, pitting, delamination, and surface decomposition. Although the metallic hemiresurfacing components made of Vitallium (a cobalt, chromium, and molybdenum alloy still in use) were more durable, bone fixation was not reliable. In addition, the early metal components did not wear well on the cartilage counterface, leading to progressive articular degeneration with clinical conditions such as pain, stiffness, and acetabular bone erosion.

The first attempts at metal-on-metal and metal-on-polyethylene resurfacing were performed with cemented components. The metal-on-polyethylene concept did not perform well, in contrast to the successful Charnley hip replacements in the 1980s, because of high rates of polyethylene wear. The resultant polyethylene particulate debris caused abundant granuloma formation, bone loss, and component loosening.[46-48] Once again, the metal-on-metal articulations available in the 1970s and 1980s provided a more durable articulation; however, the cemented fixation proved inadequate due to the higher frictional torque of the metal-on-metal bearings.[49,50] Deformation of the acetabular components and equatorial wear related to suboptimal clearance and sphericity also led to the early failure of many of these components.

In the late 1990s designers of hip resurfacing components and engineers studying the tribology of metal on metal components made major breakthroughs in design that led to the re-emergence of hip resurfacing after more than a decade of hiatus after the failure of the metal-on-polyethylene devices.[31,32,51,52] The two important advances were the ability to apply a porous surface to a cobalt-chromium monoblock socket with an inner bearing surface, and the enhanced ability to manufacture a high-quality metal bearing that would satisfy the requirements necessary to potentially achieve a fluid-film lubrication regimen in vivo.[53,54] These requirements included the recognition that a high carbon cobalt-chromium alloy was necessary along with optimized sphericity, surface roughness, head diameter, and clearance.[55] The ability to combine all of these variables into the manufactured parts provided enhanced lubrication and bearing function leading to a new era of more successful devices.[56]

Several other design variables have been debated over the past decade without resolution. These variables include the optimal surgical instrumentation for cup and head implantation with a myriad of systems and positioning tools, including computer navigation currently in use by more than a dozen implant systems

3: Hip

available around the world. Other variables include the thickness of the components, with thinner components currently in favor because of the belief that they might lead to less bone removal.

This concept is countered by the concern that thinner components might deflect enough during implantation to interfere with free movement of the bearing, causing bearing seizure in the worst-case scenario. Other design features being discussed include the optimal circumference of the acetabular component, the optimal articular surface area of the acetabular component, how low the clearance can be safely designed, whether the centering pin on the femoral component should be cemented, and whether that pin should be size specific. Likewise, certain details of the technique remain variable and nonstandard across systems, including whether low-viscosity cement or doughy cement is optimal and which surgical approach is the safest.

Another important realization for designers of devices is that the past decade of experience has exposed some unanticipated outcomes that will likely lead to design improvements and new innovations. The most prominent among these issues is the emergence of outliers in bearing function leading to adverse soft-tissue reaction. It is becoming clear that not all of the metal resurfacing bearings function in vivo in the same way that they function in wear simulator systems, with unintended wear modes perhaps leading to higher local metal levels. These observations have led to a renewed emphasis on restoration of hip mechanics, optimal surgical technique, and improvements in bearing function to achieve the lowest possible burden of metal ions. New concepts in controlling corrosion, using the potential benefits of differential hardness bearings and even using ceramic materials in hip resurfacing, are on the horizon.

Technique

Design of the components is only one part of three important variables that are critical to achieving an optimal outcome in hip resurfacing. Clinical results and retrieval studies[57] have demonstrated that surgical technique[5,58] and appropriate indications are the other two critical variables.

Templating can provide a roadmap for a successful biomechanical reconstruction. Given that the acetabular and femoral components are matched in resurfacing systems, templating serves to illustrate the implications for the sequence of steps, the implant position, and the implant size. In total hip replacement, any size of acetabular component can be matched with any size femoral component. In hip resurfacing, there is often only one size option for any given socket and head combination (there are two options in some implant systems). The key point is that the surgeon must not inadvertently implant an acetabular component that is linked with a femoral component too small for the patient's femoral neck. Likewise, the surgeon should not choose

a femoral component that is so small that it requires an acetabular component that will not fit or so large that excess acetabular bone must be resected to accommodate the femoral size.

As reviewed in the previous section, surgical exposure can be performed using a variety of approaches, including posterior, anterolateral, and anterior. With any approach, sufficient visualization is important to achieve desired component position. The key tricks to acetabular exposure using a posterior approach are elevation of the anterior hip capsule off of the acetabular rim and sectioning of the inferior hip capsule. These maneuvers will allow gentle retraction of the femoral head and neck to a position anterior and superior to the acetabulum. Protecting the blood supply to the head is another important part of the approach along with the placement of retractors, particularly at the superior-lateral quadrant where retinacular vessels that supply the femoral head and neck are located.[35]

Once the approach to the hip is complete, the work flow is as follows: measure the femoral neck to determine the smallest femoral component allowable, prepare and place the acetabular component using a size larger than the minimum femoral component size requires, and prepare and implant the femoral component. The goal is overall restoration of length and offset to achieve desired mechanics and limit the risk of subluxation or impingement.[59]

Acetabular reaming must be concentric and exact. Reaming should be sufficient to place the acetabular component against the medial wall at the base of the fovea. Excessive medialization should be avoided because it will result in soft-tissue laxity if the hip center is medialized. Underreaming more than 2 mm may cause deformation of the acetabular shell during implantation. Acetabular bone preparation for the total resurfacing procedure is no different than standard reaming for a cementless socket in total hip replacement. However, the implant is monoblock, not modular, making placement of the hip center in the desired position even more important because there is no option for an offset or lipped liner, and neither is there an option for supplemental fixation with a standard hip resurfacing component. Thus, the important requirements for success are the creation of a spherical cavity with uniform bone-implant contact, adequate press-fit for initial stability, full seating of the implant into the prepared cavity, and placement of the prosthesis at the anatomic center of rotation.

Optimal acetabular cup position is another important requirement for success. Vertical and excessively anteverted acetabular positioning can lead to elevation in metal ion levels.[60] One tip is to place the acetabular component parallel to the transverse acetabular ligament. This position will ensure that the component is not excessively anteverted, which can lead to edge loading. Additionally, allowing a couple of bead lines (or the cup's porous coating) to show at the superior-lateral edge of the implanted shell will discourage a vertical cup position. When positioning the cup, anteversion should be set first and cup abduction second. Failure to fully seat the acetabular component is another common pitfall with monoblock components. It is not possible to see through the component because there are no screw holes and no dome hole in a resurfacing shell. To ensure that the cup is fully seated, the seated position of the last reamer or a trial to use as a visual reference should be determined. The surgeon should avoid leaving a prominent edge of bone at the outer rim of the acetabulum that will prevent full seating of the cup.

Once the acetabular component is placed, implantation of the femoral component can be performed. The two critical goals for acetabular component placement are the avoidance of femoral neck notching and proper component positioning relative to the axis of the femoral neck. The femoral neck is oval, and the neck is wider from top to bottom than it is from front to back. Thus, the anterolateral neck quadrant is most vulnerable to notching during femoral component preparation. The ideal position of the stem of the component is along the axis of the neck, not the head. The position of the natural femoral head may be markedly different from the desired position of the resurfacing component. Bone erosion from the anterior and superior head, inferior osteophytes, and varus remodeling of the proximal femur can create optical illusions and make femoral component positioning very challenging. Using navigation or instruments that reference the axis of the femoral neck will address these challenges.

Femoral head bone preparation requires several important steps: placement of a guide pin down the center of the femoral neck, proximal resection of bone, and creation of the chamfer and outer wall profile with reamers. Depending on the instrumentation system, these steps will be accomplished either sequentially or simultaneously. In every system, the first step is placing a guide pin down the axis of the femoral neck. Because most femoral heads being resurfaced will have some degree of eccentricity relative to the femoral neck, the entry point of the guide pin is often located in what appears to be a superior, anterior, and valgus position on the femoral head. The starting point for the guide pin can be navigated with computer guidance, or estimated by drawing two lines up the center of the femoral neck on the inferior and anterior quadrants. The intersection of these two lines will provide a reasonable estimate of where the guide pin should enter the femoral head. The pin will then be positioned with a guide to bisect the neck from front to back, and match the valgus angle of the neck relative to the shaft of the femur. Ideal preparation of the femoral head bone places the femoral component in slight valgus alignment with a neck-shaft angle between 130° and 140°. Whether placed by free hand, by computer, or with a pin driver, the final pin position should be checked with a stylus to reference the femoral neck. If placed centrally within the neck, the guide pin should pass unimpeded to the lateral cortex of the femur. Varus positioning should be avoided,

along with overresection or shortening of the neck, because this will alter the hip mechanics and cannot be corrected by component position.

In most systems, the femoral head reaming is performed by using cannulated reamers that pass over the central guide pin. A series of reaming or milling devices turn the femoral neck into a cylindrical shape with a chamfered proximal edge. Centering of the cylindrical head reamers not only ensures proper positioning of the femoral component, but also minimizes the risk of notching the superior and anterior surfaces of the femoral neck. The superior and anterior surfaces are the tension surfaces of the femoral neck. Notching of these surfaces could place the patient at higher risk for femoral neck fracture.[24] Another important reason to center the femoral head component is to ensure adequate clearance of the femoral neck from the acetabular rim when the hip is flexed. Anterior and superior translation of the femoral component re-creates offset, increasing the femoral neck clearance in flexion as well as abduction and external rotation. Once the bone cuts are completed, final preparation of the femoral head bone to maximize the cement interface is accomplished. This preparation includes curettage of cysts, drilling of sclerotic bone, and removal of loose or mechanically inferior bone. Aggressive removal of osteophytes, which can weaken the femoral neck and damage the blood supply, should be avoided. Removal of prominent, impinging osteophytes is acceptable. Uncovered cancellous bone should not be left below the femoral component because this situation can act as a stress riser.

Before the final component is cemented, trials should determine the fully seated position of the femoral component. The final component should be gently impacted into that predetermined position using a mallet, without excessive force that could damage the neck during insertion. Cementing the femoral component should result in an even cement mantle around the component.[61] Excess cement should not be left in the dome of the component because it interferes with complete component seating. To limit the risk of thermal necrosis of bone caused by exothermic cement polymerization, the femoral head should be cooled with saline while the cement polymerizes. Retained cement should be removed, ensuring that the femoral component is fully and concentrically seated in the acetabulum when the hip is reduced.

Recent Results
Andrew John Shimmin, MD, MBBS, FAOrthA, FRACS

The concept of hip resurfacing was attractive to the pioneers of hip arthroplasty surgery and in the 1970s, hip resurfacing hip implants became available for clinical use. Because of an unacceptably high failure rate, it was believed that hip resurfacing could not be a successful treatment for hip arthritis. This sentiment changed when it was realized that the major mode of failure was a consequence of a failure of materials (a thin polyethylene acetabular component articulating on a large metal femoral component), which caused massive osteolysis.

The concept was resurrected in the early to mid 1990s using a metal-on-metal articulation, and by the end of the decade resurfacing had recommenced in several countries around the world. The clinical results available from this 10-year period have been published by design surgeons,[31,62] independent specialist centers,[63,64] and national joint registries.[65]

The Australian Joint Arthroplasty Registry reports on more than 12,000 resurfacings since its inception in 1999. Overall, the cumulative percentage of resurfacings revised at 8-year follow-up is 5.3% compared with 4.0% for total hip replacements during the same follow-up. On the basis of registry data, the ideal patient for resurfacing is a male younger than 65 years with a primary diagnosis of osteoarthritis. Results in this group of patients were as favorable as those for conventional primary hip replacements (3.6% and 4.2%, 7-year cumulative percentage revised for resurfacing and conventional replacement, respectively). This is also the group that may later require revision of any hip implant; therefore, bone conservation on the femoral side without a significant compromise in survivorship is an attractive alternative. There are certain clinical situations where resurfacing leads to suboptimal results. With current designs, higher revision rates occur in women and in patients whose primary pathology is inflammatory arthritis, developmental dysplasia, and osteonecrosis. The Australian Registry has also revealed that small-sized components seem to perform poorly compared with larger-sized components, and this is a stronger determinant of failure than sex alone. The revision rate for femoral components with a diameter of 44 mm or less is five times that of components larger than 55 mm. The reasons for this are numerous and may be related to the acetabular implant design, increased risk of edge loading of the articulation, and the surgical technique (less margin for error in component orientation).[66] The Australian Registry has also shown significant differences in outcomes among the different available implants.

Several clinical series have been published, both from design surgeons and independent centers, with 5-year survivorship ranging from 96.3% to 99.1%. Other peer-reviewed publications emphasize the importance of patient selection and describe a SARI with significantly different survivorships when the SARI is greater than 3 compared with those hips with a SARI of 3 or less.[1] This corroborates the information presented by the Australian registry.

An unresolved issue is whether hip resurfacing can produce a better functional outcome than conventional total hip replacement. In one series, hip resurfacing was associated with a reduced range of motion[67] whereas another prospective, randomized controlled trial demonstrated no difference between total hip arthroplasty (THA) and hip resurfacing with regard to total arc of motion in all planes.[68] Currently, gait analysis has failed to show a conclusive difference between THA and hip resurfacing,[69]

Unlike conventional THA, postoperative radiologic surveillance presents unique challenges because of the inability to assess what is occurring at the bone underneath the femoral component and the inability to assess wear of the metal-on-metal articulation with conventional methods.[1,70,71] Radiologic features that should be assessed at each follow-up include changes in the angle between the femoral component peg and the femoral shaft (peg shaft angle), progressive femoral neck narrowing, and radiolucent lines around the femoral peg. The causes of femoral neck narrowing may vary from physiologic remodeling to more sinister causes such as stress shielding, osteonecrosis, or pressure effects caused by fluid generated from the adverse soft-tissue response to metal ions or particles. An implant should be considered at risk when sequential postoperative radiographs demonstrate a change in peg shaft angle, neck narrowing greater than 10% of original width that is progressive after 3 years, and progressive lucent lines around the peg of the femoral component

Some complications of hip resurfacing arthroplasty are unique to the procedure. Perioperative femoral neck fracture rates are reportedly between 1% and 12%.[1,24] These fractures usually occur within 3 months of the surgery and can be related to patient factors, including poor-quality femoral head and neck bone and obesity (which can compromise adequate surgical exposure), or surgical technique factors, such as varus femoral component implantation, superior femoral neck notching, and incomplete seating of the implant. Another cause of failure, not necessarily unique to hip resurfacing but related to the use of metal on metal articulation, is the incidence of adverse local soft-tissue responses to the presence of metal ion or wear particles. This response can present as persistence of postoperative pain, osteolysis, or with the occurrence of space-occupying solid or cystic masses.[72,73] The true incidence and the cause of this is yet to be determined, but it is believed to be caused by the generation of high local metal wear particle/ion levels or the patient's particular sensitivity to the presence of the metal ions. It has been suggested that a possible cause for this phenomena may be the unforgiving nature of acetabular component positioning, with only small errors in positioning tolerated, because metal-on-metal bearings do not tolerate edge loading of the articulation.[66,23] Acetabular cup malposition can result in implant edge loading and thereby generate high levels of metal ions.

Another unique complication of hip resurfacing is ongoing hip impingement. Because the ideal patient for hip resurfacing is the younger male, the primary pathology is often femoral acetabular impingement. If this pathology is not accurately addressed at that time of surgery, this impingement scenario can continue, leading to ongoing groin pain or subluxation of the implant, which may also create an adverse environment for the metal-on-metal bearing.

Summary

Patient selection, surgical technique, and implant design are important contributors to successful hip resurfacing. The newer generations of hip resurfacing are now thought to be a viable option for consideration in a hip arthroplasty practice. The recent results would indicate that there is a place in the young patient, especially those who because of their age and anticipated activity level are likely to outlive any current, conventional THA. There are some issues regarding surgical technique that make this procedure more challenging than a conventional THA. Acetabular component position is critical where excessive anteversion and/or abduction are associated with high wear and early failure. Although the risk of femoral neck fracture after hip resurfacing remains relatively low at 1% to 2%, techniques minimizing damage to femoral head vascularity help in preventing fracture. Surgeons need to be aware of its unique complications before contemplating the procedure.

Annotated References

1. Shimmin A, Beaulé PE, Campbell P: Metal-on-metal hip resurfacing arthroplasty. *J Bone Joint Surg Am* 2008;90(3):637-654.

    The authors present a current concepts review of hip resurfacing, history, technique, complications, and results.

2. Beaulé PE, Antoniades J: Patient selection and surgical technique for surface arthroplasty of the hip. *Orthop Clin North Am* 2005;36(2):177-185.

    Case illustrations of various hip pathologies treated with surface arthroplasty of the hip are discussed. Level of evidence: IV.

3. Silva M, Lee KH, Heisel C, Dela Rosa MA, Schmalzried TP: The biomechanical results of total hip resurfacing arthroplasty. *J Bone Joint Surg Am* 2004;86(1): 40-46.

4. Ziaee H, Daniel J, Datta AK, Blunt S, McMinn DJ: Transplacental transfer of cobalt and chromium in patients with metal-on-metal hip arthroplasty: A controlled study. *J Bone Joint Surg Br* 2007;89(3):301-305.

    The authors showed that cobalt and chromium have the ability to cross the placenta in patients with metal-on-metal hip resurfacing and in control subjects with no metal implants. Level of evidence: II.

5. Beaulé PE, Dorey FJ, LeDuff MJ, Gruen T, Amstutz HC: Risk factors affecting outcome of metal-on-metal surface arthroplasty of the hip. *Clin Orthop Relat Res* 2004;418(418):87-93.

6. Lavigne M, Rama KR, Roy A, Vendittoli PA: Painful impingement of the hip joint after total hip resurfacing: A report of two cases. *J Arthroplasty* 2008;23(7): 1074-1079.

    In one of the two cases studied, anterior neck-contouring osteoplasty restored pain-free range of motion. Reproduction of the normal femoral head-neck offset ration can restore natural hip range of motion. Level of evidence: IV.

7. Amstutz HC, Campbell PA, Le Duff MJ: Fracture of the neck of the femur after surface arthroplasty of the hip. *J Bone Joint Surg Am* 2004;86(9):1874-1877.

8. Amstutz HC, Antoniades JT, Le Duff MJ: Results of metal-on-metal hybrid hip resurfacing for Crowe type-I and II developmental dysplasia. *J Bone Joint Surg Am* 2007;89(2):339-346.

    In 51 patients with either Crowe type I or II developmental dysplasia who were treated with metal-on-metal hip resurfacing, midterm results were disappointing with respect to durability of the femoral component. Fixation of the porous-coated acetabular components without adjuvant fixation was excellent. Level of evidence: IV.

9. McBryde CW, Shears E, O'Hara JN, Pynsent PB: Metal-on-metal hip resurfacing in developmental dysplasia: A case-control study. *J Bone Joint Surg Br* 2008;90(6):708-714.

    Metal-on-metal hip resurfacing was done in 85 patients (96 hips) with developmental dysplasia. Medium-term results were encouraging but significantly worse than in a group of matched patients with osteoarthritis. Level of evidence: III.

10. Naal FD, Schmied M, Munzinger U, Leunig M, Hersche O: Outcome of hip resurfacing arthroplasty in patients with developmental hip dysplasia. *Clin Orthop Relat Res* 2009;467(6):1516-1521.

    In 24 patients (32 hips) treated with hip resurfacing arthroplasty, the failure rate was 6%, despite satisfactory outcomes in clinical scores, return to sports, and hip biomechanics. Level of evidence: IV.

11. McMinn DJ, Daniel J, Ziaee H, Pradhan C: Results of the Birmingham Hip Resurfacing dysplasia component in severe acetabular insufficiency: A six- to 9.6-year follow-up. *J Bone Joint Surg Br* 2008;90(6):713-723.

    A total of 110 dysplasia resurfacing arthroplasties were performed in 103 patients. During the mean 7.8-year follow-up, three hips were converted to a total hip replacement because of fracture of the femoral neck, collapse of the femoral head, and deep infection. There was no aseptic loosening or osteolysis of the acetabular component.

12. Beaulé PE, Amstutz HC, Le Duff MJ, Dorey F: Surface arthroplasty for osteonecrosis of the hip: Hemiresur-

3: Hip

facing versus metal-on-metal hybrid resurfacing. *J Arthroplasty* 2004;19(8, suppl 3):54-58.

13. Campbell PA, Beaulé PE, Ebramzadeh E, et al: The John Charnley Award: A study of implant failure in metal-on-metal surface arthroplasties. *Clin Orthop Relat Res* 2006;453:35-46.

    The authors studied implant failure in a group of patients with metal-on-metal surface arthroplasties. Level of evidence: IV.

14. Revell MP, McBryde CW, Bhatnagar S, Pynsent PB, Treacy RB: Metal-on-metal hip resurfacing in osteonecrosis of the femoral head. *J Bone Joint Surg Am* 2006; 88(suppl 3):98-103.

    Seventy-three hip resurfacing procedures were performed on 60 patients with osteonecrosis of the femoral head. The overall survival rate of the femoral component was 93.2% after a mean of 6.1 years. Level of evidence: IV.

15. Amstutz HC, Le Duff MJ: Hip resurfacing results for osteonecrosis are as good as for other etiologies at 2 to 12 years. *Clin Orthop Relat Res* 2010;468(2):375-381. In a comparison of the results of metal-on-metal resurfacing done for osteonecrosis of the hip with those of resurfacing done for other reasons, the authors studied 70 patients with osteonecrosis and 768 patients in a control group. No difference in survivorship was noted between the two groups even after adjusting for femoral head size, body mass index, and defect size. The study results suggest that osteonecrosis is not a contraindication for resurfacing, even with large femoral head defects. Level of evidence: III.

16. Stulberg BN, Fitts SM, Zadzilka JD, Trier K: Resurfacing arthroplasty for patients with osteonecrosis. *Bull NYU Hosp Jt Dis* 2009;67(2):138-141.

    The authors report on a modern hip resurfacing system that was implanted in 1,148 hips; 116 hips had a preoperative diagnosis of osteonecrosis and 1,023 had osteoarthritis. Survival rates were not significantly different. Level of evidence: III.

17. Loughead JM, Chesney D, Holland JP, McCaskie AW: Comparison of offset in Birmingham hip resurfacing and hybrid total hip arthroplasty. *J Bone Joint Surg Br* 2005;87(2):163-166.

    The authors concluded that hip resurfacing does not restore hip mechanics as accurately as THA. Level of evidence: III.

18. Girard J, Lavigne M, Vendittoli PA, Roy AG: Biomechanical reconstruction of the hip: A randomised study comparing total hip resurfacing and total hip arthroplasty. *J Bone Joint Surg Br* 2006;88(6):721-726.

    The authors compared the biomechanical nature of hip reconstruction in conventional THA and surface replacement arthroplasty in 120 patients undergoing unilateral primary hip replacement. Level of evidence: I.

19. Beaulé PE, Harvey N, Zaragoza EJ, Le Duff MJ, Dorey FJ: The femoral head/neck offset and hip resurfacing. *J Bone Joint Surg Br* 2007;89(1):9-15.

    The authors studied femoral head-neck offset in 63 hips undergoing metal-on-metal resurfacing and 56 hips with nonarthritic pain occurring after femoroacetabular impingement. Level of evidence: III.

20. Wiadrowski TP, McGee M, Cornish BL, Howie DW: Peripheral wear of Wagner resurfacing hip arthroplasty acetabular components. *J Arthroplasty* 1991; 6(2):103-107.

21. Howie DW, McCalden RW, Nawana NS, Costi K, Pearcy MJ, Subramanian C: The long-term wear of retrieved McKee-Farrar metal-on-metal total hip prostheses. *J Arthroplasty* 2005;20(3):350-357.

    The authors found no association between type and distribution of wear and time in situ. Level of evidence: III.

22. Beaulé PE, Lee JL, Le Duff MJ, Amstutz HC, Ebramzadeh E, Ebramzadeh E: Orientation of the femoral component in surface arthroplasty of the hip: A biomechanical and clinical analysis. *J Bone Joint Surg Am* 2004;86-A(9):2015-2021.

23. De Haan R, Campbell PA, Su EP, De Smet KA: Revision of metal-on-metal resurfacing arthroplasty of the hip: The influence of malpositioning of the components. *J Bone Joint Surg Br* 2008;90(9):1158-1163.

    The authors present a review of 42 patients who had revision of metal-on-metal resurfacing procedures; 64% of these revisions were caused by acetabular malposition. The authors report excellent results with the revision of the femoral component to a component with a modular head. However, revision to total hip joint resurfacing with 28- and 32-mm heads led to increased risk of dislocation and re-revision. Level of evidence: IV.

24. Shimmin AJ, Back D: Femoral neck fractures following Birmingham hip resurfacing: A national review of 50 cases. *J Bone Joint Surg Br* 2005;87(4):463-464.

    A retrospective review of 50 hip fractures in 3,497 patients who had hip resurfacing as recorded by the Australian National Joint Replacement Registry is presented. The relative risk of fracture for women compared with men was 1.94961 (*P* < 0.01). Significant varus placement of the femoral component, intraoperative notching of the femoral neck, and technical problems were common factors in 85% of cases. Level of evidence: IV.

25. Zustin J, Sauter G, Morlock MM, Rüther W, Amling M: Association of osteonecrosis and failure of hip resurfacing arthroplasty. *Clin Orthop Relat Res* 2010; 468(3):756-761.

    The authors found that fracture incidence was correlated with the extent of osteonecrosis. Smaller regions of superficial osteonecrosis were observed in femoral remnants with periprosthetic fractures and in hips with failed hip resurfacing arthroplasty for reasons other than fracture. Level of evidence: III.

26. Little CP, Ruiz AL, Harding IJ, et al : Osteonecrosis in retrieved femoral heads after failed resurfacing arthro-

plasty of the hip. *J Bone Joint Surg Br* 2005;87(3):320-323.

The authors concluded that histologic evidence of osteonecrosis is common in failed resurfaced hips. Level of evidence: III.

27. Beaulé PE, Campbell PA, Hoke R, Dorey FJ: Notching of the femoral neck during resurfacing arthroplasty of the hip: A vascular study. *J Bone Joint Surg Br* 2006; 88(1):35-39.

    Study results suggest that femoral head vascularity in the presence of osteoarthritis is similar to that in the absence of arthritis, where damage of extraosseous vessels can predispose patients to osteonecrosis. Level of evidence: IV.

28. Steffen RT, Smith SR, Urban JP, et al : The effect of hip resurfacing on oxygen concentration in the femoral head. *J Bone Joint Surg Br* 2005;87(11):1468-1474.

    Study results indicate that there is some compromise or complete disruption to the femoral head blood supply during hip resurfacing arthroplasty. Level of evidence: IV.

29. Schoeniger R, Espinosa N, Sierra RJ, Leunig M, Ganz R: Role of the extraosseous blood supply in osteoarthritic femoral heads? *Clin Orthop Relat Res* 2009; 467(9):2235-2240.

    The authors concluded that intramedullary blood vessels to the femoral head do not provide measurable blood supply to the epiphysis when the medial femoral circumflex artery or retinacular vessels have been damaged. Level of evidence: IV.

30. Stulberg BN, Trier KK, Naughton M, Zadzilka JD: Results and lessons learned from a United States hip resurfacing investigational device exemption trial. *J Bone Joint Surg Am* 2008;90(Suppl 3):21-26.

    In a study of two groups of patients who had undergone either hip resurfacing (337 patients) or THA (266 patients), revision was necessary in 24 patients in the resurfacing group and 5 in the THA group. Failure of the femoral component was the most common cause of revision after resurfacing. Level of evidence: II.

31. Treacy RB, McBryde CW, Pynsent PB: Birmingham hip resurfacing arthroplasty: A minimum follow-up of five years. *J Bone Joint Surg Br* 2005;87(2):167-170.

    The authors review a consecutive series of 144 Birmingham hip resurfacing cases implanted between August 1997 and May 1998. At a minimum of 5 years, the overall survival of the implant was 98% in a patient population with a mean age of 52 years. Level of evidence: II.

32. Daniel J, Pynsent PB, McMinn DJ: Metal-on-metal resurfacing of the hip in patients under the age of 55 years with osteoarthritis. *J Bone Joint Surg Br* 2004; 86(2):177-184.

33. Beaulé PE, Campbell PA, Shim P: Femoral head blood flow during hip resurfacing. *Clin Orthop Relat Res* 2007;456:148-152.

The authors studied 10 patients (10 hips) with advanced osteoarthritis who underwent metal-on-metal hip resurfacing using a vascular-preserving surgical approach. Results indicate that femoral head reaming during hip resurfacing affects blood flow and infers that the extraosseous blood supply is important in the arthritic femoral head. Level of evidence: IV.

34. Khan A, Yates P, Lovering A, Bannister GC, Spencer RF: The effect of surgical approach on blood flow to the femoral head during resurfacing. *J Bone Joint Surg Br* 2007;89(1):21-25.

    The authors found that the posterolateral approach was associated with a significant reduction in blood supply to the femoral head during resurfacing arthroplasty in comparison with the transgluteal approach. Level of evidence: IV.

35. Beaulé PE, Campbell PA, Lu Z, et al : Vascularity of the arthritic femoral head and hip resurfacing. *J Bone Joint Surg Am* 2006;88(suppl 4):85-96.

    The authors present a well-illustrated description of the blood supply to the femoral head and its vulnerability with various surgical approaches. Level of evidence: III.

36. Ganz R, Gill TJ, Gautier E, Ganz K, Krügel N, Berlemann U: Surgical dislocation of the adult hip a technique with full access to the femoral head and acetabulum without the risk of avascular necrosis. *J Bone Joint Surg Br* 2001;83(8):1119-1124.

37. Beaulé PE, Shim P, Banga K: Clinical experience of Ganz surgical dislocation approach for metal-on-metal hip resurfacing. *J Arthroplasty* 2009;24(6, suppl): 127-131.

    The authors studied short-term results of metal-on-metal resurfacing using the vascular-preserving surgical approach by Ganz. Level of evidence: II.

38. Bal BS, Kazmier P, Burd T, Aleto T: Anterior trochanteric slide osteotomy for primary total hip arthroplasty: Review of nonunion and complications. *J Arthroplasty* 2006;21(1):59-63.

    The authors found that the incidence of hardware complications with the use of the slide osteotomy was too high to justify its routine use in preventing proximal migration of the trochanteric fragment during primary hip arthroplasty. Level of evidence: III.

39. Mont MA, Marker DR, Smith JM, Ulrich SD, McGrath MS: Resurfacing is comparable to total hip arthroplasty at short-term follow-up. *Clin Orthop Relat Res* 2009;467(1):66-71.

    The authors compared clinical and radiographic outcomes of two matched groups of 54 patients who underwent either resurfacing or conventional THA. Early outcomes of resurfacing are comparable with those of conventional THA. Level of evidence: III.

40. Masonis JL, Bourne RB: Surgical approach, abductor function, and total hip arthroplasty dislocation. *Clin Orthop Relat Res* 2002;405(405):46-53.

3: Hip

41. Benoit B, Gofton W, Beaulé PE: Hueter anterior approach for hip resurfacing: Assessment of the learning curve. *Orthop Clin North Am* 2009;40(3):357-363.

    The authors evaluated the safety and learning curve associated with Hueter hip resurfacing using an anterior approach or orthopaedic traction table. They concluded that the Hueter approach is a reasonable alternative to more extensile surgical approaches. Level of evidence: II.

42. Grigoris P, Roberts P, Panousis K, Bosch H: The evolution of hip resurfacing arthroplasty. *Orthop Clin North Am* 2005;36(2):125-134.

    The authors provide a review of current literature and experience in metal-on-metal hip resurfacing, explaining the limitations of prior technology and the evolution to newer implants and techniques. Level of evidence: III.

43. Judet J, Judet R: The use of an artificial femoral head for arthroplasty of the hip joint. *J Bone Joint Surg Br* 1950;32(2):166-173.

44. Aufranc OE: Constructive hip surgery with the vitallium mold: A report on 1,000 cases of arthroplasty of the hip over a fifteen-year period. *J Bone Joint Surg Am* 1957;39(2):237-248.

45. Smith-Petersen MN: Evolution of mould arthroplasty of the hip joint. *J Bone Joint Surg Br* 1948;30(1):59-75.

46. Capello WN, Ireland PH, Trammell TR, Eicher P: Conservative total hip arthroplasty: A procedure to conserve bone stock. Part I: Analysis of sixty-six patients. Part II: Analysis of failures. *Clin Orthop Relat Res* 1978;134 :59-74.

47. Head WC: Total articular resurfacing arthroplasty: Analysis of component failure in sixty-seven hips. *J Bone Joint Surg Am* 1984;66(1):28-34.

48. Howie DW, Cornish BL, Vernon-Roberts B: Resurfacing hip arthroplasty: Classification of loosening and the role of prosthesis wear particles. *Clin Orthop Relat Res* 1990;255(255):144-159.

49. Müller ME: The benefits of metal-on-metal total hip replacements. *Clin Orthop Relat Res* 1995;311:54-59.

50. Sieber HP, Rieker CB, Köttig P: Analysis of 118 second-generation metal-on-metal retrieved hip implants . *J Bone Joint Surg Br* 1998;81(1):46-50.

51. McMinn DJ: Development of metal/metal hip resurfacing. *Hip Int* 2003;13(suppl 2):S41-S53.

52. Beaulé PE, Le Duff M, Campbell P, Dorey FJ, Park SH, Amstutz HC: Metal-on-metal surface arthroplasty with a cemented femoral component: A 7-10 year follow-up study. *J Arthroplasty* 2004;19(8, suppl 3):17-22.

53. Dowson D, Hardaker C, Flett M, Isaac GH: A hip joint simulator study of the performance of metal-on-metal joints: Part II. Design. *J Arthroplasty* 2004;19(8, suppl 3):124-130.

54. Jin ZM, Dowson D, Fisher J: Analysis of fluid film lubrication in artificial hip joint replacements with surfaces of high elastic modulus. *Proc Inst Mech Eng H* 1996;211(3):247-256.

55. Dowson D, Hardaker C, Flett M, Isaac GH: A hip joint simulator study of the performance of metal-on-metal joints: Part I. The role of materials. *J Arthroplasty* 2004;19(8, suppl 3):118-123.

56. Isaac GH, Siebel T, Schmalzried TP, et al: Development rationale for an articular surface replacement: A science-based evolution. *Proc Inst Mech Eng H* 2006;220(2):253-268.

    This article reviews the available evidence for optimal mechanical features of modern metal-on-metal hip resurfacing. Level of evidence: III.

57. Morlock MM, Bishop N, Rüther W, Delling G, Hahn M: Biomechanical, morphological, and histological analysis of early failures in hip resurfacing arthroplasty. *Proc Inst Mech Eng H* 2006;220(2):333-344.

    The authors of this study reviewed wear, cement mantle and cement penetration, fracture and head morphology, as well as standard histology on 55 retrieved hip resurfacing implants, identifying a significant learning curve effect. Level of evidence: II.

58. Amstutz HC, Le Duff MJ, Campbell PA, Dorey FJ: The effects of technique changes on aseptic loosening of the femoral component in hip resurfacing: Results of 600 Conserve Plus with a 3 to 9 year follow-up. *J Arthroplasty* 2007;22(4):481-489.

    The authors present a review of a consecutive series of hip resurfacings by a designing surgeon emphasizing the importance of cement technique on improved outcome. Level of evidence: III.

59. Vail TP, Glisson RR, Dominguez DE, Kitaoka K, Ottaviano D: Position of hip resurfacing component affects strain and resistance to fracture in the femoral neck. *J Bone Joint Surg Am* 2008;90(9):1951-1960.

    This biomechanical cadaver study investigates the changes in femoral neck loading based on implant position and integrity of the femoral neck.

60. Brodner W, Grübl A, Jankovsky R, Meisinger V, Lehr S, Gottsauner-Wolf F: Cup inclination and serum concentration of cobalt and chromium after metal-on-metal total hip arthroplasty. *J Arthroplasty* 2004;19(8, suppl 3):66-70.

61. Campbell P, Takamura K, Lundergan W, Esposito C, Amstutz HC: Cement technique changes improved hip resurfacing longevity: Implant retrieval findings. *Bull NYU Hosp Jt Dis* 2009;67(2):146-153.

    The authors sectioned 15 retrieved hip resurfacing components and correlated the quality of the cement mantle with the surgical technique.

3: Hip

62. Amstutz HC, Beaulé PE, Dorey FJ, Le Duff MJ, Campbell PA, Gruen TA: Metal-on-metal hybrid surface arthroplasty: Two to six-year follow-up study. *J Bone Joint Surg Am* 2004;86(1):28-39.

63. Hing CB, Back DL, Bailey M, Young DA, Dalziel RE, Shimmin AJ: The results of primary Birmingham hip resurfacings at a mean of five years: An independent prospective review of the first 230 hips. *J Bone Joint Surg Br* 2007;89(11):1431-1438.

    The authors present an independent prospective review of 230 consecutive Birmingham hip resurfacings in 212 patients at a mean follow-up of 5 years (range, 4 to 6 years). Two patients, one with a loose acetabular component and the other with suspected avascular necrosis of the femoral head, underwent revision. The survivorship with the worst-case scenario was 97.8%. On radiologic review at 5 years, one patient had a progressive lucent line around the acetabular component and six had progressive lucent lines around the femoral component. A total of 18 femoral components (8%) had migrated into varus.

64. Pollard TC, Baker RP, Eastaugh-Waring SJ, Bannister GC: Treatment of the young active patient with osteoarthritis of the hip: A five- to seven-year comparison of hybrid total hip arthroplasty and metal-on-metal resurfacing. *J Bone Joint Surg Br* 2006;88(5):592-600.

    The authors compared metal-on-metal Birmingham hip resurfacing with a hybrid THA. There were 54 hips in both groups, matched for sex, age, body mass index, and activity level. Function was excellent in both groups, but the Birmingham hip resurfacings had higher UCLA activity scores and better EuroQol quality of life scores. The THAs had a revision or intention-to-revise rate of 8%, and the Birmingham hip resurfacings of 6%.

65. *Australian Orthopaedic Association National Hip and Knee Joint Replacement Registry Annual Report* 2009. Adelaide, Australia, Australian Orthopaedic Association, 2009, p 80.

    The annual report analyzes primary and revision hip replacements as recorded by the Registry over 1 year. Level of evidence: IV.

66. Shimmin AJ, Walter WL, Esposito C: The influence of the size of the component on the outcome of resurfacing arthroplasty of the hip: A review of the literature. *J Bone Joint Surg Br* 2010;92:469-476.

    The authors concluded that design and geometry of the component and orientation of the acetabular component are likely the most important contributors to failure of resurfacing arthroplasty of the hip.

67. Back DL, Dalziel RE, Young DA, Shimmin AJ: Early results of primary Birmingham hip resurfacings: An independent prospective study of the first 230 hips. *J Bone Joint Surg Br* 2005;87(3):324-329.

    The authors report early results of consecutive 230 Birmingham hip resurfacings. Survivorship was 99.14% with revision in one patient for a loose acetabular component. They also reported on the nonsurgical management of a fracture of the femoral neck

    at 6 weeks; the fracture united unremarkably after a period of no weight bearing. Level of evidence: II.

68. Vendittoli PA, Lavigne M, Roy AG, Lusignan D: A prospective randomized clinical trial comparing metal-on-metal total hip arthroplasty and metal-on-metal total hip resurfacing in patients less than 65 years old. *Hip Int* 2006;16(Suppl 4):73-81.

    The authors compared early clinical results of metal-on-metal hip resurfacing with those of metal-on-metal THA. Results indicate that short-term functional recovery is better with hip resurfacing than with THA because of proximal femoral bone preservation.

69. Mont MA, Seyler TM, Ragland PS, Starr R, Erhart J, Bhave A: Gait analysis of patients with resurfacing hip arthroplasty compared with hip osteoarthritis and standard total hip arthroplasty. *J Arthroplasty* 2007; 22(1):100-108.

    The authors report a gait analysis comparison between hip resurfacing patients, patients with unilateral osteoarthritic hips and unilateral standard THAs. Patients with resurfacing walked faster (average 1.26 m/s) and were comparable with normal subjects. There were no significant differences in hip abductor and extensor moments of patients with resurfacing compared with patients in the standard hip arthroplasty group. Level of evidence: II.

70. Hing CB, Young DA, Dalziel RE, Bailey M, Back DL, Shimmin AJ: Narrowing of the neck in resurfacing arthroplasty of the hip: A radiological study. *J Bone Joint Surg Br* 2007;89(8):1019-1024.

    The authors retrospectively determined the extent and progression of narrowing of the femoral neck in a series of 163 Birmingham hip resurfacings in 163 patients up to a maximum of 6 years. There was some narrowing of the femoral neck in 77% of the patients reviewed, and in 27.6% the narrowing exceeded 10% of the diameter of the neck. There was a significant association of narrowing with female sex and a valgus femoral neck-shaft angle. There was no significant association between the range of movement, position or size of the component or radiologic lucent lines and narrowing of the neck. The narrowing stabilized at 3 years. Level of evidence: IV.

71. Spencer S, Carter R, Murray H, Meek RM: Femoral neck narrowing after metal-on-metal hip resurfacing. *J Arthroplasty* 2008;23(8):1105-1109.

    The authors reviewed 40 Corin Cormet 2000 metal-on-metal resurfacing hips in 36 patients for the presence of femoral neck narrowing. Femoral neck narrowing was observed in 90% of hips at 2 years, no further narrowing occurred beyond this point. The authors discuss possible mechanisms for the narrowing. Level of evidence: IV.

72. Pandit H, Glyn-Jones S, McLardy-Smith P, et al: Pseudotumours associated with metal-on-metal hip resurfacings. *J Bone Joint Surg Br* 2008;90(7):847-851.

    The authors reported on 17 patients (20 hips) with metal-on-metal resurfacing who presented with pseudotumor. The common histologic features were

3: Hip

extensive necrosis and lymphocytic infiltration in 13 of the 20 hips that required revision. A possible mechanism for reaction was increased metal wear debris leading to failure of metal-on-metal articulations. Level of evidence: IV.

73. Campbell P, Shimmin A, Walter L, Solomon M: Metal sensitivity as a cause of groin pain in metal-on-metal hip resurfacing. *J Arthroplasty* 2008;23(7):1080-1085.

A case series of four patients with failure of metal-on-metal resurfacing caused by a metal allergy is discussed. Investigation and management are described. All patients had full resolution of their symptoms after revision. Level of evidence: IV.

Chapter 22

Primary Total Hip Arthroplasty Design and Outcomes

Amar S. Ranawat, MD   Morteza Meftah, MD   Chitranjan S. Ranawat, MD   Richard E. White Jr, MD
William A. Jiranek, MD, FACS

Cemented Total Hip Arthroplasty
Amar S. Ranawat, MD
Morteza Meftah, MD
Chitranjan S. Ranawat, MD

Total hip arthroplasty (THA) is one of the most successful surgical interventions of the past 50 years. Since the introduction of the concept of the low-friction arthroplasty by Sir John Charnley in the early 1960s, the use of cement for component fixation has been the "gold standard," especially for the femoral component.[1-3] Although the use of cementless fixation is on the rise, there are distinct advantages of cemented THA in terms of versatility, durability, and the ability to achieve immediate rigid fixation.

Cement Generations

Cemented THA has evolved since its inception, but has always remained technique-dependent. The literature describes four generations of cement technique.[2-5] The first cement generation involved manual digital packing of cement into the acetabulum and femur. The second generation included the use of an intramedullary distal femoral canal plug and retrograde cement filling using a cement gun. The third-generation cementing technique consisted of porosity reduction via vacuum mixing and the experimentation with different surface fin-

ishes. The fourth generation technique involved the use of high-pressure pulsatile lavage, preheated cement, pressurization of cement with both proximal and distal femoral canal occlusion, and stem centralization.[3,5]

The goal of all of these advances was to achieve an appropriate and symmetric cement mantle thickness of 2 to 5 mm, which would provide lasting fixation.[5]

Cementing Technique

The art of cement fixation is technically demanding and requires meticulous attention to detail. It begins with hypotensive anesthesia to prevent blood from interfering with the cement-bone interface. The next step involves thorough preparation of the bone, proper mixing and pressurization of the cement into the cancellous bone, and component insertion.[3,5]

Acetabular Cementing

Proper reaming of the acetabulum should expose the cancellous "blush" of the ischium and pubis and provide 80% to 100% coverage of the socket without violating the medial wall (Figure 1, A). Multiple keyholes should be placed in the cancellous bone of the superior acetabular dome and posterior column. These keyholes increase the surface area and improve fixation of the cement-bone interface (Figure 1, B). The next step involves thorough pulsatile lavage to remove blood and

Dr. Amar Ranawat or an immediate family member has received royalties from DePuy and Stryker; is a member of a speakers' bureau or has made paid presentations on behalf of DePuy and Stryker; serves as a paid consultant to DePuy and MAKO; serves as an unpaid consultant to ConforMIS; owns stock or stock options held in ConforMIS; has received research or institutional support from DePuy and Stryker; has received nonincome support (such as equipment or services), commercially derived honoraria, or other non-research–related funding (such as paid travel) from DePuy and Stryker; and serves as a board member, owner, officer, or committee member of the American Academy of Orthopaedic Surgeons and the EOA. Neither Dr. Meftah nor any immediate family member has received anything of value from or owns stock in a commercial company or institution related directly or indirectly to the subject of this article. Dr. Chitranjan Ranawat or an immediate family member has received royalties from DePuy and Stryker; is a member of a speakers' bureau or has made paid presentations on behalf of MAKO and ConforMIS; serves as a paid consultant to MAKO and ConforMIS; owns stock or stock options held in ConforMIS; and serves as a board member, owner, officer, or committee member of The Hip Society and the Eastern Orthopedic Education Foundation. Dr. White or an immediate family member has received royalties from Zimmer; serves as a paid consultant to Ardent Health Services Lovelace Medical Center; and serves as a board member, owner, officer, or committee member of the American Association of Hip and Knee Surgeons and The Hip Society. Dr. Jiranek or an immediate family member has received royalties from DePuy; serves as a paid consultant to DePuy; has received research or institutional support from Stryker; and serves as a board member, owner, officer, or committee member of the American Academy of Orthopaedic Surgeons, the American Association of Hip and Knee Surgeons, and The Knee Society.

3: Hip

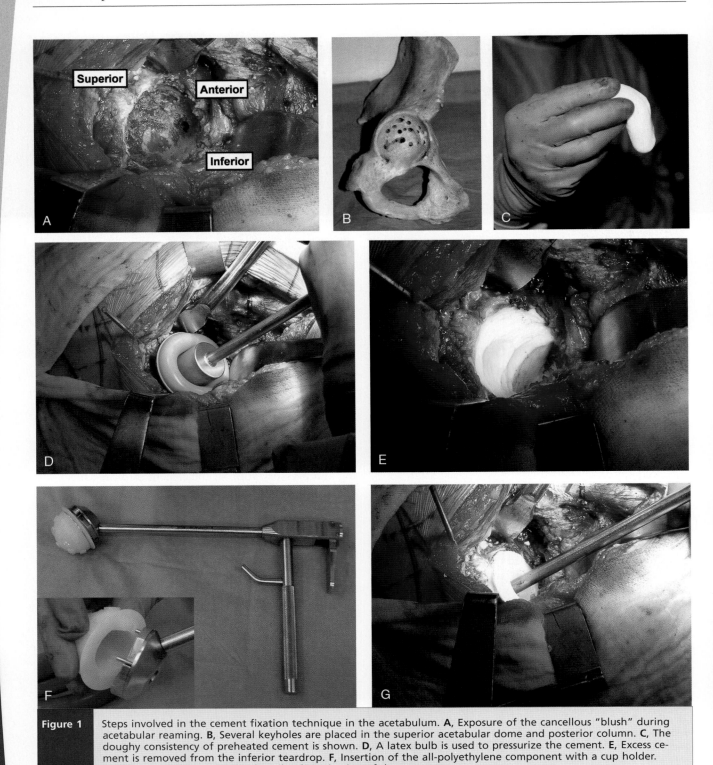

Figure 1 Steps involved in the cement fixation technique in the acetabulum. **A,** Exposure of the cancellous "blush" during acetabular reaming. **B,** Several keyholes are placed in the superior acetabular dome and posterior column. **C,** The doughy consistency of preheated cement is shown. **D,** A latex bulb is used to pressurize the cement. **E,** Excess cement is removed from the inferior teardrop. **F,** Insertion of the all-polyethylene component with a cup holder. **G,** Axial pressure is maintained until polymerization of the cement occurs.

fat debris and then careful drying of the bony bed with sponges and manual pressure.[5] Simultaneously, preheated cement is mixed and allowed to stand until it attains a doughy consistency (**Figure 1, C**). The cement is then pressurized using a latex bulb to enhance macrointerlock and microinterlock into the cancellous bone

(**Figure 1, D**). Care should be taken to remove excess cement from the inferior teardrop area before insertion of the cup to avoid cement extrusion into the pelvis (**Figure 1, E**). An all-polyethylene component is then inserted with a cup holder and held in appropriate position while excess cement around the cup is removed

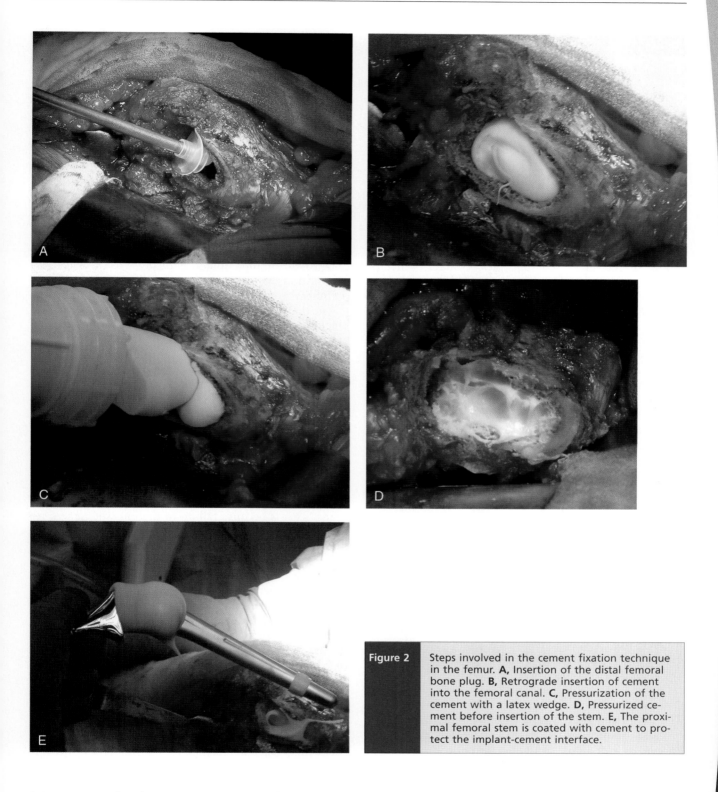

Figure 2 | Steps involved in the cement fixation technique in the femur. **A,** Insertion of the distal femoral bone plug. **B,** Retrograde insertion of cement into the femoral canal. **C,** Pressurization of the cement with a latex wedge. **D,** Pressurized cement before insertion of the stem. **E,** The proximal femoral stem is coated with cement to protect the implant-cement interface.

(Figure 1, *F*). Axial pressure is maintained on the cup until complete cement polymerization[2,3,5] **(Figure 1, *G*).**

Femoral Cementing
After broaching the femoral canal to the appropriate depth, a trial reduction is performed. Care is taken to ensure restoration of leg length, offset, and anteversion.

The trial is removed and a cement restrictor is placed approximately 1 to 2 cm beyond the tip of the femoral stem.[5] Cement powder is heated to 100°F and vacuum-mixed. The femoral canal is washed and cleaned with pressure lavage and thoroughly dried. After insertion of the distal femoral canal plug **(Figure 2, *A*),** a cement gun is used to deliver the cement into the femoral canal

3: Hip

Table 1

Long-Term Results of the Exeter Stem

Author (Year)	Hips	Follow-up (Years)	Revision Rate
Williams et al[13] (2002)	325	12	0%
Franklin et al[12] (2003)	654	10	4%
Chiu et al[10] (2005)	112	15	3.4%
Hook et al[11] (2006)	88	12.7	1.1%

in a retrograde manner (**Figure 2**, *B*). Cement is then pressurized with a latex wedge (**Figure 2**, *C* and *D*). The femoral stem is coated with cement to prevent blood or fat from coming into contact with the implant-cement interface (**Figure 2**, *E*). Insertion of the stem into the canal should be done gently, augmented by axial and lateral pressure to avoid varus positioning of the implant. Excess cement is then removed. Exposed cement around the implant is digitally pressurized and allowed to polymerize.[2,3,5]

The use of antibiotic-impregnated cement in primary THA is controversial. There are situations, however, when antibiotics may be added in selected patients with rheumatoid disease or other immunosuppressive conditions such as diabetes or cancer.

Failure Mechanisms

The mechanisms of failure of the cemented acetabulum and the femoral component are different. The common modes of failure of cemented femoral components include debonding of the stem with subsidence, loosening of the bone-cement interface, and stem fracture. Defects in the cement mantle and inappropriately thin cement predispose to early fixation failure of the stem. On the acetabular side, demarcation of the cement-bone interface occurs from fibrous membrane formation caused by a chemomediated response. Particle debris with fluid will enter this space and cause an inflammatory response of the macrophages and subsequent bone resorption. Both sides of the hip joint can fail secondary to progressive osteolysis.[1,6]

Osteolysis

The inflammatory response to wear debris that results in bone resorption at the bone-cement interface is known as osteolysis. Although initially attributed to "cement disease," the persistence of osteolysis in cementless implants has shifted attention to wear debris as the main cause of osteolysis rather than cement. Several in vivo and in vitro studies have confirmed the role of interleukin-1 (IL-1), tumor necrosis factor (TNF), and prostaglandin E_2 (PGE_2) in the development of osteolysis.[1] A more detailed discussion of the role of osteolysis in the failure of cemented THA is beyond the scope of this chapter.

Implant Design

On the acetabular side, the current standard for a cemented cup is an all-polyethylene component with adjuvant fixation lugs, spikes, and ridges to enhance fixation. Additionally, most components provided for a peripheral rim to enhance cement pressurization.

On the femoral side, implant design has focused on several issues: metallurgy, offset, modularity, collars, and surface finish. Improved metallurgy from cast cobalt-chromium and stainless steel to superalloys and forged implants has essentially eliminated component fracture.[7] Reductions in neck diameter, increased offset designs, and the introduction of head modularity have provided a balance between optimal biomechanics and decreased impingement.[4] The use of a collar is still debatable, but appears to have a role in femoral components with a satin finish. Polished stems clearly have no need for a collar because they are designed to undergo subsidence until they achieve a stable position. What is now not debatable is the continued use of roughened stems. This is because failure of the implant-cement interface and increased motion will lead to abrasion of the rough stem, rapidly generating particulate debris and resulting in osteolysis.[8,9] Smooth stems allow for micromotion, which dissipates excessive loads and protects the cement-bone interface.[9] The polished Exeter stem (Howmedica, Rutherford, NJ), consisting of a collarless, double-taper geometry, has shown excellent long-term results[10-13] (**Table 1**). There is no consensus on the optimal surface finish. Nonetheless, the literature supports the continued use of polished or satin finish stems with a Ra (the average surface roughness) of 40 microinches or less.[8,14-16]

An additional benefit of using a smooth stem is the ability to remove the stem without sacrificing the cement mantle. This enables the surgeon to use the "cement-in-cement" technique, essentially recementing a stem into the intact cement mantle, which provides improved acetabular exposure in the revision setting.[17]

Long-Term Results of Cemented Femoral Components

The accepted end point in implant survivorship should include revision surgery and clinical or radiographic failures. The radiographic evidence of loosening in a cemented femoral component includes (1) implant

Table 2

Femoral Stem Results in First-Generation Cement Techniques

Author (Year)	Hips (Final)	Follow-up (Years)	Revision Rate	Radiographic Loosening
McCoy et al[20] (1988)	100 (40)	15.3	5%	7%
Joshi et al[21] (1993)	218 (166)	16	14%	-
Schulte et al[22] (1993)	330 (98)	20	3%	7%
Wroblewski and Siney[23] (1993)	1,324 (20)	20	6%	-
Neumann et al[24] (1994)	241 (103)	17.6	8.3%	30%
Kavanagh et al[25] (1994)	333 (112)	20	16%	36%
Hook et al[11] (Exeter, 2006)	142 (88)	12.7	1.1%	1.4%
Buckwalter et al[19] (2006)	357 (52)	25	10%	17%

Table 3

Femoral Stem Results in Second-Generation Cement Techniques

Author (Year)	Hips (Final)	Follow-up (Years)	Revision Rate	Radiographic Loosening
Mulroy and Harris[27] (1990)	105	11.2	1.9%	2.9%
Barrack et al[28] (1992)	50	12	0%	2%
Mulroy et al[29] (1995)	162	15	2%	4.3%
Madey et al[30] (1997)	356	15	1%	3%
Bourne et al[31] (1998)	195	12	3%	5%
Smith et al[32] (1998)	161	18	5%	6%
Skutek et al[26] (2007)	46	22	4%	4%
Callaghan et al[33] (2008)	304	19	2.6%	4.9%

subsidence, (2) a change in implant position in the cement mantle based on serial radiographs, (3) a progressive global radiolucency, (4) cement mantle fracture, and (5) implant fracture. [5,6,18]

Table 2 summarizes the results of first-generation cement techniques.[3,11,19-25] Reported outcomes show a high incidence of aseptic loosening (30% to 40%) with a high incidence of osteolysis (5% to 16%).

Long-term survivorship of second-generation cement techniques using a femoral canal plug, pulsatile lavage, and retrograde cementing are more favorable. Improved femoral stem design with broad medial borders, rounded edges, and a distal taper resulted in improved results and less failure of fixation, with revision rates ranging from 0% to 5% and radiographic loosening from 2% to 6% after 11- to 19-years follow-ups.[3,8,26] These results[19,27-33] are summarized in Table 3.

The third-generation cement technique has a mixed medium-term follow-up (6.5 to 13.5 years). The revision rates range from 0% to 6.1%,[3,14,15,18,34-41] as shown in Table 4. One study reported results of 204 cemented THAs in 175 hips at a mean follow-up of 13.5 years.[18] The data demonstrated no revision surgery for mechanical failure, although four hips required revision surgery (two recurrent dislocations, one delayed infection, and one osteolysis). Clinically, 93.1% of the hips had good or excellent Hospital for Special Surgery hip scores. A comparison of Tables 1 through 3 shows a clear trend toward improved outcomes with improved surgical techniques.

The fourth-generation cement technique has minimal long-term follow-up. Changes in technique at this stage are relatively small and perhaps unlikely to make a significant difference. One study reported 35 cemented THAs using a fourth-generation cement technique and polished femoral stem at mean 6.4-years follow-up with no aseptic loosening.[42] Another study reported similar results of no cases of aseptic loosening in 100 primary cemented femoral components with an average of 5.7 years follow-up.[41] Longer follow-up studies are necessary to determine the effect of stem centralization on clinical survivorship.

3: Hip

Table 4

Femoral Stem Results in Third-Generation Cement Techniques

Author (Year)	Hips	Implant	Follow-up (Years)	Revision Rate for Aseptic Loosening	Radiographic Loosening
Schmalzried and Harris [39] (1993)	97	Precoat	6.5	1%	1%
Berger et al[34] (1996)	91	Precoat	8.5	1%	1.3%
Callaghan et al[35] (1996)	109	Iowa stem	9	6.1%	6.9%
Woolson and Haber[40] (1996)	121	Precoat	6	3%	8%
Harris[38] (1996)	65	Precoat	6.6	0%	0%
Dowd et al[37] (1998)	154	Harris Precoat	10	13%	15%
Goldberg et al[41] (1996)	123	Precoat	8.6	0.8%	1.6%
Clohisy and Harris[36] (1999)	100	Precoat	10	1%	3%
Rasquinha et al[18] (2003)	175	Omnifit	15	0%	0%
Firestone et al[14] (2007)	115	Iowa stem (polished)	10	0%	0%

Table 5

Long-Term Results of Cemented Acetabular Fixation

Author (Year)	Prosthesis	Hips	Follow-up (Years)	Revision Rate
DeLee and Charnley[45] (1976)	Charnley	141	10	NR
Stauffer[46] (1982)	Charnley	231	10	3
Poss et al[47] (1988)	Mixed	267	11	3.1
Ritter et al[48] (1992)	Charnley	238	10	4.6
Wroblewski and Siney[23] (1993)	Charnley	193	18	3
Kavanagh et al[25] (1994)	Charnley	112	20	16
Mulroy et al[29] (1995)	CAD, HD-2	105	10	5
Callaghan et al[49] (1998)	Charnley	93	25	19%
Smith et al[32] (1998)	CAD/Harris Design II	65	18	23%
Callaghan et al[50] (2000)	Charnley	316	25	6%
Della Valle et al[8] (2005)	Charnley	40	20	23
Rasquinha and Ranawat[44] (2004) [patients 60 to 80 years old]	Charnley	160	20	5.6%
Callaghan et al[51] (2004)	Charnley	27	30	12%
Allami et al[43] (2006)	Charnley	485	10	6.2%

Long-Term Results of Cemented Acetabular Components

Cemented acetabular fixation has proved to be a durable, reproducible, and cost-effective fixation method. The long-term results of cemented acetabula with all-polyethylene sockets are encouraging. Based on the defined criteria for failure, recent data regarding the long-term revision rate for cemented acetabular fixation vary between 0.8% and 23% at 10- to 30-years follow-ups[3,33,43-51] (Table 5).

These reported results are confounded by different designs, diagnoses, and definition of failure, which have led to questioning of the durability of cemented cups. By eliminating 32-mm heads, metal backed sockets, dysplasia, rheumatoid arthritis, and revisions from consideration, the long-term results become even better. One study reported 88% survivorship of 236 hips with cemented all-polyethylene cups at 15 years follow-up for all diagnoses, which improved to 98% of 160 hips at 20 years for osteoarthritis alone in patients 60 to 80 years old.[44] These results in part are the result of lower polyethylene wear rates with cemented fixation compared with cementless fixation.[44]

Current Indications for Cementing

In the hands of an experienced surgeon, cemented THA is a reproducible, durable, and cost-effective procedure that can be used in most patients. Nonetheless, it is being directly challenged by the growth of cementless fixation. Understanding the surgeon, patient, and implant factors specific to cemented THA will help define its appropriate indications.

Cementless Femoral Component
Richard E. White Jr, MD

Most so-called second-generation cementless femoral components were designed to address problems discovered in first-generation designs. First-generation, proximally coated, canal-filling implants had design faults including noncircumferential porous material, inadequate surface area of porous material, and stem instability. Studies conducted before 2004 confirmed that clinical results from second-generation implants were improved both in proximally coated, extensively coated, canal-filling, and tapered designs.

Clinical outcome results since 2004 have several focuses. Long-term follow-up studies of first-generation implants as well as intermediate and long-term follow-up studies of second-generation implants were published. Emphasis was also placed on important demographic factors such as age and obesity. Multiple studies also looked at the success of cementless femoral components in different diagnoses to confirm the applicability of this fixation in various patient groups.

Prosthetic design changes and innovations focused on modifications of first-generation stems rather than completely new prosthetic designs. Implant modifications included appropriate porous material distribution, increasing stem stability, and increased offset and leg length options. New component designs included the concepts of a second modular junction at the stem-neck location in addition to the head-neck modular junction. A second new stem concept was that of a much shorter femoral stem length.

Clinical Outcomes Research for Canal-Filling Stems

Long-term results of first-generation implants were best with extensively coated implants such as the Anatomic Medullary Locking (AML) implant (DePuy, Warsaw, IN). Results were equivalent in extensively coated stems regardless of stem diameter.[52] These long-term good results of extensively coated stems were also confirmed in both young (age 45 years or younger) and older patients.[53]

Many first-generation, proximally coated implants such as the HGP-1 (Zimmer, Warsaw, IN), Porous-Coated Anatomic (PCA) (Howmedica, Mahwah, NJ), and Trilock (Biomet, Warsaw, IN) had less successful results. The incidence of femoral component loosening, polyethylene wear, and osteolysis was not acceptable. In a long-term report at 18- to 24-years follow-up, the incidence of femoral loosening with the PCA was 34%.[54]

Clinical results of second-generation, proximally coated, cementless femoral components were much improved. Both straight stems[55] (Multilock, Zimmer) and curved or anatomic stems[56] (Anatomic, Zimmer) produced improved survival curves and decreased rates of osteolysis.

Although the extensively coated AML had excellent clinical results and survival curves, the Prodigy implant (DePuy) was designed to address the concerns of stress shielding and stem rigidity. Reports showed the Prodigy to have excellent results both at short-term[57] and intermediate[58] follow-up.

The Effect of Age and Obesity on Canal-Filling Stems

Initial reluctance to abandon cement fixation in older patients encouraged clinical research to evaluate the important demographic age factor. As expected, the results were uniformly good in younger patients as confirmed by meta-analysis[59] and by individual studies in proximally coated[60] and extensively coated[53] stems.

The role for cementless femoral components in older patients is less defined. Numerous studies have shown good clinical results in older patients.[61] A contradictory study from the New Zealand Joint Registry revealed a higher incidence of femoral component revision of cementless primary femoral components when compared with cement fixation in patients older than 65 years.[62]

The effect of obesity (body mass index greater than 30) is a topic of great interest. A study of 2,026 patients showed no difference in implant survival or patient satisfaction between the obese and nonobese (body mass index less than 30) groups, but, the nonobese group had better pain and functional scores.[63]

The Effect of Diagnosis on Canal-Filling Stems

Many studies evaluated the clinical success of canal-filling stems in different diagnosis groups. Reports supported the use of cementless fixation in diagnoses to include juvenile rheumatoid arthritis, Paget disease, displaced femoral neck fractures, reversal of previous hip fusion, hip dysplasia, and rapidly destructive arthropathy.

The use of cementless stems in osteonecrosis continues to be controversial. At midterm follow-up of 8 years, the overall results have been satisfactory but not as good as in patients with osteoarthritis.[64] Another study emphasized superior results in patients with osteonecrosis but without systemic disease (100% 10-year survival rate) compared with patients with systemic disease (68% 10-year survival rate).[65]

Total hip replacement in patients with ankylosing spondylitis is associated with high rates of femoral

3: Hip

component loosening (14%) and complications at mid-term follow-up of only 8.5 years.[66]

New Component Designs in Primary Total Hip Replacement

The concept of a second modular junction in a cementless femoral component is not new. Several revision systems incorporate this design feature. In these revision systems, the second modular junction is in the metaphyseal area, which allows for reconstruction of different shapes and sizes of proximal bone deficiency.

Only the S-ROM (DePuy) revision system is also frequently used in primary total hip replacement. A new location of the second modular junction is at the neck-stem junction. This concept has been incorporated in the Profemur (Wright Medical, Arlington, TN) and Kinectiv (Zimmer) hip systems. The obvious advantage of such a system is to allow more prosthetic combinations to achieve more complete restoration of leg length, femoroacetabular offset, and version. These systems allow independent correction of these three parameters and also make intraoperative corrections to increase range of motion, avoid impingement, and correct muscle tension.

In a templating study with the Kinectiv system, limb-length discrepancy and offset were completely corrected in 85% of cases; in an identical femoral stem with only a single head-neck junction (ML Taper, Zimmer), both parameters could only be completely corrected in 60% of cases. Moreover, the anteversion or retroversion options were used in 28% of cases with the Kinectiv system.

The Kinectiv system has not been available long enough to generate even short-term (less than 2 years) clinical data. The Profemur System has been available longer but has no peer-reviewed publications in primary cases.

The design concept using two modular junctions raises several mechanical concerns. With two modular junctions, the potential for third-body wear debris may be doubled. With larger offset and neck-length options, there may be an increased risk of femoral neck implant fracture. Neither system has sufficient data to address the increased wear debris issue, but Wright Medical has issued an implant adverse event report that revealed 35 femoral neck implant fractures.[67] These theoretic concerns and the fracture report suggest careful evaluation of in vitro testing data. The magnitude of these concerns and future clinical data should be considered when deciding to use the attractive clinical utility of this concept in restoring biomechanical parameters.

Acetabular Component Design
William A. Jiranek, MD, FACS

Acetabular components currently used in THA include designs intended for cemented fixation and those intended for cementless fixation. Cementless acetabular components were first introduced in the mid 1980s, and their use has steadily grown throughout the world because of excellent clinical results and relative ease of insertion. Cementless components now comprise more than 90% of all acetabular components implanted in the United States. Cemented cups are used more often in other countries. For example, in Sweden from 1992 to 2007, cementless cups represented only 10% of total cup usage. However, uncemented cup use is on the rise because of increasing evidence of poorer survival of cemented cups and difficulty with insertion.[68]

The earliest cemented acetabular components were produced as one-piece all-polyethylene cups. In an attempt to improve survival, metal backing was added to the second generation of cemented cups in an effort to improve stress distribution at the interface. The survival rate of the metal-backed cups was not as good as that of the all-polyethylene components,[33,69-75] and current cemented cups are once again one piece and all polyethylene, usually constructed with pegs on the bone side to ensure an optimal cement mantle, which has been shown in several studies to be between 2 and 4 mm thick.

Cementless acetabular components may be differentiated by the presence or absence of modularity, the substrate (for example, titanium, cobalt chromium, tantalum), geometry (both internal and external surfaces), type of porous coating, adjuvant fixation, and type of articulation and locking mechanisms, as well as type of shell liner (polyethylene, metal, or ceramic).

Modularity

Most modern cementless acetabular components are designed with modular liners that allow the surgeon to select the optimal liner independent of the shell. This allows the use of different inner diameter liners to mate with different femoral head sizes, as well as different liner substrates such as polyethylene, ceramic, and metal. Many different strategies are used to lock these liners to the shell, and these will be discussed later. With increasing evidence that dislocation risk is inversely related to head size, some manufacturers have recently produced one-piece nonmodular cups to accommodate very large femoral head sizes.

Because cemented metal-backed components had higher rates of loosening than all-polyethylene components, there are no metal-backed cemented cups currently marketed in the United States, and thus, no modular cemented acetabular components.

Substrate

Titanium has been the substrate used most often in cementless components because of excellent clinical results, in vitro and animal model evidence of decreased cell toxicity, and more rapid bone apposition compared with cobalt-chromium substrates. However, these differences have not translated into improved clinical outcome, with several cobalt-chromium cup designs having results comparable with those of titanium cups with

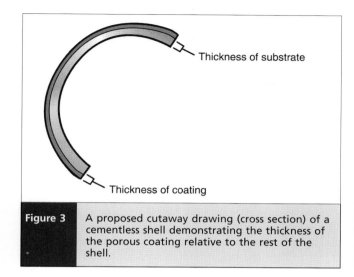

Figure 3 A proposed cutaway drawing (cross section) of a cementless shell demonstrating the thickness of the porous coating relative to the rest of the shell.

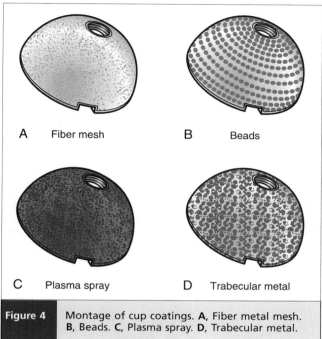

Figure 4 Montage of cup coatings. **A**, Fiber metal mesh. **B**, Beads. **C**, Plasma spray. **D**, Trabecular metal.

regard to fixation.[76] Because titanium is a poor bearing surface, several one-piece cups intended for large head metal-on-metal total hip replacement recently have been constructed of cobalt-chromium. In addition, the development of more highly porous metals that more closely approximate the modulus of elasticity of trabecular bone has led to the use of other substrates such as tantalum, although most of the highly porous cups currently use titanium as the substrate.

External Geometry

The most successful geometry has been the hemispheric design. Variations on this theme such as the dual radius cup and the extruded rim cup are more difficult to implant, and the clinical results have not been as good as those with hemispheric cups.[77] Early cementless cups were almost a complete hemisphere (180°), but recent one-piece cup designs have decreased this arc to as little as 150° in some cases. The attendant decreases in fixation area and uncoverage of the femoral head raises concerns of fixation failure and soft-tissue impingement in the bearing. Certain cup geometries have been clearly less successful than hemispheric designs. Threaded ("screw in") cups have had an unacceptable failure rate.[78-81] Results using conical shaped cups (for example, Freeman) have not been as good as results with hemispheric cups.[82]

Internal Geometry

Most current cup designs have a hemispheric inner design that mirrors the shape of the outer surface of the cup. However, some early cups had a more angular inner geometry to add stability to the locking mechanism, but this led to relatively thin areas of polyethylene near the rim, resulting in wear and failure[83] (**Figure 3**). The internal surface finish has varied from smooth to grit blasted, but there is some evidence that the rougher finishes may have contributed to backside wear. The liner articulation with the rim of the shell has varied between designs, with some liners extending beyond the

rim of the cup. For polyethylene liners this effectively led to a "bumper" effect that prevented contact of the metal neck of the femoral component with the rim of the shell. In contrast, one manufacturer stopped the liner short of the acetabular rim to prevent impingement of the neck of the femoral component with the rim of the ceramic liner.

Cup Thickness

There is evidence that cup thickness is related to cup deformation, with some of the newer designs of thin-walled cups (less than 3 mm in thickness) associated with significant reduction in the cup's opening diameter during impaction. This phenomenon has significance for hard-on-hard bearings.[84] The current range of cup thickness is between 3 and 6 mm. The drawback of thicker acetabular components is less room for the acetabular liner and greater bone removal during insertion. The advantage is less insertional deformation.

Type of Porous Coating

The ingrowth surfaces of early cementless cups were made of the same material as the cup itself, and comprise three different configurations: beads, wire mesh, and plasma spray (**Figure 4**). These coatings are bonded onto the substrate under conditions of high heat and pressure, or applied by a fine spray, also under conditions of high heat and pressure. Although the bond is quite strong, fatigue separation of small amounts of the coating from the substrate is sometimes seen in loose cups. All three types of coatings have been associated with durable fixation and similar patterns of bony remodeling. In vitro and animal model research has demonstrated that the spacing between coating elements

3: Hip

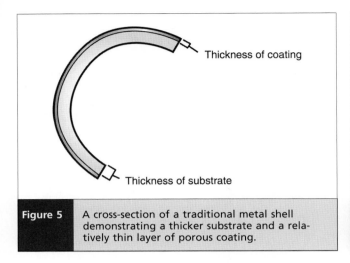

Figure 5 A cross-section of a traditional metal shell demonstrating a thicker substrate and a relatively thin layer of porous coating.

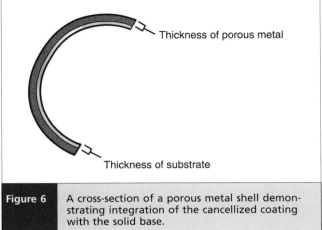

Figure 6 A cross-section of a porous metal shell demonstrating integration of the cancellized coating with the solid base.

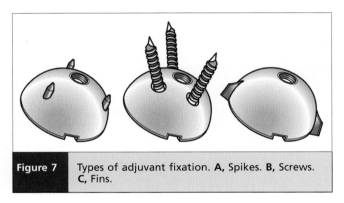

Figure 7 Types of adjuvant fixation. **A**, Spikes. **B**, Screws. **C**, Fins.

("pores") to allow optimal bony ingrowth is between 150 and 450 μ.

Newer highly porous coatings have a configuration that is closer to cancellous bone. The depth of the cancellous portion varies among the different cup designs, from near-complete in porous tantalum components to a 1.5-mm thickness for some roughened titanium surfaces. Because the "cancellized" portion is part of the entire metal substrate (as opposed to a bonded coating), the elastic modulus of the shell is lower than a shell with a solid substrate and an applied coating (Figures 5 and 6). The surface roughness of these components is considerably greater than that of earlier designs, which theoretically may contribute to more stable initial fixation. A second theoretic advantage of these more porous components is that they are less stiff, with moduli of elasticity closer to that of bone, and the hope is that there will be less stress shielding, although that has not been demonstrated in any clinical study.

In addition, some manufacturers have explored the possibility of adding osteoconductive coatings to the fixation surface of cementless sockets, with the goal of decreasing radiolucent lines and improving overall implant fixation. Prior analyses of retrieved clinically well-fixed cementless sockets have demonstrated bone ingrowth in less than 20% of the surface area. Although greater ingrowth would intuitively seem desirable, there

is no evidence that greater ingrowth is associated with superior clinical function. The most common osteoconductive coating has been hydroxyapatite added by solution deposition to promote bony ingrowth. Thus far, the fixation and clinical survival results are no better than those of cups without hydroxyapatite.[85-87] However, there are data demonstrating that hydroxyapatite coating in the absence of a roughened porous surface is associated with inferior clinical results and higher failures caused by aseptic loosening.[88]

Adjuvant Fixation

Several cup designs have used extensions from the cup to either fix the cup or to augment the press-fit fixation. Examples include pegs, spikes, fins, and screws (**Figure 7**). The results of cups with these different forms of augmentation have been roughly equivalent.[89] The disadvantage of fixed spikes, fins, or pegs is that it is difficult to adjust the cup position once it is impacted, and these designs can sometimes prevent complete seating of the component. The advantage of screws is that they tend to pull the cup to the interface, and there are numerous options for their placement, allowing the surgeon to place them in the best quality bone. The disadvantage of cups designed for use with screws is that the screw holes provide access for particulate debris to the interface, with risk of osteolysis.[90] Although this certainly remains a cause for concern, screw-hole osteolysis has not been described with newer cross-linked polyethylene bearings. Another disadvantage of screws is the risk of penetrating vascular structures adjacent to the acetabulum with the potential for severe bleeding. Most contemporary cementless cups are implanted by underreaming the socket by 2 to 4 mm relative to the cup diameter with the goal of firm interference fit at the rim. Although some clinical studies have demonstrated a high degree of cup fixation with press-fit implantation without adjuvant fixation,[91,92] it is difficult to gauge the stability of a press-fit shell. Because the best reported clinical results of acetabular shells are for those placed with screws, the sur-

Table 6

Clinical Results of Cementless Acetabular Components

Author	Year	N	F/U (yrs)	Survival	Component
Della Valle et al[101]	2009	900	20	96%	HGP
Della Valle et al[102]	2004	142	15	99%	HGP (Ti)
Anseth et al[103]	2010	60	17.2	87.7%	HGP (Ti)
Chen et al[57]	2006	157	5	99%	Duraloc (Ti)
Dearborn and Murray[104]	1998	86	7.8	100%	Arthropor (Ti)
Demmelmeyer et al[105]	2010	102	12	93%	Wagner (Ti)
Smith et al[76]	1998	72	12	96%	ARC (CC)
Zenz et al[106]	2009	82	10	97.5%	Allofit (Ti)
Hallan et al[100]	2010	9113	20	81 to 92%	Multiple types

CC, cobalt-chromium substrate; Ti, titanium substrate

geon should have a low threshold for using them if component stability is in question.

Locking Mechanisms

There has been a steady evolution in liner locking mechanisms. Design intent has been to improve lever strength, as some of the first-generation cups had a modest incidence of liner displacement. Improved locking strength is particularly important when a constrained liner is used to manage instability. Retrieval studies have revealed that motion at the backside of the acetabular liner is a substantial source of component wear;[93,94] thus, design efforts have also focused on reducing micromotion. Many cup designs have used a locking ring at the rim of the cup to address both of these problems. Two manufacturers have used a Morse taper locking mechanism, analogous to that used to attach modular femoral heads to femoral components.

Acetabular Liners

The design of acetabular liners has evolved to accommodate improvements in locking mechanisms, different bearing surfaces, and the desire to use head sizes as large as possible to reduce dislocation risk. With the introduction of cross-linked polyethylene, manufacturers have reduced their minimum polyethylene thickness, allowing the use of larger head sizes in smaller cups than was previously possible. Because of failure of numerous types of cross-linked polyethylene liners with thin liners,[95-99] an emerging consensus has suggested the minimum allowable polyethylene thickness at the rim of the liner to be 5 mm. Metal liners, on the other hand, can be thinner (3 mm) because of markedly decreased wear properties and improved strength and stiffness compared with their polyethylene counterparts. For strength considerations, it is generally believed that ceramic liners need to be thicker than metal inserts.

Design Considerations for Cementless Cup Insertion

There is considerable evidence that initial stability of the cementless shell is correlated with stable long-term fixation. Early implantation techniques reamed line-to-line and maximized initial stability through the placement of dome screws (screws placed through preformed holes in the shell into the ilium). Currently, the preferred technique in the United States is to underream the acetabular bed to maximize rim contact and therefore minimize micromotion. Supplementary screws are added if the surgeon is unsure of the fixation. Concern for screw holes serving as a conduit for particulate debris has led most manufacturers to decrease the number of holes in the shells, concentrating them in one area that is intended to be oriented to the "safe zone" of the acetabulum, the posterior superior quadrant. Currently it is unknown if fixation rates of hemispheric shells placed without screws will equal those placed with screws.

Most surgical technique manuals suggest the degree of underreaming of between 1 and 4 mm less than the outer diameter of the cementless shell. The degree of underreaming must take into account the patient's age and bone quality as well as the characteristics of the porous coating of the shell. Some of the highly porous shells are designed for insertion without underreaming (line-to line), so the surgeon must consult the manufacturer's recommendations.

Clinical Results of Acetabular Cups

Cementless Cups

The clinical track record of cementless cups[57,76,100-106] is presented in Table 6.

In general, most designs have survival rates of more than 90% at up to 15 years, with most failures caused by polyethylene wear and secondary osteolysis. With improvements in the wear properties of polyethylene, it is possible that these survival rates will improve.

3: Hip

Table 7

Results of Acetabular Components in National Registries (Cemented and Cementless)

Source	Early (< 5 yrs) Failure Rate (%)	10-Year Survival Shell
Swedish National Arthroplasty Register Report, 2007	0.5% to 7%	90% to 96%
Norwegian Arthroplasty Register Report, 2008	1% to 6%	89% to 96%
Australian Orthopaedic Association Arthroplasty Registry Report, 2008	2.4% to 8.3%	91% to 96%
New Zealand Orthopaedic Association 10-Year Report, 2008	0.5% to 1.5%	90% to 96%
National Joint Registry for England and Wales, Annual Report, 2009	2% to 2.4% (cementless) 1.2 % to 1.4% (cemented)	NA

Table 8

Clinical Results of Cemented Acetabular Components

Author	Year	N	F/U (yrs)	Survival	Component
Callaghan et al[33]	2008	304	19-20	92%	Spectron (CC - MB)
Chen et al[70]	1998	86	10	91%	Spectron (CC - MB)
Markel et al[71]	1995	115	7		55 AP, 60 MB
Peraldi et al[72]	1997	124	< 2	96%	PSA (Ti -MB)
Ziegler and Lachiewicz[75]	1996	70	9	81% MB 95% AP	Triad (CC-MB and AP)
Altenburg et al[69]	2009	500	20	79%	TiBac (MB)

Ti, titanium substrate; CC, cobalt-chromium substrate; MB, metal backed, AP, all polyethylene

The national joint registries that examine implant survival have suggested a higher early failure rate than the single center results mentioned previously. Table 7 reviews current published data from these registries. When 10-year survival rates are examined, it appears that fixation rates are high for cementless acetabular components; however, the survival rate is somewhat lower because of polyethylene wear, osteolysis, and dislocation. For example, in a review of 9,113 primary cementless sockets from Norway, the survival free of revision for any reason was 81% to 92% compared with a survival free of revision for aseptic loosening of 87% to 100%.[100]

In Scandinavia, however, cemented cups have had a better survival than the first-generation cementless cups (Swedish Hip Arthroplasty Register Report, 2007). Nonetheless, in Sweden there has been a progressive increase in the use of uncemented cups in the first decade of the 21st century, perhaps reflecting the improved survival of the more recent cup designs and the increased versatility and ease of insertion of cementless acetabular components.

Cemented Cups

Compared with that of cemented femoral components, the long-term survival rate of cemented acetabular components[33,69-72,75] has been low (Table 8). The survival of cementless acetabular components in the United States has generally been much better than that of cemented cups, with some series reporting failure rates of cemented cups of up to 40% at 10 years.[76,107,108] This finding, in addition to a perception of greater difficulty inserting and adjusting cemented cups, has led American surgeons to largely abandon cemented acetabular components. In Europe, however, where national registries reported higher early failure rates for first-generation cementless components than cemented components, cemented acetabular components predominate (65% cemented sockets, and 35% cementless sockets), although the trend is toward increasing use of cementless devices. The Swedish Hip Register has reported survival of most of the cemented acetabular components used in Sweden of approximately 90% at 10 years and 80% at 20 years (Swedish Hip Arthroplasty Register Report, 2007).

There is no clear advantage of metal-backed versus all-polyethylene cemented sockets in the literature, with some reports showing a higher failure rate of metal-backed components. A review of a consecutive nonselected series of metal-backed cemented acetabular components implanted by a single surgeon at 19- to 20-year follow-up found loosening of the acetabular component in 30% of cases, although only 8% of these cups had been revised.[33] A similar pattern of revision was found in 9% of the cemented acetabular components, but there was evidence of loosening in 32% at a mean follow-up of 9 years in a series of 86 primary total hip replacements.[70] Because of the similarity in survival and the fact that all-polyethylene components are considerably less expensive, they are the most commonly used acetabular component in Sweden.

Annotated References

1. Brown TE, Cui Q, Mihalko WM, Saleh KJ: *Arthritis and Arthroplasty: The Hip.* Philadelphia, PA, Saunders, 2009, pp 93-103.

   This book offers expert guidance on preoperative planning to surgical approaches and techniques with clear, evidence-based coverage details for cemented primary and revision THAs.

2. Callaghan JJ, Rosenberg AG, Rubash H: *The Adult Hip,* ed 2. Philadelphia, PA, Lippincott, 2007, pp 917-946.

   This book offers updated details on preoperative planning, surgical approaches, and cementing techniques for the acetabulum and femur, with clear, evidence-based data.

3. Ranawat CS, Rasquinha VJ, Rodriguez JA: Results of cemented total hip replacement, in Pellicci PM, Tria AJ, Garvin KL, eds: *Orthopaedic Knowledge Update: Hip and Knee Reconstruction 2.* Rosemont, IL, American Academy of Orthopaedic Surgeons, 2000, pp 181-195.

4. Middleton RG, Howie DW, Costi K, Sharpe P: Effects of design changes on cemented tapered femoral stem fixation. *Clin Orthop Relat Res* 1998;355:47-56.

5. Ranawat CS, Ranawat AS, Rasquinha VJ: Mastering the art of cemented femoral stem fixation. *J Arthroplasty* 2004;19(4, suppl 1):85-91.

6. Jewett BA, Collis DK: Radiographic failure patterns of polished cemented stems. *Clin Orthop Relat Res* 2006;453:132-136.

   This article retrospectively reviewed 1,031 THAs with four different polished femoral stems. Revision rate was 0.6% for aseptic loosening with no obvious difference in loosening rates or radiographic failure patterns among the four stem geometries. Level of evidence: IV.

7. Baumann B, Hendrich C, Barthel T, et al: 9- to 11-year results of cemented titanium mueller straight stem in total hip arthroplasty. *Orthopedics* 2007;30(7):551-557.

   This retrospective study reviewed 9- to 11-year results after THA with cemented titanium stems. Revisions for aseptic loosening were performed in 4%. No significant differences were found in sex, size, or type of stem, Harris Score, heterotopic ossification, or body mass index.

8. Della Valle AG, Zoppi A, Peterson MG, Salvati EA: A rough surface finish adversely affects the survivorship of a cemented femoral stem. *Clin Orthop Relat Res* 2005;436:158-163.

   One hundred seventy-five patients with rough stems and 138 total hips with satin finish were followed up for 4 to 8 years. A rough, textured stem of this design is more likely than a satin surface stem to fail at intermediate follow-up. Level of evidence: III.

9. Collis DK, Mohler CG: Comparison of clinical outcomes in total hip arthroplasty using rough and polished cemented stems with essentially the same geometry. *J Bone Joint Surg Am* 2002;84-A(4):586-592.

10. Chiu KH, Shen WY, Cheung KW, Tsui HF: Primary exeter total hip arthroplasty in patients with small femurs: A minimal of 10 years follow-up. *J Arthroplasty* 2005;20(3):275-281.

    Seventy-five hips with primary cemented THA with an Exeter stem, average follow-up of 12.8 years, were studied. Stem subsidence occurred in 9.3% with no evidence of loosening. The survival rate was 93.3% and 86% at 10 and 15 years, respectively.

11. Hook S, Moulder E, Yates PJ, Burston BJ, Whitley E, Bannister GC: The Exeter Universal stem: A minimum ten-year review from an independent centre. *J Bone Joint Surg Br* 2006;88(12):1584-1590.

    This article reports on 88 primary cemented THAs followed for a minimum of 10 years. The rate of revision for femoral components was 1.1% for aseptic loosening and osteolysis. The acetabular failure rate was 37.5%.

12. Franklin J, Robertsson O, Gestsson J, Lohmander LS, Ingvarsson T: Revision and complication rates in 654 Exeter total hip replacements, with a maximum follow-up of 20 years. *BMC Musculoskelet Disord* 2003;4:6.

13. Williams HD, Browne G, Gie GA, Ling RS, Timperley AJ, Wendover NA: The Exeter universal cemented femoral component at 8 to 12 years: A study of the first 325 hips. *J Bone Joint Surg Br* 2002;84(3):324-334.

14. Firestone DE, Callaghan JJ, Liu SS, et al: Total hip arthroplasty with a cemented, polished, collared femoral stem and a cementless acetabular component: A follow-up study at a minimum of ten years. *J Bone Joint Surg Am* 2007;89(1):126-132.

    The authors present a retrospective review of 115 hips treated with primary cemented THA with a polished surface finish at a minimum of 10-year follow-up. Although no hips were revised because of aseptic loosening, distal femoral osteolysis was observed in 5.4%, demonstrating excellent durability. Level of evidence: III.

15. Fowler JL, Gie GA, Lee AJ, Ling RS: Experience with the Exeter total hip replacement since 1970. *Orthop Clin North Am* 1988;19(3):477-489.

16. Rasquinha VJ, Ranawat CS, Dua V, Ranawat AS, Rodriguez JA: A prospective, randomized, double-blind study of smooth versus rough stems using cement fixation: Minimum 5-year follow-up. *J Arthroplasty*

3: Hip

2004;19(7, Suppl 2):2-9.

17. Ajmal M, Ranawat AS, Ranawat CS: A new cemented femoral stem: A prospective study of the Stryker accolade C with 2- to 5-year follow-up. *J Arthroplasty* 2008;23(1):118-122.

    This prospective study evaluates the short-term results of cemented femoral stems in 100 all-cemented and 100 hybrid THAs in the 2-year study group. Good to excellent results were obtained in 96%.

18. Rasquinha VJ, Dua V, Rodriguez JA, Ranawat CS: Fifteen-year survivorship of a collarless, cemented, normalized femoral stem in primary hybrid total hip arthroplasty with a modified third-generation cement technique. *J Arthroplasty* 2003;18(7, suppl 1):86-94.

19. Buckwalter AE, Callaghan JJ, Liu SS, et al: Results of Charnley total hip arthroplasty with use of improved femoral cementing techniques: A concise follow-up, at a minimum of twenty-five years, of a previous report. *J Bone Joint Surg Am* 2006;88(7):1481-1485.

    This study is a prospective report of 357 hips with primary cemented Charnley THA at 20 years. The revision rate was 2.8% for aseptic loosening, demonstrating the remarkable durability of the femoral fixation obtained with the polished flatback Charnley prosthesis. Level of evidence: IV.

20. McCoy TH, Salvati EA, Ranawat CS, Wilson PD Jr: A fifteen-year follow-up study of one hundred Charnley low-friction arthroplasties. *Orthop Clin North Am* 1988;19(3):467-476.

21. Joshi AB, Porter ML, Trail IA, Hunt LP, Murphy JC, Hardinge K: Long-term results of Charnley low-friction arthroplasty in young patients. *J Bone Joint Surg Br* 1993;75(4):616-623.

22. Schulte KR, Callaghan JJ, Kelley SS, Johnston RC: The outcome of Charnley total hip arthroplasty with cement after a minimum twenty-year follow-up: The results of one surgeon. *J Bone Joint Surg Am* 1993; 75(7):961-975.

23. Wroblewski BM, Siney PD: Charnley low-friction arthroplasty of the hip: Long-term results. *Clin Orthop Relat Res* 1993;292(292):191-201.

24. Neumann L, Freund KG, Sørenson KH: Long-term results of Charnley total hip replacement: Review of 92 patients at 15 to 20 years. *J Bone Joint Surg Br* 1994; 76(2):245-251.

25. Kavanagh BF, Wallrichs S, Dewitz M, et al: Charnley low-friction arthroplasty of the hip: Twenty-year results with cement. *J Arthroplasty* 1994;9(3):229-234.

26. Skutek M, Bourne RB, Rorabeck CH, Burns A, Kearns S, Krishna G: The twenty to twenty-five-year outcomes of the Harris design-2 matte-finished cemented total hip replacement: A concise follow-up of a previous report. *J Bone Joint Surg Am* 2007;89(4):814-818.

    This article is a prospective follow-up of 195 matte-finished Harris design-2 THAs. At 25 years, the Kaplan-Meier analysis revealed 86% survivorship for the femoral component and 93% for the acetabular component. Level of evidence: IV.

27. Mulroy RD Jr, Harris WH: The effect of improved cementing techniques on component loosening in total hip replacement: An 11-year radiographic review. *J Bone Joint Surg Br* 1990;72(5):757-760.

28. Barrack RL, Mulroy RD Jr, Harris WH: Improved cementing techniques and femoral component loosening in young patients with hip arthroplasty: A 12-year radiographic review. *J Bone Joint Surg Br* 1992;74(3): 385-389.

29. Mulroy WF, Estok DM, Harris WH: Total hip arthroplasty with use of so-called second-generation cementing techniques: A fifteen-year-average follow-up study. *J Bone Joint Surg Am* 1995;77(12):1845-1852.

30. Madey SM, Callaghan JJ, Olejniczak JP, Goetz DD, Johnston RC: Charnley total hip arthroplasty with use of improved techniques of cementing: The results after a minimum of fifteen years of follow-up. *J Bone Joint Surg Am* 1997;79(1):53-64.

31. Bourne RB, Rorabeck CH, Skutek M, Mikkelsen S, Winemaker M, Robertson D: The Harris Design-2 total hip replacement fixed with so-called second-generation cementing techniques: A ten to fifteen-year follow-up. *J Bone Joint Surg Am* 1998;80(12):1775-1780.

32. Smith SW, Estok DM II , Harris WH: Total hip arthroplasty with use of second-generation cementing techniques: An eighteen-year-average follow-up study. *J Bone Joint Surg Am* 1998;80(11):1632-1640.

33. Callaghan JJ, Liu SS, Firestone DE, et al: Total hip arthroplasty with cement and use of a collared matte-finish femoral component: Nineteen to twenty-year follow-up. *J Bone Joint Surg Am* 2008;90(2):299-306.

    This study demonstrates the durability of a cemented, matte-finish, collared femoral component at 20 years postoperatively, with a rate of revision of 2.6% caused by aseptic loosening. Level of evidence: IV.

34. Berger RA, Kull LR, Rosenberg AG, Galante JO: Hybrid total hip arthroplasty: 7- to 10-year results. *Clin Orthop Relat Res* 1996;333:134-146.

35. Callaghan JJ, Tooma GS, Olejniczak JP, Goetz DD, Johnston RC: Primary hybrid total hip arthroplasty: An interim followup. *Clin Orthop Relat Res* 1996; 333:118-125.

36. Clohisy JC, Harris WH: Primary hybrid total hip replacement, performed with insertion of the acetabular component without cement and a precoat femoral component with cement: An average ten-year follow-up study. *J Bone Joint Surg Am* 1999;81(2): 247-255.

37. Dowd JE, Cha CW, Trakru S, Kim SY, Yang IH, Rubash HE: Failure of total hip arthroplasty with a precoated prosthesis: 4- to 11-year results. *Clin Orthop Relat Res* 1998;355:123-136.

38. Harris WH: Hybrid total hip replacement: Rationale and intermediate clinical results. *Clin Orthop Relat Res* 1996;333:155-164.

39. Schmalzried TP, Harris WH: Hybrid total hip replacement: A 6.5-year follow-up study. *J Bone Joint Surg Br* 1993;75(4):608-615.

40. Woolson ST, Haber DF: Primary total hip replacement with insertion of an acetabular component without cement and a femoral component with cement: Follow-up study at an average of six years. *J Bone Joint Surg Am* 1996;78(5):698-705.

41. Goldberg VM, Ninomiya J, Kelly G, Kraay M: Hybrid total hip arthroplasty: A 7- to 11-year followup. *Clin Orthop Relat Res* 1996;333:147-154.

42. Kim YH, Kim JS, Cho SH: A comparison of polyethylene wear in hips with cobalt-chrome or zirconia heads: A prospective, randomised study. *J Bone Joint Surg Br* 2001;83(5):742-750.

43. Allami MK, Fender D, Khaw FM, et al: Outcome of Charnley total hip replacement across a single health region in England: The results at ten years from a regional arthroplasty register. *J Bone Joint Surg Br* 2006; 88(10):1293-1298.

    Using a regional arthroplasty register, outcome at 5 years of 1,198 primary Charnley THAs showed the rate of aseptic loosening, deep infection, dislocation, and revision was 2.3%, 1.4%, 5.0%, and 3.2%, respectively.

44. Rasquinha VJ, Ranawat CS: Durability of the cemented femoral stem in patients 60 to 80 years old. *Clin Orthop Relat Res* 2004;419:115-123.

45. DeLee JG, Charnley J: Radiological demarcation of cemented sockets in total hip replacement. *Clin Orthop Relat Res* 1976;121:20-32.

46. Stauffer RN: Ten-year follow-up study of total hip replacement. *J Bone Joint Surg Am* 1982;64(7):983-990.

47. Poss R, Brick GW, Wright RJ, Roberts DW, Sledge CB: The effects of modern cementing techniques on the longevity of total hip arthroplasty. *Orthop Clin North Am* 1988;19(3):591-598.

48. Ritter MA, Faris PM, Keating EM, Brugo G: Influential factors in cemented acetabular cup loosening. *J Arthroplasty* 1992;7(Suppl):365-367.

49. Callaghan JJ, Forest EE, Olejniczak JP, Goetz DD, Johnston RC: Charnley total hip arthroplasty in patients less than fifty years old: A twenty to twenty-five-year follow-up note. *J Bone Joint Surg Am* 1998;80(5): 704-714.

50. Callaghan JJ, Albright JC, Goetz DD, Olejniczak JP, Johnston RC: Charnley total hip arthroplasty with cement: Minimum twenty-five-year follow-up. *J Bone Joint Surg Am* 2000;82(4):487-497.

51. Callaghan JJ, Templeton JE, Liu SS, et al: Results of Charnley total hip arthroplasty at a minimum of thirty years: A concise follow-up of a previous report. *J Bone Joint Surg Am* 2004;86-A(4):690-695.

52. Engh CA Jr, Mohan V, Nagowski JP, Sychterz Terefenko CJ, Engh CA Sr: Influence of stem size on clinical outcome of primary total hip arthroplasty with cementless extensively porous-coated femoral components. *J Arthroplasty* 2009;24(4):554-559.

    The authors reported 97% AML femoral implant survival at 15 years; there was no difference in revision, loosening, or pain between large- and small-diameter implants.

53. Kang JS, Moon KH, Park SR, Choi SW: Long-term results of total hip arthroplasty with an extensively porous coated stem in patients younger than 45 years old. *Yonsei Med J* 2010;51(1):100-103.

    In patients younger than 45 years, there was no AML stem loosening at 12-years follow-up.

54. Ferrell MS, Browne JA, Attarian DE, Cook C, Bolognesi MP: Cementless porous-coated anatomic total hip arthroplasty at Duke: 18- to 24-year follow-up. *J Surg Orthop Adv* 2009;18(3):150-154.

    At an average follow-up of 20.2 years (range, 18 to 24 years), the rate of PCA femoral component revision was 34%.

55. Surdam JW, Archibeck MJ, Schultz SC Jr, Junick DW, White RE Jr: A second-generation cementless total hip arthroplasty mean 9-year results. *J Arthroplasty* 2007; 22(2):204-209.

    In 258 Multilock components at a mean follow-up of 9 years (range, 5 to 14 years), the rate of aseptic femoral component survivorship was 98% (two stems loose and revised, one stem loose and not revised). No distal femoral osteolysis was reported.

56. Butler JB, Lansky D, Duwelius PJ: Prospective evaluation of total hip arthroplasty with a cementless, anatomically designed, porous-coated femoral implant: Mean 11-year follow-up. *J Arthroplasty* 2005;20(6): 709-716.

    In 91 anatomic stems at a minimum follow-up of 10 years, only one femoral component was loose and revised.

57. Chen CJ, Xenos JS, McAuley JP, Young A, Engh CA Sr: Second-generation porous-coated cementless total hip arthroplasties have high survival. *Clin Orthop Relat Res* 2006;451:121-127.

    In a retrospective review of 157 consecutive THAs to determine if design modifications led to improved clinical performance compared with first-generation components, data indicated that clinical results were good.

3: Hip

In 145 Prodigy stems at an average of 6.7 years follow-up, only two hips (1.4%) were revised for loosening. No distal femoral osteolysis was noted.

58. Hennessy DW, Callaghan JJ, Liu SS: Second-generation extensively porous-coated THA stems at minimum 10-year followup. *Clin Orthop Relat Res* 2009;467(9):2290-2296.

    In 82 Prodigy hips at an average follow-up of 11.4 years (range, 10 to 12 years), there were no femoral revisions and all stems were bone ingrown. No distal femoral osteolysis was noted.

59. Springer BD, Connelly SE, Odum SM, et al: Cementless femoral components in young patients: Review and meta-analysis of total hip arthroplasty and hip resurfacing. *J Arthroplasty* 2009;24(6, suppl):2-8.

    In 6,408 hip implants in 22 studies in young patients at an average follow-up of 8.4 years, a meta-analysis revealed a pooled mechanical failure rate of 1.3%.

60. Archibeck MJ, Surdam JW, Schultz SC Jr, Junick DW, White RE Jr: Cementless total hip arthroplasty in patients 50 years or younger. *J Arthroplasty* 2006;21(4):476-483.

    In 100 Multilock implants in patients at an average age of 39 years (range, 14 to 50 years) and average follow-up of 9 years (range, 5 to 13 years), there was no femoral mechanical failure (aseptic femoral component survival rate was 100%).

61. Dutton A, Rubash HE: Hot topics and controversies in arthroplasty: Cementless femoral fixation in elderly patients. *Instr Course Lect* 2008;57:255-259.

    The authors discuss excellent results with cementless femoral fixation in elderly patients, and its use is recommended in elderly patients with good bone quality.

62. Hooper GJ, Rothwell AG, Stringer M, Frampton C: Revision following cemented and uncemented primary total hip replacement: A seven-year analysis from the New Zealand Joint Registry. *J Bone Joint Surg Br* 2009;91(4):451-458.

    In 42,665 primary total hip replacements in the New Zealand Joint Registry, cementless femoral components had a lower revision rate in patients younger than 65 years and a higher revision rate in patients older than 65 years.

63. Jackson MP, Sexton SA, Yeung E, Walter WL, Walter WK, Zicat BA: The effect of obesity on the mid-term survival and clinical outcome of cementless total hip replacement. *J Bone Joint Surg Br* 2009;91(10):1296-1300.

    In 2,026 consecutive cementless primary total hip replacements, survival rates and overall satisfaction were equivalent in obese (body mass index greater than 30) and nonobese (body mass index less than 30) patients. Harris hip score and range of motion were higher in the nonobese group.

64. Hungerford MW, Hungerford DS, Jones LC: Outcome of uncemented primary femoral stems for treatment of femoral head osteonecrosis. *Orthop Clin North Am* 2009;40(2):283-289.

    In 158 cases of four generations of PCA implants at a mean follow-up of 103 months (range, 20 to 235 months), there were 14 revisions (8.9%) for loosening and/or osteolysis.

65. Radl R, Egner S, Hungerford M, Rehak P, Windhager R: Survival of cementless femoral components after osteonecrosis of the femoral head with different etiologies. *J Arthroplasty* 2005;20(4):509-515.

    Fifty-five cementless total hip replacements were performed for osteonecrosis. Seventeen patients with no systemic disease had no revisions (100% survival) and 38 cases associated with a systemic disease had eight revisions (68% survival) at an average of 6.4 years (range, 2 to 12 years).

66. Bhan S, Eachempati KK, Malhotra R: Primary cementless total hip arthroplasty for bony ankylosis in patients with ankylosing spondylitis. *J Arthroplasty* 2008;23(6):859-866.

    In 92 cementless total hip replacements for bony ankylosis secondary to ankylosing spondylitis, 13 hips (14%) were revised for loosening at 8.5 years follow-up.

67. *A Safety Alert: The Use of Modular Necks in Total Hip Replacement.* Arlington, TN, Wright Medical Technology, Inc, 2008.

68. Callaghan JJ, Kim YS, Brown TD, Pedersen DR, Johnston RC: Concerns and improvements with cementless metal-backed acetabular components. *Clin Orthop Relat Res* 1995;311:76-84.

69. Altenburg AJ, Callaghan JJ, Yehyawi TM, et al: Cemented total hip replacement cable debris and acetabular construct durability. *J Bone Joint Surg Am* 2009;91(7):1664-1670.

    The authors demonstrated a higher polyethylene wear rate and decreased cup survival in the cohort that had trochanteric osteotomy repaired with braided cables as opposed to monofilament stainless steel wires.

70. Chen FS, Di Cesare PE, Kale AA, et al: Results of cemented metal-backed acetabular components: A 10-year-average follow-up study. *J Arthroplasty* 1998;13(8):867-873.

71. Markel DC, Huo MH, Katkin PD, Salvati EA: Use of cemented all-polyethylene and metal-backed acetabular components in total hip arthroplasty: A comparative study. *J Arthroplasty* 1995;10(Suppl):S1-S7.

72. Peraldi P, Vandenbussche E, Augereau B: Bad clinical results of cemented caps with metal-backed acetabular components: 124 cases with 21 months follow-up. *Rev Chir Orthop Reparatrice Appar Mot* 1997;83(6):561-565.

73. Ritter MA, Keating EM, Faris PM, Brugo G: Metal-backed acetabular cups in total hip arthroplasty.

3: Hip

J Bone Joint Surg Am 1990;72(5):672-677.

74. Rorabeck CH, Bourne RB, Mulliken BD, et al: The Nicolas Andry award: Comparative results of cemented and cementless total hip arthroplasty. *Clin Orthop Relat Res* 1996;325:330-344.

75. Ziegler BS, Lachiewicz PF: Survivorship analysis of cemented total hip arthroplasty acetabular components implanted with second-generation techniques. *J Arthroplasty* 1996;11(6):750-756.

76. Smith SE, Estok DM II, Harris WH: Average 12-year outcome of a chrome-cobalt, beaded, bony ingrowth acetabular component. *J Arthroplasty* 1998;13(1):50-60.

77. Van Flandern GJ, Bierbaum BE, Newberg AH, Gomes SL, Mattingly DA, Karpos PA: Intermediate clinical follow-up of a dual-radius acetabular component. *J Arthroplasty* 1998;13(7):804-811.

78. Yahiro MA, Gantenberg JB, Nelson R, Lu HT, Mishra NK: Comparison of the results of cemented, porous-ingrowth, and threaded acetabular cup fixation: A meta-analysis of the orthopaedic literature. *J Arthroplasty* 1995;10(3):339-350.

79. Simank HG, Brocai DR, Reiser D, Thomsen M, Sabo D, Lukoschek M: Middle-term results of threaded acetabular cups: High failure rates five years after surgery. *J Bone Joint Surg Br* 1997;79(3):366-370.

80. Clarius M, Jung AW, Raiss P, Streit MR, Merle C, Aldinger PR: Long-term results of the threaded Weill cup in primary total hip arthroplasty: A 15-20-year follow-up study. *Int Orthop* 2010;34(7):943-948.

   At a mean follow-up of 17 years, the revision rate of the Weill threaded cup with a smooth surface treatment was 24%.

81. Clarius M, Jung AW, Streit MR, Merle C, Raiss P, Aldinger PR: Long-term results of the threaded Mecron cup in primary total hip arthroplasty: A 15-20-year follow-up study. *Int Orthop* 2010;34(8):1093-1098.

   Of 221 threaded smooth cups followed for a mean of 17 years, the revision rate for the acetabular component was 41%.

82. Journeaux SF, Morgan DA, Donnelly WJ: Poor results of the Freeman uncemented metal-backed acetabular component: Five-to-nine-year results. *J Bone Joint Surg Br* 2000;82(2):185-187.

83. Puolakka TJ, Pajamäki KJ, Pulkkinen PO, Nevalainen JK: Poor survival of cementless Biomet total hip: A report on 1,047 hips from the Finnish Arthroplasty Register. *Acta Orthop Scand* 1999;70(5):425-429.

84. Squire M, Griffin WL, Mason JB, Peindl RD, Odum S: Acetabular component deformation with press-fit fixation. *J Arthroplasty* 2006;21(6, suppl 2):72-77.

   The authors show that in one type of cementless acetabular component there is consistent deformation of the shell on the order of 0.16 mm. In one-piece cups this amount of deformation may exceed the tolerance of hard-on-hard bearings.

85. Eskelinen A, Remes V, Helenius I, Pulkkinen P, Nevalainen J, Paavolainen P: Uncemented total hip arthroplasty for primary osteoarthritis in young patients: A mid- to long-term follow-up study from the Finnish Arthroplasty Register. *Acta Orthop* 2006;77(1):57-70.

   This study looked at a subset of the Finnish Arthroplasty Register. All patients younger than 55 years who had uncemented total hip replacement between 1980 and 2003 were evaluated. At 13-year mean follow-up, the fixation survival of the acetabular components was greater than 90%, but revision for any reason (polyethylene wear, dislocation) was 80%.

86. Coathup MJ, Blackburn J, Goodship AE, Cunningham JL, Smith T, Blunn GW: Role of hydroxyapatite coating in resisting wear particle migration and osteolysis around acetabular components. *Biomaterials* 2005;26(19):4161-4169.

   The authors implanted total hip replacement with acetabular components of various cementless coatings, including one group with hydroxyapatite. They reported significantly greater bony ingrowth in the hydroxyapatite-coated implants compared with the noncoated porous components and that this prevented particle migration to a greater degree than the cemented cup control group.

87. Thanner J: The acetabular component in total hip arthroplasty: Evaluation of different fixation principles. *Acta Orthop Scand Suppl* 1999;286:1-41.

88. D'Angelo F, Molina M, Riva G, Zatti G, Cherubino P: Failure of dual radius hydroxyapatite-coated acetabular cups. *J Orthop Surg Res* 2008;3:35.

   The authors reported a retrospective review of dual radius design acetabular cups with a smooth surface and hydroxyapatite coating. The revision rate was 11% at a mean 10-year follow-up, mainly because of aseptic loosening.

89. Archibeck MJ, Showalter D, Kavanaugh TS, Camarata D, White RE Jr: A comparison of cementless acetabular components of the same design: Spiked versus supplemental screws. *J Arthroplasty* 2003;18(7, suppl 1):122-125.

90. Schmalzried TP, Brown IC, Amstutz HC, Engh CA, Harris WH: The role of acetabular component screw holes and/or screws in the development of pelvic osteolysis. *Proc Inst Mech Eng H* 1999;213(2):147-153.

91. Schmalzried TP, Wessinger SJ, Hill GE, Harris WH: The Harris-Galante porous acetabular component press-fit without screw fixation: Five-year radiographic analysis of primary cases. *J Arthroplasty* 1994;9(3):235-242.

3: Hip

92. Ng FY, Zhu Y, Chiu KY: Cementless acetabular component inserted without screws: The effect of immediate weight-bearing. *Int Orthop* 2007;31(3):293-296.

The authors retrospectively report 2- to 6-year results for 74 cementless cups inserted without screws and with an immediate weight-bearing protocol and reported no migration or other signs of loosening.

93. Krieg AH, Speth BM, Ochsner PE: Backside volumetric change in the polyethylene of uncemented acetabular components. *J Bone Joint Surg Br* 2009;91(8):1037-1043.

This report examined 35 retrieved acetabular liners (retrieved during revision surgery for failure of the femoral component) that demonstrated that backside volumetric wear was only 3% of the front side or articular volumetric wear, although it was higher in loose components. The authors concluded that in well-fixed acetabular components, backside wear was unlikely to be an osteolytic concern.

94. Kurtz SM, Edidin AA, Bartel DL: The role of backside polishing, cup angle, and polyethylene thickness on the contact stresses in metal-backed acetabular components. *J Biomech* 1997;30(6):639-642.

95. Berry DJ, Barnes CL, Scott RD, Cabanela ME, Poss R: Catastrophic failure of the polyethylene liner of uncemented acetabular components. *J Bone Joint Surg Br* 1994;76(4):575-578.

96. Furmanski J, Anderson M, Bal S, et al: Clinical fracture of cross-linked UHMWPE acetabular liners. *Biomaterials* 2009;30(29):5572-5582.

The authors report four cases of fracture of highly cross-linked polyethylene acetabular liners, all of different designs, where analysis revealed that the fracture originated in an area of unsupported polyethylene in the rim of an elevated liner.

97. Engh CA Jr, Hopper RH, Engh CA, McAuley JP: Wear-through of a modular polyethylene liner: Four case reports. *Clin Orthop Relat Res* 2001;383:175-182.

98. Gross AE, Dust WN: Acute polyethylene fracture in an uncemented acetabular cup. *Can J Surg* 1997;40(4):310-312.

99. Tower SS, Currier JH, Currier BH, Lyford KA, Van Citters DW, Mayor MB: Rim cracking of the cross-linked longevity polyethylene acetabular liner after total hip arthroplasty. *J Bone Joint Surg Am* 2007;89(10):2212-2217.

This report analyzed four highly cross-linked acetabular liners that failed between 7 and 27 months and concluded that risk factors for cracking of the liners were thin polyethylene and vertical position of the acetabular shell.

100. Hallan G, Dybvik E, Furnes O, Havelin LI: Metal-backed acetabular components with conventional polyethylene: A review of 9113 primary components with a follow-up of 20 years. *J Bone Joint Surg Br* 2010;92(2):196-201.

This report from the Norwegian Arthroplasty Register at up to 20-year follow-up reports that intermediate-term fixation was 87% to 100%, but because of wear, osteolysis, and dislocation, revision for any reason was 81% to 92%. In a study of 9,113 primary uncemented acetabular components, the authors found that most performed well up to 7 years.

101. Della Valle CJ, Mesko NW, Quigley L, Rosenberg AG, Jacobs JJ, Galante JO: Primary total hip arthroplasty with a porous-coated acetabular component: A concise follow-up, at a minimum of twenty years, of previous reports. *J Bone Joint Surg Am* 2009;91(5):1130-1135.

The authors evauated the longer-term outcomes of primary THAs with a porous-coated acetabular component at minimum 20-year follow-up. Rate of survival at 20 years was 96%.

102. Della Valle CJ, Berger RA, Shott S, et al: Primary total hip arthroplasty with a porous-coated acetabular component: A concise follow-up of a previous report. *J Bone Joint Surg Am* 2004;86-A(6):1217-1222.

103. Anseth SD, Pulido PA, Adelson WS, Patil S, Sandwell JC, Colwell CW Jr: Fifteen-year to twenty-year results of cementless Harris-Galante porous femoral and Harris-Galante porous I and II acetabular components. *J Arthroplasty* 2010;25(5):687-691.

In a study of long-term survivorship of primary THA using cementless Harris-Galante porous femoral and Harris-Galante porous I or II acetabular components, the overall survival rate was 87.7%.

104. Dearborn JT, Murray WR: Arthopor 2 acetabular component with screw fixation in primary hip arthroplasty: A 7- to 9-year follow-up study. *J Arthroplasty* 1998;13(3):299-310.

105. Demmelmeyer U, Schraml A, Hönle W, Schuh A: Long-term results of the standard Wagner cup. *Int Orthop* 2010;34(1):33-37.

Clinical and radiographic follow-up of 102 Wagner cup implants over a 12-year period revealed an overall survival rate of 93.1%.

106. Zenz P, Stiehl JB, Knechtel H, Titzer-Hochmaier G, Schwagerl W: Ten-year follow-up of the non-porous Allofit cementless acetabular component. *J Bone Joint Surg Br* 2009;91(11):1443-1447.

Results indicated that the nonporous titanium acetabular component led to a high survival rate (97.5%) after 11.9 years.

107. Clohisy JC, Harris WH: Matched-pair analysis of cemented and cementless acetabular reconstruction in primary total hip arthroplasty. *J Arthroplasty* 2001;16(6):697-705.

108. Dorr LD: Fixation of the acetabular component: The case for cementless bone ingrowth modular sockets. *J Arthroplasty* 1996;11(1):3-5, discussion 5-6.

Chapter 23

Revision Total Hip Arthroplasty

Paul T. H. Lee, MB BCh, MA, FRCS (Eng), FRCS (Orth)   Allan E. Gross, MD, FRCSC, O.Ont
James A. Browne, MD   David G. Lewallen, MD   Steven H. Weeden, MD   Craig J. Della Valle, MD

Acetabulum
Paul T. H. Lee, MB BCh, MA, FRCS (Eng), FRCS (Orth)
Allan E. Gross, MD, FRCSC, O.Ont
James A. Browne, MD
David G. Lewallen, MD

The main challenges of revision acetabular surgery include adequate exposure, safe implant removal, navigating bone defects, obtaining immediate mechanical implant stability, and achieving joint stability. Equalization of leg lengths, an anatomic hip center, and restoration of bone stock are desirable but secondary goals.

Classification

Classification of acetabular bone defects in revision surgery helps direct treatment options and guides expectations in outcome, facilitates communication, and allows comparison of treatment outcomes for similar defect types. Clinical results are dependent on the extent of bone stock damage and more importantly, the bone remaining to support the revision component (rim, columns, superior dome, medial wall, and ischium).

Commonly used systems for classification of bone stock damage based on AP radiographs focus on characterization of defects. The three most widely used classifications are those of Paprosky, D'Antonio et al, and Saleh and Gross.[1-3] The Saleh and Gross classification is based on the actual acetabular bone stock remaining at final reaming after implant/cement/debris removal—type I defect: no significant bone loss; type II: contained cavitary defects, rim and column intact; type III: uncontained segmental defects involving less than 50% of the acetabulum and one column; type IV: uncontained segmental defects involving more than 50% of the acetabulum and both columns; and type V: defects with pelvic discontinuity. Two studies have reported excellent reproducibility and validity[4,5] (Figure 1). Furthermore, the classification is prognostic, simple to communicate, and focuses on reconstructive potential. This classification will be discussed in this chapter unless stated otherwise.

Surgical Approach

The approach chosen is usually dependent on the reason for revision, the need to address bone loss, previous

Dr. Lee or an immediate family member has received research or institutional support from The Royal College of Surgeons of England, the British Orthopaedic Association, and the John Charnley Trust. Dr. Gross or an immediate family member has received royalties from Zimmer; is a member of a Speakers' bureau or has made paid presentations on behalf of Zimmer; is a paid consultant for or is an employee of Zimmer; and serves as a board member, owner, officer, or committee member of the Canadian Orthopaedic Association, the Knee Society, and the Hip Society. Dr. Lewallen or an immediate family member has received royalties from Orthosonics, Osteotech, and Zimmer and is a board member, owner, officer, or committee member of the merican Joint Replacement Registry, the Hip Society, the MidAmerica Orthopaedic Association, and the Orthopaedic Research and Education Foundation. Dr. Della Valle or an immediate family member is a paid consultant for or an employee of Biomet, Convatec, and Smith & Nephew; is an unpaid consultant for CD Diagnostics; has received research or institutional support from Pacira, Smith & Nephew, and Zimmer; and serves as a board member, owner, officer, or committee member of the American Association of Hip and Knee Surgeons and the Arthritis Foundation. Neither Dr. Browne nor any immediate family member has received anything of value from or owns stock in a commercial company or institution related directly or indirectly to the subject of this chapter.

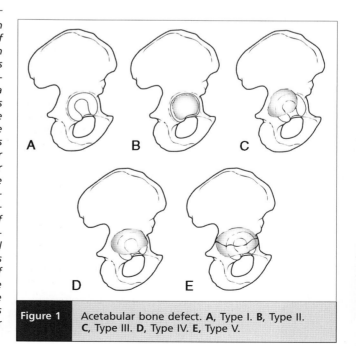

Figure 1 Acetabular bone defect. **A,** Type I. **B,** Type II. **C,** Type III. **D,** Type IV. **E,** Type V.

3: Hip

surgical incision and approach, and the training and preference of the surgeon. A standard approach, for example, the (modified) transgluteal approach (**Figure 2**) for primary hip arthroplasty may suffice for liner exchange but should be more extensile to accommodate unforeseen cup or stem loosening or bone loss that needs to be treated. Revision of one or both components, extensive osteolysis, deep infection, periprosthetic fracture, and recurrent dislocation usually require revision approaches for adequate exposure. This

will facilitate removal of implants/cement/debris with minimal bone loss or risk of periprosthetic fracture. Soft-tissue function, especially in recurrent dislocators, should be preserved.

The traditional anterior approaches (Smith-Peterson, Watson-Jones) may compromise soft-tissue function without adequate exposure and are nonextensile.

The posterior approach provides good exposure to the acetabulum and femur and is extensile. It preserves abductors but compromises external rotators and posterior capsule integrity, especially with leg lengthening during revision, and is associated with higher dislocation rates. A trochanteric osteotomy provides excellent circumferential exposure to the acetabulum and proximal femur but is associated with trochanteric nonunion, avulsion, escape, and abductor impairment. A trochanteric sliding osteotomy was developed as an extensile approach for the posterior approach. It maintains vastus lateralis attachment to the trochanteric fragment to oppose gluteus medius pull and decrease the risks of trochanteric avulsion and escape. However, the external rotators and posterior capsule are still compromised and concerns with posterior hip dislocation remain.

The modified trochanteric sliding osteotomy[6] (**Figure 3**) was developed to maintain the integrity of the external rotators and posterior capsule by leaving a posterior sleeve of the greater trochanter on the proximal femur, flipping the trochanteric fragment anteriorly with the gluteus medius and vastus lateralis attached, and using an anterior capsulectomy for access into the joint. Goodman et al[6] reported a decrease in dislocation rate from 14.8% (n = 27) to 3.3% (n = 30) by converting

Figure 2	Drawing of the acetabulum showing that care must be taken to avoid excessive splitting of the gluteus medius during a modified anterolateral approach to prevent damage to the superior gluteal nerve.

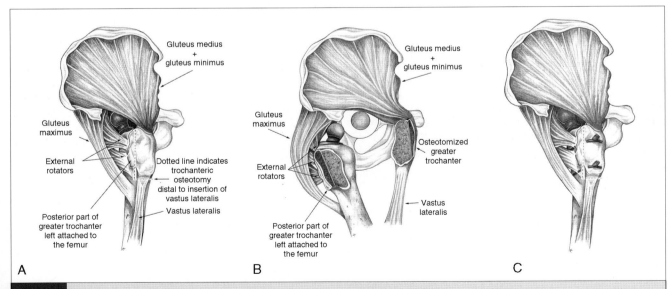

Figure 3	Diagrams of the right hip. **A**, The planned plane of osteotomy, immediately anterior to the insertion of the short external rotators, exiting just distal to the origins of the vastus lateralis. **B**, The osteotomy was performed, and the hip was dislocated. **C**, The osteotomy was fixed back in place with two cerclage wires. (Reproduced with permission from Lakstein D, Backstein D, Safir O, Kosashvili Y, Gross AE: Modified trochanteric slide for complex hip arthroplasty. *J Arthroplasty* 2010;25:363-368. http://www.sciencedirect.com/science/journal/08835403.)

from a traditional trochanteric slide to the modified trochanteric slide technique for revision hip surgery.

The extended sliding trochanteric osteotomy was used as an extensile approach for the posterior approach to allow more extensive exposure to the femoral shaft while maintaining the integrity of the abductor and vastus lateralis on the trochanteric fragment. The modified extended sliding trochanteric osteotomy, similar to the modified trochanteric slide, preserves external rotators and posterior capsule integrity by leaving a posterior sleeve of greater trochanter on the proximal femur and approaching the joint anteriorly. It allows greater posterior stability over the traditional extended sliding trochanteric osteotomy and higher union rates over the modified sliding trochanteric osteotomy because of a larger surface area for better bony opposition and repair.

Removing an intrapelvic prosthesis or cement requires optimal exposure with a revision approach to minimize risks to intrapelvic neurovascular structures, which include perforation and traction injuries caused by reactive fibrous adhesions to cup and cement. A preoperative CT angiogram of the iliac vessels is advised when the protrusion is substantial.

Removal of Components

The goal of component removal in acetabular revision is to minimize iatrogenic bone loss. The approach to component extraction depends on the type of implant and method of fixation to host bone.

Well-fixed cemented cups are generally removed by first separating the polyethylene component from the underlying cement. Various gouges and osteotomes may be used for this purpose. The underlying cement may then be removed in piecemeal fashion with osteotomes and a burr. All-polyethylene cups may also be removed with the use of a reamer or threaded extractor.

The successful removal of well-fixed cementless components has historically been very challenging, often resulting in significant bone loss. After removal of the modular liner and screws, curved gouges have traditionally been used to divide the bone-implant interface. Several other techniques, including the use of pneumatic impact wrenches, have been described. Recently, cup extraction systems with curved blades specific to the diameter of the cup (such as the Explant Acetabular Removal System; Zimmer, Warsaw, IN) have been developed to assist with this process. Short and long blades are attached to a ball and rotating handle; they are used consecutively to first penetrate dense peripheral bone and create a channel and subsequently to free the dome of the cup from bone. Multiple diameters of the pivot ball are available to center the device and cutting blade within the polyethylene liner. In the presence of adjunctive dome screws, the liner must first be removed to allow screw removal. Trial liners and bipolar trials may also be used to provide centralization of the instrument if the liner is damaged, atypically sized, or absent (such as with a large-diameter hip resurfacing

acetabular component). Recent clinical studies have confirmed this technique to be simple and efficacious in preservation of host bone stock.[7,8]

Treatment Algorithm
Contained Defects
Type I defects can be treated using the standard cemented or uncemented primary-type cup with midterm results similar to those of uncemented primary hip arthroplasty. Type II defects are contained and represent most acetabular defects. Most contained defects can be treated with morcellized bone graft with uncemented cups, especially when there is more than 50% host bone contact. Larger defects can be treated with impaction grafting with mesh and a cemented cup.[9] If there is host bone contact superiorly and inferomedially, satisfactory results have been reported using morcellized bone graft with either a jumbo uncemented cup and multiple screws or a roof reinforcement ring and cemented cup. For global defects, morcellized bone graft protected by reconstruction cage contact and a cemented cup has been used as an alternative approach if mechanical support for traditional uncemented cups is inadequate. Overall midterm to long-term survivorship rates are in the 85% to 95% range. Recently, early success has been reported with porous tantalum cups for larger contained defects with less than 50% host bone contact,[10] leading some to extend the indications for uncemented cup use.

Uncontained Defects
Type III, IV, and V defects present an increasing surgical challenge. Treatment of type III defects includes high hip center arthroplasty, oblong or eccentric cups, jumbo cups, minor column structural allografts, or porous tantalum cups and augments with good to excellent short-term to midterm results. Type IV and V defects are most challenging and options are few. Treatment options include major column structural allograft with reconstruction cages or custom-made triflange cups and Trabecular Metal (Zimmer) cup-cage constructs. Short-term to midterm results are encouraging given the degree of complexity and higher rates of complication. Excision arthroplasty may be inevitable in some but is reserved as a last resort because of poor functional outcomes.

Hemispherical Porous-Coated Components
The hemispherical uncemented cup is the most common component used in revision total hip arthroplasty (THA). With supportive host bone and a reliable ingrowth surface, these cups can be used to treat most acetabular revisions. Initial stability is often obtained with a press-fit and supplemental screw fixation. Morcellized bone grafting of osteolytic cavitary defects is typically performed with reliable radiographic incorporation. More complex reconstruction methods may be required in patients with significant bone loss.

Multiple studies from different institutions and the use of various implant designs have demonstrated a

3: Hip

low incidence of revision for aseptic loosening of these implants at medium-term follow-up. Recent long-term studies demonstrate good survivorship. A report on 77 acetabular revisions at a minimum of 20 years indicated a 95% survivorship with revision of the shell for aseptic loosening as the end point. With revision of the acetabular component for any reason as the end point, survivorship still remained 82% at 20 years.[11]

Jumbo Components

The use of extra-large porous-coated acetabular components is one approach to obtaining mechanical stability in the presence of acetabular bone deficiency. The large surface area of host bone contact is beneficial for mechanical stability, bone ingrowth, and load transfer to the pelvis. Extra-large sockets also tend to normalize the center of rotation of the hip, avoid bony impingement, allow for a large femoral head, and improve soft-tissue tension. Disadvantages include the sacrifice of bone, inability to reconstitute bone stock, and impingement on soft-tissue structures including the iliopsoas. When the superoinferior dimension is much greater than the anteroposterior dimension, a jumbo cup may require excessive reaming of the anterior and posterior columns and a different approach may be required.

There is no universally accepted definition of a jumbo cup. The authors of one study used a diameter greater than 65 mm, whereas authors in another study used a diameter of 66 mm in males and 62 mm in females.[12,13] From a technical standpoint, use of these cups is fairly straightforward and familiar to most surgeons, although care must be taken to avoid excessive reaming of the superior and posterior bone. Sufficient bone stock for good initial press fit and stability is a prerequisite for successful use of these implants, and multiple screws are typically used.

Results of jumbo cup reconstructions have generally been satisfactory, with survival rates greater than 90% at midterm follow-up.[12,13] A recent follow-up of 12 patients at a mean of 13.9 years revealed no revisions for aseptic loosening and no radiographic evidence of loosening.[14]

Oblong Components

In an attempt to obtain implant stability on viable host bone, oblong components have been developed to accommodate commonly encountered bone defects. Loose acetabular implants will often migrate superiorly, leaving an oblong defect that is greater from superior to inferior than from anterior to posterior. A hemispherical shape can be difficult to obtain without reaming away the anterior and posterior columns. This situation is most commonly encountered in smaller (often female) patients, in whom the anteroposterior dimension is limited. By matching the shape of this oblong defect to the shape of the cup, intimate bone contact and cup stability can theoretically be obtained with a porous-coated component. The bone defect is filled with metal to obviate the need for structural bone

graft, and the hip center is restored to the anatomic position.

The use of these implants may be technically challenging. Special reamers are often required, and appropriate component position may be difficult to obtain. Simultaneous restoration of an appropriate hip center of rotation, contact on host bone, and proper version and inclination can be difficult. In the past, these challenges have led to the selection of a structural bone graft for structural support instead. In many centers, the more recent use of a modular porous metal augment system has reduced the use of oblong and structural grafts in these cases.

Clinical results with midterm follow-up have been variable. In a recent study of 35 longitudinal oblong revision cups, 14% of the acetabular components had migrated and required revision at a mean of 6.3 years.[15] A second study of an oblong revision cup suggested that better results correlate with restoring the hip center of rotation and reducing limb-length discrepancy. The clinical data are sparse, with only a few studies limited to a small number of patients, multiple implant designs, and short-term follow-up.

High Hip Center Arthroplasty

A high hip center method involves placing the uncemented acetabular component superiorly against remaining bone of the ilium to achieve implant stability. This has been referred to as "chasing the good bone." A small-diameter acetabular component is often needed given the restraints of the bony anatomy. Although this technique is fairly straightforward, there are significant biomechanical disadvantages related to abductor function, and a large proportion of these patients will experience a significant limp postoperatively. Hip stability may also be compromised because of bony impingement as well as the small femoral head size dictated by the small cup. Femoral revision is required when using this method to restore soft-tissue tension and leg length. High-offset femoral components may increase the bending moment on the stem and lead to loosening.

Several studies have shown good intermediate-term survival with porous-coated implants placed at a high hip center.[16] A recent study revealed a survival rate of 93% at a mean of 16.8 years with revision of the acetabular shell because of aseptic loosening as the end point.[17] The need for isolated cup revision in the presence of a well-fixed stem may make this technique problematic because of hip instability from impingement and shortening of the limb. Given the disadvantages noted, the high hip center technique has seen decreasing popularity in favor of other techniques.

Impaction Bone Grafting

Unlike many methods of dealing with bone loss, impaction bone grafting is a biologic technique that offers the attractive potential for bone stock reconstitution. This method involves the closure of segmental bone defects with metal wire mesh followed by the replacement of cavitary bone defects with morcellized allograft bone. Stability is conferred through the use of dense impaction and cement. Recent histologic studies have suggested that survival of the construct depends on graft incorporation, suggesting that host bone may play an important role in the success of this technique.

Impaction grafting is a technically demanding procedure. The method of graft preparation has been shown to be important for mechanical stability of the cup. The choice of bone graft is controversial and the topic of several recent articles in the literature. A recent Cochrane Database systematic review found insufficient evidence to recommend processed (freeze dried or irradiated) bone in comparison with fresh frozen (unprocessed) bone for impacting grafting of the acetabulum.[18] Proponents have suggested that grafting be done with large size cancellous particulate graft (7 to 10 mm).

Results of this technique for cavitary defects have generally been good, with survival approaching 85% to 90% at 20 years.[5,19] However, a recent report on 23 hips with uncontained segmental acetabular defects included two patients with early mechanical failure and an overall survival rate with further revision as an end point of 90.8% at an average of 36 months. Mesh rupture was seen in three hips, and significant migration of the cup was seen in all patients.[20] Another recent study demonstrated a poor survival rate with severe bone defects (AAOS type III or IV).[21] These reports suggest that this technique is an excellent option for patients with small or moderate-sized acetabular defects with no discontinuity. The use of this method in the treatment of larger segmental defects and pelvic discontinuities remains challenging and has led some groups to investigate the use of structural support such as porous metal augments as an adjunct to impaction grafting.

Structural Allografts

Structural allograft in the treatment of uncontained acetabular defects can be used to restore host bone stock, physiologic hip center, and leg length. It provides adequate support for primary implant fixation stability and potentially converts uncontained to contained defects to facilitate future revision surgery. The disadvantages of this technique are lack of universal availability, technical difficulties, the potential for disease transmission, and the possibility of late graft resorption and collapse.

Minor column or shelf allograft is used to describe a structural graft that provides 50% or less support to the new acetabular component (**Figure 4**). The midterm results with the use of minor column (shelf) allograft for defects involving less than 50% of the acetabulum and only one column (type III) are encouraging, with approximately 75% cup survivorship for aseptic loosening at a mean follow-up of 10 years.[22,23] The results for the use of bulk femoral head, acetabular, or distal femur allografts were similar.

Despite concerns with long-term graft resorption, collapse, and failure, midterm to long-term studies have shown that during rerevision surgery, most of the bulk

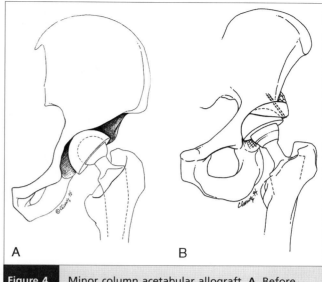

Figure 4 — Minor column acetabular allograft. **A,** Before surgery. **B,** After surgery. (Reproduced with permission from Woodgate I, Gross AE: Minor column structural acetabular allografts in revision hip arthroplasty. *Clin Orthop Relat Res* 2000;371: 75-85.)

allograft remained intact with host-graft boundaries obscured, enabling cup-only exchanges. One recent report showed an 80% Kaplan-Meier graft survivorship for aseptic loosening at 15 and 20 years follow-up.[24]

It is important to separate the results of structural allograft for type III from type IV or V defects because the results for type III defects are generally better than those for type IV or V defects. This is an understandable finding because segmental defects involving more than 50% of the acetabulum and both columns (type IV) with pelvic discontinuity (type V) are difficult to treat. Major column allograft is used to describe a structural graft that provides more than 50% support to the new acetabular component (**Figure 5**). The use of major column allografts without support by an antiprotrusio ilioischial cage has been met with poor results, with short-term to midterm survivorship rates of 45% to 60%.[3,25] When major column structural allografts were supported by reconstruction cages securely fixed to the ilium and ischium in conjunction with cemented cups, the results were more encouraging with survivorship rates of approximately 77% to 87%.[26] The cage protects the structural graft by providing pelvic stability in spanning across the ilium and ischium and offloading the graft until bony interdigitation occurs.

Higher rates of dislocation and sciatic nerve palsy have been associated with the use of bulk structural allograft in conjunction with ilioischial cages. These rates can be improved by slotting the inferior flange of the cage into the ischium to provide a more stable fixation and more horizontal position, and preventing exposure of the sciatic nerve.

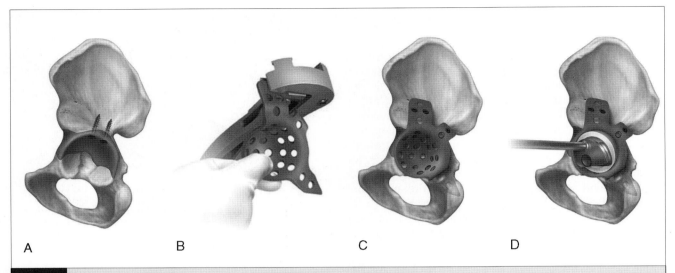

Figure 5 Treatment of a major column defect with an ilioischial cage. **A,** Major column allograft, used for uncontained acetabular defect and more than 50% for acetabulum, is fixed with screws. **B,** The iliac flanges of the ilioischial cage are contoured. **C,** The ischial flange is slotted into the ischium and the iliac flanges fixed with screws to the ilium. **D,** The acetabular component is cemented into the cage in a position that is independent to the cage position. (Reproduced with permission from Gross AE, Goodman S: The current role of structural grafts and cages in revision arthroplasty of the hip. *Clin Orthop Relat Res* 2004;429:193-200.)

Porous Tantalum Cups and Augments

Porous tantalum, also known as Trabecular Metal, has high volumetric porosity (75% to 85%) and high frictional characteristics (40% to 75% higher than traditional porous coatings) that make it conducive to biologic fixation with extensive bony ingrowth. It is safe, biocompatible, and has a modulus of elasticity (3 MPa) similar to that of subchondral bone to allow better physiologic load transfer and yet a higher endurance limit and yield and ultimate strength. In acetabular revision, its use as a cup component has shown encouraging early results and its use as an augment may serve as a structural bone graft substitute. Disadvantages include notch sensitivity, brittleness, expense, and the lack of host bone stock restoration.

Trabecular Metal cups without augments have been used in type I and II defects with excellent early results. Authors of a 2009 study reported a cup survivorship of 96% (n = 53) using Trabecular Metal cups without augments for contained defects involving more than 50% of the acetabulum at a mean follow-up of 3.8 years (range, 2.0 to 5.9 years).[10]

The use of Trabecular Metal cups with the optional use of augments in type III, IV, and V defects has also shown good early results.[27-29] One study reported a cup survivorship of 96.4% (n = 28) using Trabecular Metal cups and augments for type III defects at a mean follow-up of 3.1 years (range, 1 to 4 years).[28] Another study reported a cup survivorship of 98% with the use of Trabecular Metal cups and augments for 33 type III and 10 type V defects at a mean follow-up of 2.8 years (range, 2 to 4 years).[29] The initial success using porous tantalum has prompted several other manufacturers to

develop porous metal acetabular components, generally fabricated of highly porous titanium. Results of such newer devices are not yet available.

Porous Tantalum Cup-Cage Construct

The use of ilioischial cages without support by structural allograft in type IV or V defects has been met with mechanical failures because traditional cages were not made with materials that promoted bone ongrowth or ingrowth for permanent fixation and succumbed to loosening or fatigue fractures. With current technology, it is not possible to incorporate Trabecular Metal into reconstructive cages because of its brittleness or to coat the cage flanges with Trabecular Metal because of notch sensitivity. Furthermore, the risk of junctional fatigue fractures persists if the cage is not supported by host bone stock or structural graft.

The use of the Trabecular Metal cup-cage construct was first described in 2005.[30] The main indications for this construct are for type IV and V defects but also large global type II defects, where cup contact with host bone is inadequate to acquire rigid screw fixation for the uncemented cup for initial stable cup fixation. The construct involves filling the deficient acetabular floor with morcellized bone graft, impacting or securing a large trabecular metal cup over the defect with screws into the ilium, placing an antiprotrusio ilioischial cage over the cup, and cementing a polyethylene liner into the cage (**Figure 6**). The cage is fixed to the ilium with screws and to the ischium by slotting the inferior flange into the ischium. The rationale for the construct is for the well-secured ilioischial cage to initially protect and offload the Trabecular Metal cup to

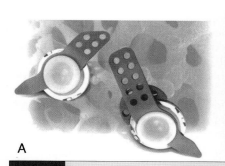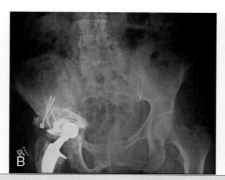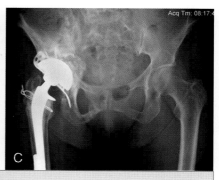

Figure 6 **A,** Illustration of the Trabecular Metal cup-cage construct. **B,** Radiograph showing a failed cemented acetabular component associated with massive bone loss, pelvic discontinuity, and component protrusion into the pelvis. **C,** Cup-cage acetabular device with porous metal acetabular shells and modular wedges. (Reproduced with permission from Boscainos PJ, Kellett CF, Maury AC, Backstein DJ, Gross AE: Management of periacetabular bone loss in revision hip arthroplasty. *Clin Orthop Relat Res* 2007;465:159-165.

allow time for bony ingrowth and cup stabilization. This will also allow incorporation and remodeling of morcellized graft placed beneath the cup. Subsequently, the stabilized cup will help support the cage to prevent fatigue.

Early results for these difficult conditions are encouraging. A 2009 study reported a cup survivorship of 88.5% for aseptic loosening with the use of the Trabecular Metal cup-cage construct for massive segmental bone defects associated with pelvic discontinuity at a mean follow-up of 3.7 years (range, 2.0 to 5.7 years).[31]

Femur
Steven H. Weeden, MD
Craig J. Della Valle, MD

The combination of today's aging population and the acceptance of THA in younger patients has resulted in an incremental increase in the revision rates for THA.[32] The revision surgeon must have a thorough understanding of the surgical techniques required to safely remove the existing implant while preserving bone stock. Knowledge of various revision implant systems and the appropriate indications for each is essential.

Indications for Femoral Revision

Patients under consideration for revision THA represent a complex diagnostic challenge. The symptoms associated with a failed THA may include startup pain, instability, or the presence of new leg-length inequality. In patients with infection, symptoms may include pain at rest, constitutional symptoms, and occasional localized inflammation or even drainage. Care must be taken to differentiate these findings from nonhip sources such as mechanical low back pain, radiculopathy, abdominopelvic pathology, soft-tissue injury, or greater trochanteric bursitis.

To identify the source of the discomfort, the evaluation must include a thorough history and physical examination. Any pain should be carefully recorded in terms of location, severity, character, and precipitating and relieving activities. The presence or absence of a postoperative pain-free interval and duration of symptoms are noted. A comprehensive physical examination should include an evaluation of gait and range of motion of both hips and knees, and a neurologic examination. Radiographic studies should include at minimum an AP and lateral view of the femur and an AP pelvic radiograph.[33] These radiographic views are evaluated to determine the overall stability of the implants, evidence of instability, and presence of fractures, wear, or osteolysis. The criteria for the assessment of cemented component loosening, including the presence and extent of radiolucent lines, implant migration, and cement mantle fracture, has been delineated.[34] Similarly, cementless stem fixation can be evaluated using the criteria of Engh et al.[35] Major signs of loosening include the absence of spot welds and implant migration. Minor signs of loosening include calcar hypertrophy, the absence of stress shielding, bead shedding, or pedestal formation. Other studies—including CT, bone scan, ultrasound, and MRI—and aspiration are used when indicated. Laboratory studies, including complete blood count, C-reactive protein, and erythrocyte sedimentation rate, should be obtained in an attempt to rule out occult infection. In patients with metal-on-metal articulations, cobalt-chromium blood levels and a metal artifact reduction sequence MRI may be considered.

Prior to femoral revision, the patient should have demonstrated one or more of the indications for surgical intervention: aseptic loosening, severe femoral osteolysis, malposition, severe thigh pain, metal sensitivity, or infection. Intraoperative indications for femoral revision include excessive damage to the Morse taper at the time of revision, inadequate exposure during acetabular revision, instability after revision of the acetabular component with inadequate neck length or offset options, and monoblock stem mismatch of the femoral head or damage to a monoblock stem femoral head.[36-40]

Femoral Component Extraction

Preoperative radiographs should establish whether or not the femoral component is well fixed.[35,41] Extraction of a well-fixed cemented or cementless femoral component can be time consuming and may incur significant damage to the remaining host bone. Removal of loose components is usually less arduous and destructive to the host bone.

Cemented Femoral Component Removal

In most instances, the removal of cemented femoral components includes the disruption of the implant-cement interface, removal of the component, and subsequent extraction of retained cement. As with all surgical procedures, visualization is paramount, especially the entire proximal portion of the femoral component (including the lateral shoulder). This procedure is routinely performed with the use of a high-speed pencil-tip burr or an osteotome. A loose component that has undergone subsidence may have bone overgrowth in the vicinity of the collar; thus, medial calcar bone may need to be resected before implant removal.

Femoral stems that are highly polished or that have debonded from their cement mantle may be removed with a retrograde blow via a tamp, an implant-specific femoral component extractor, or a universal extraction device. A carbide-tipped burr may be used to notch the femoral neck to enhance purchase of the universal extraction device to the prosthesis.

Well-fixed textured, porous coated, and precoated components commonly require disruption of the implant-cement interface before disimpaction. Disruption of this interface can be performed with the use of flexible osteotomes. However, use of these devices increases the risk of femoral fracture or perforation. A high-speed pencil-tip burr is effective for this task and reduces the risk of fracture during disruption of the implant-cement interface. If a collar impedes access medially, a carbide-tipped metal cutting burr may be used to notch or remove the collar and allow access to the medial implant surface.

Highly textured, well-fixed cemented femoral stems are not easily removed. The previously described techniques only afford access to the metaphyseal region of the stem. If the prosthesis-cement enhancement extends beyond the metaphysis, an extended proximal femoral osteotomy may be required.[42] An extended proximal femoral osteotomy is indicated when there is well-bonded distal cement, varus or valgus remodeling of the proximal femur, or when cement extends past the apex of the anterior bow of the femur. Alternatively, a femoral window can be used. An oval window is created anteriorly using a combination of drill holes and high-speed burr. Once the window is removed, a high-speed pencil-tip burr may be used to disrupt the distal cement-implant interface. Once the proximal and distal cement-implant interfaces are disrupted, a carbide-tipped punch and mallet may be used to extricate the component with retrograde blows. When cement removal is completed, the window is replaced and fixed with cables. This technique is not commonly used because most revision physicians are comfortable performing an extended proximal femoral osteotomy.

Once a cemented component is extracted, the quality of the residual cement mantle is evaluated. Recementing a femoral component into a preexisting intact cement mantle has been described.[43,44] If no significant cement voids are identified and the bone-cement interface is well maintained, the cement surface is roughened using high-speed burrs. Care must be taken to prevent perforation of the distal cement mantle. Consideration should be given to the use of an ultrasonic tool.[44] A new, smaller prosthesis is then cemented into the modified cement mantle.

It is often preferable to remove the entire cement mantle. This process is undertaken in a stepwise fashion, moving from proximal to distal. Metaphyseal cement may be debulked with a high-speed burr and then split longitudinally into segments with a standard osteotome or special T or V cementatome. The cement is then removed with a reverse hook, curet, or pituitary rongeur. It is imperative to clear the proximal femur before proceeding distally to provide adequate visualization of the femoral canal. When an extended trochanteric osteotomy (ETO) has been performed, the proximal cement is easily removed under direct vision. The cement may be sectioned with a high-speed burr and then removed with special osteotomes. If present, the distal cement plug is then removed. An ETO allows a more direct approach to the distal cement plug. Alternatively, controlled perforation has been described with good results; however, fracture through the perforation is a major concern.[45]

Often a distal bony pedestal is present. The bony pedestal should be perforated with a long drill or an X osteotome. The remaining bony pedestal is removed by applying a retrograde force to a reverse hook placed through the pedestal perforation. Alternatively, sequential flexible reamers may be used to "ream away" the pedestal. This reaming may be performed with the use of fluoroscopy or radiographic assistance if desired.

Upon completion of cement removal, the femoral canal must be assessed to ensure that a perforation has not occurred. Intraoperative radiographs help ensure complete cement removal and the absence of cortical defects or fractures.

If a controlled perforation is undertaken, the revision stem must bypass the last perforation by at least two cortical diameters or 5 cm.[45] If a cemented stem is to be replaced, compression over the holes using a sterile glove or similar device is required to prevent cement extrusion. One study reported 219 cases using the controlled perforation technique with 9 femoral fractures, only one occurring through a perforation site.[45]

Cementless Stem Removal
Proximally Coated Femoral Implants
If the component is loose, disimpaction of the prosthesis with a universal femoral component extractor or

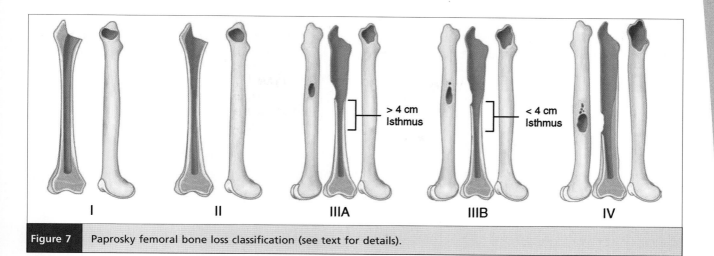

Figure 7   Paprosky femoral bone loss classification (see text for details).

with an implant-specific extraction device may be necessary. In contrast, if a proximally coated femoral implant is well fixed, the bone-implant interface must be divided. Either flexible osteotomes or a high-speed burr may be used. If a collar prevents access to the proximal-medial interface, a carbide-tipped burr may be used to notch or remove the collar. If the prosthesis does not dislodge with moderate retrograde force, an ETO to allow distal interface access and division should be considered.

Proximally coated, nontapered stems are commonly removed without the use of an osteotomy, unless there is evidence of trochanteric overgrowth (in which case an osteotomy may be performed in an attempt to preserve bone stock). In contrast, the removal of a well-ingrown proximally porous-coated tapered stem frequently requires the use of an extended femoral osteotomy.[46] The geometry of the tapered stem design makes access to the bone-implant interface with an osteotome difficult. Moreover, large metaphyseal-filling femoral stems also allow little space for the insertion of flexible osteotomes or a burr. One may elect to perform an ETO for removal of wedge-shaped and metaphyseal-filling femoral components.[39] Ideally, 4 to 6 cm of diaphyseal femoral bone should remain beyond the ETO to allow satisfactory support for the revision stem.

Fully Porous-Coated Stems
A well-fixed fully porous-coated stem is particularly difficult to remove.[36] The use of an ETO is recommended. The osteotomy length is determined preoperatively and is based on several factors including preservation of host bone, stem length, and femoral anatomy. The porous-coated surface must be exposed to the level of the cylindrical portion of the implant. Once the osteotomy is completed, removal techniques are similar to those described previously. Three to five disimpaction blows are attempted to free the femoral component. If the component does not easily disengage from the femur, the femoral stem should be transected at the

distal level of the osteotomy along with trephination of the remaining retained component. Care is taken to ensure that only the femoral component is cut. Modular cementless femoral components may be extremely difficult to extricate. It is important to have component-specific extraction instruments from the manufacturer available during removal. The same techniques described for cementless femoral stem removal are then used to remove these modular components.

Revision Implants Based on Femoral Defect
The most commonly used classification for femoral defects is that described by Paprosky[47] (Figure 7). This widely used classification facilitates communication among clinicians and allows for meaningful scientific comparison of various revision techniques for various degrees of bone stock damage. Because it correlates with surgical complexity, it is useful for patient education and also for determining if a given case lies within a revision surgeon's comfort zone.

With a comprehensive understanding of this classification system, the surgeon can anticipate the intraoperative pathology and the appropriate reconstruction options (Table 1, Figure 8). Type I defects typically have normal femoral bone stock and are associated with acetabular revisions or a failed cup arthroplasty (resurfacing) implant. In a type II defect, there is loss of cancellous bone in the metaphysis region that precludes the use of a standard length cemented femoral component. The metaphysis, however, is still supportive and can sometimes be relied on for fixation. Common reconstructive options include a modular, metaphyseal-engaging stem with a proximal sleeve, a diaphyseal-stabilizing stem, or a fully porous-coated implant. If the porous-coated implant is selected, the stem should be of adequate length to engage at least 4 cm of the femoral isthmus; a 6-inch stem is typically adequate during type II reconstruction. Type III defects are characterized by metaphyseal and diaphyseal damage. The metaphysis is no longer supportive and there is variable damage to the remaining isthmus. Type III defects are subdi-

3: Hip

Table 1

Femoral Reconstruction Based on Paprosky Defect

Defect Type	Femoral Pathology	Reconstruction Options
I	Condition similar to primary THA Minimal bone loss	Implant similar to one used in primary THA Fully porous-coated, diaphyseal engaging stem
II	Metaphyseal compromised bone Minimal diaphyseal damage	Fully porous-coated, diaphyseal engaging stem (bowed) Modular, metaphyseal engaging stem with a proximal sleeve and diaphyseal stabilizing stem
III A	Significant proximal and metadiaphyseal femoral bone loss Minimum 4-cm scratch-fit is obtainable at isthmus	Fully porous-coated, diaphyseal engaging stem (modular or monoblock) Modular tapered implant. Consider particularly if canal diameter > 18 mm and/or if torsional remodeling of the femur is present
III B	Extensive metaphyseal and diaphyseal bone loss Less than 4 cm available for scratch fit; fixation must be obtained more distally	Modular tapered implant Impaction bone grafting
IV	Extensive femoral metadiaphyseal damage (up to or past isthmus) with thin cortices and widened canals	Modular tapered implant Impaction bone grafting Allograft prosthetic component Low-demand patients requiring minimal surgical time: long-stem cemented femoral component or proximal femoral replacement (tumor prosthesis)

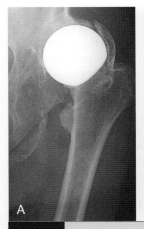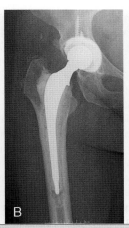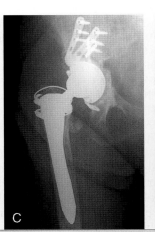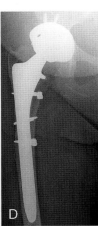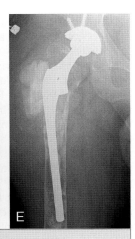

Figure 8 Paprosky femoral defect classification system. **A**, Type I. **B**, Type II. **C**, Type IIIA. **D**, Type IIIB. **E**, Type IV.

vided into types A and B based on the amount of isthmus remaining for distal fixation. Type IIIA femurs have at least 4 cm of intact isthmus available for distal fixation, whereas type IIIB femurs have less than 4 cm of intact isthmus. This differentiation is based on a clinical series in which a higher rate of failed ingrowth or fibrous ingrowth was seen in patients with less than 4 cm of intact isthmus.[48] In a type IIIA femur, a fully porous-coated, diaphyseal-engaging stem may be used. Appropriate stem length is based on the principle that a minimum of 4 cm of isthmus is engaged by the revision component (**Figure 9**). Surgeons should keep in mind

that the technical complexity of the reconstruction increases with longer stem length secondary to the bow of the femur. In general, the shortest stem that allows for adequate distal fixation should be chosen. Possible limitations to the use of a fully porous-coated, cementless implant for type IIIA femurs include a canal diameter greater than 18 mm, as reports have shown a higher rate of failure as compared to a titanium modular tapered stem.[49] A modular revision stem is also preferred in patients with torsional remodeling of the femur (usually into retroversion), a situation commonly encountered during revision of a loose femoral component. The use of a monolithic stem, in this situation, may lead to component retroversion, instability, or a proximal femoral insertional fracture as the surgeon attempts to force the stem into appropriate anteversion.

Type IIIB defects are most commonly treated with a titanium modular tapered revision implant. Impaction grafting is an alternative and may be theoretically attractive in younger patients with a contained femoral defect as bone stock restoration may be achieved. However, the technique of impaction grafting is challenging.[50] The North American experience with this method has been mixed; it is both time- and resource-intensive (secondary to the need for large amounts of bone graft), and is associated with a substantial risk of both intraoperative and early postoperative periprosthetic fracture, stem subsidence, and failure. A contemporary retrospective study of 69 revision THAs using impaction grafting demonstrated mild to moderate subsidence in 14.5% and massive subsidence in 7.2%. However, upon further analysis, patients with Endo-Klinik class III bone demonstrated a 76.6% incidence of subsidence and demonstrated that a higher Endo-Klinik class was the only independent predictor of early subsidence.[51]

In a type IV femoral defect, both the metaphysis and diaphysis are severely damaged and nonsupportive. The remaining isthmus is inadequate for distal fixation, making any type of cementless fixation extremely challenging. If the proximal femoral defect is contained, impaction grafting is an appealing option. If the proximal femoral defect is noncontained, a proximal femoral allograft-prosthetic composite or a proximal femoral replacement can be used.[41,42] Although an allograft-prosthetic composite offers the potential benefit of better soft-tissue attachment, the surgical technique is more complex than a proximal femoral replacement prosthesis. Abductor reattachment in either technique is unpredictable with a resultant high risk of instability postoperatively. A constrained acetabular liner or tripolar component may be required.[52,53] Cemented long-stemmed components are another potential solution if the femoral defect is contained and the patient is low demand. The use of modular tapered stems is another potential option; however, with no isthmus available for distal fixation, it may be difficult to gain adequate initial component stability for osseointegration to occur.

Revision With Fully Porous-Coated, Monolithic Stems

Monoblock, fully porous-coated stems continue to be the workhorse implant for most femoral revisions. The surgical technique is straightforward and familiar, and the published results have been excellent. Results are less satisfactory if less than 4 cm of isthmus is available for distal fixation, the isthmic diameter is larger than 18 mm, or the femur has undergone substantial remodeling into retroversion. Adequate diaphyseal stability must be obtained at the time of implant insertion and is typically achieved by underreaming the femoral isth-

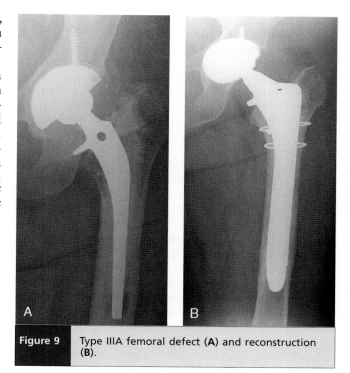

Figure 9 Type IIIA femoral defect (**A**) and reconstruction (**B**).

mus by 0.5 mm or line-to-line reaming. To assess the long-term survivorship of fully porous-coated monoblock femoral stems in a revision setting, a retrospective analysis of 905 femoral revisions was performed from 1980 through 2006.[54] The rerevision rate was 2.2%, with the indications including aseptic loosening (1.3%), infection (0.4%), and stem fracture (0.3%). All revisions were within the first 10 years from the index revision surgery, with a Kaplan-Meier survivorship curve of 95.9% at 10 years. Further analysis of the rerevisions (again revised with fully coated nonmodular implants) was performed. There were 13 patients available for study (mean follow-up, 9.8 years).[55] Two patients reported moderate to severe thigh pain, one had a fibrous ingrowth fixation, and all others had evidence of bone ingrowth. In this subset of patients, no further revision surgery was required.

Femoral component revision with extensively coated femoral components have yielded stable fixation with good to excellent long-term outcomes. However, the issues of thigh pain and stress-shielding remain concerning. Modification to the coating material has been attempted to address these concerns. Hydroxyapatite coating of implants has demonstrated increased bone ingrowth in revision, as well as decreased stress-shielding in primary cases.[56] A retrospective analysis of 59 femoral revisions with hydroxyapatite-coated femoral implants was performed, with an average follow-up of 3.3 years. The results demonstrated a 2% mechanical failure rate when excluding complication for fracture (6%) or infection (4%).[57] The advantages of hydroxyapatite coatings in femoral revision will require further study.

3: Hip

Titanium Modular Tapered Stems

The initial experience with tapered revision femoral components, such as the Wagner stem, showed osseointegration without stress shielding in a high percentage of cases.[58] However, subsidence, leg-length inequality, abductor weakness, and instability were common because it is difficult to determine level of implant seating at which axial stability will be obtained with a tapered monoblock stem. To address these issues, modular tapered stems were introduced, which allow for impaction of the distal portion of the stem until axial stability is achieved (rotational stability is obtained via flutes), and then leg length, offset, and anteversion can be recreated independently with modular proximal bodies. Although this solution potentially addresses on problems encountered with nonmodular tapered revision femoral components, the addition of modularity itself has theoretic and real disadvantages. These systems add expense, complexity, and the potential for both corrosion and breakage at the modular junction. Factors associated with implant fracture include proximal bone loss resulting in an unsupported proximal segment, use of an extended offset body, large body habitus, and a tapered, corundumized stem.[59] The modular junctions of these contemporary designs have been strengthened to decrease the risk of fracture. Although modern titanium alloy modular connections are stronger than similar monoblock cobalt-chromium implants, the potential for corrosion still exists.

A 2010 study reported early to midterm follow-up of 43 revision THAs with the use of a modular cementless implant. Subsidence was noted in 25.5% of the revisions using the modular femoral stems, all of which appeared to be undersized radiographically. Surprisingly, only 9% require rerevision surgery.[60] Another 2010 study reported a subsidence rate greater than 5 mm in 8% of revisions performed, yet all became stable and none required further revision surgery.[61] In a prospective cohort study using the ZMR prosthesis (Zimmer), an average subsidence of 4.4 mm occurred, whereas only 13% had an incidence of subsidence greater than 5 mm.[62] In that study, the incidence of subsidence was associated with a smaller stem-canal ratio on the postoperative radiographs (0.78 versus 0.93). However, the usefulness of an intraoperative radiograph to access stem-canal ratio has not been demonstrated.

Retrospective review of modular femoral revision stems at midterm to long-term follow-up demonstrates excellent survivorship with revision for aseptic loosening as the end point. A retrospective review with 5- to 10-year follow-up with Profemur-R (Wright Medical, Memphis, TN) modular revision stem demonstrated 96% survivorship at 10 years, with no re-revisions after 20 months.[63] The subsidence rate was noted to be 14.3%, with 6.1% greater than 5 mm. Similar survival results were reported for the ZMR femoral revision system (93.8% at 10 years).[64]

A retrospective comparison of procedures performed between 2000 and 2006 using either titanium modular stems or fully porous coated stems measured improvements in quality of life, restoration of bone stock, and complication rates.[65] Preoperative analysis demonstrated no statistically significant difference in preoperative diagnosis; however, patients who underwent revision with the modular implants had statistically higher femoral defects (Paprosky types IIIB and IV). Even with severe femoral defects, patients who underwent reconstruction with modular implants demonstrated statistically higher Western Ontario and McMaster Universities Arthritis Index pain and stiffness scores, Oxford hip scores, and overall satisfaction scores. Intraoperative fractures were seen in both groups at similar frequencies (even with the addition of an ETO). Radiographic analysis demonstrated statistically significant restoration of bone stock and a decreased incidence of bone loss in the modular revision cohort. Implant fractures were seen in both groups; four fractures (2%) in the modular group and two (1%) in the monolithic cohort (3% of the entire revision group). All modular fractures were associated with first-generation modular junction design.[65]

Summary

The keys to success in revision of THA include careful preoperative evaluation, adequate exposure, safe implant removal, familiarity with a variety of implants and techniques to navigate around bone defects, obtaining immediate mechanical implant stability, and achieving joint stability. Obtaining equal leg lengths, anatomic hip center, and restoration of bone stock are desirable secondary objectives. The evaluation and reconstruction of patients with a failed THA continues to challenge arthroplasty surgeons. A comprehensive history, examination, and radiographic evaluation are required to identify the underlying etiology of implant failure. Preoperative planning is necessary to prevent intraoperative complications and restore femoral function. Monoblock fully porous-coated cementless stems are indispensable in revisions for Paprosky types I-IIIA femoral defects. In contrast, recent literature and experience have revealed that in cases with more advanced proximal femoral bone loss (Paprosky type IIIB and IV defects), a modular titanium stem has improved results compared with traditional monoblock stems. As the number of revision cases increases and the treatment resources decrease, the revision surgeon must continue to evaluate and assess new implants and reconstruction methods.

Acknowledgments

The authors would like to thank Hugo Sanchez, MD, PhD (orthopaedic fellow) for his assistance with this manuscript.

Annotated References

1. Paprosky WG, Perona PG, Lawrence JM: Acetabular defect classification and surgical reconstruction in revision arthroplasty: A 6-year follow-up evaluation. *J Arthroplasty* 1994;9(1):33-44.

2. D'Antonio JA: Periprosthetic bone loss of the acetabulum: Classification and management. *Orthop Clin North Am* 1992;23(2):279-290.

3. Garbuz D, Morsi E, Mohamed N, Gross AE: Classification and reconstruction in revision acetabular arthroplasty with bone stock deficiency. *Clin Orthop Relat Res* 1996;324:98-107.

4. Gozzard C, Blom A, Taylor A, Smith E, Learmonth I: A comparison of the reliability and validity of bone stock loss classification systems used for revision hip surgery. *J Arthroplasty* 2003;18(5):638-642.

5. Saleh KJ, Holtzman J, Gafni A, Saleh L, et al: Development, test reliability and validation of a classification for revision hip arthroplasty. *J Orthop Res* 2001;19(1):50-56.

6. Goodman S, Pressman A, Saastamoinen H, Gross AE: Modified sliding trochanteric osteotomy in revision total hip arthroplasty. *J Arthroplasty* 2004;19(8):1039-1041.

7. Mitchell PA, Masri BA, Garbuz DS, Greidanus NV, Wilson D, Duncan CP: Removal of well-fixed, cementless, acetabular components in revision hip arthroplasty. *J Bone Joint Surg Br* 2003;85(7):949-952.

8. Taylor PR, Stoffel KK, Dunlop DG, Yates PJ: Removal of the well-fixed hip resurfacing acetabular component: A simple, bone preserving technique. *J Arthroplasty* 2009;24(3):484-486.

   The authors discuss the use of the Explant system (Zimmer, Warsaw, IN) for component removal with minimal bone loss and reduced fracture risk.

9. Schreurs BW, Bolder SB, Gardeniers JW, Verdonschot N, Slooff TJ, Veth RP: Acetabular revision with impacted morsellised cancellous bone grafting and a cemented cup: A 15- to 20-year follow-up. *J Bone Joint Surg Br* 2004;86(4):492-497.

10. Lakstein D, Backstein D, Safir O, Kosashvili Y, Gross AE: Trabecular metal cups for acetabular defects with 50% or less host bone contact. *Clin Orthop Relat Res* 2009;467(9):2318-2324.

    The authors reported a cup survivorship of 96% (n = 53) using trabecular metal cups without augments for contained defects (type II) involving more than 50% of the acetabulum at a mean follow-up of 3.8 years (range, 2.0 to 5.9 years). Level of evidence: IV.

11. Park DK, Della Valle CJ, Quigley L, Moric M, Rosenberg AG, Galante JO: Revision of the acetabular component without cement: A concise follow-up, at twenty to twenty-four years, of a previous report. *J Bone Joint Surg Am* 2009;91(2):350-355.

    The authors reported survivorships of 82% for all causes and 95% for aseptic loosening in 77 acetabular revisions using cementless acetabular shells at a minimum follow-up of 20 years. Infection and instability were two common reasons for revision. Level of evidence: IV.

12. Dearborn JT, Harris WH: Acetabular revision arthroplasty using so-called jumbo cementless components: An average 7-year follow-up study. *J Arthroplasty* 2000;15(1):8-15.

13. Whaley AL, Berry DJ, Harmsen WS: Extra-large uncemented hemispherical acetabular components for revision total hip arthroplasty. *J Bone Joint Surg Am* 2001;83-A(9):1352-1357.

14. Hendricks KJ, Harris WH: Revision of failed acetabular components with use of so-called jumbo noncemented components: A concise follow-up of a previous report. *J Bone Joint Surg Am* 2006;88(3):559-563.

    The authors reported no cup re-revisions for aseptic loosening in 12 acetabular revisions with jumbo cups at a mean follow-up of 13.9 years (minimum 12 years). Despite some radiolucencies at the component-bone interface, none were deemed radiographically loose. Level of evidence: IV.

15. Herrera A, Martínez AA, Cuenca J, Canales V: Management of types III and IV acetabular deficiencies with the longitudinal oblong revision cup. *J Arthroplasty* 2006;21(6):857-864.

    The authors reported an 85.5% survivorship for aseptic loosening in 35 acetabular revisions (29 AAOS type III, 6 type IV) with oblong (LOR) cups at a mean follow-up of 6.3 years (range, 4 to 8 years). Failure was associated with incomplete acetabular rim contact. Level of evidence: IV.

16. Dearborn JT, Harris WH: High placement of an acetabular component inserted without cement in a revision total hip arthroplasty: Results after a mean of ten years. *J Bone Joint Surg Am* 1999;81(4):469-480.

17. Hendricks KJ, Harris WH: High placement of noncemented acetabular components in revision total hip arthroplasty: A concise follow-up, at a minimum of fifteen years, of a previous report. *J Bone Joint Surg Am* 2006;88(10):2231-2236.

    The authors reported shell survivorship of 93% for aseptic loosening and 89% for all causes in 46 acetabular revisions with acetabular high hip centers at a mean follow-up of 16.8 years. Cup survivorship for all causes was 74%. Level of evidence: IV.

3: Hip

18. Board TN, Brunskill S, Doree C, et al: Processed versus fresh frozen bone for impaction bone grafting in revision hip arthroplasty. *Cochrane Database Syst Rev* 2009;4:CD006351.

   The authors studied the clinical effectiveness of freeze dried or irradiated bone compared with unprocessed bone.

19. Schreurs BW, Slooff TJ, Gardeniers JW, Buma P: Acetabular reconstruction with bone impaction grafting and a cemented cup: 20 years' experience. *Clin Orthop Relat Res* 2001;393:202-215.

20. Buttaro MA, Comba F, Pusso R, Piccaluga F: Acetabular revision with metal mesh, impaction bone grafting, and a cemented cup. *Clin Orthop Relat Res* 2008; 466(10):2482-2490.

   The authors reported a cup survivorship with further revision as an end point of 90.8% in 23 acetabular revisions for uncontained (AAOS type III) defects using impaction grafting, mesh and cemented cups at a mean follow-up of 36 months (range, 24 to 56 months). Level of evidence: IV.

21. van Haaren EH, Heyligers IC, Alexander FG, Wuisman PI: High rate of failure of impaction grafting in large acetabular defects. *J Bone Joint Surg Br* 2007; 89(3):296-300.

   The authors reported a 72% cup survivorship for aseptic loosening in 20 acetabular revisions using impaction bone allograft at a mean follow-up of 7.2 years (range, 1.6 to 9.7 years). Of the failures, 14 (70%) had an AAOS type III or IV bone defect. Level of evidence: IV.

22. Woodgate IG, Saleh KJ, Jaroszynski G, Agnidis Z, Woodgate MM, Gross AE: Minor column structural acetabular allografts in revision hip arthroplasty. *Clin Orthop Relat Res* 2000;371:75-85.

23. Sporer SM, O'Rourke M, Chong P, Paprosky WG: The use of structural distal femoral allografts for acetabular reconstruction: Average ten-year follow-up. *J Bone Joint Surg Am* 2005;87(4):760-765.

   The authors reported a survivorship of 78.3% for aseptic loosening with revision as the end point in 23 patients who underwent acetabular revision using distal femoral allograft for Paprosky type IIIA defect at a mean follow-up of 10.3 years. Level of evidence: IV.

24. Lee PT, Raz G, Safir OA, Backstein DJ, Gross AE: Long term results for minor column allografts in revision hip arthroplasty. *Clin Orthop Relat Res* 2010; 468(12):3295-3303.

   The authors reported 15- and 20-year survivorship rates of 67% and 61% for cups and 81% for grafts, with re-revision for aseptic loosening as the end point, in 74 patients who underwent acetabular revision using minor column allograft for uncontained acetabular bone defects sized between 30% and 50% of the acetabulum at mean follow-up of 16 years. Level of evidence: IV.

25. Sporer SM, O'Rourke M, Paprosky WG: The treatment of pelvic discontinuity during acetabular revision. *J Arthroplasty* 2005;20(4, Suppl 2):79-84.

   The authors reported a survivorship of 96.4% (n = 28) using trabecular metal cups and augments for type III defects at a mean follow-up of 3.1 years (range, 1 to 4 years). Level of evidence: IV.

26. Regis D, Magnan B, Sandri A, Bartolozzi P: Long-term results of anti-protrusion cage and massive allografts for the management of periprosthetic acetabular bone loss. *J Arthroplasty* 2008;23(6):826-832.

   The authors reported a cup survivorship for aseptic loosening of 87.5% (n = 56) for acetabular revisions using major column allografts and Burch-Schneider antiprotrusio cages at a mean follow-up of 11.7 years. Level of evidence: IV.

27. Siegmeth A, Duncan CP, Masri BA, Kim WY, Garbuz DS: Modular tantalum augments for acetabular defects in revision hip arthroplasty. *Clin Orthop Relat Res* 2009;467(1):199-205.

   The authors reported a 95% survivorship for aseptic loosening in 34 patients who underwent acetabular revision using trabecular metal shells and augments for 27 uncontained and 7 contained cavitary acetabular defects at a mean follow-up of 34 months (range, 24 to 55 months). Level of evidence: IV.

28. Sporer SM, Paprosky WG: The use of a trabecular metal acetabular component and trabecular metal augment for severe acetabular defects. *J Arthroplasty* 2006;21(6, Suppl 2):83-86.

   The authors reported a cup survivorship for aseptic loosening of 96.4% (n = 28) using trabecular metal cups and augments for type III defects at a mean follow-up of 3.1 years (range, 1 to 4 years). Level of evidence: IV.

29. Weeden SH, Schmidt RH: The use of tantalum porous metal implants for Paprosky 3A and 3B defects. *J Arthroplasty* 2007;22(6, Suppl 2):151-155.

   The authors reported a cup survivorship for aseptic loosening of 98% with the use of trabecular metal cups and augments for 33 type III and 10 type IV defects at a mean follow-up of 2.8 years (range, 2 to 4 years). Level of evidence: IV.

30. Hanssen AD, Lewallen DG: Modular acetabular augments: Composite void fillers. *Orthopedics* 2005; 28(9):971-972.

31. Kosashvili Y, Backstein D, Safir O, Lakstein D, Gross AE: Acetabular revision using an anti-protrusion (ilio-ischial) cage and trabecular metal acetabular component for severe acetabular bone loss associated with pelvic discontinuity. *J Bone Joint Surg Br* 2009;91(7): 870-876.

   The authors reported a cup survivorship of 88.5% for aseptic loosening with the use of the Trabecular Metal cup-cage construct for massive segmental bone defects associated with pelvic discontinuity at a mean follow-up of 3.7 years (range, 2.0 to 5.7 years). Level of evidence: IV.

32. Manley M, Ong K, Lau E, Kurtz SM: Effect of volume on total hip arthroplasty revision rates in the United States Medicare population. *J Bone Joint Surg Am* 2008;90(11):2446-1451.

The authors studied a subset of Medicare claims data on THA revision rates and their results indicate that patients of low-volume surgeons are more at risk of arthroplasty revision at 6 months but are not at greater risk of revision at long-term follow-up. No significant association was found between hospital volume and rate of THA revisions.

33. Duffy PJ, Masri BA, Garbuz DS, Duncan CP: Evaluation of patients with pain following total hip replacement. *J Bone Joint Surg Am* 2005;87(11):2566-2575.

The authors present a systematic method for the evaluation of patients with painful THA. Physical examination pearls associated with failure of THA as well as associated etiology are presented. The use of laboratory and radiographic analysis also is discussed. Level of evidence: V.

34. O'Neill DA, Harris WH: Failed total hip replacement: Assessment by plain radiographs, arthrograms, and aspiration of the hip joint. *J Bone Joint Surg Am* 1984;66(4):540-546.

35. Engh CA, Massin P, Suthers KE: Roentgenographic assessment of the biologic fixation of porous-surfaced femoral components. *Clin Orthop Relat Res* 1990;257:107-128.

36. Glassman AH, Engh CA: The removal of porous-coated femoral hip stems. *Clin Orthop Relat Res* 1992;285:164-180.

37. Paprosky WG, Greidanus NV, Antoniou J: Minimum 10-year-results of extensively porous-coated stems in revision hip arthroplasty. *Clin Orthop Relat Res* 1999;369:230-242.

38. Taylor JW, Rorabeck CH: Hip revision arthroplasty: Approach to the femoral side. *Clin Orthop Relat Res* 1999;369:208-222.

39. Paprosky WG, Weeden SH, Bowling JW Jr: Component removal in revision total hip arthroplasty. *Clin Orthop Relat Res* 2001;393:181-193.

40. Burstein G, Yoon P, Saleh KJ: Component removal in revision total hip arthroplasty. *Clin Orthop Relat Res* 2004;420:48-54.

41. Harris WH, McGann WA: Loosening of the femoral component after use of the medullary-plug cementing technique: Follow-up note with a minimum five-year follow-up. *J Bone Joint Surg Am* 1986;68(7):1064-1066.

42. Aribindi R, Paprosky W, Nourbash P, Kronick J, Barba M: Extended proximal femoral osteotomy. *Instr Course Lect* 1999;48:19-26.

43. Lieberman JR, Moeckel BH, Evans BG, Salvati EA, Ranawat CS: Cement-within-cement revision hip arthroplasty. *J Bone Joint Surg Br* 1993;75(6):869-871.

44. McCallum JD III, Hozack WJ: Recementing a femoral component into a stable cement mantle using ultrasonic tools. *Clin Orthop Relat Res* 1995;319:232-237.

45. Sydney SV, Mallory TH: Controlled perforation: A safe method of cement removal from the femoral canal. *Clin Orthop Relat Res* 1990;253:168-172.

46. Younger TI, Bradford MS, Magnus RE, Paprosky WG: Extended proximal femoral osteotomy: A new technique for femoral revision arthroplasty. *J Arthroplasty* 1995;10(3):329-338.

47. Paprosky WG, Burnett RS: Assessment and classification of bone stock deficiency in revision total hip arthroplasty. *Am J Orthop* 2002;31(8):459-464.

48. Paprosky WG, Bradford MS, Younger TI: Hip revision surgery with cemented, cementless or hybrid prosthesis. *Chir Organi Mov* 1994;79(4):415-417.

49. Sporer SM, Paprosky WG: Femoral fixation in the face of considerable bone loss: The use of modular stems. *Clin Orthop Relat Res* 2004;429:227-231.

50. Wraighte PJ, Howard PW: Femoral impaction bone allografting with an Exeter cemented collarless, polished, tapered stem in revision hip replacement: A mean follow-up of 10.5 years. *J Bone Joint Surg Br* 2008;90(8):1000-1004.

This study looked at long-term survival of impaction grafting and notes that early subsidence (1 year) had a strong association with long-term subsidence. Survivorship at 10.5 years was 92%. Level of evidence: IV.

51. Hassaballa M, Mehendale S, Poniatowski S, Kalantzis G, Smith E, Learmonth ID: Subsidence of the stem after impaction bone grafting for revision hip replacement using irradiated bone. *J Bone Joint Surg Br* 2009;91(1):37-43.

A retrospective study of a consecutive series of 69 hips that underwent revision THA with impaction grafting is presented. Massive subsidence (>10 mm) occurred in 7.2%. Subsidence was associated with higher Endo-Klinik class and early subsidence. Level of evidence: IV.

52. Kung PL, Ries MD: Effect of femoral head size and abductors on dislocation after revision THA. *Clin Orthop Relat Res* 2007;465:170-174.

A retrospective cohort analysis of 230 patients was performed to determine the contribution of femoral head size to revision THA. Patients were grouped according to head size and quality of abductor mechanism. Results demonstrated that a 36-mm head had a greater decrease in dislocation rate than a 28-mm head with intact abductors. Level of evidence: III.

53. Levine BR, Della Valle CJ, Deirmengian CA, et al: The use of a tripolar articulation in revision total hip arthroplasty: A minimum of 24 months' follow-up. *J Arthroplasty* 2008;23(8):1182-1188.

A retrospective cohort study (at two institutions) was performed to evaluate the use of a tripolar acetabular component during revision THA in patients with intraoperative instability. Of the 31 patients in the cohort, only 2 required additional surgery for instability with a mean follow-up of 38 months. Level of evidence: III.

54. Hamilton WG, Cashen DV, Ho H, Hopper RH Jr, Engh CA: Extensively porous-coated stems for femoral revision: A choice for all seasons. *J Arthroplasty* 2007; 22(4, Suppl 1):106-110.

A retrospective review of 905 revision THAs was analyzed for femoral stem failure. Twenty femora were identified and revised with an extensively porous-coated monolithic stem. At 10-year follow-up the survivability was found to be 95.9%. Level of evidence: IV.

55. Hamilton WG, McAuley JP, Tabaraee E, Engh CA Sr: The outcome of rerevision of an extensively porous-coated stem with another extensively porous-coated stem. *J Arthroplasty* 2008;23(2):170-174.

A retrospective review of rerevision cases with repeat use of a fully porous-coated implant is presented. Level of evidence: IV.

56. Chambers B, St Clair SF, Froimson MI: Hydroxyapatite-coated tapered cementless femoral components in total hip arthroplasty. *J Arthroplasty* 2007;22(4, Suppl 1):71-74.

The authors present a comprehensive review of current literature of hydroxyapatite-coated stems, which demonstrates improved bone ingrowth, decreased stress-shielding, and improved osseous remodeling. Level of evidence: III.

57. Crawford CH III, Malkani AL, Incavo SJ, Morris HB, Krupp RJ, Baker D: Femoral component revision using an extensively hydroxyapatite-coated stem. *J Arthroplasty* 2004;19(1):8-13.

58. Böhm P, Bischel O: The use of tapered stems for femoral revision surgery. *Clin Orthop Relat Res* 2004;420: 148-159.

59. Böhm P, Bischel O: Femoral revision with the Wagner SL revision stem: Evaluation of one hundred and twenty-nine revisions followed for a mean of 4.8 years. *J Bone Joint Surg Am* 2001;83A(7):1023-1031.

60. Patel PD, Klika AK, Murray TG, Elsharkawy KA, Krebs VE, Barsoum WK: Influence of technique with distally fixed modular stems in revision total hip arthroplasty. *J Arthroplasty* 2010;25(6):926-931.

A retrospective cohort analysis of 43 femora, which underwent revision THA with a titanium modular stem with a minimum 2-year follow-up, is presented. Eleven of the 43 stems subsided with 4 requiring revision surgery. All stems with subsidence were found to be undersized on postoperative radiographs. Level of evidence: III.

61. Ovesen O, Emmeluth C, Hofbauer C, Overgaard S: Revision total hip arthroplasty using a modular tapered stem with distal fixation: Good short-term results in 125 revisions. *J Arthroplasty* 2010;25(3):348-354.

This study reported a retrospective analysis of 125 revision femora using the ZMR modular stem. Overall survivability was 94% with reoperation as the end point. Ten stem were noted to have significant subsidence greater than 5 mm, but all stabilized. Level of evidence: III.

62. Kang MN, Huddleston JI, Hwang K, Imrie S, Goodman SB: Early outcome of a modular femoral component in revision total hip arthroplasty. *J Arthroplasty* 2008;23(2):220-225.

A prospective cohort analysis of 46 femora, which underwent revision surgery with the ZMR implant, is presented. Thirty-six femora were available for radiographic analysis, which demonstrated an average subsidence of 4.4 mm. One stem was revised for subsidence with instability. Level of evidence: II.

63. Köster G, Walde TA, Willert HG: Five- to 10-year results using a noncemented modular revision stem without bone grafting. *J Arthroplasty* 2008;23(7):964-970.

The authors present a retrospective analysis of 46 revision femora that underwent revision surgery with the Pro-Femur-R implant. With a mean follow-up of 6.2 years, three stems required revision surgery, two of these for subsidence. Level of evidence: III.

64. Lakstein D, Backstein D, Safir O, Kosashvili Y, Gross AE: Revision total hip arthroplasty with a porous-coated modular stem: 5 to 10 years follow-up. *Clin Orthop Relat Res* 2010;468(5):1310-1315.

Prospective cohort analysis of 72 revision femora was performed using the ZMR implant with a mean 85-month follow-up. Overall survival rate was 93.8%. Level of evidence: II.

65. Garbuz DS, Toms A, Masri BA, Duncan CP: Improved outcome in femoral revision arthroplasty with tapered fluted modular titanium stems. *Clin Orthop Relat Res* 2006;453:199-202.

This study reviews outcomes and patient satisfaction in 220 patients treated with either a modular tapered titanium stem or a more traditional extensively porous-coated cobalt stem. The modular tapered cohort tended to score higher in most observed outcomes. Level of evidence: III.

Chapter 24

Complications of Total Hip Arthroplasty

Donald S. Garbuz, MD, MPH, FRCSC   Moritz Tannast, MD   Simon D. Steppacher, MD
Stephen B. Murphy, MD   Scott M. Sporer, MD, MS   Carlos J. Lavernia, MD

Fractures
Donald S. Garbuz, MD, MPH, FRCSC

Periprosthetic fractures after a total hip arthroplasty (THA) have been a challenge for orthopaedic surgeons[1,2] for some 50 years. The incidence of intraoperative acetabular periprosthetic fractures has been reported to be as low as 0.2% during cemented THA.[3] However, with the advent of cementless acetabular fixation this incidence has increased.[4] Postoperative acetabular fractures are also relatively uncommon.[5]

The incidence of intraoperative femoral fractures has been reported to be 0.3% in primary cemented stems but 5.4% in uncemented THAs.[5]

Revision surgery carries an even greater incidence of periprosthetic fracture, which usually occurs intraoperatively with some reports as high as 30%.[6]

Diagnosis

Intraoperative periprosthetic fractures are more likely to occur during one of the three stages of the recon-

Dr. Garbuz or an immediate family member serves as a paid consultant for or is an employee of Zimmer and has received research or institutional support from DePuy and Zimmer. Dr. Murphy or an immediate family member has received royalties from Wright Medical Technology; serves as a paid consultant for or is an employee of Wright Medical Technology; owns stock or stock options in Surgical Planning Associates; and is a board member, owner, officer, or committee member of the International Society of Computer Assisted Orthopedic Surgery. Dr. Sporer or an immediate family member serves as a paid consultant for or is an employee of Smith & Nephew and Zimmer and has received research or institutional support from Coolsystems. Dr. Lavernia or an immediate family member has received royalties from MAKO Surgical Corp; serves as a paid consultant for or is an employee of MAKO Surgical Corp; owns stock or stock options in Johnson & Johnson and Zimmer; received research or institutional support from MAKO Surgical Corp; and is a board member, owner, officer, or committee member for the American Association of Hip and Knee Surgeons. Neither of the following authors or any immediate member has received anything of value from or owns stock in a commercial company or institution related directly or indirectly to the subject of this chapter: Dr. Tannast and Dr. Steppacher.

struction: removal of a preexisting implant; bone preparation; or new implant placement. Most postoperative periprosthetic fractures are obvious, although clinical suspicion is necessary in patients with nondescript reports of pain around the implant, especially if there is evidence of osteolysis.

Comprehensive radiographic evaluation is essential, and comparison with previous radiographs is also helpful. More specialized imaging, such as CT and MRI, is rarely required.

Classification

Management of periprosthetic fractures is optimized when the surgeon has a thorough grasp of the problem and is appropriately prepared with the necessary implants and instruments. This is facilitated by the use of a classification system.

Acetabular Fractures

The anterior and posterior columns are the basis for describing fracture patterns of the acetabum.[7] Subsequent modifications[8] subclassified the fractures into the elementary group, including posterior wall, posterior column, anterior wall, anterior column, and transverse injuries, and the associated group, including both-column, transverse plus posterior wall, anterior wall/column plus posterior hemitransverse, posterior column plus posterior wall, and T-shaped injuries.

Another modification includes fractures of the medial wall and classification according to the stability of the acetabular component: type 1 if stable and type 2 if unstable.[9]

Femoral Fractures

The most widely used system for classifying periprosthetic femoral fractures is the Vancouver classification.[10] This system is based on the three most important factors that influence outcome: the site of the fracture, the stability of the stem, and the quality of the bone available for reconstruction (**Table 1**).

Subsequently, the system was modified so that it could be applied to intraoperative femoral fractures.[11] The anatomic designations A, B, and C are subdivided

3: Hip

Table 1

The Vancouver Classification for Postoperative Periprosthetic Femoral Fractures[10]

Fracture Type and Subtype	Location of Fracture
A_G	Greater trochanteric area
A_L	Lesser trochanteric area
B_1	Around or just distal to the prosthesis but implant stable
B_2	Around or just distal to the prosthesis but implant unstable with good bone stock
B_3	Around or just distal to the prosthesis but implant unstable with poor bone stock
C	Below the implant

into subtype 1, representing a simple cortical perforation; subtype 2, representing a nondisplaced linear fracture; and subtype 3, representing a displaced or unstable fracture.

Treatment

Acetabular Fractures

Stable intraoperative acetabular fractures that occur during insertion of an uncemented component require no additional fixation. Unstable fractures may require additional screw fixation of the shell alone, followed by a period of no weight bearing postoperatively. To gain fracture stability, additional fixation outside of the shell occasionally will be required with or without autograft.[12] Postoperative minimally displaced acetabular fractures with a stable acetabular component that has been augmented with screw fixation may be treated nonsurgically.[13] If there is significant fracture displacement, revision of the component and reduction and stabilization of the fracture will be necessary. Fracture stability can be achieved by plating the posterior column together with bone grafting and insertion of an uncemented acetabular component with additional screw fixation.

Patients with pelvic discontinuity pose a difficult problem for surgeons. Fractures in these patients can be treated with a cemented cup with or without an antiprotrusio cage, or with an uncemented cup with a posterior column plate to stabilize the pelvis.[5]

Femoral Fractures

Type A Intraoperative Fractures of the Greater or Lesser Trochanter

Cortical perforations can be ignored because they are unlikely to affect the primary fixation of the femoral stem. With small, nondisplaced cracks, a cerclage wire should be sufficient and should be applied before stem insertion to prevent its propagation. If the fracture does propagate and becomes unstable, then a distally fitting, diaphyseal stem can be used to bypass the area.[14]

If a type A_3 fracture involves the calcar, a diaphyseal fitting uncemented stem is the implant of choice. Displaced fractures of the greater trochanter can be reduced and held with cerclage wires or cables, or a trochanteric claw plate and cables. Good results have been achieved with this method of fixation, although the fixation hardware may cause discomfort.[15]

Type B Intraoperative Fractures

Cortical perforations of the diaphysis (B_1) should be managed with a longer stem to bypass the affected area by a minimum of two diaphyseal diameters.[16] Before stem insertion, it would be sensible to place a prophylactic cable to prevent fracture propagation as the stem is impacted into the femur. In those few instances where the perforation extends below the tip of the longest stem, a cortical strut allograft should be used to bypass the area together with filling of the perforation with bone graft.

B_2 fractures can be treated with a cerclage wire or cable and the fracture bypassed with a longer stem. If the fracture cannot be bypassed because it is too distal, a cortical strut graft or a plate and screws can be used to bypass the fracture. Cortical strut grafts are favored in the setting of poor bone stock because this type of graft has been shown to increase cortical strength and is associated with a good clinical outcome.[17]

Type B_3 fractures that have a spiral or oblique pattern can be reduced and held with cerclage wires; for transverse fractures, one or two cortical strut grafts should be used. Alternatively, a plate and cables can be used with one cortical strut graft. Once the fracture has been reduced and fixed, a femoral stem should be implanted that bypasses the fracture by at least two diaphyseal diameters.

Type C Intraoperative Fractures

Cortical perforations (C_1) distal to the tip of the stem are uncommon. Bone grafting and onlay cortical strut grafts should be used to avoid a possible stress riser and risk of additional fracture in the future. Nondisplaced linear fractures distal to the tip of the stem can be treated with cerclage wires with or without a cortical strut graft. Displaced fractures that are distal to the stem and that cannot be bypassed by a longer stem should be treated with open reduction and internal fixation. Recent encouraging results have been published with the use of the Less Invasive Stabilization System or LISS plate (Synthes, West Chester, PA). With this implant, unicortical screws can be used proximally at the level of the femoral stem and bicortical screws distally. For additional proximal fixation, cerclage wires or cables can be used to augment the unicortical screw fixation.[18]

Postoperative Fractures

When managing a THA with a postoperative periprosthetic fracture, it is prudent to exclude the possibility of infection. Because the inflammatory markers (erythrocyte sedimentation rate [ESR] and C-reactive protein [CRP] level) tend to be at high levels in the presence of a fracture, a needle aspiration should be done.

Type A Postoperative Fractures
Fractures of the greater trochanter are usually stable and can be treated nonsurgically if they are displaced less than 2 cm. Protected weight bearing and avoidance of abduction are advised until fracture union is evident, which can take 6 to 12 weeks.

If fractures are displaced more than 2 cm, or if painful trochanteric nonunion with weak abduction with or without instability develops after a period of nonsurgical management, these fractures should be reduced and fixed.

Isolated fractures of the lesser trochanter are uncommon. If they are relatively small and the implant is stable they can be treated nonsurgically. If the fracture involves a significant part of the calcar, the stability of the implant will be compromised and will need revision.

Type B Postoperative Fractures
Type B$_1$ fractures should be treated with a plate and screws, supplemented with cerclage wire or cable fixation if needed. An alternative approach is a cortical on-lay graft[19] fixed securely with cerclage wires or cables, often in combination with a plate.[20] The use of locking plates with unicortical screws as well as cerclage wires avoids the risk of compromising stem stability. An approach such as the minimally invasive percutaneous plate osteosynthesis technique, which avoids unnecessary soft-tissue stripping by the use of indirect reduction, can be used and has achieved good results.[21]

Type B$_2$ fractures require revision of the femoral component to a longer stem, bypassing the distal extent of the fracture by at least two diaphyseal diameters. Successful outcomes have been achieved with uncemented as well as cemented implants with or without impaction grafting.[22] If an uncemented stem is used, additional rotational stability can be achieved by using a strut graft with cerclage wires or cables.[23]

Type B$_3$ fractures often can necessitate the use of a structural allograft of the proximal femur.[24] However, the use of segmental allografts requires protected weight bearing until host-allograft union occurs. This is a significant disadvantage, paticularly in elderly patients. Alternatively, in this patient group a proximal femoral replacement[25] may be indicated. Another option is to use a distally fixed, fluted, tapered modular stem to bypass the proximal femur and then to reduce the fracture around the implant proximally to form a stable construct. Provisional results have been encouraging.[26]

Type C Postoperative Fractures
Because these fractures are distal to the tip of the femoral component, they can be treated with open reduction and internal fixation following standard AO principles as described for intraoperative fractures. The LISS or LISS femoral locking plate has considerable potential in the treatment of this type of fracture.[27]

The early results with the LISS plate are encouraging; however, the series reported to date are small. Larger series with similar fracture patterns are needed to fully evaluate the contribution that the LISS plate has in the management of periprosthetic fractures.

Causes of Dislocation After THA
Moritz Tannast, MD
Simon D. Steppacher, MD
Stephen B. Murphy, MD

Dislocation is one of the most common complications to occur after THA, with a reported incidence ranging from less than 1% to as high as 10% after primary THA[28-32] and up to 27% after revision THA.[33] Most initial dislocations occur early, with approximately 60% to 70% within the first 4 to 6 weeks after the surgery.[28,34] The causes of dislocation are most often multifactorial (Table 2). A comprehensive analysis of risk factors is crucial for the successful treatment of recurrent dislocations after THA.

Patient-Related Factors
Demographics
The risk of dislocation has been shown to be higher in women.[28,32,35] The reason for this predisposition is unknown. It ia suspected that an increased prevalence of dysplastic hips together with an increased range of motion (ROM) and more compliant soft tissue in women may contribute to this higher risk of dislocation.[32,35,36]

Age has also been shown to be a risk factor.[35] However, the higher incidence of dislocation in elderly patients may be confounded by other risk factors such as neuromuscular and cognitive deficits, comorbidities, or fractures.[29,37] Body height and weight have not been shown to be risk factors.[37] A preoperative American Society of Anesthesiologists score of 3 or 4 also contributes to the risk of instability.[35]

Preoperative Diagnosis and Previous Surgery
The only preoperative diagnoses associated with a higher risk of dislocation are trauma (particularly femoral neck fractures),[35] developmental dysplasia of the hip,[30] osteonecrosis,[35,38] and rheumatoid arthritis.[31,35] Possible explanations include the lack of stabilizing capsular fibrosis, a different preoperative and postoperative leg length/offset, soft-tissue tension, and possible injuries to the stabilizing short external rotators.[37,39] Previous hip surgery (such as acetabular fracture fixation) increases the risk of dislocation of a subsequent prosthetic hip by a factor of two.[32] Patients who had had previous surgical treatment may also have bone loss or deformity, abductor dysfunction, or insufficient external rotator muscles.[32]

3: Hip

Table 2

Factors Associated With Hip Dislocations After THA

Category	Parameter
Patient-Related	
Demography	Female
	Older than 80 years
	Previous surgery
Preoperative diagnosis	Hip trauma
	Hip dysplasia
	Rheumatoid arthritis
Neuromuscular dysfunction	Muscle dystrophy
	Cerebral palsy
	Morbus Parkinson disease
	Epilepsy
Cognitive dysfunction	Dementia
	Alcoholism
	Psychosis
Implant-Related	
Geometry	Head-neck offset
	Head size
	Liner profile
Wear	Deformation of polyethylene
Surgery-Related	
Surgical approach	Anterior
	Anterolateral
	Direct lateral
	Transtrochanteric
	Posterior
	Superior capsulotomy
Implant orientation/position	Excessive/deficient cup version
	Excessive/deficient cup inclination
	Excessive/deficient stem torsion
	Decreased leg length
Extra-articular impingement	Bone-to-bone impingement
	Bone-to-prosthesis impingement
	Secondary bony impingement (heterotopic ossification)
Surgical experience	

Neuromuscular Function

Patients with muscle dystrophy, cerebral palsy, and other neurologic diseases such as Parkinson disease or epilepsy have a higher risk of instability because of contractures, poor muscle control, altered muscle balance or altered unfavorable body mechanics.[28,30,34,40]

Cognitive Dysfunction

Patients with cognitive dysfunction independent of etiology (dementia, alcoholism, psychosis) have a higher prevalence of dislocation.[41,42] In these patients, the increased risk might be attributable to lack of ability to comply with activity restrictions or a lack of coordination or imbalance.

Implant-Related Factors

Head-Neck Offset

Prosthetic impingement results when the femoral neck and the acetabular rim come into contact during ROM. The mechanism of dislocation is that the impingement point acts as a fulcrum about which the femoral component rotates as it subluxates. For the same prosthetic femoral neck diameter, larger prosthetic femoral head sizes (increased head-neck offset) provide a greater impingement-free ROM (**Figure 1, *A***). In experimental studies with physical testing of implants, an increased head-neck offset led to a larger ROM before impingement occurred, whereas the use of femoral head components with reinforcing skirts resulted in a decreased impingement-free ROM[43,44] (**Figure 1, *B* and Figure 2**). Nonetheless, larger heads (28 and 32 mm) have not yet been proven to be superior with regard to dislocation rate in primary THA.[28,32] However, in revision THA for unstable hips a significant benefit of 28- or 32-mm heads has been demonstrated.[45]

Head Size

Larger femoral heads are seated deeper within the acetabular liner and require greater displacement to dislocate[46] (**Figure 1, *C***).

Liner Profile

Theoretically, elevated acetabular liner rims improve hip stability by providing additional support. Nevertheless, this benefit was not demonstrated when elevated and standard liners were compared at midterm follow-up.[47] Drawbacks of elevated liners include decreased impingement-free ROM (which may even cause dislocation), additional wear, and loosening[46] (**Figure 1, *D***).

Wear and Deformation of the Polyethylene

Polyethylene wear with deformation has been proposed as a reason for late dislocation.[48,49] Deeper head penetration into the socket theoretically increases the risk of prosthetic impingement (**Figure 1, *E***).

Surgery-Related Factors

Surgical Approach

The prevalence of unstable THA is strongly dependent on the surgical approach chosen. An intact posterior cap-

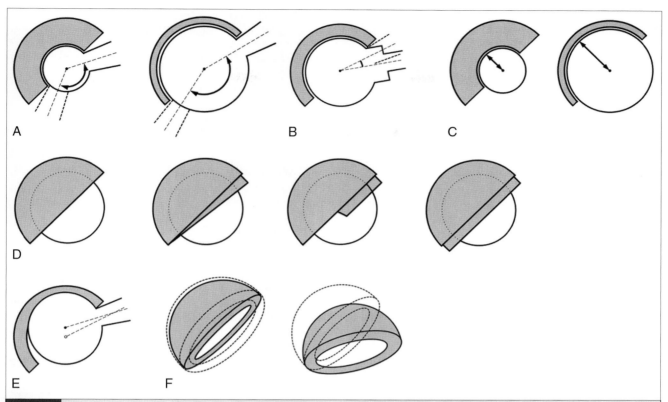

Figure 1 Drawings showing factors associated with hip dislocations after THA. **A,** Smaller femoral head sizes result in decreased head-neck offset. **B,** Femoral head components with reinforcing skirts result in decreased head-neck offset. **C,** Femoral heads with increased diameters are seated deeper within the acetabular liner, requiring greater displacement to dislocate. **D,** Elevated acetabular liners result in a decreased impingement-free ROM. **E,** Polyethylene wear with deformation increases the risk of prosthetic impingement. **F,** Excessive acetabular version or deficient cup abduction increases the risk of dislocation.

sule and short external rotators are of utmost importance in preventing instability because 75% to 90% of dislocations are in the posterior direction.[50] Preservation of the posterior capsule and the short external rotators is associated with a lower risk of dislocation. A meta-analysis involving more than 13,000 procedures found a dislocation rate of 3.2% after a posterior approach compared with 0.6% after a direct lateral approach,[51] 0.6% after a direct anterior approach,[52] 2.2% after an anterolateral approach,[51] 1.3% after a transtrochanteric approach,[32,51] or 0.5% using the superior capsulotomy.[53] However, for the posterior approach, the risk of dislocation can be lowered by a meticulous repair of the short external rotators and/or capsulorrhaphy.[35,54-57]

Implant Positioning
Both orientation and position of the acetabular and femoral components contribute to hip stability. The acetabular orientation is described by cup version and inclination. Excessive acetabular anteversion or retroversion results in anterior or posterior dislocation, respectively[35] (**Figure 1,** *F* and **Figure 2**). Similarly, excessive inclination predisposes to lateral dislocation with the hip adducted. In contrast, deficient cup abduction may lead to impingement-related dislocations (**Fig-**

ure 1, *F* and **Figure 2**). A safe zone for cup inclination of 40° ± 10° and cup anteversion of 15° ± 10° was defined in the early 1970s and is still considered as the gold standard.[58] Novel surgical technologies such as computer navigation or sophisticated mechanical guides have the potential for increased accuracy of cup orientation with a lower dislocation rate compared with freehand positioning.[59,60] Although an excessive medialization or a high cup center theoretically decreases soft-tissue tension, no association with increased hip instability could be shown.[35,39]

On the femoral side, deficient or excessive torsion of the femoral stem is associated with hip instability.[35] Improper femoral version is, however, rarely an isolated cause of instability.[39,48,50] Decreased femoral offset results in a higher risk of dislocation, which is attributed to a loss of soft-tissue tension.[30,39] This effect can be aggravated by leg-length shortening.[35] Varus or valgus malpositioning of the femoral component did not influence the rate of dislocation but influenced the rate of aseptic loosening.[35]

Whereas improper positioning or orientation of either component alone may be acceptable, malposition of both components may contribute to the increased likelihood of dislocation.

3: Hip

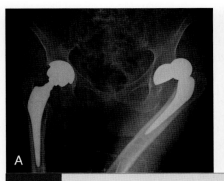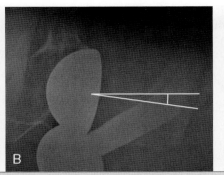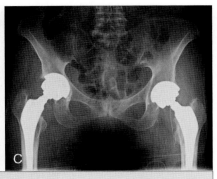

Figure 2 Radiographs from a 75-year-old woman with rheumatoid arthritis. She has a recurrent posterior hip dislocation after THA despite a large diameter bearing (**A**). Possible reasons for the dislocation include acetabular retroversion (**B**), low acetabular inclination, and an unfavorable prosthesis design (the neck reinforcing the skirt in **C**).

Extra-articular Impingement

Extra-articular impingement typically occurs at the bone-on-bone or bone-on-component interface. It can occur at the time of surgery (primary type)[39] or after the formation of heterotopic ossification (secondary type).[61] All forms have been attributed to hip instability.

Surgeon Experience

Given the impact of the numerous mentioned factors on dislocation, it is not surprising that surgeon experience is also related to the risk of dislocation.[40]

Infection
Scott M. Sporer, MD, MS

Epidemiology

Prosthetic infection after primary or revision THA is a devastating complication. The early and late infection rates continue to remain constant despite advances in prosthetic design, surgical technique, and improved compliance with prophylactic antibiotic guidelines. Medicare databases have demonstrated that the prevalence of infection within 2 years after primary hip surgery among patients older than 65 years remains 1.63%, whereas the prevalence between 2 years and 10 years is 0.59%.[62] This rate is similar to that reported from the prior 28 years (1969-1996) at the Mayo Clinic of 1.7% for primary and 3.2% for revision hip procedures.[63] Authors of a 2009 study evaluated 51,345 patients in The Healthcare Cost and Utilization Project Nationwide Inpatient Sample and demonstrated revision for infection to account for 14.8% of all revision surgeries, with an associated average length of hospital stay of 6.2 days and resulting charges for each patient averaging $54,553.[64] The rate of revision hip arthroplasty for infection is expected to rise dramatically over the next several years. Authors of a 2007 study have shown that the number of infections after revision THA was projected to increase from 3,400 in 2005 to 46,000 in 2030. The number of revision THAs

done because of deep infection was also projected to increase from 8.4% in 2005 to 47.5% in 2030.[65] Consequently, deep infection has the potential to become the most frequent failure mode for THA in the United States within the next two to three decades.

Risk Factors

The etiology of prosthetic infection is multifactorial and includes host factors, environmental factors, surgical technique, and associated perioperative medical management. All surgical wounds are colonized upon the completion of a hip arthroplasty procedure despite the best efforts of the surgical team. The goal at the time of surgery is to decrease the number of pathogens to a level below that required to initiate sepsis. A retrospective review of Medicare patients undergoing THA demonstrated that a preoperative Charlson comorbidity index greater than 5 was shown to result in an increased odds ratio of 2.20 for subsequent postoperative infection,[62] In another study of more than 8,000 joint arthroplasties, obesity (body mass index > 50), diabetes, and younger age were all found to be independent risk factors for infection.[66] Similarly, patients admitted directly from a healthcare facility have an increased odds ratio of 4.35 for the development of a surgical site infection,[67] whereas a lower socioeconomic status also results in a greater risk of infection.[62,68]

The environment of the hospital and operating room undoubtedly contributes to the rate of infection. Greater hospital and surgeon volumes have been shown to result in lower rates of infection in both primary and revision procedures.[69] The exact etiology remains unknown, yet is likely because of improved efficiencies in the operating room that lead to minimal soft-tissue damage, decreased surgical time, and early patient mobilization. Laminar airflow, ultraviolet light, and body exhaust suits also have been studied extensively as a method of reducing the risk of infection. Charnley was one of the pioneers not only in joint arthroplasty but also in modalities to decrease infection. He was able to reduce the infection rate from 7% to 0.5% through the use of laminar airflow, double gloves, and reinforced surgical gowns.[70] Subsequent studies corroborated these findings with a decreased incidence of infection from 1.5% to 0.6% when laminar airflow was used.[71] Although these operating room modalities are unlikely detrimental, their clinical significance remains largely unproven because most of these historic studies were retrospective and uncontrolled.

Appropriately administered antibiotic prophylaxis has been shown to decrease the prevalence of infection during both primary as well as revision hip surgery. A first-generation cephalosporin administered within 1 hour of the surgical incision remains the antibiotic of choice. Recent hospital screening programs for methicillin-resistant *Staphylococcus aureus* (MRSA) have shown that the prevalence of MRSA in the community is approximately 3.9%.[72] Preoperative nasal decolonization with mupirocin resulted in decreased rates of infection of approximately 50% among patients undergoing elective joint arthroplasty.[73,74] Vancomycin should be considered as a prophylactic agent among patients testing positive for MRSA colonization. Appropriate postoperative medical management has also been shown to decrease the risk of infection. Poor glycemic control during the perioperative period has been shown to result in a higher incidence of infection. The authors of a 2009 study examined approximately 1 million patients who had undergone primary joint arthroplasty. Patients were categorized into those with uncontrolled diabetes, controlled diabetes, and no diabetes. Patients with uncontrolled diabetes had a 2.28 odds ratio of wound infection along with increased rates of stroke, urinary tract infection, ileus, and death.[75] The significance of allogeneic blood resulting in greater infection rates remains controversial. Allogeneic blood results in suppression of cell-mediated immunity. Although infection rates remain higher among patients receiving a transfusion, the use of white blood cell–filtered blood may decrease the potential of immunosuppression in patients receiving allogeneic versus autologous blood.[76]

S aureus and *Staphylococcus epidermidis* remain the most common pathogens seen in postoperative joint infection.[77] These organisms have the ability to produce a glycocalyx biofilm that allows adhesion of the bacteria to solid surfaces. This bacterial cell wall property results in greater difficulty in eradicating an infection because of restricted penetration of antimicrobial agents into the biofilms, decreased bacterial growth rates, and expression of biofilm-specific resistance genes. There has also been a recent prevalence of more resistant bacterial strains. The emergence of MRSA and vancomycin-resistant strains is of great concern.[78] These bacteria are especially difficult to eradicate and demonstrate a much higher incidence of recurrent infection even after a two-stage exchange.[79] Polymicrobial infections also have been reported. Successful clinical treatment is less likely in patients with these infections than with a monomicrobial infection because of the high prevalence of MRSA and anaerobes.[80]

Clinical Evaluation

Infection must always be ruled out in a patient with a painful THA. A thorough history with reports of delayed postoperative wound healing, prolonged postoperative antibiotics, recent remote infection, or multiple medical comorbidities in an institutionalized patient should raise the suspicion of deep infection. The diagnosis of acute infection will be obvious in a patient with a fever and associated draining sinus, erythema, and indurated tissue. However, most patients with chronic infection present with vague reports of pain and intermittent sweating.

Laboratory Evaluation

ESR and CRP level should be assessed in every patient with a painful total joint arthroplasty. These studies remain an excellent screening tool for infection, with the ESR and CRP level having a sensitivity and a negative predictive value of greater than 95%.[81] In other words, these tests will be elevated in almost all patients with infection, whereas infection is extremely unlikely if these laboratory results are normal. Noninfectious causes of an elevated ESR or CRP level should also be considered because these serologic tests are acute phase reactants. Elevated ESR and CRP level are common after uncomplicated surgery. The ESR and CRP level have been shown to peak approximately 5 days and 2 days postoperatively, respectively. The CRP level should return to normal within 21 days, whereas the ESR can remain elevated for several months.[82] Consequently, the CRP level is more helpful in evaluating an acute postoperative infection and is especially concerning if it continues to rise after the third postoperative day. A systemic white blood cell count is rarely elevated except in the patient with sepsis and therefore is a poor screening test.

Radiographic Evaluation

Plain radiographs, including an AP view of the pelvis and AP and lateral views of the hip, should be obtained in all patients with persistent pain or in patients in whom infection is suspected. Plain radiographs are often unremarkable in patients with a septic THA unless the infection has been long-standing. Radiographic signs indicating infection include the progression of rapid osteolysis, periostitis, endosteal scalloping, or early component loosening. Most patients with septic THA demonstrate radiographic signs of well-fixed implants.

MRI and CT can be useful in some clinical situations to define a soft-tissue abscess surrounding a joint arthroplasty or extension of infection into the pelvis. These imaging modalities are currently limited by their poor resolution because of metallic artifact. Improved metal suppression algorithms may allow future use of these techniques. Ultrasound can be used to help localize abscess collections and determine capsular distention. The routine use of these advanced imaging modalities is not recommended.

3: Hip

Nuclear medicine studies remain controversial in the evaluation and diagnosis of infection. A technetium Tc 99m bone scan has a high sensitivity but a poor specificity for diagnosing infection. This test should not be used during the first year after surgery because it can remain positive even among patients who have well-fixed, noninfected components. Mechanical loosening, heterotopic ossification, inflammatory conditions, fracture, and tumors should also be considered when the test is positive because they may also demonstrate increased radioisotope uptake. However, a negative bone scan can be useful because it has a high negative predictive value. Indium-labeled leukocyte scans combined with a technetium Tc 99m bone scan have improved the sensitivity and specificity of occult infection, especially if the length of time of the scan is extended to 24 hours after infusion. These scans are helpful only if the patient has an appropriate blood supply to allow white blood cell uptake and consequently may not be helpful in patients with chronic osteomyelitis. Despite the improved positive predictive value of these combined tests, they remain unable to reliably differentiate between aseptic and septic causes of loosening. Nuclear studies may be useful in the rare situation where there is a high index of suspicion of infection yet multiple aspirations have failed to isolate a bacterial strain.

Joint Aspirate

The routine aspiration of a painful total joint arthroplasty is not recommended because of the possibility of a false-positive result.[83] However, if infection is suspected because of the patient's history, radiographic findings, or elevated ESR and CRP level, a hip aspiration is required.[84] Patients should remain off antibiotics for a minimum of 2 weeks before hip aspiration to minimize the chance of a false-negative culture. Arthrocentesis should be performed under fluoroscopic guidance and the synovial fluid should be sent for aerobic, anaerobic, and fungal cultures. A recent study evaluating 235 patients demonstrated 87% sensitivity, 92% specificity, and 91% accuracy of preoperative hip aspiration. Synovial fluid obtained at the time of aspiration should also be analyzed for the white blood cell count and differential. A synovial white blood cell count greater than 3,000 white blood cells/mL in a patient with an elevated ESR and CRP level or a white blood cell count greater than 9,000 white blood cells/mL in a patient without an elevated ESR or CRP level is highly indicative of infection. This cutoff is markedly lower than that which would be indicative of infection in a native hip.[81]

The usefulness of a Gram stain in diagnosing infection is limited. A Gram stain has a high specificity but an extremely poor sensitivity. Consequently, the current recommendation is to avoid the routine use of this test to diagnose infection.[85,86]

Tissue Biopsy

An intraoperative frozen section remains a useful test to diagnose infection. However, the accuracy of this test is heavily influenced by the experience and knowledge of the pathologist. Historically, a frozen section was considered positive if there were either 5 or 10 neutrophils per high-power field. The difficulty in comparing previous studies is that authors used varying degrees of magnification and varying definitions of "neutrophils per high-power field." Currently a frozen section is considered positive in most institutions if there are more than five neutrophils per high-power field (×400) in five or more fields. It is important for the pathologist to know that neutrophils in the surface fibrin or inflammatory exudates should be excluded. Using these criteria, the sensitivity of frozen sections is 80% to 100% with a specificity of 94% to 100%.

Sonication

Sonication is a process to dislodge adherent bacteria from explanted implants. This method may be helpful in improving the yield among bacteria with biofilms or in patients who had received antimicrobial therapy within 14 days from surgery. Of 331 patients with explanted arthroplasty implants, 14 demonstrated growth within the sonicate fluid but not by the prosthetic tissue fluid.[87] This technique may be considered when previous aspiration has demonstrated no growth.

Treatment

The treatment of a joint infection depends on many factors, including host comorbidities, duration of symptoms, and the infecting organism. The type of infection is frequently categorized into one of four categories: positive intraoperative cultures, early postoperative infection (less than 4 weeks postoperatively), chronic infection, and late hematogenous infection.[88] Most surgeons would recommend component retention, infectious disease consultation, and a course of intravenous antibiotics after revision in a patient with a positive intraoperative culture on solid media. Component retention with irrigation and débridement and modular component exchange is recommended in patients with an early postoperative infection or an acute hematogenous infection. A two-stage exchange is recommended in patients with a chronic infection or a highly virulent organism. Chronic antibiotic suppression or resection arthroplasty may be considered in the extremely frail patient who is unable to undergo surgery or in the patient in whom multiple attempts at eradication have failed.

Intravenous Antibiotics

The significance of a positive culture after revision hip arthroplasty is dependent on the associated laboratory, radiographic, and clinical findings. It is advised to obtain multiple intraoperative cultures to minimize the chance of a false-positive result. In a patient with an elevated ESR or CRP level, frozen section, or early clinical failure, the culture results are unlikely erroneous. In a study of 31 patients treated with a 6-week course of intravenous antibiotics after a positive intraoperative culture, 16% had recurrence of infection.[89] This recurrence rate is significantly lower than the rate observed among patients with a positive intraoperative culture who did not receive a 6-week postoperative course of antibiotics.[90]

Débridement and Component Retention
Débridement and retention of the components is often used in patients with acute hematogenous infections or acute postoperative infections. A radical débridement must be performed including an extensive synovectomy and removal of all nonviable soft tissue and bone. Additionally, the modular components of the hip arthroplasty should be exchanged to facilitate cleaning between these interfaces. Débridement and component retention has no role in a patient with chronic infection.[91] The success rate of component retention is variable. One study reported a 71% rate of eradication among early postoperative infections and a 50% success rate in the treatment of acute hematogenous infections.[89] Other authors have shown much poorer results with the retention of components. Results from one study demonstrated a dismal 14% rate of success and suggested débridement was unlikely to be successful if performed more than 2 weeks from the onset of symptoms.[91]

Single-Stage Exchange
Retention of the components is not advised in patients with an established infection. A single-stage exchange can be an option for a select group of patients.[92] A literature review of 12 studies suggested that factors leading to a successful direct single exchange were the absence of wound complications after the initial total hip replacement; good general health of the patient; methicillin-sensitive *S epidermidis*, *S aureus*, and *Streptococcus* species; and an organism that was sensitive to the antibiotic mixed into the bone cement. Factors that were associated with failure were polymicrobial infection, gram-negative organisms and methicillin-resistant *S epidermidis*, and group D streptococcus. The authors also suggest that revision with cementless implant may be a contraindication.[93] In this review the success rate of a single-stage exchange was 83% at an average follow-up of 4.8 years.

Two-Stage Exchange
A two-stage exchange remains the gold standard in the United States to treat a chronic hip infection or a failure of an early postoperative or hematogenous infection. The infected hip implant must be removed in its entirety and a thorough synovial débridement and excision of nonviable bone must be performed. It is imperative that all hardware and retained cement be removed because this foreign material can serve as a nidus for infection. An extended trochanteric osteotomy can be

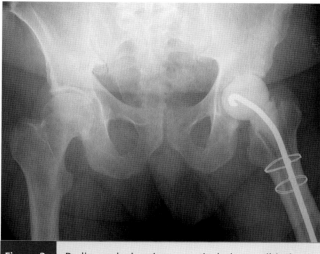

| Figure 3 | Radiograph showing an articulating antibiotic spacer fashioned over a bent Rush rod. |

safely used during a two-stage exchange because this technique has not been shown to result in a higher risk of osteomyelitis or recurrent infection.[94,95] Once the implant has been removed, either an articulating or nonarticulating spacer can be placed. Theoretic advantages of an articulating spacer include improved ambulation, maintenance of soft-tissue tension, easier motion, and the prevention of soft-tissue contractures. The prosthesis with antibiotic-loaded acrylic cement (PROSTALAC, DePuy, Warsaw, IN) consists of a cemented all-polyethylene constrained acetabular component and femoral stem with a metal-on-polyethylene articulation. All surfaces except the articular surfaces are covered with antibiotic-loaded polymethyl methacrylate bone cement. The acetabular component is cemented into the pelvis near the end of polymerization while the femoral component is press-fit once the stem is removed from the mold. Alternative articulating spacers include premanufactured hip spacers, self-made intraoperative spacers, and those that use a disposable mold system (**Figure 3**). Advantages to using the latter two methods include the ability to adjust the amount and type of antibiotic in the cement. Static antibiotic spacers are suggested in patients with extensive bone loss if there is concern about further compromise of host bone with ambulation. In this situation an antibiotic puck can be placed in the acetabulum while an antibiotic dowel can be placed in the femur (**Figure 4**).

The most commonly used combination of antibiotics is 3.6 g of tobramycin and 1.5 g of vancomycin for each package of cement. The antibiotic dosage may be adjusted depending on the infecting organism and patient comorbidities. The peak concentration and elution of vancomycin and tobramycin from the cement occurs between 3 and 18 hours after implantation. The concomitant use of vancomycin and tobramycin has been shown to improve the elution of each antibiotic by 68% and 103%, respectively. A minimum 6-week

3: Hip

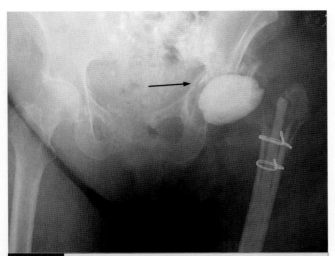

Figure 4 Radiograph showing a static antibiotic spacer, which is useful in situations of severe bone loss or pelvic discontinuity. Note the separation of the superior and inferior hemipelvis.

course of intravenous antibiotics is suggested after placement of the antibiotic spacer. During this time, the ESR and CRP level should be monitored for a downward trend. The ideal time before second-stage reimplantation is controversial, with some surgeons recommending 1 year. There has been a recent trend to earlier reimplantation and the current recommendations are to wait 8 to 12 weeks before the second-stage reimplantation. It is important to examine the overall trend of the serum markers (ESR/CRP) while the patient is off antibiotics for at least 2 weeks. A precipitous rise in either the ESR/CRP or associated wound erythema immediately before surgery is concerning for residual sepsis. Several recent studies have shown that ESR and CRP level frequently have not completely normalized at the time of the second stage, yet the hip is sterile.

The clinical success of a two-stage exchange has been reported to be between 85% and 95% among many different institutions.[96-98] Initially it was believed that cementless reconstructions had a higher incidence of recurrence. However, recent studies would suggest that cementless acetabular and femoral components used at the time of reconstruction result in a similar low rate of recurrence and a high rate of bone ingrowth.[99,100] However, contemporary resistant organisms may be a cause for alarm. Authors of a 2009 study examined the results of infection caused by methicillin-resistant staphylococcal strains.[79] In this select group of patients, a two-stage exchange was successful in only 75% of patients. The authors suggest that alternative novel techniques for infection control are needed.

Resection Arthroplasty

Resection arthroplasty remains an option to treat infection in patients with limited ambulatory capacity, severe medical comorbidities, or failed multiple two-stage procedures. A Girdlestone procedure can effectively eliminate pain and eradicate infection in most patients.[101] Limb shortening of up to 10 cm can be expected, and patients will require support for ambulation. Older female patients tend to have greater residual pain and more difficulty with ambulation.[102] Extensive preoperative discussion is required when considering this surgical option.

Persistent Infection

A two-stage exchange is still recommended in any patient who had undergone a prior failed attempt at component salvage with irrigation and débridement for an acute postoperative or hematogenous infection. The clinical success rate for a two-stage exchange in this scenario continues to be approximately 90%. However, recurrent hip infection after a failed two-stage exchange can be an extremely difficult problem to manage. A study of 34 patients who underwent a two-stage exchange after recurrent infection showed a 38% rate of reinfection.[103] These patients need to be counseled preoperatively that there is a high probability that they will require chronic antibiotic suppression or a resection arthroplasty.

Implant Failure
Carlos J. Lavernia, MD

The causes of implant failure are extremely complex but their understanding is essential for implant design, clinical decision making, and the development of sound healthcare policy. The term implant failure encompasses a wide range of scenarios that can be divided into two broad categories: clinical and material failure. The first type includes the type of failures seen in most patients with aseptic loosening and encompasses malposition, incorrect sizing, and improper fixation. The second type includes true implant failure caused by improper material selection, design flaws, manufacturing problems, and in vivo changes of material properties. When these failures occur in a large number of patients, implant recalls are triggered by the government agency in charge of regulating implant use, for example, the Food and Drug Administration (FDA). Distinguishing between these failure modes is a complex process clouded by medicolegal and economic factors.

The Durom (Zimmer, Warsaw, IN) and the Inter-op (Sulzer, Austin, TX) acetabular components were recently recalled by the manufacturers because of an excessive revision rate at 12 to 24 months postoperatively. Initially, in both recall notices, the companies attributed the problems that occurred to poor surgical technique. Subsequent analysis demonstrated that in the Inter-op recall a step in the manufacturing process was the cause for the early failure. The manufacturers eliminated a "cleaning" step and residue of a mineral oil used during manufacturing was left on the implants. An adverse tissue reaction to the mineral oil ensued and there were numerous revisions because of pain and loosening. The company that manufactured the implant is no longer in business. Liability issues and large punitive damages make corporations reluctant to accept design or material problems in their products, causing them to almost always shift the blame to the surgical technique.[104] Surgeons performing revision surgery are often hesitant to pinpoint in the operative report the exact cause of the failure for similar reasons. Punitive damages in cases in which technical errors are the main cause of reintervention often reach tens of millions of dollars. Damages in cases in which the companies are at fault reach the hundred-million-dollar range.[105] These issues cloud the literature and most discussions of the true causes of revision surgery and material failure.

The only timely way surgeons can learn of large numbers of implant failures within the United States is during professional meetings. The FDA previously kept an online database of failed implants that was available for surgeons to review. The process of reporting medical device failure was abandoned in 1996. A medical device recall database was created in 2002 by the FDA and is now updated as items become available. [106]

Most developed countries have national implant registries that serve to provide an early warning of catastrophic implant failures that affect thousands of patients. In England, the case of the 3M Capital cemented hip stem (3M Health Care, Leicestershire, UK) illustrates the effectiveness of such a mechanism. Based on registry data a rapid and early failure rate was identified and the National Health Service removed the implant from the market.[107] No such registry is currently available in the United States. The American Association of Hip and Knee Surgeons in conjunction with the American Academy of Orthopaedic Surgeons is actively pursuing the creation of a national registry in the United States. Having aggregate information early would allow surgeons to stop using problematic implants.

Clinical Implant Failure

According to a 2009 study, the most common causes of revision in the first 8 years after implantation are instability/dislocation (22.5%) and mechanical loosening (19.7%).[64] Male sex, an age of 59 years or younger, and a high Charlson comorbidity index (more than two disease categories) have been identified as predictors of THA aseptic loosening failure.[108] In a significant number of these cases, loosening of either component can be attributed to a combination of biomechanical, biologic, and genetic factors. Rarely is the cause of failure simple to pinpoint. Furthermore, several groups have identified patient-specific characteristics that make the reason for revision even more confusing. Recently, gene polymorphisms have been associated as risk factors of early implant failure, specifically the promoter of the matrix metalloproteinase-1 gene, whose product (a fibroblast-type collagenase) performs an important function in collagen degradation. Single nucleotide

polymorphisms in the mannose-binding lectin (a liver-derived serum protein that apparently plays an important role in the innate immune system and possibly in chronic inflammation) have also been positively associated with early loosening of THA components.[109] Failures in some of these series have occurred with adequately sized and properly positioned implants. The basic components in a successful THA are material composition, design of the implant, and surgical technique. These factors are intertwined and often a failure is the result of a combination of these factors.

In a significant number of revision cases, the principal cause of failure is technical error. A classic example of a technical problem is the placement of a cemented stem in varus. A varus cemented stem will cause increased loads in the cement mantle with subsequent fragmentation of the material. The particles will then become engulfed by macrophages that then release cytokines, leading to loosening and early revision surgery. Another common error observed on the femoral side is the undersizing of the implant, a common cause of failure in the early history of porous coating.[110,111]

The Durom recall will eventually demonstrate technical failure as the main reason for the early revision of these components. This cup was recently removed from the market in the United States because of an extremely high revision rate in the first 24 months after implantation. The implantation technique recommended and published by the manufacturer caused incomplete seating of the cups, which resulted in a lack of bony surface contact with the porous coating and led to early revision in a large number of cases.[112]

Material Implant Failure

In the development stages of THA, true material failures were common. In the early history of THA, Teflon was used as the first bearing surface, with catastrophic consequences. The wear properties of Teflon in the laboratory were excellent, but the biologic reaction to the material was catastrophic when implanted in the body.[113,114] This finding illustrated the importance of limited controlled clinical trials in the development of biomaterials that are used in hip arthroplasty.

In the second generation of cemented THA almost 6% of the stems implanted in males fractured.[115] Stainless steel had a poor fatigue life and the specific alloy used at the time proved to be inadequate for repeated load bearing. In the United States in 2009, broken stems and cups were extremely uncommon.[64] True "material failures" of contemporary implants are rare and usually are the result of design factors or late biologic reactions. The success of an implant is a combination of material, design, and surgical technique. Surgery in younger patients (age 50 years and younger) places a significant physical demand on these materials.[116,117] A 50-year-old patient will probably subject a THA to 5 million cycles annually. No modern-day machine or appliance is expected to last 150 million cycles. True material failure might be defined as an implant that re-

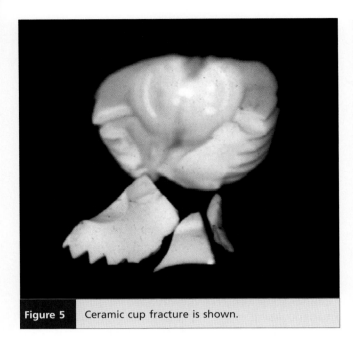

Figure 5 | Ceramic cup fracture is shown.

quires revision within the first 5 years of reasonable use. Reasonable use consists of necessary activities of daily living.

Material failure in a component can be subdivided into three broad types: the bearing articulation, the surface coating, or the substrate. Bearing surface failures and porous coating failures produce excess wear debris and, over the long term, loosening of the implants. Substrate failures are rare catastrophic events that usually require immediate surgical intervention. Success of the bearing surfaces is dependent on the specific material combination used. The metal-on-plastic couple continues to be the most used articulation worldwide and remains the gold standard in primary THA. This bearing combination is historically known for producing osteolysis in some patients. This phenomenon has been the subject of many basic and clinical studies.

Osteolytic induction enhanced by wear particles is one of the most widely studied phenomena. The osteolysis process is related to the number, size, and type of particles produced. As a result of extensive research, there has been a continuous evolution of the manner in which ultra-high-molecular-weight polyethylene is manufactured, sterilized, and stored. Certain changes have resulted in material failures. In the early 1990s, heat-pressed ultra-high-molecular-weight polyethylene and cobalt-chromium emerged as the dominant bearing couple. Severe delamination and subsurface cracking caused early catastrophic failure and rapidly eliminated this material from use for arthroplasty. Oxidation at the bearing surface causes increased wear rates, subsurface cracking, and delamination. In some of the most important papers of modern-day material science, sterilization in an inert environment proved to provide the optimal manufacturing process for these plastic articular surfaces.[118-120] In addition, increased cross linking of polyethylene produces materials with very low wear rates. Highly cross-linked polyethylene is currently used in more than 80% of primary arthroplasties performed in the United States. The use of this material has reduced the head penetration rate to less than 0.08 mm per year. In clinical studies these reductions in wear have been confirmed at 7-year follow-up. The rate of osteolysis observed in these series is a fraction of that reported in series using polyethylene sterilized in air. Highly cross linking the polyethylene significantly weakens the plastic and decreases the fracture toughness of the material. The clinical significance of this reduction measured in the laboratory remains unclear. Early failures of these liners with fracture of the peripheral rim around the polyethylene inserts represent material failures. In most of these cases the cups were implanted too vertical, causing increased rim loading. A new type of potential type of material failure has been recently identified.[121] These authors reported data on the increased rate of oxidation observed ex vivo after exposure of the plastic to a precursor of cholesterol. This lipid adheres to the surfaces and increases the oxidation rate. New methodologies, including postradiation remelting and addition of vitamin E to the polyethylene, are now being developed that further reduce this oxidation pathway and prevent the lipids from adhering to the plastic. The metal-on-metal bearing surface couple was introduced in the United States in the 1960s and was quickly abandoned because of high frictional torque that produced early failures. The metal-on-metal bearing surface was reintroduced in the American marketplace over the past 10 years after the development of newer manufacturing techniques and newer alloy combinations. Metal-on-metal surfaces initially generated substantial interest because of a very low wear rate. A significant number of surgeons continue to allow patients receiving metal-on-metal THAs to return to impact loading activities such as marathons and boxing. The high cost of metal-on-metal THAs and recent reports of increased ion levels in the blood and urine as well as pseudotumor formation around some of these implants and aseptic lymphocytic vasculitis-associated lesions have led to a decrease in their use in recent months.[122] The development of these pseudotumors continues to be an unresolved matter. Although infrequent, they are extremely destructive and their true incidence remains uncertain.

The other commonly used bearing couple, ceramic-on-ceramic, has had significant material-related problems. Early liner and head fracture, although uncommon, were catastrophic for both the patient and the surgeon (**Figure 5**). Revisions were quite challenging. The large amount of very "hard" debris" made the revision very difficult. The trunnion on these well-fixed stems was severely damaged after the liner or the head fractured, mandating the revision of well-fixed stems. Newer developments in the microstructure of the ceramic materials used and better designs in the socket-liner couples have made these failures rare. Although ceramic-on-ceramic articulations have been reported to significantly reduce wear rates, they are not widely used because of their high cost and the squeaking reported in some series. In addition, investigators have identified a unique type of wear in ceramic-on-ceramic articulations (stripe wear).[123,124] The etiology of this wear pattern remains elusive and the long-term consequences of squeaking and this new wear pattern remain disconcerting.

Coatings have been used in stems and sockets for more than 30 years. In the 1980s, the cementless revolution swept the world of hip surgery. Plasma spray and beaded and wire mesh surfaces were being applied to more than 85% of the stems implanted worldwide. Early on, true material failures dampened enthusiasm for their use. "Bead shedding" became a common occurrence in primary hip cases. These beads came loose because of inadequate metallurgy processing, resulting in loosening and third-body wear. Most of the companies making these surfaces had significant problems with the metallurgy of the application process. The manufacturing techniques used to apply these coatings caused either improper bonding of the beads (leading to bead shedding) or weakening of the substrate where the beads were placed (leading to stem fractures). Substrate failures, which had almost been eliminated from primary arthroplasty, began to occur once again.[111] The authors reported a high incidence of fractures in stems smaller than 13.5 mm. These stems were fabricated as cast materials and a porous coating was then applied to them, yielding a substrate that was significantly weakened. Bead shedding, although for the most part eliminated, continues to plague some manufacturers. **Figure 6** shows a stem manufactured in 2005 in which the shedding process was ongoing.

Substrate failure remains a rare cause for revision. Fracture of the stems and cups, although common in the earlier years of hip replacement, was quite infrequent in 2009. Failures of the substrates of modular components, however, have become the modern-day equivalent of the fractured stainless steel stems that were seen in the early days of THA. In the early stages of THA, corrosion, particularly fretting and crevice corrosion, were commonly seen in the head-neck junction of modular devices. Through advances in manufacturing techniques (computer-aided design and manufacturing) and the tighter tolerances currently used, crevice corrosion has become rare. However, with the use of increased modularity for primary hip replacements, a new wave of fractures has been identified.

Recently, failures of modular necks at the neck-body junction have been reported. In these new modular neck body designs such as the Kinectiv Technology (Zimmer M/L Taper Hip Prosthesis, Zimmer) several types of neck lengths and angulations can be matched with the femoral component. These can then be matched with each stem body, giving the surgeon multiple intraoperative choices. Authors of a 2009 study reported a fracture and moderate to marked corrosion on devices of

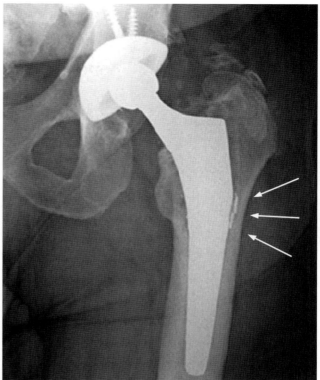

Figure 6	Radiograph of the hip of a young, active patient in whom coating was improperly applied, which in turn caused bead shedding and early failure of a stem (arrows).

this type.[125] These devices had a fracture originating at the distal taper junction in the necks. These surfaces were very corroded. There was no evidence of corrosion at the proximal hip-neck connection in the same cases. This led to the conclusion that unfavorable mechanics and perhaps crevice corrosion are the main mechanisms causing the fatigue failure identified.

Body fluids affect the material properties of implants and on occasion cause changes that were not predicted in the laboratory testing process; such an example is the newly identified mechanisms of increased oxidation of the surface of plastic after the adherence of cholesterol precursors.

Summary

Both intraoperative and postoperative periprosthetic fractures after total hip replacement remain a challenge for orthopaedic surgeons. Using a classification system to evaluate the preoperative radiographs to help create a preoperative plan is essential to successful management of these fractures. The etiology of hip instability after THA is often multifactorial, involving several patient-, implant-, and surgery-related factors (**Table 1**). It is important for the orthopaedic surgeon to assess the preoperative risk, choose the appropriate implant and approach, and detect potential causes of dislocation in patients with hip instability. The gold standard for the treatment of chronic prosthetic joint infection remains a two-stage exchange that includes prosthetic component removal and débridement of nonviable tissue, with the subsequent placement of a temporary antibiotic-laden spacer. Irrigation and débridement should not be performed in patients with chronic infection.

Annotated References

1. Charnley J: The healing of human fractures in contact with self-curing acrylic cement. *Clin Orthop Relat Res* 1966;47:157-163.

2. Scott RD, Turner RH, Leitzes SM, Aufranc OE: Femoral fractures in conjunction with total hip replacement. *J Bone Joint Surg Am* 1975;57(4):494-501.

3. McElfresh EC, Coventry MB: Femoral and pelvic fractures after total hip arthroplasty. *J Bone Joint Surg Am* 1974;56(3):483-492.

4. MacKenzie JR Jr, Callaghan JJ, Pedersen DR, Brown TD: Areas of contact and extent of gaps with implantation of oversized acetabular components in total hip arthroplasty. *Clin Orthop Relat Res* 1994;298:127-136.

5. Berry DJ, Lewallen DG, Hanssen AD, Cabanela ME: Pelvic discontinuity in revision total hip arthroplasty. *J Bone Joint Surg Am* 1999;81(12):1692-1702.

6. Meek RM, Garbuz DS, Masri BA, Greidanus NV, Duncan CP: Intraoperative fracture of the femur in revision total hip arthroplasty with a diaphyseal fitting stem. *J Bone Joint Surg Am* 2004;86(3):480-485.

7. Letournel E: Fractures of the acetabulum: A study of a series of 75 cases. J de Chirurgie 82:47-87, 1961 (translated and substantially abridged). *J Orthop Trauma* 2006;20(1, suppl)S15-S19.

   A review of a large case series of acetabular fractures from a recognized expert in the field is presented. Level of evidence: IV.

8. Letournel E, Judet RF: Fractures of the acetabulum, in Elson RA, ed: *Les Fractures du Cotyle*. New York, NY, Springer, 1993.

9. Peterson CA II, Lewallen DG: Periprosthetic fracture of the acetabulum after total hip arthroplasty. *J Bone Joint Surg Am* 1996;78(8):1206-1213.

10. Duncan CP, Masri BA: Fractures of the femur after hip replacement. *Instr Course Lect* 1995;44:293-304.

11. Masri BA, Meek RM, Duncan CP: Periprosthetic fractures evaluation and treatment. *Clin Orthop Relat Res* 2004;420:80-95.

12. Sharkey PF, Hozack WJ, Callaghan JJ, et al: Acetabular fracture associated with cementless acetabular component insertion: A report of 13 cases. *J Arthroplasty* 1999;14(4):426-431.

13. Callaghan JJ: Periprosthetic fractures of the acetabulum during and following total hip arthroplasty. *Instr Course Lect* 1998;47:231-235.

14. Mont MA, Maar DC: Fractures of the ipsilateral femur after hip arthroplasty: A statistical analysis of outcome based on 487 patients. *J Arthroplasty* 1994;9(5):511-519.

15. Zarin JS, Zurakowski DF, Burke DW: Claw plate fixation of the greater trochanter in revision total hip arthroplasty. *J Arthroplasty* 2009;24(2):272-280.

    A retrospective review of patients treated with the trochanteric claw plate is presented. Level of evidence: IV.

16. Larson JE, Chao EY, Fitzgerald RH: Bypassing femoral cortical defects with cemented intramedullary stems. *J Orthop Res* 1991;9(3):414-421.

17. Haddad FS, Duncan CP: Cortical onlay allograft struts in the treatment of periprosthetic femoral fractures. *Instr Course Lect* 2003;52:291-300.

18. Currall V, Thomason K, Eastaugh-Waring S, Ward AJ, Chesser TJ: The use of LISS femoral locking plates and cabling in the treatment of periprosthetic fractures around stable proximal femoral implants in elderly patients. *Hip Int* 2008;18(3):207-211.

    A retrospective review of patients with Vancouver type C fractures treated with the LISS system is presented. Level of evidence: IV.

19. Haddad FS, Duncan CP, Berry DJ, Lewallen DG, Gross AE, Chandler HP: Periprosthetic femoral fractures around well-fixed implants: Use of cortical onlay allografts with or without a plate. *J Bone Joint Surg Am* 2002;84(6):945-950.

20. Garbuz DS, Masri BA, Duncan CP: Periprosthetic fractures of the femur: Principles of prevention and management. *Instr Course Lect* 1998;47:237-242.

21. Ricci WM, Bolhofner BR, Loftus T, Cox C, Mitchell S, Borrelli J Jr: Indirect reduction and plate fixation, without grafting, for periprosthetic femoral shaft fractures about a stable intramedullary implant: Surgical technique. *J Bone Joint Surg Am* 2006;88(suppl 1, pt 2):275-282.

    A review of a consecutive series of patients with a Vancouver type B$_1$ fracture treated with the minimally invasive percutaneous plate osteosynthesis technique is presented. Level of evidence: IV.

22. Tsiridis E, Narvani AA, Haddad FS, Timperley JA, Gie GA: Impaction femoral allografting and cemented revision for periprosthetic femoral fractures. *J Bone Joint Surg Br* 2004;86(8):1124-1132.

23. Tower SS, Beals RK: Fractures of the femur after hip replacement: The Oregon experience. *Orthop Clin North Am* 1999;30(2):235-247.

24. Gross AE: Revision arthroplasty of the hip using allograft bone, in Czitrom AA, Gross AE, eds: *Allografts in Orthopaedic Practice.* Baltimore, MD, Williams & Wilkins, 1992, pp 147-173.

25. Malkani AL, Paiso JM, Sim FH: Proximal femoral replacement with megaprosthesis. *Instr Course Lect* 2000;49:141-146.

26. Garbuz DS, Toms AF, Masri BA, Duncan CP: Improved outcome in femoral revision arthroplasty with tapered fluted modular titanium stems. *Clin Orthop Relat Res* 2006;453:199-202.

    A cross-sectional study comparing a modular, tapered, fluted stem with a cylindrical extensively coated design is presented. Level of evidence: III.

27. Kobbe P, Klemm R, Reilmann H, Hockertz TJ: Less invasive stabilisation system (LISS) for the treatment of periprosthetic femoral fractures: A 3-year follow-up. *Injury* 2008;39(4):472-479.

    A midterm report on the functional outcome of patients with a periprosthetic fracture treated with the LISS system is presented. Level of evidence: IV.

28. Ali Khan MA, Brakenbury PH, Reynolds IS: Dislocation following total hip replacement. *J Bone Joint Surg Br* 1981;63(2):214-218.

29. Ekelund A, Rydell N, Nilsson OS: Total hip arthroplasty in patients 80 years of age and older. *Clin Orthop Relat Res* 1992;281:101-106.

30. Fackler CD, Poss R: Dislocation in total hip arthroplasties. *Clin Orthop Relat Res* 1980;151:169-178.

31. Mallory TH, Lombardi AV Jr, Fada RA, Herrington SM, Eberle RW: Dislocation after total hip arthroplasty using the anterolateral abductor split approach. *Clin Orthop Relat Res* 1999;358:166-172.

32. Woo RY, Morrey BF: Dislocations after total hip arthroplasty. *J Bone Joint Surg Am* 1982;64(9):1295-1306.

33. Kavanagh BF, Fitzgerald RH Jr: Multiple revisions for failed total hip arthroplasty not associated with infection. *J Bone Joint Surg Am* 1987;69(8):1144-1149.

34. Lindberg HO, Carlsson AS, Gentz CF, Pettersson H: Recurrent and non-recurrent dislocation following total hip arthroplasty. *Acta Orthop Scand* 1982;53(6):947-952.

35. Kim YH, Choi Y, Kim JS: Influence of patient-, design-, and surgery-related factors on rate of dislocation after primary cementless total hip arthroplasty. *J Arthroplasty* 2009;24(8):1258-1263.

    In their series of 1,268 patients (1,648 hips), the authors found a 3% prevalence of posterior dislocation; significant risk factors included female sex, advanced age, and a high American Society of Anesthesiologists score.

36. Coventry MB: Late dislocations in patients with Charnley total hip arthroplasty. *J Bone Joint Surg Am* 1985;67(6):832-841.

37. Sanchez-Sotelo J, Berry DJ: Epidemiology of instability after total hip replacement. *Orthop Clin North Am* 2001;32(4):543-552, vii.

38. Barrack RL: Modularity of prosthetic implants. *J Am Acad Orthop Surg* 1994;2(1):16-25.

39. Soong M, Rubash HE, Macaulay W: Dislocation after total hip arthroplasty. *J Am Acad Orthop Surg* 2004;12(5):314-321.

40. Hedlundh U, Ahnfelt L, Hybbinette CH, Weckstrom J, Fredin H: Surgical experience related to dislocations after total hip arthroplasty. *J Bone Joint Surg Br* 1996;78(2):206-209.

41. Paterno SA, Lachiewicz PF, Kelley SS: The influence of patient-related factors and the position of the acetabular component on the rate of dislocation after total hip replacement. *J Bone Joint Surg Am* 1997;79(8):1202-1210.

42. Woolson ST, Rahimtoola ZO: Risk factors for dislocation during the first 3 months after primary total hip replacement. *J Arthroplasty* 1999;14(6):662-668.

43. Amstutz HC, Lodwig RM, Schurman DJ, Hodgson AG: Range of motion studies for total hip replacements: A comparative study with a new experimental apparatus. *Clin Orthop Relat Res* 1975;111:124-130.

44. Krushell RJ, Burke DW, Harris WH: Range of motion in contemporary total hip arthroplasty: The impact of modular head-neck components. *J Arthroplasty* 1991;6(2):97-101.

45. Alberton GM, High WA, Morrey BF: Dislocation after revision total hip arthroplasty: An analysis of risk factors and treatment options. *J Bone Joint Surg Am* 2002;84(10):1788-1792.

46. Scifert CF, Brown TD, Lipman JD: Finite element analysis of a novel design approach to resisting total hip dislocation. *Clin Biomech (Bristol, Avon)* 1999;14(10):697-703.

47. Cobb TK, Morrey BF, Ilstrup DM: The elevated-rim acetabular liner in total hip arthroplasty: Relationship to postoperative dislocation. *J Bone Joint Surg Am* 1996;78(1):80-86.

48. Daly PJ, Morrey BF: Operative correction of an unstable total hip arthroplasty. *J Bone Joint Surg Am* 1992;74(9):1334-1343.

3: Hip

49. Gioe TJ: Dislocation following revision total hip arthroplasty. *Am J Orthop (Belle Mead NJ)* 2002;31(4): 225-227.

50. Morrey BF: Instability after total hip arthroplasty. *Orthop Clin North Am* 1992;23(2):237-248.

51. Masonis JL, Bourne RB: Surgical approach, abductor function, and total hip arthroplasty dislocation. *Clin Orthop Relat Res* 2002;405:46-53.

52. Bhandari M, Matta JM, Dodgin D, et al; Anterior Total Hip Arthroplasty Collaborative Investigators: Outcomes following the single-incision anterior approach to total hip arthroplasty: A multicenter observational study. *Orthop Clin North Am* 2009;40(3):329-342.

    This multicenter study shows the overall dislocation rates with a single-incision anterior approach to the hip for THA.

53. Murphy SB, Ecker TM, Tannast M: THA performed using conventional and navigated tissue-preserving techniques. *Clin Orthop Relat Res* 2006;453:160-167.

    This article shows the dislocation rates of a modern, tissue-preserving approach in combination with sophisticated computer-assisted techniques.

54. Goldstein WM, Gleason TF, Kopplin M, Branson JJ: Prevalence of dislocation after total hip arthroplasty through a posterolateral approach with partial capsulotomy and capsulorrhaphy. *J Bone Joint Surg Am* 2001;83(pt 1, suppl 2)2-7.

55. Pellicci PM, Bostrom M, Poss R: Posterior approach to total hip replacement using enhanced posterior soft tissue repair. *Clin Orthop Relat Res* 1998;355:224-228.

56. Tsai SJ, Wang CT, Jiang CC: The effect of posterior capsule repair upon post-operative hip dislocation following primary total hip arthroplasty. *BMC Musculoskelet Disord* 2008;9:29.

    This article emphasizes the necessity of a meticulous posterior capsule repair for reducing the risk of dislocation with the posterior approach.

57. White RE Jr, Forness TJ, Allman JK, Junick DW: Effect of posterior capsular repair on early dislocation in primary total hip replacement. *Clin Orthop Relat Res* 2001;393:163-167.

58. Lewinnek GE, Lewis JL, Tarr R, Compere CL, Zimmerman JR: Dislocations after total hip-replacement arthroplasties. *J Bone Joint Surg Am* 1978;60(2):217-220.

59. Murphy SB: The hip sextant: Navigation of acetabular component orientation using a mechanical instrument, in Davies BL, ed: *Computer Assisted Orthopaedic Surgery.* Berlin, Germany, Pro Business, 2009, pp 149-151.

    The author discusses how novel technical advancements in the field of acetabular cup positioning can be used to optimize the cup orientation in THA.

60. Sugano N, Nishii T, Miki H, Yoshikawa H, Sato Y, Tamura S: Mid-term results of cementless total hip replacement using a ceramic-on-ceramic bearing with and without computer navigation. *J Bone Joint Surg Br* 2007;89(4):455-460.

    This article shows in a comparative setup the benefit of computer-assisted methods in placement of the acetabular component.

61. Feinblatt JS, Berend KR, Lombardi AV Jr: Severe symptomatic heterotopic ossification and dislocation: A complication after two-incision minimally invasive total hip arthroplasty. *J Arthroplasty* 2005;20(6):802-806.

    This is one of the few publications that relate a hip dislocation after THA directly to extra-articular heterotopic ossification.

62. Ong KL, Kurtz SM, Lau E, Bozic KJ, Berry DJ, Parvizi J: Prosthetic joint infection risk after total hip arthroplasty in the Medicare population. *J Arthroplasty* 2009;24(6, suppl)105-109.

    This study examines the incidence and risk factors associated with early onset and delayed periprosthetic joint infection in the Medicare patient population.

63. Hanssen AD, Rand JA: Evaluation and treatment of infection at the site of a total hip or knee arthroplasty. *Instr Course Lect* 1999;48:111-122.

64. Bozic KJ, Kurtz SM, Lau E, Ong K, Vail TP, Berry DJ: The epidemiology of revision total hip arthroplasty in the United States. *J Bone Joint Surg Am* 2009;91(1): 128-133.

    The authors present the most common reasons for revision hip arthroplasty in the US Medicare population.

65. Kurtz SM, Ong KL, Schmier J, et al: Future clinical and economic impact of revision total hip and knee arthroplasty. *J Bone Joint Surg Am* 2007;89(suppl 3): 144-151.

    The authors provide a prediction of the impact that prosthetic infection will have in future years. Infection will quickly become one of the most common reasons for revision and have a large economic impact within the United States.

66. Malinzak RA, Ritter MA, Berend ME, Meding JB, Olberding EM, Davis KE: Morbidly obese, diabetic, younger, and unilateral joint arthroplasty patients have elevated total joint arthroplasty infection rates. *J Arthroplasty* 2009;24(6, Suppl)84-88.

    The authors report their experience on risk factors for infection following joint arthroplasty. Obesity and diabetes were significant risk factors for postoperative infection. Level of evidence: IV.

67. Lee J, Singletary R, Schmader K, Anderson DJ, Bolognesi M, Kaye KS: Surgical site infection in the elderly following orthopaedic surgery: Risk factors and outcomes. *J Bone Joint Surg Am* 2006;88(8):1705-1712.

The authors demonstrate that patients who reside in a health care facility before surgery have a higher rate of infection.

68. Webb BG, Lichtman DM, Wagner RA: Risk factors in total joint arthroplasty: Comparison of infection rates in patients with different socioeconomic backgrounds. *Orthopedics* 2008;31(5):445.

    The authors demonstrate a higher incidence of infection after total joint arthroplasty among patients of a lower socioeconomic background.

69. Katz JN, Phillips CB, Baron JA, et al: Association of hospital and surgeon volume of total hip replacement with functional status and satisfaction three years following surgery. *Arthritis Rheum* 2003;48(2):560-568.

70. Charnley J: Postoperative infection after total hip replacement with special reference to air contamination in the operating room. *Clin Orthop Relat Res* 1972;87:167-187.

71. Lidwell OM, Elson RA, Lowbury EJ, et al: Ultraclean air and antibiotics for prevention of postoperative infection: A multicenter study of 8,052 joint replacement operations. *Acta Orthop Scand* 1987;58(1):4-13.

72. Robicsek A, Beaumont JL, Paule SM, et al: Universal surveillance for methicillin-resistant Staphylococcus aureus in 3 affiliated hospitals. *Ann Intern Med* 2008;148(6):409-418.

    The authors report the decline in the rate of MRSA infection when a universal screening program was instituted.

73. Hacek DM, Robb WJ, Paule SM, Kudrna JC, Stamos VP, Peterson LR: Staphylococcus aureus nasal decolonization in joint replacement surgery reduces infection. *Clin Orthop Relat Res* 2008;466(6):1349-1355.

    The authors demonstrate that a program of S aureus nasal decolonization can reduce the rate of surgical site infections. Level of evidence: III.

74. Rao N, Cannella B, Crossett LS, Yates AJ Jr, McGough R III: A preoperative decolonization protocol for staphylococcus aureus prevents orthopaedic infections. *Clin Orthop Relat Res* 2008;466(6):1343-1348.

    The authors demonstrate that a program of S aureus nasal decolonization can reduce the rate of sugical site infections. Level of evidence: II.

75. Marchant MH Jr, Viens NA, Cook C, Vail TP, Bolognesi MP: The impact of glycemic control and diabetes mellitus on perioperative outcomes after total joint arthroplasty. *J Bone Joint Surg Am* 2009;91(7):1621-1629.

    The authors demonstrate that patients with poor glycemic control are at a greater risk of infection.

76. Innerhofer P, Klingler A, Klimmer C, Fries D, Nussbaumer W: Risk for postoperative infection after transfusion of white blood cell-filtered allogeneic or autologous blood components in orthopedic patients undergoing primary arthroplasty. *Transfusion* 2005;45(1):103-110.

    The authors demonstrate that there is an increased risk of postoperative infection in patients receiving allogenic and autologous blood. White blood cell filtration has been recommended.

77. Moran E, Masters S, Berendt AR, McLardy-Smith P, Byren I, Atkins BL: Guiding empirical antibiotic therapy in orthopaedics: The microbiology of prosthetic joint infection managed by debridement, irrigation and prosthesis retention. *J Infect* 2007;55(1):1-7.

    The authors report their microbiologic profile of patients with an infected joint arthroplasty. Coagulase-negative staphylococci and methicillin-senstive S aureus were the most common, followed by MRSA. Level of evidence: IV.

78. Parvizi J, Ghanem E, Azzam K, Davis E, Jaberi F, Hozack W: Periprosthetic infection: Are current treatment strategies adequate? *Acta Orthop Belg* 2008;74(6):793-800.

    The authors suggest that the current method of treatment of resistant organisms is inadequate and that alternative methods of treatment are needed: Level of evidence: IV.

79. Parvizi J, Azzam K, Ghanem E, Austin MS, Rothman RH: Periprosthetic infection due to resistant staphylococci: Serious problems on the horizon. *Clin Orthop Relat Res* 2009;467(7):1732-1739.

    The authors report the results of treatment of methicillin-resistant staphylococcal strains. The treatment results are inferior to those of other organisms, especially in patients with medical comorbidities. Level of evidence: IV.

80. Marculescu CE, Cantey JR: Polymicrobial prosthetic joint infections: Risk factors and outcome. *Clin Orthop Relat Res* 2008;466(6):1397-1404.

    The authors discuss risk factors for polymicrobial infection and demonstrate poorer results after two-stage exchange. Level of evidence: III.

81. Schinsky MF, Della Valle CJ, Sporer SM, Paprosky WG: Perioperative testing for joint infection in patients undergoing revision total hip arthroplasty. *J Bone Joint Surg Am* 2008;90(9):1869-1875.

    The authors describe the utility of synovial fluid to diagnose infection. A white blood cell count greater than 3,000 cells/mL in a patient with an elevated ESR and CRP level is indicative of infection. Level of evidence: IV.

82. Larsson S, Thelander U, Friberg S: C-reactive protein (CRP) levels after elective orthopedic surgery. *Clin Orthop Relat Res* 1992;275:237-242.

83. Barrack RL, Harris WH: The value of aspiration of the hip joint before revision total hip arthroplasty. *J Bone Joint Surg Am* 1993;75(1):66-76.

3: Hip

84. Lachiewicz PF, Rogers GD, Thomason HC: Aspiration of the hip joint before revision total hip arthroplasty: Clinical and laboratory factors influencing attainment of a positive culture. *J Bone Joint Surg Am* 1996; 78(5):749-754.

85. Morgan PM, Sharkey P, Ghanem E, et al: The value of intraoperative Gram stain in revision total knee arthroplasty. *J Bone Joint Surg Am* 2009;91(9):2124-2129.

    The authors review their experience with Gram stain to identify infection. The results suggest that this test should not be routinely used in revision surgery. Level of evidence: IV.

86. Spangehl MJ, Masterson E, Masri BA, O'Connell JX, Duncan CP: The role of intraoperative gram stain in the diagnosis of infection during revision total hip arthroplasty. *J Arthroplasty* 1999;14(8):952-956.

87. Trampuz A, Piper KE, Jacobson MJ, et al: Sonication of removed hip and knee prostheses for diagnosis of infection. *N Engl J Med* 2007;357(7):654-663.

    The authors describe a technique to improve the bacterial yield following explantation of a joint. This technique may allow improved recovery of fastidious organisms in patients who are receiving antibiotics. Level of evidence: IV.

88. Segawa H, Tsukayama DT, Kyle RF, Becker DA, Gustilo RB: Infection after total knee arthroplasty: A retrospective study of the treatment of eighty-one infections. *J Bone Joint Surg Am* 1999;81(10):1434-1445.

89. Tsukayama DT, Estrada R, Gustilo RB: Infection after total hip arthroplasty: A study of the treatment of one hundred and six infections. *J Bone Joint Surg Am* 1996;78(4):512-523.

90. Dupont JA: Significance of operative cultures in total hip arthroplasty. *Clin Orthop Relat Res* 1986;211:122-127.

91. Crockarell JR, Hanssen AD, Osmon DR, Morrey BF: Treatment of infection with débridement and retention of the components following hip arthroplasty. *J Bone Joint Surg Am* 1998;80(9):1306-1313.

92. Callaghan JJ, Katz RP, Johnston RC: One-stage revision surgery of the infected hip: A minimum 10-year followup study. *Clin Orthop Relat Res* 1999;369:139-143.

93. Jackson WO, Schmalzried TP: Limited role of direct exchange arthroplasty in the treatment of infected total hip replacements. *Clin Orthop Relat Res* 2000;381:101-105.

94. Levine BR, Della Valle CJ, Hamming M, Sporer SM, Berger RA, Paprosky WG: Use of the extended trochanteric osteotomy in treating prosthetic hip infection. *J Arthroplasty* 2009;24(1):49-55.

    The authors review their results of an extended trochanteric osteotomy when used in a patient with a septic total hip replacement. This surgical technique can be used safely without an increased risk of infection or failed healing of the osteotomy. Level of evidence: IV.

95. Morshed S, Huffman GR, Ries MD: Extended trochanteric osteotomy for 2-stage revision of infected total hip arthroplasty. *J Arthroplasty* 2005;20(3):294-301.

    The results of an extended trochanteric osteotomy used in a patient with a septic total hip replacement are presented. This surgical technique can be used safely without an increased risk of infection or failed healing of the osteotomy. Level of evidence: IV.

96. Masri BA, Panagiotopoulos KP, Greidanus NV, Garbuz DS, Duncan CP: Cementless two-stage exchange arthroplasty for infection after total hip arthroplasty. *J Arthroplasty* 2007;22(1):72-78.

    The authors report their results of a PROSTALAC spacer to treat a chronic hip infection. Of those studied, 90% of patients had resolution of their infection. Level of evidence: IV.

97. Sanchez-Sotelo J, Berry DJ, Hanssen AD, Cabanela ME: Midterm to long-term followup of staged reimplantation for infected hip arthroplasty. *Clin Orthop Relat Res* 2009;467(1):219-224.

    The average 7-year results of a two-stage exchange demonstrate a 7% recurrence of infection. The method of reconstruction did not correlate with the risk of recurrence. Level of evidence: IV.

98. Toulson C, Walcott-Sapp S, Hur J, et al: Treatment of infected total hip arthroplasty with a 2-stage reimplantation protocol: Update on "our institution's" experience from 1989 to 2003. *J Arthroplasty* 2009;24(7):1051-1060.

    The authors review their results of a two-stage exchange on multidrug-resistant organisms. They suggest that a two-stage protocol is effective at treating resistant organisms including MRSA. Level of evidence: IV.

99. Fink B, Grossmann A, Fuerst M, Schäfer P, Frommelt L: Two-stage cementless revision of infected hip endoprostheses. *Clin Orthop Relat Res* 2009;467(7):1848-1858.

    The authors report their results of cementless two-stage exchange for infected total hip arthoplasty. They show good clinical success with this method of treatment. Level of evidence: IV.

100. Haddad FS, Muirhead-Allwood SK, Manktelow AR, Bacarese-Hamilton I: Two-stage uncemented revision hip arthroplasty for infection. *J Bone Joint Surg Br* 2000;82(5):689-694.

101. Ballard WT, Lowry DA, Brand RA: Resection arthroplasty of the hip. *J Arthroplasty* 1995;10(6):772-779.

102. Grauer JD, Amstutz HC, O'Carroll PF, Dorey FJ: Resection arthroplasty of the hip. *J Bone Joint Surg Am* 1989;71(5):669-678.

103. Pagnano MW, Trousdale RT, Hanssen AD: Outcome after reinfection following reimplantation hip arthroplasty. *Clin Orthop Relat Res* 1997;338(338):192-204.

104. Cohen R, Orr JS: A hip maker's billion-dollar mistake. *The Star-Ledger*. August 13, 2002. http://www.nj.com/specialprojects/index.ssf?/specialprojects/implants/implants3.html. Accessed May 26, 2011.

105. Company News: Sulzer Medica Says Judge Approves Implant Settlement. *The New York Times*. May 9, 2002. http://www.nytimes.com/2002/05/09/business/company-news-sulzer-medica-says-judge-approves-implant-settlement.html. Accessed May 26, 2011.

106. *US Food and Drug Administration List of Device Recalls. http://www.fda.gov/medicaldevices/safety/recallscorrectionsremovals/listofrecalls/default.htm. Accessed May 25, 2011.*

107. Faulkner JK: Regulating human implant technologies in Europe: Understanding the new era in medical device regulation. *Health Risk Soc* 2002;4(2):189-209.

108. Johnsen SP, Sørensen HT, Lucht U, Søballe K, Overgaard S, Pedersen AB: Patient-related predictors of implant failure after primary total hip replacement in the initial, short- and long-terms: A nationwide Danish follow-up study including 36,984 patients. *J Bone Joint Surg Br* 2006;88(10):1303-1308.

   The article examined the association between patient-related factors and the risk of initial, short-, and long-term implant failure after primary THA using the Danish Hip Arthroplasty Registry and found that advanced age was associated with increased risk of failure.

109. Malik MH, Bayat A, Jury F, Kay PR, Ollier WE: Genetic susceptibility to total hip arthroplasty failure: Positive association with mannose-binding lectin. *J Arthroplasty* 2007;22(2):265-270.

   This study on mannose-binding lectin compared patients with aseptic loosening or deep infection to those with clinically and radiologically well-fixed THAs. Immunologic response may be involved in the biologic cascade of events initiated by wear debris and bacterial infection around loosened THAs.

110. Aldinger PR, Jung AW, Pritsch M, et al: Uncemented grit-blasted straight tapered titanium stems in patients younger than fifty-five years of age: Fifteen to twenty-year results. *J Bone Joint Surg Am* 2009;91(6):1432-1439.

   A series of 154 THAs, mean follow-up 17 years, was reported. Survivorship of the stem for any reason was 90%; for aseptic loosening, 95%. The main mode of failure was a periprosthetic fracture or late aseptic loosening in undersized femoral implants.

111. Engh CA, Bobyn JD, Glassman AH: Porous-coated hip replacement: The factors governing bone ingrowth, stress shielding, and clinical results. *J Bone Joint Surg Br* 1987;69(1):45-55.

112. Long WT, Dastane M, Harris MJ, Wan Z, Dorr LD: Failure of the Durom Metasul acetabular component. *Clin Orthop Relat Res* 2010;468(2):400-405.

   The authors prospectively studied 181 patients (207 hips) in whom a large-diameter articulation was implanted and found that revision rate and quality of clinical results were unacceptable compared with those of historic control subjects. Level of evidence: IV.

113. Charnley J: The long-term results of low-friction arthroplasty of the hip performed as a primary intervention. *J Bone Joint Surg Br* 1972;54(1):61-76.

114. Charnley J: Surgery of the hip-joint: Present and future developments. *Br Med J* 1960;1(5176):821-826.

115. Charnley J: Fracture of femoral prostheses in total hip replacement: A clinical study. *Clin Orthop Relat Res* 1975;111:105-120.

116. Archibeck MJ, Surdam JW, Schultz SC Jr, Junick DW, White RE: Cementless total hip arthroplasty in patients 50 years or younger. *J Arthroplasty* 2006;21(4):476-483.

117. Kearns SR, Jamal B, Rorabeck CH, Bourne RB: Factors affecting survival of uncemented total hip arthroplasty in patients 50 years or younger. *Clin Orthop Relat Res* 2006;453:103-109.

   The authors retrospectively reviewed 221 patients younger than 50 years who underwent 299 uncemented THAs in an assessment of 5- to 10-year survival with revision as the end point. Uncemented femoral stems had a 90% survival rate at 15 years.

118. Hopper RH Jr, Young AM, Orishimo KF, Engh CA Jr: Effect of terminal sterilization with gas plasma or gamma radiation on wear of polyethylene liners. *J Bone Joint Surg Am* 2003;85(3):464-468.

119. McKellop H, Shen FW, Lu B, Campbell P, Salovey R: Effect of sterilization method and other modifications on the wear resistance of acetabular cups made of ultra-high molecular weight polyethylene: A hip-simulator study. *J Bone Joint Surg Am* 2000;82(12):1708-1725.

120. Sychterz CJ, Orishimo KF, Engh CA: Sterilization and polyethylene wear: Clinical studies to support laboratory data. *J Bone Joint Surg Am* 2004;86(5):1017-1022.

121. Muratoglu OK, Wannomae KK, Rowell SL, Micheli BR, Malchau H: Ex vivo stability loss of irradiated and melted ultra-high molecular weight polyethylene. *J Bone Joint Surg Am* 2010;92(17):2809-2816.

   The authors concluded that cyclic loading and absorption of lipids may alter the oxidative stability of ultra-high-molecular-weight polyethylene in vivo.

122. Glyn-Jones S, Pandit H, Kwon YM, Doll H, Gill HS, Murray DW: Risk factors for inflammatory pseudotumour formation following hip resurfacing. *J Bone Joint Surg Br* 2009;91(12):1566-1574.

3: Hip

The purpose of this study was to determine the incidence and risk factors for pseudotumors serious enough to require revision. There were 1,419 metal-on-metal resurfacings. Incidence at 8 years: 4%, revision rate: 1.8%. Significant risk factors were female sex, age younger than 40 years, small components, and dysplasia.

123. Jarrett CA, Ranawat AS, Bruzzone M, Blum YC, Rodriguez JA, Ranawat CS: The squeaking hip: A phenomenon of ceramic-on-ceramic total hip arthroplasty. *J Bone Joint Surg Am* 2009;91(6):1344-1349.

The authors report that the incidence of squeaking in association with ceramic-on-ceramic bearings may be higher than previously reported, and causes and implications of squeaking have not yet been determined.

124. Taylor S, Manley MT, Sutton K: The role of stripe wear in causing acoustic emissions from alumina ceramic-on-ceramic bearings. *J Arthroplasty* 2007;22(7, suppl 3):47-51.

The authors concluded that wear stripes caused by edge loading may be associated with bearing noise that can occur during edge loading or normal articulation.

125. Rodrigues DC, Urban RM, Jacobs JJ, Gilbert JL: In vivo severe corrosion and hydrogen embrittlement of retrieved modular body titanium alloy hip-implants. *J Biomed Mater Res B Appl Biomater* 2009;88(1):206-219.

The surface of three designs of retrieved hip implants modular body titanium alloy interfaces in the stem were studied for evidence of severe corrosion and precipitation of brittle hydrides. Severe corrosion was present, with evidence of etching, pitting, delamination, and surface cracking.

Chapter 25

Total Hip Arthroplasty Registry: Lessons Learned

Fabian von Knoch, MD, PhD   Anthony Marchie, MD, MPhil, FRCS(C)   Henrik Malchau, MD, PhD

Introduction

National joint registries have become useful and powerful surveillance systems for monitoring and improving the outcomes of contemporary total joint arthroplasty. The Swedish Knee Registry was the first in 1976, followed by the Swedish Hip Registry in 1979.[1,2] Since that time, other countries have followed suit with their own national registries, including Australia, Canada, Denmark, England, Wales, Finland, New Zealand, Norway, Romania, Slovakia, and Malawi.[3,4] Registries that span beyond national boundaries have been created, and the Nordic Arthroplasty Registry Association is one such example.[5]

As the number of joint surgeries performed in the United States easily eclipses those of other nations, it is natural that an American national joint registry be established, and the foundation has already been laid. The United States alone accounts for more than 200,000 primary total hip arthroplasties (THAs) done annually in patients older than 80 years,[6] and the figure is expected to reach 600,000 by the year 2030.[7] Not surprisingly, the incidence of revision procedures has also risen and will continue to increase exponentially, doubling in the next two decades.[8,9] This projected increase in surgical cases and the growth in implant technology demand a regular and objective method of monitoring and feedback.[10]

The mechanisms inherent within national registries enable improvement of quality, outcomes, and cost effectiveness of joint surgeries[11] by (1) providing timely feedback to both surgeons and industry; (2) providing a sentinel to potential complications; (3) warning of early implant failure; (4) reducing the economic burden of patient morbidity; and (5) monitoring the performance of surgical technique and implant design on a real-time basis.

It is important to review the logistics of operating a national registry, share the lessons that have been learned, discuss their limitations, and speculate on what the future might hold for joint registries.

Logistic Factors: The Necessary Components of a Successful Joint Registry

Since the advent of the first national joint registries in Sweden, there are now a handful of registries of comparable scope around the world, each with its own unique framework, degree of influence, and effectiveness. The formative years of these registries were largely a process of trial and error, and their similarities and differences highlight particular factors that are universally shared among those that are cost effective and have high participation rates. The four components required of a registry include organizational control and funding, participation, data management, and feedback mechanisms.

Organizational Control and Funding

In order for a registry to be accepted by surgeons, industry, and the general public, its information and analyses must be credible and unbiased. This credibility is partly derived from where the executive control resides. Most registries are managed by national orthopaedic associations, with the bulk of funding given by their respective national governments.[4] The Swedish Hip Registry, one of the most successful registries, belongs to the Swedish Orthopaedic Association, and yet it is financed entirely by taxpayers through Sweden's Board of Health and Welfare. In contrast, Canadian, English, and Finnish registries are wholly managed and funded by government institutions. The National Joint Registry of England and Wales is run by the United Kingdom Atomic Energy Authority. A recent survey of 405 British orthopaedic surgeons revealed that there was serious concern regarding the lack of joint arthroplasty expertise, physicians, and surgeons on the steering

Dr. Malchau or an immediate family member is a board member, owner, officer, or committee member for RSA Biomedical; has received royalties from Smith & Nephew; is a paid consultant to or an employee of Smith & Nephew and Biomet; and has received research or institutional support from Zimmer, Smith & Nephew, and Biomet. Neither of the following authors or any immediate family members has received anything of value from or owns stock in a commercial company or institution related directly or indirectly to the subject of this chapter: Dr. von Knoch and Dr. Marchie.

3: Hip

committee of the United Kingdom Atomic Energy Authority.[12] The Registry's management in its current form raised additional concern about the use of data for the production of any league table used for comparison between hospitals and regions. Overwhelmingly, the consensus was for a surgeon-peer–run national registry.

The source of funding is an important aspect of registry management, and is critical to its success or failure. The German National Registry was initially funded through grants by implant manufacturers and surgeons, but these grants eventually were not able to keep pace with the costs.[4] Both the Danish and Canadian registries were also marred by financial challenge at their inception, and the expenditures were gradually assumed by their respective government agencies. It has been suggested that an implant tax could be raised to help fund these registries. As in most other scenarios, 'who pays what' remains an issue of contention. Nevertheless, it seems evident that the long-term success of any registry will require government support in one form or another.

Voluntary Participation

In democratic societies, participation should be voluntary or the registry would not likely be well received and information would be only reluctantly surrendered. Participation is indeed voluntary in most countries, including Australia, Canada, New Zealand, Norway, Romania, and Sweden.[4] Because the participation rate has been low in Canada, there is current discussion of "piggybacking" participation with reimbursement fees. In Finland, Slovakia, and Denmark, mandatory participation in these registries by hospitals has been enacted into law. Generally, it is believed that participation needs to be a minimum of 85% to reach an adequate level of confidence to avoid bias or skewed results from unreported revisions and complications.

Data Management

The three important aspects of registry data management are data collection, validation of accuracy and completeness, and analysis.

Collection of patient, implant, and surgeon data is, of course, premised on confidentiality and data security. Traditionally, data have been prospectively collected and submitted in hard-copy format, and more recently, electronic means of data gathering and reporting have been the norm. In Sweden, recent figures indicate that more than 90% of primary and 75% of revision hip replacements are now reported immediately online, and most of the remaining cases are reported within a few weeks.[13]

Beyond data on primary and revision joint procedures, joint registries typically include information on a patient identifier, surgeon (normally deidentified), hospital, and basic details of the operation (date of surgery, diagnosis, procedure, surgical approach, laterality, implant specification, type of cement).[4] There is now a

movement toward the inclusion of patient-derived outcomes as well as radiographs to improve the sensitivity of outcome assessment. The inclusion of more data may, however, compromise surgeon and hospital participation rates. Also of note is the use of a standardized patient identifier that is essential to the success of long-term follow-up, and the lack of such a standardized identifier has already led to problems in both the Swiss and German national registries.[14] In the United States, a person's social security number may be used as such an identifier in the nation's developing registry.

The utility and applicability of registry data moreover depend on their accuracy and completeness. Hence, data need to be regularly validated. At the initial stage of data collection and entry, there must be qualified personnel using well-established routines to help minimize error. Once data have been collected and stored, registry personnel are required to verify the external validity of cross sections of collected information and to periodically review the quality control mechanisms for incoming data to ensure that there is no undue bias or misinformation. Validation exercises for the Norwegian Arthroplasty Registry (NAR) indicate that there was an error rate of 1.1%, and these errors included incorrect surgery dates and even the wrong side of surgery.[15] Most of these errors were attributed to illegible penmanship and were based on information collected from 1983 to 2003 (the data were deemed to be complete only from years 1999 to 2002).[16] In the Danish Hip Registry,[17] for example, it was found that the rate of data completeness was lower in academic centers (91%) than in community hospitals, and lower in low-volume centers (92%) than in high-volume units (96%). Certain diagnoses were often unavailable and were only confirmed in a third of cases, with postoperative complications confirmed in two thirds of cases. This 'incompleteness' of data emphasizes the caution that is required when interpreting such analyses.

Only when data have been validated and confirmed to be complete can they be used for analysis. The end point for implant failure is commonly defined as the need for revision surgery. Data are normally presented as survival analyses, with the time to first revision based on the Kaplan-Meier statistical method. Practicing surgeons should realize, however, that failure of an implant often does not require revision surgery because some patients choose to tolerate pain and poor function. Such patients would not be captured by the 'revision' definition of implant failure, and thus there is the aforementioned need for patient-derived outcomes and radiographs to be included in the analyses. These broadened criteria for success or failure of surgery would increase outcome sensitivity and be more likely to accurately represent the cost effectiveness and utility of implants, techniques, and other surgical considerations.[13] Patient-derived data are already being included in the national registries of Finland, New Zealand, and Sweden, with clinical scores used in Denmark, and radiographic data in Romania. Only the

Swiss registry contains both patient-derived outcomes and radiographic information.

Feedback Mechanism

The ultimate objective of a joint registry is to continually inform surgeons, industry, and the general public on the performance of various surgical practices and implant designs. By doing so, best practices and implant designs are allowed to perpetuate, while suboptimal approaches and components can be discontinued early and their harm minimized. Naturally, this feedback mechanism needs to be done in a timely manner to permit quick action and encourage surgeon participation and reflection. The feedback needs to be unbiased and objective, and not perceived to be punitive to underperformers. Only then can participants be uninhibited in their participation and analysis, and treat the reports in a constructive and helpful manner. Most reports are compiled annually or published periodically in scientific journals, and are generally accessible via the Websites of the various national registries (http://www.jru.orthop.gu.se).[4]

Joint Registries: Moving Toward Evidence-Based Medicine for Joint Arthroplasty Surgeries

Joint registries help define the epidemiology of replacement surgeries. Information relating to the surgeries, such as diagnosis, number of primary and revision surgeries, age and sex distribution, cemented versus cementless fixation, and implant designs, is taken in real time.

The Danish Arthroplasty Registry,[18] for example, revealed that there was significant regional variation for primary and revision hip surgery. Oddly, there was no correlation with local demographics at all; the ratio of patients to surgeons, proportion of patients with primary osteoarthritis and preoperative hip function, or population density could not account for the differences.

The Nordic registries[19] also showed that the overall incidence of hip replacement surgery was remarkably similar across Denmark, Finland, Iceland, Norway, and Sweden, but that there were sex differences, and a discordance between the types of implants used. In Norway, two women on average underwent surgery for every man who did, whereas replacement surgery was evenly divided between men and women in all the other countries. The use of uncemented components and hybrid hip replacement surgery was also much more common in Finland and Denmark than elsewhere.

As national demographics evolve, one would expect these changes to be reflected in the findings of the registries, and help to forecast future needs and trends. From 1996 to 2002 in Denmark, the incidence of primary and revision hip replacements increased by 30% and 10%, respectively, and were especially higher in patients 50 to 59 years old. With these figures and projections of those who will reach this age group, it has been forecasted that the rate of replacement surgery will increase by at least 210% by 2020.[20] These types of projections allow governments to plan ahead and prepare the necessary resources to meet the impending demand.

Improving Overall Surgical Outcomes

The use of registries has also helped improve outcomes of joint surgeries in five major categories: determining prognostic factors, refining indications for surgery, monitoring the effectiveness of various surgical techniques, following the performance of different implant designs; and scrutinizing perioperative complications.

Prognostic Indicators

The large sample size of registries, along with their prospective outlook, afford a powerful tool for studying predictors of surgical outcome. For example, European registries have already helped identify sex, age, body mass index, preoperative functional status, postoperative physical activity, and particular diagnoses as such predictors of outcome.

Using data from 1995 to 2002, the Danish Hip Arthroplasty Registry[21] looked at the outcomes of patients over three different follow-up time frames: 0 to 30 days, 31 days to 6 months, and 6 months to 8 years. The authors reported that male patients who had a high comorbidity index score were likely to do poorly at all times of follow-up; that during the first 30 days, patients who were older than 80 years and had undergone hip replacement for trauma, osteonecrosis, or hip dysplasia had high failure rates; and that those who were younger than 60 years had a high likelihood of failure over long-term follow-up.

Preoperative function also has been used as a prognostic factor for outcome by the International Documentation and Evaluation System (IDES), based on data from the European Hip Registry[22] from 1967 to 2002. Preoperative function was defined along the categories of pain, mobility, and range of motion, and studied in patients with a mean follow-up of 4 years (range, 29 days to 10 years). Predictably, those with poor preoperative walking capacity or a hip flexion contracture were likely to fare worse postoperatively in walking and hip range of motion. There was no association between preoperative pain level and postoperative pain relief, as there was generally excellent pain relief after surgery.

The NAR[23] has revealed that patients in the top quartile of body mass index were 2.5 times more likely to experience femoral stem loosening. Men were also twice as likely as women to have an unstable stem. Men who had vigorous physical activity postoperatively were almost five times more likely to undergo a revision for acetabular cup loosening. In the multivariate analysis adjusted for physical activity, there was only a weak correlation between patient age at the time of primary total hip replacement and the risk of later

3: Hip

revision caused by aseptic loosening.

The Finnish Arthroplasty Registry[24] studied the effect of age on outcomes, and in particular looked at relatively young patients (younger than 55 years) who had undergone primary THA. Survivorship analyses of the components implanted between 1991 and 2001 showed that 90% of second-generation cementless stems (that is, proximally porous or hydroxyapatite coated) were still in good position at 10-year follow-up in patients with primary osteoarthritis, but that certain designs of these cementless components had high polyethylene wear or poor liner locking mechanisms, leading to an unacceptably high incidence of aseptic loosening and low survival rates. Also revealed in the same registry,[25] between 1980 and 2003, patients who were younger than 55 years and had rheumatoid arthritis were 2.4 times more likely to have aseptic loosening if they had a cemented stem versus that of a proximally circumferential porous-coated stem. By contrast, in the same group of patients, those who had cemented polyethylene acetabular components were at lower risk for undergoing revision than those with uncemented cups.

At the other end of the spectrum, for those older than 80 years, Finnish Registry[26] data between 1980 and 2004 showed that the prevalence of aseptic loosening was lower than in younger patients. Recurrent dislocation, periprosthetic fracture, and infection were found to be more common complications in the elderly, and cemented stems had better long-term results overall than cementless fixation.

Refining Indications for THA Surgery

Registries have permitted studies of patient subsets relating to particular preoperative diagnoses. Recent examples have included the use of THA for arthritis secondary to childhood hip disorders, conversion of hemiarthroplasty to THA, and the use of THA after femoral neck fractures.

The Danish Hip Arthroplasty Registry[27] has reported that there were no significant differences in revision risk between THAs for primary osteoarthritis versus childhood hip disorders, including developmental dysplasia of the hip, Legg-Calve-Perthes disease, and epiphysiolysis. These 55,820 patients were followed from 1995 to 2005, and had follow-up ranging from 6 months to 12 years. There was, however, a 2.8-fold increased risk of revision for dislocation during the first 6 months of follow-up for patients who had acetabular dysplasia. Similarly, the NAR[28] compared the outcomes of patients from 1987 to 2003 who had THA for primary osteoarthritis (N = 59,774) versus those for developmental dysplasia of the hip (N = 7,135). After adjusting for age and the recent popularity of cementless femoral stems, there was no significant difference in outcomes between the two groups.

For patients with failed hemiarthroplasties who underwent conversion to THA, the NAR[29] reported that there was a lower subsequent revision risk (RR, 0.4) when the femoral stem was replaced. This finding was based on follow-up of 595 patients who were older than 60 years: 122 of whom had retained the original femoral stem at the conversion surgery, and 473 who had the stem exchanged. This finding was attributed to poor initial femoral position in the patients with the retained component.

For those patients who underwent THA after an acute or old femoral neck fracture, there was an increased RR (1.6 and 1.3, respectively) compared with patients who had THA for primary osteoarthritis.[30] For patients who had THA for an old and healed femoral neck fracture, the risk of dislocation or periprosthetic fracture was twice that of those who had a hip replacement for primary osteoarthritis.[30]

Surgical Approach and Outcomes

The sheer number of patients followed by registries enables analysis of the superiority of particular approaches. The NAR[31] revealed that there was a lower RR (0.6) when a lateral approach with trochanteric osteotomy was used in primary THA than other surgical approaches. It has also reconfirmed the increased RR (1.9) caused by hip dislocation when a posterolateral approach was used.

The NAR[32] compared the outcomes of patients who had isolated liner exchange hip revisions with those who had a complete acetabular component exchange and found that the former had a higher risk of subsequent revision than the latter. The most common cause of subsequent revision was dislocation (28%). It was noted, however, that confounders were not well controlled, and the results should therefore be interpreted with caution. Nevertheless, this finding would suggest that the threshold for acetabular component revision (even in the presence of a well-fixed cup) should be lowered, particularly when there is liner wear and osteolysis.

Performance of Implant Design and Fixation Technique

An important aspect of any registry is its ability to monitor the success of different implant techniques and types. For example, in Europe, cemented implant fixation is preferred, whereas in North America cementless fixation is favored.[33] In Europe, Finnish and Danish surgeons are more likely to use cementless or hybrid fixation in THA. The European registries have shed light on the debate regarding fixation technique. After following 14 different femoral stem designs used in 11,516 THAs between 1987 and 2005,[34] it was found that the overall performance of cementless stems was good. There were, however, significant differences in the popularity and survivorship of the different designs, ranging from 29% to 97% survival at 15 years with stem revision as the end point. It was also concluded that a minimum of 7 years of follow-up was necessary to detect poor-performing femoral implants. Generally, men had an increased risk of revision compared with women (RR, 1.3), although age and preoperative diagnosis did not have an effect on outcome. A more recent

NAR study[35] of the 10 most commonly used implants in 62,305 primary cemented THAs from 1987 to 2007 found significantly inferior results in some of the newer implants.

The New Zealand Registry[36] analyzed patients who had primary THAs using cementless (N = 10,898), cemented (N=16,005), reverse hybrid (N = 573), or hybrid (N = 15,189) fixation techniques. The revision rate was generally lowest for patients with cemented implants. However, for those younger than 65 years, cementless implants had the lowest revision rate. Cementless acetabular components (in cementless or hybrid hip arthroplasties) had a lower revision rate than if they were cemented. As for femoral fixation, there was significantly less revision in patients who were older than 75 years and who had cemented components. Infection as a cause of revision was more common in those younger than 65 years, and who had either hybrid or cemented THAs. Dislocation was nevertheless the most common reason for revision and was especially associated with cementless acetabular components.

The Finnish Arthroplasty Registry[37] similarly compared cementless, hybrid, and cemented fixation techniques in primary THAs for primary osteoarthritis. The authors reported that there were no significant differences in long-term survival between cementless and cemented THAs, but that younger patients (55 to 74 years old) who had straight, porous-coated cementless stems had better implant survival than those with cemented stems. Polyethylene liner wear in cemented modular cups was, however, a common cause for revision in this age group. The Danish Hip Arthroplasty Registry[38] has also compared the revision rates in 7,907 patients who had hydroxyapatite-coated stems versus those who did not, and found no difference in overall outcome.

With rapidly advancing and proliferating implant technology, registries serve as a method of quality control of new designs and implants. One such example was the likely lipid contamination of components manufactured by Sulzer Orthopaedics in 2000, leading to unacceptably high revision rates. In the United States alone, an estimated 17,500 such components were implanted, 3,000 of which were later revised.[39]

Scrutinizing Perioperatvie and Postoperative Complications

Registries have also recently analyzed the outcomes of treatments of intraoperative fractures in primary THA, and periprosthetic fractures after both primary and revision hip replacement. Compared with primary THAs without intraoperative fracture, there was an almost sixfold increased risk for later revision during the first 6 months of follow-up for patients who had undergone open reduction and internal fixation for their intraoperative fracture.[40] Patients should be made aware of this finding after such fractures. The increased risk for revision was attributed mainly to subsequent dislocation caused by implant instability. There was no signif-

icant difference in RR for those who were able to reach the 6-month to 11-year follow-up period. Based on this observation, the recommendation was made to include change to larger diameter stems with distal fixation during repair of these intraoperative fractures, and to be judicious with the patient's weight-bearing restrictions.

For 321 patients with periprosthetic fractures from 1999 to 2000, the Swedish Hip Registry[41] reported that most of these fractures were caused by minor trauma. Most patients had an unstable femoral stem at the time of fracture (66% of patients after a primary THA, and 51% after a revision hip replacement); most of these periprosthetic fractures (88%) were around the implant distal to the lesser trochanter but proximal to the stem tip (Vancouver type B). There was a high failure rate (almost 75%) for the first 5 years after a periprosthetic fracture (that is, 33% nonunion, 24% refracture, 13% femoral stem loosening), especially if reoperation only included open reduction and internal fixation of the fracture (as the diagnosis of a loose implant may be unrecognized). Thus, testing implant stability after such fracture repair and having close clinical and radiographic follow-up would be essential to detecting these loose implants. Particular implant designs were also associated with increased risk of periprosthetic fracture, including the Charnley and the Exeter stems.

The New Zealand National Registry[42] reported that patients who underwent revision surgery between 1999 and 2004 for a periprosthetic fracture had poorer functional outcomes than those who had revisions for other reasons. Most seriously, the 6-month mortality rate was seven times higher (7.3% versus 0.9%), with an almost threefold increased risk (7.3% versus 2.6%) of further revision surgery after the index revision operation.

Recent Examples of Registry Feedback and Improved Outcome

Regular feedback is a cornerstone of any registry, and has already had tremendous impact over the decisions of both surgeon and industry. During the late 1990s, there was a significant resurgence in hip resurfacing procedures as detected by the Australian National Joint Registry.[43] The popularity of hip resurfacing steadily increased until 2006 when it accounted for almost 9% of all THAs in Australia (versus 5.6% in 2001). Patients who were younger than 55 years represented the demographic group in which this increase was most pronounced (29% underwent hip resurfacing in 2005 compared with 20% in 2001). These implants were continually analyzed by the national registry, and noted to have a higher revision rate than conventional THAs. Women who had a resurfacing procedure and smaller implant sizes in general had a twofold increased revision rate compared with women with standard THAs (4.2% versus 2.0%). This recognition of sex-related failure and increased revision rate was disseminated quickly throughout the Australian orthopaedic community, and since 2007, has led to consecutive annual de-

3: Hip

clines in both the proportion and absolute number of hip resurfacing procedures performed.[44] Proportionally, there has also been a shift away from resurfacing arthroplasties in women (from 28.8% in 2007 to 23.6% in 2009) and certain types of implant systems used. Three implant systems, with more than twice the risk of revision compared with all the other resurfacing systems combined, have been identified; one such system has already been discontinued. Clearly, the Australian registry played a pivotal role in acting as a warning system for the unacceptably high revision rates; helped refine the indication for the procedure for a particular subset of patients; and identified implant systems that had high failure rates.

In 2005, the Swedish Hip Registry[45] identified one of its participating hospitals as having an unusually high revision rate due to recurrent dislocation (4.8% versus the national average of 1.4%) secondary to component malposition. The Registry organized a site-specific program that included elements of patient education, patient selection, preoperative templating, use of cup-positioning guides, larger femoral heads, and capsular and piriformis tendon repair for a posterior hip approach. Since the implementation of the program in 2006, there have been no further revisions due to dislocation caused by cup malpositioning. This example is but the tip of the iceberg in Sweden, as the national hip and knee registries have had a tremendous influence on overall outcome, helping to reduce the national revision burden by 2.5 times (from 17% in 1979 to 7% in 1997).[46]

Socioeconomic Implication of National Registries

The revision burden on both patients and the overall economy is significantly lower in registry-driven countries such as Norway and Sweden, in comparison with the United States, which does not yet have a national registry database (**Figure 1**). From 1992 to 2000, 16.9% of American patients who were older than 65 years with a THA required revision surgery, whereas only 6.4% of Swedes in the same age group required surgery. It is estimated that each percentage reduction in revision procedures corresponds to a range of $42.5 million to $112.6 million annually in the United States.[6] Thus, a decrease of 10% in the US revision rate (which would approach the Swedish rate) could potentially save upward of $1 billion each year.

Limitations and Future Outlook for Joint Registries

Despite the wealth of information that registry databases offer, there are inherent limitations: (1) a national participation rate of less than 85% may skew results due to unreported revisions[11]; (2) registry findings do not purport to answer the 'why' and the 'how' of the observations; (3) the use of revision as an outcome end

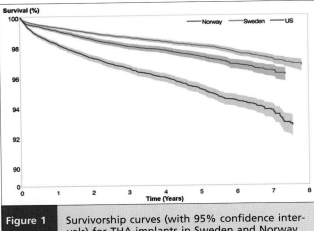

Figure 1   Survivorship curves (with 95% confidence intervals) for THA implants in Sweden and Norway (national joint replacement registry established) compared with those in the United States (no national joint replacement registry established). (Reproduced with permission from Kurtz SM, Ong KL, Schmier J, et al: Future clinical and economic impact of revision total hip and knee arthroplasty. *J Bone Joint Surg Am* 2007;89(suppl 3):144-151.)

point may be reliable but inadequate;[47] (4) level 1 registry data lack sensitivity to detect failure; and (5) as cohort data, confounding variables are difficult to control.[34]

Provided that compliance is good, and one is aware that registries address primarily the what, when, and where, then the potential to improve on contemporary registry designs exists. Revision surgery is indicated based on a host of factors, namely, functional and radiographic signs of failure. These indications can vary depending on surgeon, hospital, and regional practices. Academic hospitals are also known to have higher revision rates than community centers,[48] and this may be because of referral patterns to tertiary and quaternary services, where care for the high-risk patient and sub-specialized surgical skill are offered. In a community hospital, a patient with radiographic signs of implant failure may have surgery postponed because of significant comorbidity or lack of revision expertise. When revision is used as an end point, these nuances are not detected, and neither can one differentiate whether failure is related to the patient, the surgeon, or the implant system. A potential solution is to go beyond level 1 data retrieval, and consider factors relating to patient selection, surgeon experience, case volume of the surgeon and hospital, and revision policy.[11] These are variables that can be controlled to help minimize confounding effect. To improve the sensitivity of registries at detecting failure, data on clinical outcome (for example, mental health, hip function, and quality-of-life scores) and radiographic signs should also be included.[49] Currently, unless there is a revision operation, all patients, including those who are dissatisfied, have poor function, or have radiographic signs of failure, would still be considered to have a successful outcome. Clearly, these limitations and others intrinsic to any cohort study indicate that there remains an important role for prospective, blinded, randomized controlled trials.

In the United States, most THAs are performed by surgeons who do fewer than 20 THAs per year.[50] Half of all revision hip arthroplasties are performed in centers where fewer than 10 revision cases are done annually.[50] Most of the hip arthroplasty research is conducted by subspecialized high-volume surgeons in tertiary or quaternary centers. The results of these centers therefore are unlikely to be an accurate representation of general hip arthroplasty outcome in the nation.[51] A national registry database would provide a warning system for unsafe outliers, and more importantly, provide ongoing feedback to surgeons and industry on the quality of care and implant systems. As such, a registry would supply data for evidence-based management and may help align best practices to physician remuneration, which is already the case in Switzerland, Germany, the United Kingdom, the Netherlands, Japan, and Canada.

Summary

National joint registries have had a strong positive impact on the outcomes of hip and knee arthroplasties. Registries have helped define their respective national epidemiology for joint arthroplasties, identified prognostic indicators, the outcomes of surgical techniques, the performance of various prosthetic implants and biomaterials, and their associated complications. Registries have played a critical role in serving as a close to real-time warning system with regular feedback to surgeons, industry, and the general public. Registries have ultimately helped to integrate the principles of evidence-based medicine with arthroplasty surgery, leading into improved patient outcomes and cost effectiveness on a macroeconomic scale. With the forecasted exponential rise in demand for both primary and revision total hip and knee replacement surgeries in the near future, the use of joint registries and their information will be more important than ever.

Annotated References

1. Herberts P, Ahnfelt L, Malchau H, Strömberg C, Andersson GB: Multicenter clinical trials and their value in assessing total joint arthroplasty. *Clin Orthop Relat Res* 1989;249:48-55.

2. Ahnfelt L, Herberts P, Malchau H, Andersson GB: Prognosis of total hip replacement: A Swedish multicenter study of 4,664 revisions. *Acta Orthop Scand Suppl* 1990;238:1-26.

3. Lubega N, Mkandawire NC, Sibande GC, Norrish AR, Harrison WJ: Joint replacement in Malawi: Establishment of a National Joint Registry. *J Bone Joint Surg Br* 2009;91(3):341-343.

   This study reports on the early results of total hip replacement in Malawi analyzing data from a recently established national arthroplasty registry.

4. Kolling C, Simmen BR, Labek G, Goldhahn J: Key factors for a successful National Arthroplasty Register. *J Bone Joint Surg Br* 2007;89(12):1567-1573.

   The authors performed an international survey of 15 national arthroplasty registries to determine key factors required for a functional national joint registry.

5. Havelin LI, Fenstad AM, Salomonsson R, et al: The Nordic Arthroplasty Register Association: A unique collaboration between 3 national hip arthroplasty registries with 280,201 THRs. *Acta Orthop* 2009;80(4): 393-401.

   This study introduces the concept of the Nordic Arthroplasty Register and reports on preliminary data analysis showing different demographics, implant fixation, and implant survival for the contributing countries of Denmark, Sweden, and Norway.

6. Kurtz S, Mowat F, Ong K, Chan N, Lau E, Halpern M: Prevalence of primary and revision total hip and knee arthroplasty in the United States from 1990 through 2002. *J Bone Joint Surg Am* 2005;87(7):1487-1497.

   This study evaluated the National Hospital Discharge Survey and United States Census data from 1990 and 2002 and determined that the number and prevalence of primary THA, primary total knee arthroplasty, revision THA, and revision total knee arthroplasty increased by 46%, almost 150%, 60%, and 166%, respectively.

7. Kurtz S, Ong K, Lau E, Mowat F, Halpern M: Projections of primary and revision hip and knee arthroplasty in the United States from 2005 to 2030. *J Bone Joint Surg Am* 2007;89(4):780-785.

   Based on the National Inpatient Sample and United States Census data from 1990 to 2003, the demand for primary and revision THA as well as primary and revision total knee arthroplasty were projected to increase by 174%, 137%, 673%, and 601%, respectively.

8. Kurtz SM, Lau E, Ong K, Zhao K, Kelly M, Bozic KJ: Future young patient demand for primary and revision joint replacement: National projections from 2010 to 2030. *Clin Orthop Relat Res* 2009;467(10):2606-2612.

   Using the National Inpatient Sample, the projected future demand of primary and revision THA and total knee arthroplasty in patients younger than 65 years was determined to increase up to 50% by 2030 for different regression models using variable or constant procedure rates. Level of evidence: II.

9. Bozic KJ, Kurtz SM, Lau E, Ong K, Vail TP, Berry DJ: The epidemiology of revision total hip arthroplasty in

3: Hip

the United States. *J Bone Joint Surg Am* 2009;91(1): 128-133.

This level II prognostic study analyzed the epidemiology of revision THA in the United States utilizing the National Inpatient Sample database. THA instability, mechanical loosening, and infection were identified as the main reasons for revision.

10. Kurtz SM, Ong KL, Schmier J, et al: Future clinical and economic impact of revision total hip and knee arthroplasty. *J Bone Joint Surg Am* 2007;89(suppl 3): 144-151.

This study determined the historic and projected numbers of periprosthetic hip and knee infections and associated future socioeconomic burden in the Medicare population.

11. von Knoch F, Malchau H: Why do we need a national joint replacement registry in the United States? *Am J Orthop (Belle Mead NJ)* 2009;38(10):500-503.

This review text summarizes the current evidence in support of joint registries and provides a rationale for implementing such a national joint replacement registry in the United States.

12. Philipson MR, Westwood MJ, Geoghegan JM, Henry AP, Jefferiss CD: Shortcomings of the National Joint Registry: A survey of consultants' views. *Ann R Coll Surg Engl* 2005;87(2):109-112.

A survey of a large number of orthopaedic consultants on The National Joint Registry for England and Wales revealed that most participants support their national registry but share concerns related to the lack of orthopaedic representation on the steering committee.

13. Malchau H, Garellick G, Eisler T, Kärrholm J, Herberts P: Presidential guest address: The Swedish Hip Registry. Increasing the sensitivity by patient outcome data. *Clin Orthop Relat Res* 2005;441:19-29.

The founders of the Swedish Hip Registry present an extract of the most recent annual report and report their preliminary experience with patient-delivered outcome and cost-utility analyses.

14. Pitto RP, Lang I, Kienapfel H, Willert HG: The German Arthroplasty Register. *Acta Orthop Scand Suppl* 2002;73(305):30-33.

15. Arthursson AJ, Furnes O, Espehaug B, Havelin LI, Söreide JA: Validation of data in the Norwegian Arthroplasty Register and the Norwegian Patient Register: 5,134 primary total hip arthroplasties and revisions operated at a single hospital between 1987 and 2003. *Acta Orthop* 2005;76(6):823-828.

This study confirmed the validity and reliability of data from the NAR by its comparison with data from a local hospital.

16. Espehaug B, Furnes O, Havelin LI, Engesaeter LB, Vollset SE, Kindseth O: Registration completeness in the Norwegian Arthroplasty Register. *Acta Orthop* 2006;77(1):49-56.

Registration completeness of the NAR from 1999 to 2002 was analyzed and found to be high for primary and exchange total joint replacement but low for less common joint replacements and removal revisions.

17. Pedersen A, Johnsen S, Overgaard S, Søballe K, Sørensen HT, Lucht U: Registration in the danish hip arthroplasty registry: Completeness of total hip arthroplasties and positive predictive value of registered diagnosis and postoperative complications. *Acta Orthop Scand* 2004;75(4):434-441.

18. Pedersen AB, Johnsen SP, Overgaard S, Søballe K, Sørensen HT, Lucht U: Regional variation in incidence of primary total hip arthroplasties and revisions in Denmark, 1996-2002. *Acta Orthop* 2005;76(6):815-822.

This study evaluated data from the Danish Hip Arthroplasty Registry and demonstrated substantial regional differences in the incidence rates of total hip replacement in Denmark that were not associated with various patient- and health care system–related variables.

19. Lohmander LS, Engesaeter LB, Herberts P, Ingvarsson T, Lucht U, Puolakka TJ: Standardized incidence rates of total hip replacement for primary hip osteoarthritis in the 5 Nordic countries: Similarities and differences. *Acta Orthop* 2006;77(5):733-740.

The authors analyzed national registry data from Denmark, Finland, Iceland, Norway, and Sweden and found a comparable incidence of THA between these countries but substantially different ratios between women and men, and in the use of different implant types.

20. Pedersen AB, Johnsen SP, Overgaard S, Søballe K, Sørensen HT, Lucht U: Total hip arthroplasty in Denmark: Incidence of primary operations and revisions during 1996-2002 and estimated future demands. *Acta Orthop* 2005;76(2):182-189.

This study analyzed data from the Danish Hip Arthroplasty Registry and found that the incidence rates of primary and revision THA in Denmark increased from 1996 to 2002 and is estimated to further increase until 2020 beyond current national capacities.

21. Johnsen SP, Sørensen HT, Lucht U, Søballe K, Overgaard S, Pedersen AB: Patient-related predictors of implant failure after primary total hip replacement in the initial, short- and long-terms: A nationwide Danish follow-up study including 36,984 patients. *J Bone Joint Surg Br* 2006;88(10):1303-1308.

The authors studied data from the Danish Hip Arthroplasty Registry at three follow periods and found that male sex and a high Charlson comorbidity index score were time-independent predictors of implant failure, whereas patient age and surgical diagnosis predicted failure dependent on the period of follow-up.

22. Röder C, Staub LP, Eggli S, Dietrich D, Busato A, Müller U: Influence of preoperative functional status on outcome after total hip arthroplasty. *J Bone Joint Surg Am* 2007;89(1):11-17.

This level II prognostic study on data from the IDES European hip registry identified limited preoperative walking capacity and hip flexion as risk factors associated with suboptimal functional outcome after THA. In contrast, the authors did not find a correlation between preoperative pain and postoperative pain reduction. Level of evidence: II.

23. Flugsrud GB, Nordsletten L, Espehaug B, Havelin LI, Meyer HE: The effect of middle-age body weight and physical activity on the risk of early revision hip arthroplasty: A cohort study of 1,535 individuals. *Acta Orthop* 2007;78(1):99-107.

    This study reports on matched data from the NAR and data collected at a cardiovascular screening and found that upper quartile body weight and increased physical activity before total hip replacement negatively affected implant survival.

24. Eskelinen A, Remes V, Helenius I, Pulkkinen P, Nevalainen J, Paavolainen P: Uncemented total hip arthroplasty for primary osteoarthritis in young patients: A mid to long-term follow-up study from the Finnish Arthroplasty Register. *Acta Orthop* 2006;77(1):57-70.

    The authors report on national registry data of cementless THA in patients younger than 55 years in Finland and conclude that both modern cementless stems with proximal circumferential coating and press-fit cups have a favorable outcome at 10-year follow-up with respect to aseptic loosening. However, cup survival was low due to liner revisions that were common in this patient population and were mainly related to polyethylene wear and unfavorable locking mechanisms.

25. Eskelinen A, Paavolainen P, Helenius I, Pulkkinen P, Remes V: Total hip arthroplasty for rheumatoid arthritis in younger patients: 2,557 replacements in the Finnish Arthroplasty Register followed for 0-24 years. *Acta Orthop* 2006;77(6):853-865.

    In this survival analysis of data from the Finnish Arthroplasty Register on primary THA in patients with rheumatoid arthritis and younger than 55 years, cementless proximally circumferentially coated stems and cemented all-polyethylene cups demonstrated superior implant survival compared with cement stem and cementless cup designs.

26. Ogino D, Kawaji H, Konttinen L, et al: Total hip replacement in patients eighty years of age and older. *J Bone Joint Surg Am* 2008;90(9):1884-1890.

    The authors studied the outcome of primary total hip replacement in patients 80 years of age or older recorded in the Finnish Arthroplasty Register, and found the prevalence of aseptic loosening was lower than reported in younger patients but instability, periprosthetic infection, and fracture were more common. Cemented stem fixation provided superior long-term implant survival. Level of evidence: II.

27. Thillemann TM, Pedersen AB, Johnsen SP, Søballe K, Danish Hip Arthroplasty Registry: Implant survival after primary total hip arthroplasty due to childhood hip disorders: Results from the Danish Hip Arthroplasty Registry. *Acta Orthop* 2008;79(6):769-776.

    This study on data from the Danish Hip Arthroplasty Registry demonstrated a comparable survival of primary THA due to childhood hip disorders and those patients with primary hip osteoarthritis. However, patients with acetabular dysplasia revealed an increased risk of revision because of dislocation during the first 6 months after surgery.

28. Engesaeter LB, Furnes O, Havelin LI: Developmental dysplasia of the hip—good results of later total hip arthroplasty: 7135 primary total hip arthroplasties after developmental dysplasia of the hip compared with 59774 total hip arthroplasties in idiopathic coxarthrosis followed for 0 to 15 years in the Norwegian Arthroplasty Register. *J Arthroplasty* 2008;23(2):235-240.

    Using data from the NAR, the authors found a comparable implant survival of total hip replacement for developmental dysplasia of the hip and primary osteoarthritis when multivariate analysis was adjusted for younger patients and use of more cementless implants in patients with developmental dysplasia of the hip.

29. Figved W, Dybvik E, Frihagen F, et al: Conversion from failed hemiarthroplasty to total hip arthroplasty: A Norwegian Arthroplasty Register analysis of 595 hips with previous femoral neck fractures. *Acta Orthop* 2007;78(6):711-718.

    The authors analyzed data from the NAR and demonstrated that conversion from failed hip hemiarthroplasty to THA is associated with a lower implant survival when the stem is retained compared with conversion procedures with stem exchange.

30. Gjertsen JE, Lie SA, Fevang JM, et al: Total hip replacement after femoral neck fractures in elderly patients: Results of 8,577 fractures reported to the Norwegian Arthroplasty Register. *Acta Orthop* 2007;78(4):491-497.

    The authors used data from the NAR to demonstrate that THA after femoral neck fractures is associated with good implant survival but an increased risk of early dislocation and periprosthetic fractures compared with patients undergoing THA for osteoarthritis.

31. Arthursson AJ, Furnes O, Espehaug B, Havelin LI, Söreide JA: Prosthesis survival after total hip arthroplasty: Does surgical approach matter? Analysis of 19,304 Charnley and 6,002 Exeter primary total hip arthroplasties reported to the Norwegian Arthroplasty Register. *Acta Orthop* 2007;78(6):719-729.

    This study on data of primary THAs from the NAR showed that the lateral approach with trochanteric approach resulted in a lower revision risk compared with the lateral approach without the trochanteric approach or the posterolateral approach.

32. Lie SA, Hallan G, Furnes O, Havelin LI, Engesaeter LB: Isolated acetabular liner exchange compared with complete acetabular component revision in revision of primary uncemented acetabular components: A study of 1649 revisions from the Norwegian Arthroplasty

Register. *J Bone Joint Surg Br* 2007;89(5):591-594.

The authors used data from the NAR to determine that isolated acetabular liner exchange is associated with a higher risk of subsequent cup revision than revision of the entire acetabular component (both for loose and well-fixed cups).

33. Mäkelä K, Eskelinen A, Pulkkinen P, Paavolainen P, Remes V: Cemented total hip replacement for primary osteoarthritis in patients aged 55 years or older: Results of the 12 most common cemented implants followed for 25 years in the Finnish Arthroplasty Register. *J Bone Joint Surg Br* 2008;90(12):1562-1569.

The authors analyzed the Finnish Arthroplasty Register and concluded that the long-term survival of cementless versus cemented total hip replacement in patients 55 years of age or older is comparable. However, in patients between 55 and 74 years of age, survival of cementless stems was superior compared with that of cemented stems. Level of evidence: III.

34. Hallan G, Lie SA, Furnes O, Engesaeter LB, Vollset SE, Havelin LI: Medium- and long-term performance of 11,516 uncemented primary femoral stems from the Norwegian arthroplasty register. *J Bone Joint Surg Br* 2007;89(12):1574-1580.

This study used data from the NAR and demonstrated that a variety of modern cementless stems performed well overall with aseptic loosening as the end point at 10- to 15-year follow-up.

35. Espehaug B, Furnes O, Engesaeter LB, Havelin LI: 18 years of results with cemented primary hip prostheses in the Norwegian Arthroplasty Register: Concerns about some newer implants. *Acta Orthop* 2009;80(4):402-412.

The authors analyzed the long-term survival of the 10 most common implant combinations for cemented primary THAs in Norway and found clinically significant differences between implants. Inferiorly performing implants were identified.

36. Hooper GJ, Rothwell AG, Stringer M, Frampton C: Revision following cemented and uncemented primary total hip replacement: A seven-year analysis from the New Zealand Joint Registry. *J Bone Joint Surg Br* 2009;91(4):451-458.

This study on data from the New Zealand Joint Registry showed cemented THA had a lower rate of revision for any reason at short-term follow-up, whereas cementless hip replacement had a lower rate of revision for aseptic loosening in patients younger than 65 years.

37. Mäkelä KT, Eskelinen A, Pulkkinen P, Paavolainen P, Remes V: Total hip arthroplasty for primary osteoarthritis in patients fifty-five years of age or older: An analysis of the Finnish arthroplasty registry. *J Bone Joint Surg Am* 2008;90(10):2160-2170.

This analysis of the Finnish Arthroplasty Register revealed that long-term survival of cementless versus cemented THA was comparable in patients age 55 years or older; straight porous-coated cementless stems had superior survival compared with cemented stems in patients age 55 to 74 years; and excessive polyethylene wear was a significant problem associated with modular cementless cups in all age groups.

38. Paulsen A, Pedersen AB, Johnsen SP, Riis A, Lucht U, Overgaard S: Effect of hydroxyapatite coating on risk of revision after primary total hip arthroplasty in younger patients: Findings from the Danish Hip Arthroplasty Registry. *Acta Orthop* 2007;78(5):622-628.

The authors found that in patients younger than 70 years the use of hydroxyapatite-coated acetabular and femoral implants did not result in a significantly lower risk of revision after primary total hip replacement compared with noncoated implants.

39. Lefevre G: Hip replacement patients may face more surgery: 17,500 hip units recalled. CNN Website. http://archives.cnn.com/2001/HEALTH/17/hip.replacement/index.html. Published January 17, 2001. Accessed November 15, 2009.

This online news article reports on the lipid contamination of Sulzer Orthopaedics components implanted in the United States, 3,000 of which were later revised.

40. Thillemann TM, Pedersen AB, Johnsen SP, Søballe K: Inferior outcome after intraoperative femoral fracture in total hip arthroplasty: Outcome in 519 patients from the Danish Hip Arthroplasty Registry. *Acta Orthop* 2008;79(3):327-334.

Using data from the Danish Hip Arthroplasty Registry the authors found that intraoperative femoral periprosthetic fracture in primary total hip replacement is associated with an increased risk of revision during the first 6 months after surgery.

41. Lindahl H, Garellick G, Regnér H, Herberts P, Malchau H: Three hundred and twenty-one periprosthetic femoral fractures. *J Bone Joint Surg Am* 2006;88(6):1215-1222.

This prognostic level II analysis of the Swedish Hip Registry demonstrated that most periprosthetic femoral fractures after THA were caused by minor trauma, were classified as Vancouver type B, resulted in an unstable femoral stem, and had a high failure rate of almost 75% for the first 5 years after a periprosthetic fracture. Level of evidence: II.

42. Young SW, Walker CG, Pitto RP: Functional outcome of femoral peri prosthetic fracture and revision hip arthroplasty: A matched-pair study from the New Zealand Registry. *Acta Orthop* 2008;79(4):483-488.

The authors studied data from the New Zealand National Registry and found that revision THA for periprosthetic fracture is associated with poorer functional outcome and higher mortality compared with revision THA for aseptic loosening.

43. Buergi ML, Walter WL: Hip resurfacing arthroplasty: The Australian experience. *J Arthroplasty* 2007;22(7, suppl 3):61-65.

The authors analyzed the Australian National Joint Registry and observed a significant resurgence in hip resurfacing procedures during the late 1990s, and a steady increase in the popularity of hip resurfacing until 2006 (9% of all THAs versus 5.6% in 2001). Patients who were younger than 55 years represented the demographic group in which this increase was most pronounced.

44. Australian Orthopaedic Association: *2009 Annual Report: Hip and Knee Replacement*. Sydney, Australia, Australian Orthopaedic Association, 2009, pp 48-49.

The 2009 Annual Report as well as previous reports of the Australian National Joint Registry revealed a higher revision of certain implant types of hip resurfacing arthroplasty as well as hip resurfacing in women and those patients with smaller implant sizes compared with conventional total hip replacement. This resulted in a shift away from certain hip resurfacing implant types and hip resurfacing arthroplasties in women.

45. Kärrholm J, Garellick G, Herberts P: *Swedish Hip Arthroplasty Register: Annual Report 2006*. Gothenburg, Sweden, Department of Orthopaedics, Sahlgrenska University Hospital, August 2007, pp 44-45.

The Annual Report 2005 of the Swedish Hip Registry identified one of its participating hospitals as having an unusually high revision rate due to recurrent dislocation secondary to component malposition. The Registry organized a site-specific program to address this problem. The Annual Report 2006 showed since the implementation of this program there have been no further revisions due to dislocation caused by cup malposition. This underlines the strong influence of national joint registries on total hip replacement outcomes.

46. Herberts P, Malchau H: How outcome studies have changed total hip arthroplasty practices in Sweden. *Clin Orthop Relat Res* 1997;344:44-60.

47. Hulleberg G, Aamodt A, Espehaug B, Benum P: A clinical and radiographic 13-year follow-up study of 138 Charnley hip arthroplasties in patients 50-70 years old: Comparison of university hospital data and registry data. *Acta Orthop* 2008;79(5):609-617.

This study compared university hospital data and NAR data to demonstrate that revision-based registry studies are limited. The authors conclude a more complete evaluation of implant function requires additional assessment of hip joint-specific functional outcome, patient satisfaction, quality of life, and radiographic outcome.

48. Espehaug B, Havelin LI, Engesaeter LB, Vollset SE: The effect of hospital-type and operating volume on the survival of hip replacements: A review of 39,505 primary total hip replacements reported to the Norwegian Arthroplasty Register, 1988-1996. *Acta Orthop Scand* 1999;70(1):12-18.

49. Rolfson O, Dahlberg LE, Nilsson JA, Malchau H, Garellick G: Variables determining outcome in total hip replacement surgery. *J Bone Joint Surg Br* 2009; 91(2):157-161.

The authors analyzed data from the Swedish Hip Arthroplasty Register, including data from the EuroQol-System (EQ-5D), to determine that the preoperative EQ-5D anxiety/depression dimension was a strong predictor of pain relief and patient satisfaction after THA.

50. Katz JN, Losina E, Barrett J, et al: Association between hospital and surgeon procedure volume and outcomes of total hip replacement in the United States Medicare population. *J Bone Joint Surg Am* 2001; 83(11):1622-1629.

51. Katz JN, Phillips CB, Baron JA, et al: Association of hospital and surgeon volume of total hip replacement with functional status and satisfaction three years following surgery. *Arthritis Rheum* 2003;48(2):560-568.

Index

in implants, 42, 43*f*
types of, 43
Lysis. *See also* Osteolysis
anteversion and, 5
detecting, 3, 19

M

Magnetic resonance angiography, 10–11, 10*f*
Magnetic resonance arthrography (MRA), 281–282, 282*f*
Magnetic resonance imaging (MRI). *See also under imaging under various diagnoses*
with computer-assisted TKA, 128–131
CT vs., 282
detecting osteolysis, 3, 194
detecting osteonecrosis, 60, 60*f*, 64
general principles of, 8–10, 9*f*, 10*f*, 11
in THA, 273
in TKA, 6
Mako Tactile Guidance System, 126–127, 126–127*t*, 128*f*
Malalignment
in minimally invasive TKA, 140, 144, 147
in TKA, 124, 151, 166*t*, 191
Malignancy
infections and, 202*t*
metal implant carcinogenicity, 44–45
Malnutrition, wound complications after TKA and, 179
Malunion. *See* nonunion
Manipulation. *See* physical therapy
Marrow stimulation for cartilage lesions, 101–102
Martell method, 18, 19
Mayo Clinic
bulk allograft study, 170
clinical score with ROBODOC, 125
hip dislocation study, 272–273
infection study, 206, 210
TKA study/experiences, 5, 155, 178, 181, 182
Mechanical antithrombic devices, 36
Medial collateral ligament (MCL)
iatrogenic injury to, 184
rupture of, 146
Medial compartment arthritis, treatment for, 99
Medial wall displacement osteotomy for hip dysplasia, 237
Medical Expenditure Panel Survey: COX inhibitor study, 97
Medical Outcomes Study 36-Item Short Form Health Survey (SF-36)
acetabular fracture treatment, 254
femoral reconstruction, 240
knee arthritis, 99
measuring TKA outcomes with, 151, 153, 208

Megaprostheses, infections and, 202*t*
Meniscal tear, 110
Meniscectomy
high tibial osteotomy and, 99
need for, 103
Meniscus
high flexion and biomechanics of, 87, 90*f*
mobile-bearing TKA and, 153
removal of, 113
Merle d'Aubigné scale with osteochondral allografts, 103
Mesenchymal stem cells, osteonecrosis and, 59, 62
Metal metaphyseal cones in revision TKA, 170–172, 171*f*
Metal-on-metal implants. *See* Implants, biologic response to
Metastatic carcinoma, 64
Methicillin-resistant *Staphylococcus aureus* (MRSA), 202, 205, 207*f*, 208, 349, 352
Methicillin-resistant *Staphylococcus epidermidis* (MRSE), 202
Methotrexate, 205
Methylprednisolone, 59
Methylprednisolone acetate (MPA), 98
Microfracture
autologous chondrocyte implantation vs., 103
marrow stimulation and, 101
Miller-Galante implant system for UKA, 109
Minimally invasive surgery (MIS)
fixed-bearing TKA, 152
total hip arthroplasty, 263–273
total knee arthroplasty, 139–147
Mini-medial parapatellar approach for TKA, 139, 143–144, 143*f*, 146
Mini-midvastus approach for TKA, 139, 142–143, 143*f*, 145–146
Mini-subvastus approach for TKA, 139–142, 141*f*, 142*f*, 146, 147
Modified sliding trochanteric osteotomy, 328
Modular blocks/wedges in revision TKA, 170
Moore posterior approach (THA), 272
Morcellized cancellous allograft. *See also* Allografts
in revision TKA, 169
in THA, 247, 250*f*, 251, 252, 253, 254
Morphine, 76
Mosaicplasty
autologous chondrocyte implantation vs., 102–103
for cartilage lesions, 101
in chrondrocyte transplantation, 102
Multiple myeloma, 64
Mupirocin, 349
Muscle dystrophy, 346, 346*t*

Muscle ischemia, risk of, 131
Muscular atrophy, 73–74
Musculoskeletal Function Assessment, 254
Mycobacterium, 202
Myocardial infarction
beta blocker usage and, 177
NSAID/COX therapy and, 97

N

Naproxen, with proton pump inhibitor, 97
Narcotics, in rehabilitation, 73, 76
National Health Service (England), implant warning, 353
National Institutes of Health, Consensus Statement on Total Knee Replacement, 205
National Joint Registry of England and Wales, 320*t*, 363–364
National Nosocomial Infection Surveillance System, 202
National Patient Safety Goals. *See under* Joint Commission
Nationwide Inpatient Sample
computer-navigated TKA and cardiac complications, 122
infection rates, 348
Navigation. *See* Computer-assisted arthroplasty
Necrosis. *See* Periprosthetic necrosis
Nerve conduction velocity, 246
Nerve injury
with ROBODOC, 125
in THA, 233
Netherlands joint registry, 369
Neurapraxia, after THA, 268
Neuroma, in TKA, 166*t*
Neuromodulatory agents, 76, 77*t*
New Zealand National (Joint) Registry, 315, 364, 367
New Zealand Orthopaedic Association, 320*t*
Nonsteroidal anti-inflammatory drugs (NSAIDs)
HA vs., 98
for knee arthritis, 97, 103
for osteonecrosis, 64
for pain relief, 76, 77*t*
with proton pump inhibitor, 103
wound complications after TKA and, 179
Nonunion
of acetabular fractures, 241, 243, 251
in arthrodesis, 210
bulk allograft and, 169–170
in hip resurfacing, 298*t*, 299
in ORIF, 244*f*, 246*f*
pelvic nonunion, 252
of periprosthetic fractures, 183, 367
risk of, 100, 328